HANDBOOK OF PAIN ASSESSMENT

Handbook of
PAIN ASSESSMENT

THIRD EDITION

EDITED BY

DENNIS C. TURK
RONALD MELZACK

THE GUILFORD PRESS
New York   London

© 2011 The Guilford Press
A Division of Guilford Publications, Inc.
72 Spring Street, New York, NY 10012
www.guilford.com

Printed in the United States of America

This book is printed on acid-free paper.

Last digit is print number: 9   8   7   6   5   4   3   2   1

Library of Congress Cataloging-in-Publication Data

Handbook of pain assessment / edited by Dennis C. Turk, Ronald Melzack.–3rd ed.
   p. ; cm.
  Includes bibliographical references and index.
  ISBN 978-1-60623-976-6 (hardcover: alk. paper)
  1. Pain—Measurement—Handbooks, manuals, etc.   I. Turk, Dennis C.
II. Melzack, Ronald.
  [DNLM: 1. Pain—diagnosis. 2. Pain—psychology. 3. Pain
Measurement.   WL 704 H243 2011]
  RB127.H355 2011
  616.'0472—dc22
                                                            2010016505

About the Editors

Dennis C. Turk, PhD, is the John and Emma Bonica Professor of Anesthesiology and Pain Research and Director of the Center for Pain Research on Impact, Measurement, and Effectiveness at the University of Washington School of Medicine. His research focuses on the assessment and treatment of a range of chronic pain conditions, clinical trial design, comparative effectiveness research, subgroup identification and treatment matching, and coping and adaptation. Dr. Turk is a recipient of the John C. Liebeskind Award for Career Contribution to Pain Research from the American Academy of Pain Management and the Wilbert E. Fordyce Clinical Investigator Award from the American Pain Society.

Ronald Melzack, PhD, is Professor Emeritus of Psychology at McGill University. He developed the McGill Pain Questionnaire, a widely used measurement tool for research on pain in human subjects. In recognition of his breakthrough research on pain, Dr. Melzack has received numerous awards from groups including the Canadian Psychological Association, Canadian Pain Society, Canada Council for the Arts, American Academy of Pain Management, and American Society of Regional Anesthesia. In 2009, he was inducted into the Canadian Medical Hall of Fame.

Contributors

Khush A. Amaria, PhD, Divisional Center for Pain Management and Pain Research, Department of Anesthesia and Pain Medicine, The Hospital for Sick Children, Toronto, Ontario, Canada

Karen O. Anderson, PhD, Department of Symptom Research, University of Texas M. D. Anderson Cancer Center, Houston, Texas

Frank Andrasik, PhD, Department of Psychology, University of Memphis, Memphis, Tennessee

Nadine Attal, MD, PhD, Center for the Evaluation and Treatment of Pain, Ambroise-Pare Hospital, Boulogne, France

Didier Bouhassira, MD, PhD, Center of Evaluation and Treatment of Pain, Ambroise-Pare Hospital, Boulogne, France

Jennifer Brennan Braden, MD, MPH, Department of Psychiatry and Behavioral Sciences, University of Washington, Seattle, Washington

Lynn M. Breau, PhD, School of Nursing, Dalhousie University, Halifax, Nova Scotia, Canada

Emily Brede, RN, Department of Psychology, University of Texas at Arlington, Arlington, Texas

Dawn C. Buse, PhD, Department of Neurology, Albert Einstein College of Medicine, and Clinical Health Psychology Doctoral Program, Ferkauf Graduate School of Psychology, Yeshiva University, Bronx, New York

Annmarie Cano, PhD, Department of Psychology, Wayne State University, Detroit, Michigan

Andrew J. Cook, PhD, Mental Health and Behavioral Medicine, Olin E. Teague VA Medical Center, Central Texas Veterans Health Care System, Temple, Texas

Kenneth D. Craig, PhD, Department of Psychology, University of British Columbia, Vancouver, British Columbia, Canada

Douglas E. DeGood, PhD, Department of Psychiatry and Neurobehavioral Sciences, University of Virginia Health System, Charlottesville, Virginia

Robert H. Dworkin, PhD, Departments of Anesthesiology, Neurology, Oncology, and Psychiatry, University of Rochester Medical Center, Rochester, New York

James A. Fauerbach, PhD, Department of Psychiatry and Behavioral Sciences, Johns Hopkins University School of Medicine, Baltimore, Maryland

Herta Flor, PhD, Department of Cognitive and Clinical Neuroscience, Central Institute of Mental Health, University of Heidelberg, Mannheim, Germany

Lucia Gagliese, PhD, School of Kinesiology and Health Science, York University; Psychosocial Oncology and Palliative Care Research Division, Behavioral Sciences and Health Research Division, Department of Anesthesia and Pain Management, University Health Network; Departments of Anesthesia and Psychiatry, University of Toronto, Toronto, Ontario, Canada

Robert J. Gatchel, PhD, ABPP, Department of Psychology, University of Texas at Arlington, Arlington, Texas

Lynn R. Gauthier, PhD, MA, School of Kinesiology and Health Science, York University, Toronto, Ontario, Canada

Ian Gilron, MD, MSc, Departments of Anesthesiology and Pharmacology and Toxicology, Queen's University, Kingston, Ontario, Canada

Ruth E. Grunau, PhD, Department of Pediatrics, University of British Columbia, Vancouver, British Columbia, Canada

Thomas Hadjistavropoulos, PhD, ABPP, FCAHS, Department of Psychology and Centre on Aging and Health, University of Regina, Regina, Saskatchewan, Canada

Jennifer A. Haythornthwaite, PhD, Department of Psychiatry and Behavioral Sciences, Johns Hopkins University School of Medicine, Baltimore, Maryland

Mark P. Jensen, PhD, Department of Rehabilitation Medicine, University of Washington, Seattle, Washington

Paul Karoly, PhD, Department of Psychology, Arizona State University, Tempe, Arizona

Joel Katz, PhD, Department of Psychology, York University, Toronto, Ontario, Canada

Francis J. Keefe, PhD, Department of Psychiatry and Behavioral Sciences, Duke University Medical Center, Durham, North Carolina

Alyssa Lettich, MD, Department of Neurology, Albert Einstein College of Medicine, Bronx, New York

Shawn T. Mason, PhD, Department of Psychiatry and Behavioral Sciences, Johns Hopkins University School of Medicine, Baltimore, Maryland

Patricia A. McGrath, PhD, Divisional Center for Pain Management and Pain Research, Department of Anesthesia and Pain Medicine, The Hospital for Sick Children, Toronto, Ontario, Canada

Ronald Melzack, PhD, Department of Psychology, McGill University, Montreal, Quebec, Canada

Patric Meyer, PhD, Department of Cognitive and Clinical Neuroscience, Central Institute of Mental Health, Mannheim, Germany

Alec B. O'Connor, MD, MPH, Department of Medicine, University of Rochester Medical Center, Rochester, New York

Peter B. Polatin, MD, MPH, The Rehabilitation and Research Centre for Victims of Torture, Copenhagen, Denmark

Kenneth M. Prkachin, PhD, Psychology Program, University of Northern British Columbia, Prince George, British Columbia, Canada

James P. Robinson, MD, PhD, Department of Rehabilitation Medicine, University of Washington, Seattle, Washington

Joan M. Romano, PhD, Department of Psychiatry and Behavioral Sciences, University of Washington, Seattle, Washington

Danielle A. Ruskin, PhD, Divisional Center for Pain Management and Pain Research, Department of Anesthesia and Pain Medicine, The Hospital for Sick Children, Toronto, Ontario, Canada

Karen B. Schmaling, PhD, Office of Academic Affairs, Washington State University, Vancouver, Washington

Suzanne J. Smith, PhD, Department of Psychology, Cleveland Veterans Administration Medical Center and Department of General Internal Medicine, Case School of Medicine, Cleveland, Ohio

Tamara J. Somers, PhD, Department of Psychiatry and Behavioral Sciences, Duke University Medical Center, Durham, North Carolina

Mark D. Sullivan, MD, PhD, Department of Psychiatry, University of Washington, Seattle, Washington

Dennis C. Turk, PhD, Department of Anesthesiology and Pain Medicine, University of Washington, Seattle, Washington

Michael Von Korff, ScD, Group Health Research Institute, Group Health Cooperative, Seattle, Washington

Fay F. Warnock, PhD, School of Nursing, University of British Columbia, Vancouver, British Columbia, Canada

Paul J. Watson, PhD, FCSP, Department of Health Sciences, University of Leicester, Leicester, United Kingdom

David A. Williams, PhD, Department of Psychiatry, University of Michigan, Ann Arbor, Michigan

Whitney E. Worzer, MA, Department of Psychology, University of Texas at Arlington, Arlington, Texas

Preface

Pain is ubiquitous—it is an integral part of life and has an important protective function. It is also the primary symptom that prompts people to seek medical attention. Uncontrolled, prolonged pain produces depression, inability to work, and persistent stress. It thus becomes a disease itself. People's beliefs and emotions can amplify or diminish the experience substantially. Prolonged pain is also influenced by the social environment, particularly how significant others, including health care providers, respond to reports of pain. All of these factors—individual, sociocultural, health care, and compensation systems—have been shown to have a profound influence on perceived pain intensity, response to treatments, and disability. Persistent pain greatly compromises quality of life and has become a growing concern of health care.

Despite the prevalence of pain, there remains much that we do not understand about it. Pain has many perplexing characteristics. Why do two people with ostensibly the same degree of physical pathology sometimes report strikingly different intensities of pain? Why do patients treated by the same methods to control pain show different results? Why are so many chronic pain syndromes more prevalent in women? Increased insights into the contributions of genetic factors, neurophysiology, plasticity of the nervous system, and individual learning histories are shedding important insights on the subject and suggesting some explanations, but a great deal remains unknown.

Pain is a perception that is experienced by a conscious person. According to the definition accepted by the International Association for the Study of Pain (IASP) (Merskey, 1986), "Pain is an unpleasant sensory and emotional experience associated with actual or potential tissue damage or described in terms of such damage" (p. 51). This definition underscores the inherent subjectivity of pain and acknowledges the importance of emotional as well as sensory factors.

To understand and to treat pain adequately, we must be able to measure it. This seems at first to be a quite simple task. All that is required is that the individual respond to the question "How much does it hurt?" Unfortunately, as is illustrated throughout this volume, the problem is not simple. Many factors contribute to the individual's response to the question. This is our primary rationale for this volume. There does not appear to be a simple relationship between the amount of pain and the extent of tissue damage. As noted in the IASP definition, psychological factors are involved in the pain experience. Pain is influenced by cultural, economic, social, demographic, and environmental factors. The individual's personal history, situational factors, interpretation of the symptoms and resources, current psychological state, as well as physical pathology, all contribute to the patient's response to the question "How much does it hurt?"

The complexity of pain has been revealed in recent decades. Investigators and clinicians have learned that a diverse range of factors need to be examined in the hope of understanding the response to the simple question of how much it hurts. In the two previous editions of this volume, spanning over 20 years, we asked a group of internationally acknowledged experts to provide a description of the available instruments and procedures for assessing people with pain. In addition, we asked contributors to evaluate existing methods and to provide practical information about their merits, and to thereby assist clinical investigators or health care providers in making informed decisions regarding the most appropriate methods to assess the person who is experiencing pain. We also included contributions that provided more general discussion of issues that need to be considered in selecting from the array of available instruments and procedures. From the first edition to the present volume, our knowledge of pain has increased exponentially. Many of the advances have been directly related to improved methods of assessment. This edition is designed to be a status report and to serve as a guide for future developments.

This handbook is organized into five sections, with an Introduction and Conclusion by the editors (Dennis C. Turk & Ronald Melzack). The first section, Self-Report Measures of Pain, includes chapters that address the assessment of pain per se. This section includes general chapters that focus specifically on self-report scales used with adults (Mark P. Jensen & Paul Karoly, Joel Katz & Ronald Melzack) and a chapter on methods of assessing other components of the pain (e.g., attitudes, beliefs, coping, mood) that are essential for understanding the pain experience. Measures of pain are not highly associated with physical pathology. It appears that cognitive interpretation and mood modulate the experience of pain and are important factors that must be included as part of a comprehensive assessment. Douglas E. DeGood and Andrew J. Cook describe the use of interviews and standardized measures to assess these influential components of the pain experience. The final chapter in this section draws attention to the important consideration of people with pain within the broader social context. People respond to others experiencing pain and can provide important insights about how the person with pain is responding and adapting to his or her condition. Moreover, significant others are also influenced by the person who is in pain. Joan M. Romano, Annmarie Cano, and Karen B. Schmaling provide important insights into strategies to assess couples and family with chronic pain.

The second section focuses on Measures of Pain Not Dependent on Self-Report. In addition to self-report, other important modes of communicating are characterized by facial expressions, nonverbal sounds (e.g., sighs, moans), and characteristic movements, postures, and soothing efforts (e.g., rubbing a painful body part)—all observable behaviors. Chapters in this section focus on surrogate measures of pain, including facial expressions (Kenneth D. Craig, Kenneth M. Prkachin, & Ruth E. Grunau), the overt expressions of pain using observation measures (Francis J. Keefe, Tamara J. Somers, David A. Williams, & Suzanne J. Smith), psychophysiological measures (Herta Flor & Patric

Meyer), and medical examination (Peter B. Polatin, Whitney E. Worzer, Emily Brede, & Robert J. Gatchel). Craig and colleagues provide a discussion of the use of features of facial expression to make inferences about pain. Facial expressions (action patterns) are universal in humans, and specific patterns appear to be unique to the experience of pain. Thus, they provide a more objective measure of pain than self-report measures that are open to distortion by a range of biases and may be consciously manipulated. The chapter by Keefe and colleagues describes methods to observe, record, and quantify a range of movements, in addition to facial expression and nonverbal sounds, called pain behaviors. What is of central importance here is that not only can these behaviors be carefully monitored and assessed by health care providers, but they are also observable by patients' significant others. These behaviors not only communicate about the subjective experience of pain, but they are also capable of eliciting responses. Thus, in contrast to facial action patterns of pain that appear to be relatively hardwired, pain behaviors are subject to the changing influences of environmental contingencies. The chapter by Flor and Meyer underscores the potential of physical factors, in particular, psychophysiological correlates of pain, to assist in assessment and provides practical information about traditional and innovative methods for using physiological data to assess persistent pain. Polatin and colleagues describe the use of a detailed protocol to quantify function and relate this to the *International Classification of Functioning, Disability and Health* (World Health Organization, 2001). This section closes with a chapter by Dennis C. Turk and James P. Robinson, who describe a comprehensive approach to illustrate how medical, psychosocial, and behavioral methods can be integrated when assessing people with chronic pain.

The third section deals with the Assessment of Special Populations: infants, children, and adolescents (Danielle A. Ruskin, Khush A. Amaria, Fay F. Warnock, & Patricia A. McGrath); older adults (Lynn R. Gauthier & Lucia Gagliese); and those who are unable to communicate verbally due to physical or mental limitations (Thomas Hadjistavropoulos, Lynn M. Breau, & Kenneth D. Craig). These chapters provide important insights into strategies needed to access the unique characteristics of these groups that represent a significant portion of the population. The authors describe creative strategies that have been developed to provide comprehensive assessments.

The fourth section addresses Assessment of Specific Pain Conditions and Syndromes. It includes chapters that describe unique features of diagnosing and assessing patients with acute pain in order to assess patient satisfaction (Shawn T. Mason, James A. Fauerbach, & Jennifer A. Haythornthwaite) and the most prevalent chronic pain syndromes: back pain (Paul J. Watson); myofasical pain, whiplash, and fibromyalgia (James P. Robinson & Dennis C. Turk); neuropathic pain (Ian Gilron, Nadine Attal, Didier Bouhassira, & Robert H. Dworkin); headache (Frank Andrasik, Dawn C. Buse, & Alyssa Lettich); and pain associated with cancer (Karen O. Anderson).

The fifth section, Special Issues and Applications, covers three important areas where assessment plays an important role in clinical decision making. There is a high prevalence of comorbid psychiatric disorders in people with chronic pain. The issue of cause and effect may be of scientific interest, but in clinical practice, both must be treated. Mark D. Sullivan and Jennifer Brennan Braden review the most prevalent psychiatric disorders observed in people with chronic pain, describing the criteria for diagnosis of each of these disorders. James P. Robinson covers the difficult and controversial topic of disability evaluation. He describes the intricacies of different compensation systems and provides useful suggestions regarding how an evaluator can conduct impairment and disability evaluations that address ambiguities while meeting the demands inherent in these imperfect compensation systems.

A number of advanced surgical and neuroaugmentation procedures have been developed since the publication of the two previous editions of this volume. Despite technical advances, there is growing evidence that psychosocial factors have an important role to play in treatment response. Detailed assessment methods have been developed to screen patients prior to receiving these treatments. There has also been an expanded interest in issues associated with use and misuse of opioids and whether it is possible to predict aberrant behaviors. Robert J. Gatchel describes the importance of comprehensive assessment of patients in an attempt to improve prediction of treatment response.

The fifth section also includes chapters on important methodological topics that transcend the topic of assessment. Michael Von Korff provides an updated and expanded discussion of epidemiological and survey methods. Features inherent in epidemiological research limit types of data that can be obtained. Heavy reliance is based on relatively brief self-reports, and Von Korff discusses both retrospective reporting and the growing interest in electronic diaries and "real-time" data capture. Von Korff also describes a strategy for redefining chronic pain that, rather than depending solely on duration, includes prognosis.

Alec B. O'Connor and Robert H. Dworkin discuss the importance of health-related quality of life as an outcome in clinical trials. They describe the efforts of the Initiative on Methods Meaurement and Pain Assessment in Clinical Trials (IMMPACT) to create consensus among investigators related to assessment outcome domains and measures in clinical trials, and strategies to evaluate existing measures and develop new ones as a means of advancing knowledge of treatment effects.

In our introductory and concluding chapters, we have provided an overview of concepts of pain assessment and have attempted to identify current trends as well as future directions. This volume reflects the advances in assessment methods that have contributed so much to the increased understanding of pain, the person with pain, and the evaluation of new treatments. Furthermore, our intent for this edition is to (1) provide a practical guide to currently available instruments and procedures, (2) suggest areas in which current procedures are inadequate, and (3) serve as an impetus for research to improve on existing instruments and procedures. The achievement of these goals should further enhance our understanding of pain and lead to more successful treatment. Our ultimate aim in this volume is to decrease suffering and improve the quality of life of those who experience pain.

DENNIS C. TURK
RONALD MELZACK

REFERENCES

Merskey, H. (Ed.). (1986). Classification of chronic pain syndromes and definitions of pain terms. *Pain* (Suppl. 3), S1–S225.

World Health Organization. (2001). *International classification of functioning, disability and health*. Geneva: Author.

Contents

INTRODUCTION

CHAPTER 1

The Measurement of Pain and the Assessment of People Experiencing Pain

DENNIS C. TURK
RONALD MELZACK

Just as "my pain" belongs in a unique way only to me, so I am utterly alone with it. I cannot share it. I have no doubt about the reality of the pain experience, but I cannot tell anybody what I experience. I surmise that others have "their" pain, even though I cannot perceive what they mean when they tell me about them. I am certain about the existence of their pain only in the sense that I am certain of my compassion for them. And yet, the deeper my compassion, the deeper is my certitude about the other person's utter loneliness in relation to his experience.
—IVAN ILLICH (1976, pp. 147–148)

. . . the investigator who would study pain is at the mercy of the patient, upon whose ability and willingness to communicate he is dependent.
—LOUIS LASAGNA (1960, p. 28)

Pain is ubiquitous and essential for survival; however, it is a prevalent and costly problem. One in four adult Americans reports an episode of pain during the last month that persisted more than 24 hours (National Center for Health Statistics [NCHS], 2006). Nearly 50% of Americans see a physician with a primary complaint of pain each year (Mayo Clinic, 2001). Pain appears to be equally prevalent in children and adolescents (Perquin et al., 2000). The NCHS (2006) estimated that approximately 25% of the U.S. population has chronic or recurrent pain, that 1 person in 10 reported pain that lasted a year or more, and that 40% stated the pain had a moderately or severely degrading impact on their lives. Data from the National Health Interview Survey (Lethbridge-Cejku & Vickerie, 2005) indicates that during the 3 months prior to the survey, 15% of adults had experienced a migraine or severe headache, and 15% had experienced pain in the neck area, 27% in the lower back, and 4%, in the jaw. Extrapolating to the adult U.S. population, these percentages would translate to 31,066,000 persons with migraine, 52,325,000 with low back pain, 28,401,000 with head and neck pain, and 9,535,000 with jaw pain. In the U.S. population-based study by the Gallup Organization, 14.7% of eligible women (773/5,263, 1 in 7) reported pelvic pain in the prior 3 months, 15% of employed women with chronic pelvic pain reported that they lost time from work, and 45% reported reduced work productivity due to their pain (Mathias, Kuppermann, Liberman, Lipschurz, & Steefe, 1996).

It is hardly surprising that pain is among the most common symptoms leading U.S. patients to consult a physician (Hing, Cherry, & Woodwell, 2006), accounting for 2.3% of all visits or approximately 17.4 million visits/year (Cherry, Burt, & Woodwell., 2001). The statistics cited earlier are derived from physician and hospital records, but they probably reflect only the tip of the iceberg when it comes to the prevalence of pain. Many people who experience pain self-manage their pain without seeking medical attention.

Comparable prevalence statistics have been reported internationally. For example, a World Health Organization (WHO) survey of primary care patients in 15 countries reported that 22% of patients reported pain present for 6 months or longer that required medical attention, medication, or interfered significantly with daily activities (Gureje, 1998). A population survey in the United Kingdom found that 25% of adults experienced back or neck (spinal) pain in the prior month, with half reporting chronic pain (Webb et al., 2003). Migraine has an estimated worldwide prevalence of approximately 10% (Sheffield, 1998).

Considering all sources of expenditures, chronic pain is projected to cost the U.S. economy roughly $100 billion each year ("Employer Health Care Strategy Survey," 2003; Washington Business Group on Health and Watson Wyatt Worldwide, 2003). Lost productive time from common pain conditions among workers cost an estimated $61.2 billion/year. The majority (76.6%) of the lost productive time was explained by reduced performance while at work, not work absence (Stewart, Ricci, Chee, Morganstein, & Lipton, 2003).

We can consider several persistent pain problems to illustrate the cost and impact on society. Over $12.5 billion is spent annually on the medical treatment of arthritis alone in the United States (Cantor, 2002). Estimates of the financial impact (e.g., lost productivity, uncompensated lost wages, loss in household services and tax revenues, social security benefits) of back pain range from $45 billion to $54 billion/year (National Academies of Sciences & Institute of Medicine, 2001). According to the National Headache Foundation (2005) more than 45 million American experience chronic headaches, with losses of $50 billion a year due to absenteeism and medical expenses, and an excess of $4 billion spent on over-the-counter medications. The estimated cost of annual lost productive work time from arthritis in the U.S. workforce was $7.11 billion, with 65.7% of the cost attributed to the 38% of workers with pain exacerbations (Ricci et al., 2005).

Given the statistics cited here, it might be expected that pain would be well treated. Unfortunately, this is not the case. Most forms of chronic pain are poorly understood, and even when they are understood, the severity may not be adequately managed. Despite advances since our previous editions (Turk & Melzack, 1992, 2001), a central impediment to increased understanding and appropriate treatment of pain continues to be the inherent subjectivity of pain. This problem has been noted as far back as the early 1960s, as indicated by the Lasagna quote earlier. In the absence of objective methods to assess pain, we are dependent on people's responses and their attempts to communicate what they are experiencing or have experienced at some time in the past.

Many of the epidemiological data outlined earlier are based on patients' ability to retrieve information from memory, even though memory of subjective experiences can be notoriously faulty (Broderick et al., 2008). This observation has led some to suggest that more accurate information can be obtained from patients' daily diaries or from real-time data using technology rather than relying on recall. However, this issue remains controversial, and it appears that recall of, at least, relatively short duration (days and even weeks) can be reasonably accurate (e.g., Broderick et al., 2008; Jamison, Raymond, Slawsby, McHugo, & Baird, 2006) although it may deteriorate over more extended periods (e.g., many months). However, average pain over the past 6 months may be as important, if not more important, in some studies than average pain over the past week, which may not be representative of a patient's usual pain. Retrospective reports might also be expected to vary in accuracy depending on a multitude of factors discussed in some detail by Mason, Fauerbach, and Haythornthwaite (Chapter 14) and Von Korff (Chapter 23) in this volume.

It is difficult to describe pain, which is a subjective experience, a complex perceptual phenomenon. Thus, by its very nature, pain can only be assessed indirectly by what people in pain tell us verbally; by their overt behavior (see Keefe, Somers, Williams, & Smith, Chapter 7, in this volume), including facial expressions (see Craig, Prkachin, & Grunau, Chapter 6, this volume); or by physiological correlates (see Flor & Meyer, Chapter 8, this volume). However, in order for patients, clinicians, and researchers, and policymakers to communicate, there needs to be a common language and a classification system that can be used in a meaningful and consistent fashion (Turk & Okifuji, 2001).

CLASSIFYING PAIN

One common way to classify pain is to consider it along a continuum of duration. Thus, pain associated with tissue damage, inflammation, or a disease process that is of relatively brief duration (i.e., hours, days, or even weeks), regardless of its intensity, is frequently referred to as *acute pain* (e.g., postsurgical pain; see Mason et al., Chapter 14, this volume). Pain that persists for extended periods of time (i.e., months or years), that accompanies a disease process (e.g., rheumatoid arthritis), or that is associated with an injury that has not resolved within an expected period of time (e.g., myofascial pain syndromes, neuropathic pain; see Chapter 16 by Robinson & Turk, and Chapter 17 by Gilron, Attal, Bouhassira, & Dworkin, this volume) is referred to as *chronic pain*. This duration continuum is inadequate, because it does not include acute recurrent pain (e.g., migraine headaches, sickle cell disease); it tends to ignore pain associated with progressive diseases, such as chronic obstructive pulmonary disease and metastatic cancer. In the case of acute recurrent pain, people may suffer from episodes of acute pain interspersed with periods of being totally pain-free (see Chapter 18 by Andrasik, Buse, & Lettich, this volume). In the case of pain associated with progressive diseases, certain unique features of the pain are influenced by the nature of the disease and need to be considered (see Anderson, Chapter 19, this volume). Finally, in the laboratory, a number of contextual factors need to be considered before extrapolations can be made to

the clinical context. Using these five discrete classifications of pain (i.e., acute, acute recurrent, chronic, chronic progressive, and laboratory-induced) comprises a categorical approach to classification rather than a simple continuum based on duration. Another way to classify pain is based on diagnosis, such as back pain (see Watson, Chapter 15, this volume), fibromyalgia syndrome (see Robinson & Turk, Chapter 16, this volume), and somatization disorders (see Sullivan & Braden, Chapter 20, this volume). Related to diagnosis, but more specific, are recent calls for classification based on underlying mechanisms (see, e.g., Woolf et al., 1998).

A common way to classify pain is to use severity as a linear dimension—measured on categorical scales (e.g., "Mild," "Moderate," and "Severe"), numerical rating scales (e.g., 0, "No pain" to 10, "Worst pain possible"), visual analogue scales (a point along a 10-cm line; see Jensen & Karoly, Chapter 2, this volume)—or to use some adjectival descriptors (see Katz & Melzack, Chapter 3, this volume). Although intensity and descriptive characteristics are critical features of pain that demand attention, they are not sufficiently broad features to provide an adequate classification of the experience of even acute pain (see Mason et al., Chapter 14, this volume).

Yet another continuum is based on ages of the individuals affected. For example, there has been much debate as to whether infants and children experience pain in the same way as adults do (see Ruskin, Amaria, Warnock, & McGrath, Chapter 11, this volume). At the other end of the lifespan, there has been considerable discussion regarding alterations in sensory sensitivity of people in the later stages of life, and the impact of age-related physical changes on pain perception (see Gauthier & Gagliese, Chapter 12, this volume).

The dimensions of intensity, duration, descriptive characteristics, diagnoses, or age are not completely satisfactory in predicting persistence of pain and the associated disability. One strategy is to develop a classification based on a combination such as intensity and degree of disability to create a prognostic index (see Von Korff, Chapter 23, this volume). More extensive assessment may be particularly relevant for clinical decision making (see Turk & Robinson, Chapter 10, this volume). So, no single system for classifying pain patients has been universally accepted by clinicians or researchers.

PURPOSES OF ASSESSMENT

The measurement of pain is essential for the study of pain mechanisms and the evaluation of methods to control pain. The procedures and measures used in the assessment of pain, and people who experience pain, depend on the purpose(s) of the assessment and the unique characteristics of the population being assessed (e.g., age, educational levels, ability to communicate verbally), and the context of the assessment (e.g., acute postsurgical, emergency department/ trauma, chronic, cancer; medicolegal). The objectives of assessment can be varied and generally categorized as clinical outcomes, epidemiological, and quality improvement. Although it is important for all measures to meet basic psychometric properties of reliability (internal consistency, stability over time) and validity (for the intended use), the purposes of assessment influence number, nature, and content of measures selected.

From the clinical perspective, the intent of the assessment may be to make a differential diagnosis; to predict response to treatment; to evaluate the characteristics of pain and the impact of pain on patients' lives; to assist in disability determination and establishment of limitation of physical capacity; to monitor progress following initiation of treatment; and to evaluate the effectiveness of treatment, along with the need to continue or modify a treatment regimen, among others. When the issue is treatment success, it is important to consider who determines success. Patients, providers, managed care organizations, and workers' compensation carriers may have different criteria for judging the success of a treatment. For the patient, success might be defined by reduction in pain severity. Whereas a provider may consider both pain reduction and functional outcomes as being important, a managed care organization may base success on reduction in health care utilization, and a workers' compensation carrier may care little about pain reduction but prioritize the ability of a treatment to return workers to gainful employment.

High-quality outcomes research is based on methodological rigor with a careful study design but varying goals, from assessing treatment efficacy compared to a placebo treatment and/or active comparator, to determining appropriate dose, side effect profile, time to effect, or maintenance of treatment effect. Careful attention to the internal validity of the study is central. Specific inclusion and exclusion criteria are essential, and psychometrically sound assessment measures are included. The measures selected for assessment must be appropriate for the sample of patients actually included in the study. For example, a measure of functional activities developed for low back pain patients might not be appropriate for a study of patients with carpel tunnel syndrome. When possible, and when they are available, disease-specific measures should be used. However, if the intent is to compare across different diagnoses, then generic measures may be appropriate (Turk et al., 2003).

Epidemiological research includes the same rigor as clinical research but focuses on identification of risk factors, determination of incidence, and prevalence of pain diagnoses in specific populations. Since epidemiological research often is conducted in multiple countries and with different cultural groups, investigators need to pay particular attention to the appropriateness of even well-developed measures that have not been validated with the target populations. For example, a measure that has gone through rigorous psychometric evaluation with an English-speaking population cannot simply be translated to another language and used with speakers of that language, because the concepts may not make sense culturally.

The emphasis on quality improvement in pain management is enhancement of the quality of pain management delivery. The results of quality improvement evaluation provide a better understanding of the extent and nature of problems in service delivery, motivation for change, and points for comparison after change has been made in a system. A thorough evaluation of quality requires examination of the structure, process, and outcomes of care. In contrast to formal research, the results of a quality assurance study are not intended to produce new knowledge of widely generalizable or universal value (Berwick, 2008).

An important consideration in selecting from the vast array of assessment measures and procedures described throughout this volume and other publications, regardless of purpose, is *patient burden*; that is how long can patients with different types of pain (e.g., postsurgical, trauma in the emergency department, chronic noncancer, and terminally ill cancer patients) be expected to respond to questions, especially complex questions? Some tradeoff must be made between quantity and quality of responses. Although it might be acceptable for a chronic noncancer patient to complete a set of questionnaires requiring 1 hour and to complete home diaries several times a day for periods of weeks, such an assessment would be inappropriate in the context of a traumatic injury or acute pain following a medical procedure. Assessment addressing substance misuse and potential abuse might be relevant for a patient with chronic pain who is being considered for long-term opioid therapy, but it would be irrelevant to assess pain following a dental extraction, with pain expected to persist for only a few days at most.

Even for patients with chronic pain, one must be concerned about the quality of responses toward the end of lengthy assessment batteries. An important and related issue that has not received sufficient attention relates to the order of questions and the influence of earlier questions on subsequent ones—a *priming effect* (Haythornthwaite & Fauerbach, 2001). For example, what is the impact of asking patients to give a global rating of how well they are doing following the implementation of a particular treatment after they have responded to a set of questions about physical and emotional functioning, and the converse?

Some pain measures are indirect and make no direct demands on the patient, in that they assess behavior, facial expression, or physiological indices, after which inferences are made about the presence, strength, and characteristics of pain. Although such methods may reduce patient burden, they raise clinician burden, another factor that has to be taken into consideration in developing an assessment protocol. Measures and procedures that do not rely on patient self-reports often require special equipment and training, which may not be feasible in quality improvement studies or in the context of clinical practice.

Given the objectives of assessment, differences in populations and samples, and extent of burden involved, it becomes obvious that no single measure is appropriate for all purposes. It is this fact that motivated us to develop this volume and its two predecessors. Regardless of the way one classifies pain and people with pain, and the purposes of assessment, there appear to be a number of commonalities that transcend the age of the affected person, the duration of pain, or the diagnosis. Many of these are discussed in chapters in this volume. However, before we can hope to understand pain, we need to consider how to measure it.

MEASUREMENT OF PAIN

There is no simple thermometer that can objectively record how much pain an individual experiences. As we have noted, all that can be determined about the intensity of a person's pain is based on what the patient verbally or nonverbally communicates about his or her subjective experience. Often patients are asked to quantify their pain by providing a single general rating of pain: "Rate your *usual* level of pain on a scale from 0 to 10, where 0 equals 'no pain' and 10 is the 'worst pain you can imagine.'" Here a patient is being asked to quantify and to average his or her experience of pain over time and situations. These ratings are retrospective, and a number of studies have reported that patients significantly overestimate and underestimate their pain when asked to recall previous levels of pain (e.g., Stone, Broderick, Shiffman, & Schwartz, 2004). Moreover, pain intensity is likely to vary over time and depends on what the individual is doing. It has also been demonstrated that present levels of pain tend to influence memory; consequently, present pain levels may serve as anchors that influence the averaging of pain (see Mason et al., Chapter 14, and Von Korff, Chapter 23, this volume). Furthermore, it is possible that patients may be unable to discriminate reliably between the points on a scale and, for some, the points may not even be considering the same dimensions. The anchor words of the scale may also influence the distribution of responses. We noted concerns about retrospective reports earlier in this chapter, and many of these points are discussed by Jensen and Karoly (Chapter 2), Mason and colleagues (Chapter 14), and Von Korff (Chapter 23) in this volume.

Despite the concerns noted, intensity of pain is without a doubt the most salient dimension of pain, and a variety of procedures have been developed to measure it. However, pain is a complex, multidimensional, subjective experience. The report of pain is related to numerous variables, such as cultural background, past experience, the meaning of the situation, personality variables, attention, arousal level, emotions, and reinforcement contingencies (see DeGood & Cook, Chapter 4; Romano, Cano, & Schmaling, Chapter 5; and Turk & Robinson, Chapter 10, this volume). Using a single dimension, such as intensity, will inevitably fail to capture the many qualities of pain. In short, pain intensity, although frequently used in clinical practice to quantify the disorder, is inadequate. Moreover, pain intensity itself does not provide a good reflection of either psychological or physical disruption caused by specific disorders (as noted in many chapters in this volume).

Considerable attention has been devoted to developing measures of physical functioning. A number of attempts have relied on people's self-reports of their abilities to engage in a range of functional activities in general (e.g., Bergner, Bobbitt, Carter, & Gilson, 1981; Millard, 1989; Pollard, 1984) or disease-specific activities (Bennett et al., 2009; Roland & Fairbank, 2000), and the pain experienced upon performance of those activities (e.g., Jette, 1987) by using verbal statements or pictorial representations of specific activities (Kugler, Wijn, Geillen, de Jong, & Vlaeyen, 1999; Turk, Robinson, Sherman, Burwinkle, & Swanson, 2008). Although many investigators are skeptical of the validity of self-report measures and prefer more objective measures, studies have revealed a high level of concordance among self-report and disease characteristics, physicians' or physical therapists' ratings of functional abilities, and objective functional performance (e.g., Deyo & Diehl, 1983; Jette, 1987). Despite obvious limitations of

bias, self-report instruments have several advantages. They are economical; they enable the assessment of a wide range of behaviors relevant to the patient that may not be directly observable or measurable by any other means; and they permit emotional, social, and mental functioning to be assessed. Investigators have also developed systematic procedures for physical examination and evaluation of functional capacity that directly assess the individual's physical limitations and capabilities (see Polatin, Worzer, Brede, & Gatchel, Chapter 9, and Watson, Chapter 15, this volume).

Despite evidence to the contrary, in an effort to avoid the many problems inherent in self-reports of pain severity, some investigators and many clinicians suggest that the report of pain should be ignored, since it is a symptom rather than an "objective" sign (which is believed to be more reliable and valid). For example, the Social Security Administration in the United States bases disability determination solely on physical examination, and on imaging and laboratory diagnostic tests. It is only when these objective findings are identified that subjective report of pain is considered (Cocchiarella & Andersson, 2001; Robinson, Turk, & Loeser, 2004).

Biomedical research and advanced technology have been used in an attempt to identify the physical basis of the report of pain. The implicit assumption of this research seems to be that there is an isomorphic relationship between the report of pain and tissue pathology. Thus, once the extent of tissue pathology is identified, the intensity of pain can be known. Using objective physical assessment, diagnostic nerve blocks and sophisticated imaging, and laboratory diagnostic procedures to identify the nature and extent of pathology is assumed to provide direct knowledge of the subjective state (see Watson, Chapter 15, this volume).

To date, biomedical research has been disappointing (see Polatin et al., Chapter 9, and Robinson, Chapter 21, this volume). Little information is available on how to integrate effectively and appropriately the information derived from multiple physical examinations, diagnostic imaging, and laboratory tests. Moreover, the relationships among pathology, physical measurements of muscle strength and range of motion, behavior, and reports of pain have not been firmly established, and these factors appear to be only weakly associated (e.g., Deyo, 1986; Waddell, 2004). A number of studies demonstrate significant pathology in individuals who have little or no pain (e.g., Boden, Davis, Dina, Patronas, & Wiesel, 1990; Hitselberger & Witten, 1968; Jensen, Brant-Zawadski, Obuchowski, Modic, & Malkasian Ross, 1994; Weishaupt, Zanetti, & Hodler, 1998; Wiesel, Tsourmas, & Feffer, 1984) but, conversely, little identifiable pathology in patients who report severe pain (e.g., Deyo, 1986).

In short, the association between physical abnormalities and patients' reports of pain is often ambiguous or weak. In addition, physical pathology has been reported not to be predictive of disability (Cats-Baril & Frymoyer, 1991; Hagglund, Haley, Reveille, & Alarcon, 1989; see Robinson, Chapter 21, this volume), of return to work after an injury (e.g., Turner, Franklin, & Turk, 2000), or of treatment outcome following surgery, other invasive procedures, or rehabilitation (e.g., Waddell, 2004). One possible factor contributing to the apparent lack of correlation among pathology, symptoms, and outcome is the observation that the reliability of many physical examination procedures is questionable (see, e.g., Hunt et al., 2000; Nitschke, Nattrass, & Disler, 1999; see also Watson, Chapter 15, this volume). In addition, although physical examination measurements such as flexibility and strength may be objective, they are influenced in many cases by the patient's motivation, effort, and psychological state.

A number of physicians who have tried to develop systematic approaches to physical assessment have suggested that sophisticated laboratory and imaging techniques should form the basis of pain assessment (see Watson, Chapter 15, this volume). However, a preponderance of research has demonstrated that there is no isomorphic association between physical pathology and pain (see Robinson & Turk, Chapter 16, this volume). Many factors seem to mediate this association in both acute (Bonica, 1990) and chronic pain (Waddell, Bircher, Finlayson, & Main, 1984), as well as pain associated with terminal illnesses (Turk & Feldman, 2009). Identification of pain-specific physiological response has also met with mixed success

(cf. Sternbach, 1968; Turk, 1989). The reliability of many psychophysiological parameters has been questioned (see, e.g., Arena, Blanchard, Andrasik, Cotch, & Meyers, 1983). As Sternbach (1968) noted, "Because of the variability of response elicited by different pain stimuli, and because of the additional variance contributed by individual differences in response-stereotype, it is difficult to specify a pattern of physiological responses characteristic of pain" (p. 259).

In many patients, objective physical findings to support their reports of pain are absent. Thus, reliable and valid measures of pain and function must be developed. Some investigators have challenged the validity of patients' self-reports of activities as inaccurate (e.g., Kremer, Block, & Gaylor, 1981); however, a number of studies have demonstrated that self-report questionnaires can be highly valid measures of functional status (see, e.g., Deyo & Diehl, 1983). Physical and laboratory measures are useful primarily to the degree that they correlate with symptoms and functional ability (see Flor & Meyer, Chapter 8, this volume). However, self-report functional status instruments seek to quantify symptoms, function, and behavior directly rather than to infer them (Deyo, 1988).

Psychologists have also been concerned with the development of assessment procedures that do not rely on self-reports to evaluate patients with pain. Fordyce (1976) provided an important contribution by emphasizing the important role of environmental contingencies on the communication of pain, distress, and suffering. Patients experiencing pain display a broad range of observable manifestations that communicate to others the fact that they are feeling pain—that they are distressed and suffering. These behaviors, termed *pain behaviors*, include verbal report, paralinguistic vocalizations, motor activity, facial expressions, gesticulations, and postural adjustments (Fordyce, 1976; see Keefe, Somers, Williams, & Smith, Chapter 7, this volume). Because pain behaviors, unlike pain per se, are observable, they are susceptible to conditioning and learning influences. Patients have many opportunities to learn that the display of pain behaviors may lead to reinforcing consequences, such as attention, and the opportunity to avoid unwanted responsibilities. In some cases, these pain behaviors may be maintained by their reinforcing consequences long after the normal healing time for injury.

According to operant theory, behavior is controlled to a great extent by its consequences. With an initial injury or pathological state, these behaviors may be reflexive responses (in the language of behavioral theory, *respondents*); however, over time, these initially reflexive responses may be maintained by reinforcement contingencies; that is, attention or financial gain may be positively reinforcing and thereby contribute to the maintenance of the behaviors long after the initial cause of pain has been resolved. These insights have led to an emphasis on the assessment of these pain behaviors (see Keefe et al., Chapter 7, this volume), as well as treatments designed to extinguish maladaptive pain behaviors and to increase activity (i.e., adaptive or well behaviors).

Typically, methods used to assess pain behaviors have relied on patients' self-reports of their activities. For example, patients have been asked to indicate in general how much time they spend in specific activities such as sitting, standing, and walking (*uptime*), or to complete daily monitoring forms that record the frequency of such activities. Keefe and his colleagues (for a review, see Chapter 7, this volume) have developed specific behavioral observation methods to assess pain behaviors that are not dependent on patients' self-reports.

Unfortunately, none of the pain behaviors appear to be uniquely or invariably associated with the experience of pain. Craig and his colleagues (Chapter 6, this volume) have made a strong case for the priority of nonverbal facial expression of pain for making judgments about the pain experienced by others. These investigators have conducted fine-grained observations of the facial musculature associated with pain. As noted previously, assessment of pain based on nonverbal communication may be particularly important for those who have restrictions in their ability to communicate.

Interestingly, Flor and Turk (1988), among others (e.g., Waddell, 1987), have found that although physical impairment is related to disability, it bears a much smaller association with self-reported pain. Council, Ahern, Follick, and Kline (1988) found that the actual physical performance of patients with back pain was best predicted by their *beliefs in their capabilities* and not by pain per se. Moreover, Vlaeyen and Linton (2000) have demonstrated that fears of pain and injury are particularly potent predictors of physical functioning. Turk and colleagues (Flor & Turk, 1988; Turk, Okifuji, Sinclair, & Starz, 1996) examined the relationship among general and specific pain-related thoughts, convictions of personal control, pain severity, and disability levels in patients with chronic back pain, rheumatoid arthritis, and fibromyalgia. The general and situation-specific convictions of uncontrollability and helplessness were more highly related to pain and disability than to disease status for the patients with back pain and rheumatoid arthritis. For the patients with fibromyalgia syndrome, there was only a low correlation between what patients *said* they were able to do and their actual activities. These data suggest that it is important to assess not only how much patients report they hurt and what they say they are able to do, but also how much they actually do.

The failure to find a relationship between reported pain and pathology has resulted in the suggestion that personality factors may be the cause of pain or may influence reports of pain that are "disproportionate" to the identified pathology. The search for a "pain-prone personality" (see, e.g., Blumer & Heilbronn, 1982) and for "psychogenic pain" has proven to be futile (see Sullivan & Braden, Chapter 20, this volume). The many variables that have been perceived to be part of a personality constellation related to psychogenic pain may actually be reactions to illness, independent of psychiatric diagnosis. A number of investigators have begun to examine the predictive power of individual-difference measures to predict response to diverse treatments for pain. Many third-party payers are beginning to require presurgical screening prior to surgery or use of implantable devices (i.e., spinal cord stimulators, pumps; see Gatchel, Chapter 22, this volume), and measures have been developed in an effort to predict patients at risk for opioid misuse. However, many of the common psychological instruments have not demonstrated clear utility in diagnostic or treatment outcome predictions (Turk, 1989; Turk, Swanson, & Gatchel, 2008). This area holds promise for improving outcomes but calls for additional research to confirm the predictive validity of the assessment protocols.

A BROADER PERSPECTIVE IN THE PERSON EXPERIENCING PAIN

Over the past 45 years, major research advances have greatly increased knowledge of the anatomy and neurophysiology of nociception. The landmark papers by Melzack and his colleagues (Melzack & Casey, 1968; Melzack & Wall, 1965) formulating the *gate control* theory of pain expanded the conceptualization of pain from a purely sensory phenomenon to a multidimensional model that integrates motivational–affective and cognitive–evaluative components with sensory–physiological ones. The gate control model served as an important impetus to physiological research and research on identifying and demonstrating the modulation of pain perception by psychological variables. The gate control model emphasizes that pain is not exclusively sensory, and that simple measures of pain intensity are inadequate to understand it. In the 1970s, Melzack and colleagues (Melzack, 1975; Melzack & Torgerson, 1971) developed the first assessment instrument, the McGill Pain Questionnaire, designed to measure the three components of pain postulated by the gate control theory (see Katz & Melzack, Chapter 3, this volume).

Since Melzack and his colleagues' pioneering work on pain assessment, a number of investigators have emphasized that pain that extends over time (i.e., chronic pain, acute recurrent pain, pain associated with progressive diseases) has an important impact on all domains of the sufferer's life. Persistent pain is so prepotent that psychological factors may come to play an even greater role in influencing the subjective experience, report, and responses. Physicians have long recognized that disease categories provide minimal information about the impact of illness upon patients' experiences. A diagnosis is important, because it may identify a cause of symptoms and suggest a course of treatment. Yet within each specific diagnosis, patients differ considerably in how they are affected (see, e.g., Turk & Rudy, 1990) and how they respond to treatment. Consequent-

ly, appropriate evaluation of these patients requires assessment of much more than just the direct components of pain; it also calls for assessment of mood, attitudes, beliefs, coping efforts, resources, and the impact of pain on patients' lives (see DeGood & Cook, Chapter 4, and Turk & Robinson, Chapter 10, this volume). Moreover, because people do not live in isolation, chronic pain influences interpersonal relationships and is influenced by them. Thus, it is important to consider both contextual and individual patient characteristics (see Romano et al., Chapter 5, this volume).

In conclusion, health care providers have long considered pain as being synonymous with nociceptive stimulation and pathology. It is important, however, to make a distinction among *nociception, pain, suffering*, and *pain behavior* (Turk & Wilson, 2009). *Nociception* is the processing of stimuli that are related to the stimulation of nociceptors and capable of being experienced as pain. *Pain*, because it involves conscious awareness, selective abstraction, appraisal, ascribing meaning, and learning, is best viewed as a perceptual process that comprises the integration and modulation of a number of afferent and efferent processes (Melzack & Casey, 1968). Thus, the experience of pain should not be equated with peripheral stimulation. *Suffering*, which includes interpersonal disruption, economic distress, occupational problems, and myriad other factors associated with pain's impact on life functioning, is largely associated with the interpretive processes and subsequent response to the perception of pain. A number of studies dating back over 20 years (e.g., Reesor & Craig, 1988) have demonstrated that cognitive processes appear to amplify or distort patients' experience of pain and suffering. In sharp contrast to the nociceptive model, operant pain *behaviors* can occur in the absence of and may thus be independent of nociception.

Although biomedical factors appear to instigate the initial report of pain in the majority of cases, psychosocial and behavioral factors may serve over time to exacerbate and maintain levels of pain and subsequent disability. It is important to acknowledge that disability is not solely a function of the extent of physical pathology or reported pain severity (see, e.g., Fordyce et al., 1984; Waddell et al., 1984; see Robinson, Chapter 21, this volume). Disability is a complex phenomenon that incorporates tissue pathology, the total individual's response to that physical insult, and environmental factors that can serve to maintain the disability and associated pain even after the initial physical cause has resolved. Pain that persists over time should be viewed not as the result of either solely physical or solely psychological causes, but rather as a set of biomedical, psychosocial, and behavioral factors contributing to the total experience of pain.

CHANGES IN HEALTH CARE

Over the past few years, there has been a marked change in health care. Much greater attention is being given to evidence for not only the clinical effectiveness but also the cost-effectiveness of treatments. Health care providers are being asked—actually, challenged—to provide evidence of the effectiveness of the treatment they propose to perform, and reimbursement will be based on actual outcomes—"pay for performance." Many decisions regarding reimbursement are based on the availability of convincing data that the treatment results in positive outcomes—ones that are important to third-party payers (i.e., reduction in health care consumption, reduction in indemnity payments, return to gainful employment) and are less costly than alternatives. To be responsive to these demands, it has become incumbent on health care providers to make available information supporting the effectiveness of their treatments and demonstrating that they achieve positive outcomes in their practices. Effective dissemination of evidence of treatment outcomes is also becoming crucial. Thus, health care providers need to give greater attention to the performance of clinical trials, to program evaluation, and to effective communication of their own and others' published results of relevant outcome studies and epidemiological research (see Chapter 23 by Von Korff and Chapter 24 by O'Connor & Dworkin, this volume). In selecting measures to use for communication, for treatment decision making, for the interpretation of published results, and for the evaluation of their own practices, they need to be aware of the basic requirements of psychometrics.

SOME PROSPECTIVE CAVEATS

In this volume, detailed discussions are presented, and descriptions of a broad range of assessment techniques, methods, and measures are provided. At this point, it seems appropriate to provide some cautions that may serve to inoculate the reader. One of us (DCT) is reminded of the examination question he gave to graduate students in the course on tests and measurements he taught: "Imagine that you read a journal article describing a new assessment battery, and you believe it is the answer to your prayers for the research study that you are proposing in a grant application. Describe how you would go about convincing your collaborators and the grant reviewers that this battery is appropriate and should be used."

We must balance the tendency to focus on variables for which there are existing reliable and valid measures against the need to examine what is truly important. Clinicians and researchers should also guard against picking instruments blindly "off the shelf" simply because they are well known, popular, or have received extensive validation. It is essential that the instrument or procedure under consideration has been standardized on the population of interest and addresses the question(s) of interest in the study. We should not assume that because an instrument or procedure has been demonstrated to have good psychometric properties in one population it can be applied to another population without a demonstration of the instrument's psychometric properties in the new population.

Currently there is no single agreed-upon method for evaluating patients with pain. Many competing instruments, procedures, and methods are available. Each investigator or clinician develops his or her own set by selecting from the many available techniques or by developing personalized assessment instruments—often without giving sufficient attention to the psychometric properties of the measures used. This practice makes it difficult to compare results across studies. There needs to be some agreement with regard to what set of instruments and procedures will be used as the standards for each relevant domain of assessment. This is something of a double-edged sword, and we must be careful not to preclude using some new measures that may provide important new information.

Developing assessment instruments and procedures that have appropriate psychometric properties is necessary but not sufficient. Given the complexities inherent in the construct of subjective pain, there is a need to obtain a diversity of assessment information that must then be integrated to understand the patient's pain and to contribute to treatment decision making. Many clinical outcome studies report on the mean differences between groups that receive the treatment of interest compared to a placebo or an active comparator. Although the results tend to report on the between-group statistical significance of prespecified outcome measures (i.e., primary endpoint) such mean effects do not provide any indication of the results' clinical importance or their importance to patients. There is a growing acknowledgment of the need to report on meaningfulness of the outcomes rather than to rely solely on statistical significance; that is, with sufficient sample size, a change of one-half point on a 10-point numerical rating scale may prove to be statistically significant, but how meaningful is such a small change? A number of parameters can be used as indications of meaningfulness, such as effect sizes, number needed to treat (to produce a positive benefit or harm), and more formal approaches to determine the minimally important difference (Busse & Guyatt, 2009; see also O'Connor & Dworkin, Chapter 24, this volume).

Most of what is known about patients with chronic pain has been learned from studying patients referred to specialized pain clinics. These patients represent a very small percentage of patients who experience chronic pain—those who have gone through a selective filtering process (Turk & Rudy, 1990). The degree to which this segment of patients is representative of the larger population of people with chronic pain is highly questionable. As epidemiological surveys seem to suggest, pain clinic samples may differ in many ways from community samples. For example, the association between psychological findings and pain frequently noted in pain clinics is less frequently observed in epidemiological studies (Crook, Weir, & Tunks, 1989).

Our primary purpose in this volume is to provide a comprehensive and practical review of the advances in the measurement of pain and the assessment of patients with pain, and to recommend the most appropriate tests and procedures given the current state of knowledge. Our hope is that the reader will, upon examination of each of the contributions, be in a better situation to provide psychometrically acceptable and sufficiently comprehensive approaches to the problem to be investigated.

ACKNOWLEDGMENT

Preparation of this chapter was supported in part by Grant No. AR44724 from the National Institutes of Health (National Institute of Arthritis and Musculoskeletal and Skin Diseases) to Dennis C. Turk.

REFERENCES

Arena, J. G., Blanchard, E. B., Andrasik, F., Cotch, P. A., & Meyers, P. E. (1983). Reliability of psychophysiological assessment. *Behaviour Research and Therapy, 21,* 447–460.

Bennett, R. M., Friend, R., Jones, K., Ward, R., Han, B. K., & Ross, R. L. (2009). The revised Fibromyalgia Impact Questionnaire (FIQR): Validation and psychometric properties. *Arthritis Research and Therapy, 11,* R120.

Bergner, M., Bobbitt, R. A., Carter, W. B., & Gilson, B. S. (1981). The Sickness Impact Profile: Development and final revision of a health status measure. *Medical Care, 19,* 787–805.

Berwick, D. (2008). The science of improvement. *Journal of the American Medical Association, 299,* 1182–1184.

Blumer, D., & Heilbronn, D. (1982). Chronic pain as a variant of depressive disease: The pain-prone disorder. *Journal of Nervous and Mental Disease, 170,* 381–406.

Boden, S. D., Davis, D. O., Dina, T. S., Patronas, N. J., & Wiesel, S. W. (1990). Abnormal magnetic resonance scans of the lumbar spine in asymptomatic subjects. *Journal of Bone and Joint Surgery, 72A,* 403–408.

Bonica, J. J. (1990). Postoperative pain. In J. J. Bonica, J. D. Loeser, C. R. Chapman, & W. E. Fordyce (Eds.), *The management of pain* (pp. 461–480). Philadelphia: Lea & Febiger.

Broderick, J. E., Schwartz, J. E., Vikingstad, G., Pribbernow, M., Grossman, S., & Stone, A. A. (2008). The accuracy of pain and fatigue items across different reporting periods. *Pain, 139,* 146–157.

Busse, J. W., & Guyatt, G. H. (2009). Optimizing the use of patient data to improve outcomes for patients: Narcotics for chronic noncancer pain. *Expert Review of Pharmacoeconomics and Outcomes Research, 9,* 171–179.

Cantor, S. B. (2002). Pharmacoeconomics of coxib therapy. *Journal of Pain and Symptom Management, 24*(Suppl. 1), S28–S37.

Cats-Baril, W. L., & Frymoyer, J. W. (1991). Identifying patients at risk of becoming disabled because of low back pain: The Vermont Engineering Center Predictive Model. *Spine, 16,* 605–607.

Cherry, D., Burt, C., & Woodwell, D. (2001). *National Ambulatory Medical Care Survey: 1999 summary* [Advance Data from Vital and Health Statistics, No. 322]. Hyattsville, MD: National Center on Health Statistics.

Cocchiarella, L., & Andersson, G. B. J. (2001). *Guides to the evaluation of permanent impairment* (5th ed.). Chicago: AMA Press.

Council, J. R., Ahern, D. K., Follick, M. J., & Kline, C. L. (1988). Expectancies and functional impairment in chronic low back pain. *Pain, 33,* 323–331.

Crook, J., Weir, R., & Tunks, E. (1989). An epidemiological follow-up survey of persistent pain sufferers in a group family practice and specialty pain clinic. *Pain, 36,* 49–61.

Deyo, R. A. (1986). The early diagnostic evaluation of patients with low back pain. *Journal of General Internal Medicine, 1,* 328–338.

Deyo, R. A. (1988). Measuring the functional status of patients with low back pain. *Archives of Physical Medicine and Rehabilitation, 69,* 1044–1053.

Deyo, R. A., & Diehl, A. K. (1983). Measuring physical and psychosocial function in patients with low-back pain. *Spine, 8,* 635–642.

Employer Health Care Strategy Survey. (2003, March). *Deloitte & Touche LLP Health Magazine.*

Flor, H., & Turk, D. C. (1988). Chronic back pain and rheumatoid arthritis: Predicting pain and disability from cognitive variables. *Journal of Behavioral Medicine, 11,* 251–265.

Fordyce, W. E. (1976). *Behavioral methods for chronic pain and illness.* St. Louis, MO: Mosby.

Fordyce, W. E., Lansky, D., Calsyn, D. A., Shelton, J. L., Stolov, W. C., & Rock, D. L. (1984). Pain measurement and pain behavior. *Pain, 18,* 53–69.

Gureje, O. (1998). Persistent pain and well-being: A World Health Organization study in primary care. *Journal of the American Medical Association, 280,* 147–151.

Hagglund, K. J., Haley, W. E., Reveille, J. D., & Alarcon, G. S. (1989). Predicting individual impairment among patients with rheumatoid arthritis. *Arthritis and Rheumatism, 32,* 851–858.

Haythornthwaite, J. A., & Fauerbach, J. A. (2001). Assessment of acute pain, pain relief, and patient satisfaction. In D. C. Turk & R. Melzack (Eds.), *Handbook of pain assessment* (2nd ed., pp. 417–430). New York: Guilford Press.

Hing, E., Cherry, D. K., & Woodwell, D. A. (2006). *National Ambulatory Medical Care Survey: 2004 summary* [Advance Data from Vital and Health Statistics, No. 374]. Hyattsville, MD: National Center or Health Statistics.

Hitselberger, W. E., & Witten, R. M. (1968). Abnormal myelograms in asymptomatic patients. *Journal of Neurosurgery, 28,* 204–206.

Hunt, D. G., Zuberbier, O. A., Kozolowski, A. J., Robinson, J., Berkowitz, J., Schultz, I. Z., et al. (2001). Reliability of the lumbar flexion, lumbar extension and passive straight leg raise test in normal populations embedded within a complete physical examination. *Spine, 26,* 2714–2718.

Illich, I. (1976). *Medical nemesis: The exploration of health.* Harmondsworth, UK: Penguin Books.

Jamison, R. N., Raymond, S. A., Slawsby, E. A., McHugo, G. J., & Baird, J. C. (2006). Pain assessment in patients with low back pain: Comparison of weekly reall and momentary electronic data. *Journal of Pain, 7,* 192–199.

Jensen, M. C., Brant-Zawadski, M. N., Obuchowski, N., Modic, M. T., & Malkasian Ross, J. S. (1994). Magnetic resonance imaging of the lumbar spine in people with back pain. *New England Journal of Medicine, 331,* 69–73.

Jette, A. M. (1987). The Functional Status Index: Reliability and validity of a self-report functional disability measure. *Journal of Rheumatology, 14*(Suppl. 14), 15–19.

Kremer, E. F., Block, A., & Gaylor, M. S. (1981). Behavioral approaches to treatment of chronic pain: The inaccuracy of patient self-report measures. *Archives of Physical Medicine and Rehabilitation, 62,* 188–191.

Kugler, K., Wijn, J., Geillen, M., de Jong, D., & Vlaeyen, J. W. (1999). *The photograph series of daily activities (PHODA).* CD-ROM version 1.0. Heerlen, The Netherlands: Institute for Rehabilitation Research and School for Physiotherapy.

Lasagna, L. (1960). Clinical measurement of pain. *Annals of the New York Academy of Sciences, 86,* 28–37.

Lethbridge-Cejku, M., & Vickerie, J. (2005). Summary health statistics for U.S. adults: National Health Interview Survey, 2003. National Center for Health Statistics. *Vital Health Statistics, 10*(225).

Mathias, S. D., Kuppermann, M., Liberman, R.

F., Lipschurz, R. C., & Steegle, J. F. (1996). Chronic pelvic pain: Prevalence, health-related quality of life, and economic correlates. *Obstetrics and Gynecology, 87,* 321–327.

Mayo Clinic. (2001). Managing pain: Attitude, medication and therapy are keys to control. Mayo Clinic website. Retrieved September 19, 2001, from *www.mayoclinic.com/invoke.cfm?id=HQO/055.*

Melzack, R. (1975). The McGill Pain Questionnaire: Major properties and scoring methods. *Pain, 1,* 277–299.

Melzack, R., & Casey, K. L. (1968). Sensory, motivational, and central control determinants of pain: A new conceptual model. In D. Kenshalo (Ed.), *The skin senses* (pp. 423–443). Springfield, IL: Thomas.

Melzack, R., & Torgerson, W. S. (1971). On the language of pain. *Anesthesiology, 34,* 50–59.

Melzack, R., & Wall, P. D. (1965). Pain mechanisms: A new theory. *Science, 150,* 971–979.

Millard, R. W. (1989). The Functional Assessment Screening Questionnaire: Application for evaluating pain-related disability. *Archives of Physical Medicine and Rehabilitation, 70,* 303–307.

National Academies of Sciences & Institute of Medicine. (2001). *Musculoskeletal disorders and the workplace: Low back pain and upper extremities.* Washington, DC: National Academies Press.

National Center for Health Statistics [NCHS]. (2006). *Health, United States, 2006 with chartbook on trends in the health of Americans.* Hyattsville, MD: Author.

National Headache Foundation. (2005). Fact Sheet, January 1, 2003. Retrieved September 22, 2006, from *www.headaches.org/consumer/presskit/factsheet.pdf.*

Nitschke, J. E., Nattrass, C. L., & Disler, P. B. (1999). Reliability of the American Medical Association guides' model for measuring spinal range of motion. *Spine, 24,* 262–268.

Perquin, C. W., Hazebroek-Kampscheur, A. A., Hunfeld, J. A., Bohnen, A. M., van Suijlekom-Smit, L. W. A. Passchier, J., et al. (2000). Pain in children and adolescents: A common experience. *Pain, 87,* 51–58.

Pollard, C. A. (1984). Preliminary study of the Pain Disability Index. *Perceptual and Motor Skills, 59,* 974.

Reesor, K. A., & Craig, K. D. (1988). Medically incongruent chronic back pain: Physical limitations, suffering, and ineffective coping. *Pain, 32,* 35–45.

Ricci, J. A., Stewart, W. F., Chee, E., Leotta, C., Foley, K., & Hochberg, M. C. (2005). Pain exacerbating as a major source of lost productive time in U.S. workers with arthritis. *Arthritis and Rheumatism, 53,* 673–681.

Robinson, J. P., Turk, D. C., & Loeser, J. D. (2004). Pain, impairment, and disability in the AMA guides. *Journal of Law, Medicine, and Ethics, 32,* 315–326.

Sheffield, R. E. (1998). Migraine prevalence: A literature review. *Headache, 38,* 595–601.

Sternbach, R. (1968). *Pain: A psychophysiological analysis.* New York: Academic Press.

Stewart, W. F., Ricci, J. A., Chee, E., Morganstein, D., & Lipton, R. (2003). Lost productive time and cost due to common pain conditions in the workforce. *Journal of the American Medical Association, 290,* 2443–2454.

Stone, A. A., Broderick, J. E., Shiffman, S. S., & Schwartz, J. E. (2004). Understanding recall of weekly pain from a momentary assessment perspective: Absolute agreement, between- and within-person consistency, and judged change in weekly pain. *Pain, 107,* 61–69.

Turk, D. C. (1989). Assessment of pain: The elusiveness of latent constructs. In C. R. Chapman & J. D. Loeser (Eds.), *Advances in pain research and therapy: Vol. 12. Issues in pain measurement* (pp. 267–279). New York: Raven Press.

Turk, D. C., Dworkin, R. H., Allen, R. R., Bellamy, N., Brandenburg, N., Carr, D. B., et al. (2003). Core outcomes domains for chronic pain clinical trials: IMMPACT recommendations. *Pain, 106,* 337–345.

Turk, D. C., & Feldman, C. F. (2009). Cognitive-behavioral approaches to symptom management in palliative care: Augmenting somatic interventions. In H. M. Chochinov & W. Breitbart, (Eds.), *Handbook of psychiatry in palliative medicine* (2nd ed., pp. 470–489). New York: Oxford University Press.

Turk, D. C., & Melzack, R. (Eds.). (1992). *Handbook of pain assessment.* New York: Guilford press.

Turk, D. C., & Melzack, R. (Eds.). (2001). *Handbook of pain assessment* (2nd ed.). New York: Guilford Press.

Turk, D. C., & Okifuji, A. (2001). Pain terms and taxonomies. In J. D. Loeser, C. R. Chapman, S. D. Butler, & D. C. Turk (Eds.), *Bonica's management of pain* (3rd ed., pp. 17–25). Philadelphia: Lippincott Williams & Wilkins.

Turk, D. C., Okifuji, A., Sinclair, J. D., & Starz, T. W. (1996). Pain, disability, and physical functioning in subgroups of fibromyalgia patients. *Journal of Rheumatology, 23,* 1255–1262.

Turk, D. C., Robinson, J. P., Sherman, J. J., Burwinkle, T. M., & Swanson, K. S. (2008). Assessing fear in patients with cervical pain: Development and validation of the Pictorial Fear of Activity Scale—Cervical (PFActS-C). *Pain, 139,* 55–62.

Turk, D. C., & Rudy, T. E. (1990). Neglected factors in chronic pain treatment outcome studies: Referral patterns, failure to enter treatment, and attrition. *Pain, 43*, 7–26.

Turk, D. C., Swanson, K. S., & Gatchel, R. J. (2008). Predicting opioid misuse by chronic pain patients: A systematic review and literature synthesis. *Clinical Journal of Pain, 24*, 497–508.

Turk, D. C., & Wilson, H. D. (2009). Pain, suffering, pain-related suffering: Are these constructs inextricably linked? [Editorial]. *Clinical Journal of Pain, 25*, 353–355.

Turner, J. A., Franklin, G., & Turk, D. C. (2000). Predictors of long-term disability in injured workers: A systematic literature synthesis. *American Journal of Industrial Medicine, 38*, 707–722.

Vlaeyen, J. W. S., & Linton, S. J. (2000). Fear-avoidance and its consequences in chronic musculoskeletal pain: A state of the art. *Pain, 85*, 317–332.

Waddell, G. (1987). A new clinical method for the treatment of low back pain. *Spine, 12*, 632–644.

Waddell, G. (2004). *The back pain revolution* (2nd ed.). Edinburgh, UK: Churchill Livingstone.

Waddell, G., Bircher, M., Finlayson, D., & Main, C. J. (1984). Symptoms and signs: Physical disease or illness behavior? *British Medical Journal, 289*, 739–741.

Washington Business Group on Health and Watson Wyatt Worldwide. (2003). *Creating a sustainable health care program* [Eighth annual Washington Business Group on Health/Watson Wyatt Survey Report]. Washington, DC: Author.

Webb, R., Brammah, T., Lunt, M., Urwin, M., Allison, T., & Symmons, D. (2003). Prevalence and predictors of intense, chronic and disabling neck and back pain in the UK general population. *Spine, 28*, 1195–1202.

Weishaupt, D., Zanetti, M., & Hodler, J. (1998). MR imagining of the lumbar spine: Prevalence of intervertebral disk extrusion and sequestration, nerve root compression, and end plate abnormalities, and osteoarthritis of the facet joints in asymptomatic volunteers. *Radiology, 209*, 661–666.

Wiesel, S. W., Tsourmas, N., & Feffer, H. (1984). A study of computer-assisted tomography: 1. The incidence of positive CAT scans in an asymptomatic group of patients. *Spine, 9*, 549–551.

Woolf, C., Bennett, G. J., Doherty, M., Dubner, R., Kidd, B., Koltzenburg, M., et al. (1998). Towards a mechanism-based classification of pain [Editorial]. *Pain, 77*, 227–229.

PART I

SELF-REPORT MEASURES OF PAIN

CHAPTER 2

Self-Report Scales and Procedures for Assessing Pain in Adults

MARK P. JENSEN
PAUL KAROLY

Because feelings of pain and suffering are private, internal events that cannot be directly observed by clinicians or indexed via bioassays, their assessment is frequently built upon the use of patient self-report. Our purpose in this chapter is to evaluate critically the major types of self-report indices currently being employed to assess the subjective experiences of pain. Our aim is to assist clinicians and researchers to select the procedures that best serve their purposes. We begin with a brief discussion of some key issues to consider when selecting self-report pain scales, then critically evaluate the methods currently available for assessing pain experience.

EXPERIENTIAL DIMENSIONS OF CHRONIC PAIN

At least four dimensions or categories of the pain experience can be assessed in nearly all pain patients: pain intensity, pain affect, pain quality, and pain location.

Pain intensity may be defined as *how much* a person hurts. Patients are usually able to provide quantitative pain intensity estimates relatively quickly, and most measures of pain intensity tend to be closely related to one another statistically (e.g., Jens-

en, Karoly, & Braver, 1986; Jensen, Karoly, O'Riordan, Bland, & Burns, 1989). Pain intensity is a fairly homogeneous dimension that is relatively easy for adults to identify.

Pain affect, on the other hand, is more complex than pain intensity. Pain affect is the degree of emotional arousal or the changes in action readiness caused by the sensory experience of pain. Pain-related affect is often felt as distressing or frightening, and can lead to interference with daily activities, habitual modes of response, and/or regulatory efficiency. Pain affect is, thus, a mental state triggered by an implicit or explicit appraisal of threat. In chronic pain, the emotional aspects (or fear appraisals) can come to dominate the clinical picture.

Measures of pain affect are statistically distinct from measures of pain intensity, yet they are rarely completely independent (Fernandez & Turk, 1992; Gracely, 1992; Huber et al., 2007). Furthermore, measures of pain affect are not as homogeneous as measures of pain intensity (i.e., they are less likely to be strongly related to one another). This finding indicates that the affective component of pain consists of a variety of emotional reactions (Clark et al., 2003; Morley, 1989; Morley & Pallin, 1995). The complexity of affective pain experience makes it similar to other sensory-perceptual experiences, and it often requires more than a single word or number to describe it adequately.

Pain quality refers to the specific physical sensations associated with pain. Because pain can be felt (and described) in so many ways, this category of pain contains a variety of constructs, such as perceived temperature (e.g., "cold" to "hot"), and sharpness (e.g., "dull" to "sharp"), among many others (see Katz and Melzack, Chapter 3, this volume).

Pain location can be defined as the perceived location(s) of pain sensation that patients experience on or in their bodies. Clinicians have learned to pay attention to several aspects of patient descriptions of pain location. The sites and the number of locations indicated, and the way in which patients describe the location(s) of their pain, all appear to be related to physical and psychosocial functioning.

ON THE MULTIPLE CONTEXTS OF PAIN MEASUREMENT

The pain context model (Karoly, 1985, 1991; Karoly & Jensen, 1987) directs an assessor's attention to the degree to which the pain experience is embedded in its surroundings. When we talk of "objective" measures or "quantifiable" indices, the reader should understand that we do not intend to depict pain as a static, all-or-none, body-centered occurrence that exists somehow independent of time, place, the patient's states of consciousness, or the observer's presuppositions. Clearly, there is no single best way to interpret pain, and we can probably serve our patients better if we acknowledge that we are jointly engaged in creating the pain dimensions we seek to measure (Karoly & Jensen, 1987, p. 7). Moreover, it is important to remember that thought, action, and emotion are inextricably bound together in the sentient organism—and they are separable only for the sake of convenience. Moreover, pain experience *emerges* from the dynamic interplay of thought, action, and emotion in context.

Research from a number of sources and with different populations provides strong evidence that many factors influence communication about pain. For example, Levine and De Simone (1991) placed college stu-

dents in the presence of an attractive male or female while immersing one hand in ice water and providing a rating of their pain. Based on gender role expectations, Levine and De Simone predicted that males would report less pain in the presence of the female as opposed to the male experimenter. This is exactly what they found. Female students, on the other hand, were not significantly influenced by the gender of the experimenter (see also Kállai, Barke, & Voss, 2004). In another study, Craig and Weiss (1971) found that modeling of pain tolerance influences the report of pain. Subjects who observed people displaying high pain tolerance reported higher pain tolerance (in response to electric shock) than subjects who observed people modeling low pain tolerance. Dworkin and Chen (1982) showed that changing the environment influences pain report. Their subjects reported that tooth pulp stimulation hurt more when administered in a dental clinic rather than a research laboratory setting. Even a person's history of injury can alter how he or she responds to painful stimuli (Dar, Ariely, & Frank, 1995).

There are several implications of the previous findings for assessing and interpreting self-report pain data. First, the findings illustrate that self-reports of pain do not stand in a one-to-one relationship to *nociception* (defined as the activation of sensory transduction in receptors or nerves that convey information about tissue damage). In addition, although it is likely that people attempt to report their subjective pain experience honestly in most situations, there are no guarantees that what people say about their pain accurately reflects their current or past pain experience. These considerations have caused some clinicians and investigators to advocate the elimination of self-report data. Although we do not agree with such an extreme position, we nonetheless strongly advise clinicians and researchers to be wary of relying solely on decontextualized subjective pain reports when attempting to understand an individual's pain problem.

A key implication of this body of research is that clinicians and researchers should take into account the factors known to influence self-report of pain. The conditions under which self-reports of pain are made should be as similar as possible between comparison groups or between assessment periods.

Attempts should be made, for example, to have patients rate their pain at the same time of day, in the same place, and in the presence of the same people at each assessment period. It is also necessary to use the same measures, with the same endpoint descriptors across time. A decision to aggregate multiple measures across time and/or across measures (e.g., taking the average of several pain measures) will help to minimize the influence of extraneous or irrelevant contextual factors, and may have a greater impact on increasing the reliability and validity of pain assessment than any other decision a clinician or researcher may make, including decisions about specific pain measures. In support of this practice, aggregated pain measures have been shown to be more reliable (Andrasik & Holroyd, 1980; Jensen & McFarland, 1993; Jensen, Turner, Romano, & Fisher, 1999) and more sensitive to treatment effects (Max, 1991) than single items. It is also possible to allow the respondent him- or herself to aggregate pain experience by providing a rating of "average" pain over the course of a specific time period (say, during the past week). Although such estimates are adequately valid in many situations (Jensen, Turner, Turner, & Romano, 1996; Salovey, Smith, Turk, Jobe, & Willis, 1993), memory of previous pain is biased (to some degree) by current pain experience (i.e., people tend to rate their previous pain as worse if they are experiencing more pain at the time they are asked to recall previous pain than if they are experiencing less pain when rating previous pain) (Jensen et al., 1996; Salovey et al., 1993). Therefore, more accurate estimates of actual average pain can be obtained by averaging multiple measures (of current pain) over time than by asking patients to recall and rate their average pain (Jensen et al., 1996).

OBTAINING SELF-REPORTS IN REAL TIME AND IN THE NATURAL ENVIRONMENT: PAIN DIARY METHODS

A growing number of clinicians and researchers have elected to make use of daily pain diaries (typically electronic devices; e.g., cell phones, pagers, or personal digital assistants [PDAs]) that require patients to record their pain levels, along with pain-related thoughts, feelings, or activities, on multiple occasions over the course of a day and to repeat the process for an extended period of time (several weeks to several months). Alternatively called *experience sampling, time sampling, intensive momentary recording, real-time data capture, ecological momentary assessment*, or simply *diary methods*, this set of procedures is characterized by attempts to model the causal dynamics underlying sampled moments of people's lives by means of electronic cueing and recording (Bolger, Davis, & Rafaeli, 2003; Shiffman, Stone, & Hufford, 2008). The use of diaries in the domain of pain has grown in recent years not only because of clinicians' desires to transcend retrospective recall biases but also because the momentary diary recordings reported in the literature have been relatively brief (typically involving 20 or so responses per occasion), have been completed with remarkably high levels of compliance and minimal shifts in pain levels due to recording (reactivity), and have been accompanied by impressive ratings of user satisfaction (see Burton, Weller, & Sharpe, 2007; Stone et al., 2003).

Although there are significant costs to the use of electronic diaries (discussed below), there are also some real advantages that justify the serious consideration of the diary methodology where feasible, and especially when there is a need to understand the pattern of interrelationships between pain and other key variables over time. Understanding the repeatable pain patterns that influence a patient's life as it unfolds at home, at work, or at play, as well as gauging how personally meaningful interpersonal and intrapsychic events impact the day-to-day experience of pain could mean the difference between an informed (data-driven) and successful intervention and an unsuccessful one. Nonetheless, the design of pain diary protocols, like the design of self-report questionnaires or response scales, requires careful attention to numerous practical and conceptual considerations. First, although how much a person is hurting (pain intensity level), for how long, and at what bodily location(s) can all be diary targets, the assessor must first decide upon the exact purpose of measurement. If the goal, for example, is to identify the situational triggers of pain, then the assessment might initially focus on *where* and *when* the pain happens, and *who* is present when the pain occurs. In such a case, a time-based sampling strategy (i.e., having an electronic diary randomly emit a signal [a "beep"] to indicate that now is the time to respond) might be used for tracking events that fluctuate over the course of a day. If we discover that pain flares are most apt to happen in the presence of a spouse, then we might later elect to employ an event-sampling procedure wherein the person enters his or her pain-related data only in the company of the presumed interpersonal trigger. Diary pain assessments can also use a combination of time- and event-based sampling. What is critical, of course, is that the sampling be *context sensitive*—situated in time and place—and, therefore, not so obviously prone to the usual memory distortions that tend to occur with retrospective recall.

Another consideration centers on the *burden* imposed by the number of diary responses called for per sampling occasion and the extent of the technical training necessary to ensure accuracy and persistence of data entry. Although minimizing such burdens goes a long way toward facilitating high-quality reporting, skimping on participant training should be avoided. There are also a host of other decisions pertaining to which diary platforms to purchase, which software to use, and precisely how to assemble and analyze the large datasets produced (even from a single pain patient) (see Christensen, Feldman Barrett, Bliss-Moreau, Lebo, & Kaschub, 2003; Piasecki, Hufford, Solhan, & Trull, 2007).

On the other hand, diary measures are susceptible to four significant weaknesses or drawbacks that should be kept in mind (Jensen, 2010). First, the hardware and software required for electronic data capture are expensive to obtain and maintain, and may exceed the budget of some investigators or clinical practitioners. Second, diary data require more time and effort than do simple recall ratings, yet it is not obvious how many times per day patients need to report pain to capture their usual pain experience adequately. Although some procedures require only one assessment per day (e.g., Gaertner, Elsner, Pollmann-Dahmen, Radbruch, & Sabatowski, 2004; Heiberg et al., 2007; Palermo, Valenzuela, & Stork, 2004), it is more common to ask patients to provide three

(Stinson et al., 2008) or even more (e.g., four to six times; Evans et al., 2007; Litcher-Kelly, Kellerman, Hanauer, & Stone, 2007; Roelofs, Peters, Patijn, Schouten, & Vlaeyen, 2006) daily ratings. Multiple ratings require a significant effort on the part of patients. A third problem with diary data is that this approach can result in missing data. The reported percentages of missing data points from electronic diary studies range from 6 (Stone et al., 2003) to 17% (Peters et al., 2000). The reported rates of study participants who provide incomplete data (i.e., at least some missing data during the study period) range from 17 (Evans et al., 2007) to 46% (Gaertner et al., 2004). The primary reported reason for missing electronic data is that the patient did not hear the alarm or cue signaling the assessment (Aaron, Mancl, Turner, Sawchuk, & Klein, 2004). When data are missing, investigators need either to remove subjects from the analyses (which limits the generalizability of the findings, and runs the risk of overstating the impact of treatment) or to use some method to impute the missing data (i.e., to estimate what the missing ratings might have been had all subjects provided complete data). Regardless of the approach used, imputed data are estimates only, and no evidence currently exists that the error associated with data imputation is any less then the error in recall ratings.

A final problem is that the use of automated data collection can potentially limit the subjects who can participate in a study. For example, in one electronic diary study, of the 52 possible participants, six refused participation outright, one did not have the motor ability to hold the computer stylus, and five had visual problems that interfered with their ability to read the computer display (Gaertner et al., 2004). By restricting the participants in clinical trials to those who are able and willing to employ electronic diaries, the use of experience sampling procedures in these trials could potentially limit the generalizability of the study findings.

It is particularly important to remember that research supports the conclusion that recall ratings possess adequate validity for measuring average pain in clinical pain trials. Although both peak and end effects may distort recall ratings, these effects tend to be small (Jensen, Mardekian, Lakshminarayanan, & Boye, 2008). Moreover, research indicates that the correlations between recalled average pain (in the previous 7 days) and actual average pain during that same period (as assessed by diaries) are strong (correlation coefficients range from .68 to .99; see Bolton, 1999; Jamison, Raymond, Slawsby, McHugo, & Baird, 2006; Jamison, Sbrocco, & Parris, 1989; Jensen et al., 1996; Kikuchi et al., 2006; Stone, Broderick, Kaell, DelesPaul, & Porter, 2000; Stone, Broderick, Shiffman, & Schwartz, 2004) and well within a range that indicates they carry valid variance as measures of average or usual pain. And, perhaps most critically, recall ratings have been repeatedly shown to be responsive to the effects of pain treatments.

In summary, diary ratings are best used when assessors seek to understand how change in pain over time influences, or is influenced by, other key variables. However, their use may add significant cost, bias, and error to measurement in clinical trials. It has not yet been determined if their benefits outweigh these drawbacks (Jensen et al., 2010).

Up to this point we have discussed the issues that should be considered when collecting self-report data. In the next four sections we discuss the specific measures and procedures that may be used to assess the dimensions of the pain experience introduced earlier: pain intensity, pain affect, pain quality, and pain location.

ASSESSING PAIN INTENSITY

Pain intensity is a quantitative estimate of the severity or magnitude of perceived pain. The three most commonly used methods to assess pain intensity are the verbal rating scale (VRS), the visual analogue scale (VAS), and the numerical rating scale (NRS) (see Figure 2.1). A measure originally developed for children, but which has been increasingly used in older adults, is the picture (or faces) scale.

Verbal Rating Scales

A VRS consists of a list of adjectives describing different levels of pain intensity. An adequate VRS of pain intensity should include adjectives that reflect the extremes of this dimension (e.g., from "No pain" to "Extremely intense pain") and sufficient additional adjectives to capture the gradations of pain intensity that may be experienced. Patients are asked to read over the list of adjectives, then select the word or phrase that best describes their level of pain on the scale.

VRSs usually list the adjectives in rank order of pain severity and assign each one a score as a function of its rank. In the 4-point VRS used by Seymour (1982), for example, "No pain" would be given a score of zero (0), "Mild pain" a score of one (1), "Moderate pain" a score of two (2), and "Severe pain" a score of three (3). The number as-

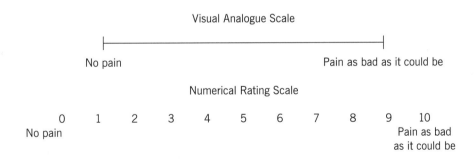

FIGURE 2.1. The visual analogue scale (VAS), numerical rating scale (NRS), and verbal rating scale (VRS).

sociated with the adjective chosen by the patient would constitute his or her pain intensity score.

A criticism frequently raised with respect to the rank-scoring method is that it assumes equal intervals between the adjectives, even though it is extremely unlikely that equal perceptual intervals exist; that is, the interval between "No pain" and "Mild pain" may be much smaller than that between "Moderate pain" and "Severe pain," yet each interval is scored as if the difference were equivalent. This characteristic of rank-scoring procedures can pose several problems when interpreting VRS data. For example, rank scores do not allow for adequate interpretations of the magnitude of any differences found. A change from 3 to 2 (on a 4-point scale) might represent a 10% change in perceived pain or a 50% change, depending on the perceived interval represented by the words on the list. In addition, some investigators have raised the objection that ranked data should not be analyzed using the more common (and usually more powerful) parametric statistics. Nonetheless, it has become increasingly recognized that most parametric techniques (e.g., analysis of variance and the t-test) are still valid when used with data that do not represent equal interval values, especially if the number of categories on the scale is five or more (Cicchetti, Showalter, & Tyrer, 1985; Philip, 1990; Rasmussen, 1989; see also Baker, Hardyck, & Petrinovich, 1966).

Cross-modality matching procedures have been used as a means of transforming VRS ratings to scale scores that are more likely to have ratio properties, that is, to scores with equivalent intervals (Gracely, McGrath, & Dubner, 1978a, 1978b). The matching procedure involves asking each patient to indicate the severity that each word represents in reference to one or more other modalities (e.g., the loudness of a tone, the length of a line, or handgrip force). The rating that the patient gives to a particular word (or the average of several, if the patient rates each word more than once) is then used as the score for that word. Because the modalities used by patients to match pain descriptors can themselves be indexed using ratio scales, the numbers or scores derived from such a procedure are believed likely to have ratio properties and to reflect actual perceived differences in magnitudes.

There are two major limitations of cross-modality matching procedures. First, the procedure is time-consuming and can be tedious, both of which can adversely affect patient compliance (Ahles, Ruckdeschel, & Blanchard, 1984). One way around this problem is to assign standardized scores for each word based on data from groups of previously tested individuals (for standardized scores for specific words, see Gracely et al., 1978a; Tursky, Jamner, & Friedman, 1982; Urban, Keefe, & France, 1984). Second, most of the standardized scores have been developed using nonpatients in response to experimental pain. There is evidence that patients with chronic pain may rate the intensity of pain words differently than do patients with acute (i.e., postoperative) pain (Wallenstein, Heidrich, Kaiko, & Houde, 1980). Even within diagnostic subgroups, the score given to a word by one patient has been shown to vary from that given by other patients, indicating that standardized scores for VRS adjectives may be less reliable than originally hoped (Urban et al., 1984).

Moreover, VRS scores obtained through cross-modality procedures may correlate so highly with those obtained using the ranking method that they contain essentially the same amount of useful information (Hall, 1981; Levine & De Simone, 1991). Similarly, VRS scores created by either of the two methods show the same patterns of associations to other pain measures, again suggesting that the information contained in the scores derived from the two methods are comparable (Jensen et al., 1989). Therefore, we recommend that the simpler ranking method be employed when relationships between pain intensity and other factors are examined. The more sophisticated cross-modality matching procedures should be used only when ratio-like scaling is needed (i.e., when one needs to know the specific magnitude of differences in pain ratings across time or between groups).

The strengths of VRSs include the ease with which they can be administered and scored, provided that scores are calculated using the ranking method or from data developed from previous cross-modality matching experiments. Because they are generally easy to comprehend, compliance rates for VRSs are quite good and often better than those for other measures of pain intensity (Jensen et al., 1986, 1989). Also, VRSs have consistently demonstrated their validity as indicants of pain intensity. They are related positively and significantly to other measures of pain intensity (e.g., Jensen et al., 1986; Kremer, Atkinson, & Ignelzi, 1981; Ohnhaus & Adler, 1975; Paice & Cohen, 1997). VRSs also consistently demonstrate sensitivity to treatments that are known to impact pain intensity (Fox & Melzack, 1976; Ohnhaus & Adler, 1975; Rybstein-Blinchik, 1979).

Despite these strengths, we hesitate to recommend VRSs as the method of choice if only one index is employed. One weakness of VRSs is that patients need to read over, or be familiar with, the entire list of pain adjectives before they can select the one that most closely describes their pain. For longer lists (e.g., 15 or more items), this requirement can make the task time-consuming, and the clinician or researcher cannot be assured that the patient or subject adequately reviewed the entire list of adjectives. Also, because VRSs require patients to select from a finite number of descriptors, patients may be unable to find one that accurately describes their perceived pain intensity (Joyce, Zutshi, Hrubes, & Mason, 1975). Among illiterate patients who must be read to, VRSs are less reliable than other pain intensity measures (Ferraz et al., 1990). Finally, a clinician or researcher using a VRS must select a scoring procedure, and, as already discussed, each scoring method has its drawbacks. Possibly because of the relative weaknesses of VRSs, and the availability of other measures of pain intensity, VRSs are being used less often than previously in pain treatment outcome research.

Visual Analogue Scales and Graphic Rating Scales

The VAS consists of a line, usually 10 cm long, whose ends are labeled as the extremes of pain (e.g., "No pain" to "Pain as bad as it could be"). A VAS may have specific points along the line that are labeled with intensity-denoting adjectives or numbers. Such scales are called graphic rating scales (GRSs). Patients are asked to indicate which point along the line best represents their pain intensity. The distance from the "No pain" end to the mark made by the patient is that patients' pain intensity score. Figure 2.1 illustrates a typical VAS.

Like VRSs, there is much evidence supporting the validity of VASs of pain intensity. Such scales demonstrate positive relations to other self-report measures of pain intensity (Jensen et al., 1986; Kremer et al., 1981; Paice & Cohen, 1997; Seymour, 1982) as well as to observed pain behavior (Gramling & Elliot, 1992; Teske, Daut, & Cleeland, 1983). They are sensitive to treatment effects (Joyce et al., 1975; Seymour, 1982; Turner, 1982) and are distinct from measures of other subjective components of pain (Ahles et al., 1984). The scores from VASs appear to have the qualities of ratio scale data for groups of people (Myles, Troedel, Boquest, & Reeves, 1999; Myles & Urquhart, 2005; Price & Harkins, 1987; Price, McGrath, Rafii, & Buckingham, 1983). Thus, differences in pain intensity (for groups, but not necessarily for individuals), as measured by VAS scales, represent actual differences in magnitude. For example, a significant change in average pain intensity from 60 to 30 in a group of individuals who received a treatment would indicate not only a decrease in pain intensity but also presumably that perceived pain intensity was halved. Another advantage over some other pain intensity scales is the high number of response categories of VASs. Since they are usually measured in millimeters, a 10 cm VAS can be considered to have 101 response levels. This high number of response categories makes the VAS potentially more sensitive to changes in pain intensity than measures with limited numbers of response categories.[1] Although research that compares the VAS to other measures indicates minimal differences in sensitivity to change most of the time, when differences are found, the VAS is usually more sensitive than other measures, especially those with a limited number of response categories (i.e., seven or less, Bolton & Wilkinson, 1998; Jensen et al., 1999; Joyce et al., 1975; Max, Schafer, Culnane, Dubner, & Gracely, 1987; Sriwatanakul et al., 1983).

One of the problems with VASs is that scoring is more time-consuming and involves more steps (therefore, more opportunity for error) than the other measures of pain intensity. To address this problem, several investigators have created mechanical VASs or computer-based VASs (see, e.g., Choinière & Amsel, 1996; Gaston-Johansson, 1996; Grossi, Borghi, Cerchiari, Della Puppa, &

Francucci, 1983; Grossman et al., 1992; Price, Bush, Long, & Harkins, 1994; Price, Patel, Robinson, & Staud, 2008; Thomas & Griffiths, 1982). Mechanical VASs usually consist of laminated paper or plastic VAS scales with a sliding marker that patients use to rate their pain intensity. Commonly, one side of the scale, which the patient sees, just lists the pain endpoints (e.g., "No pain" to "Unbearable pain"). For some mechanical VASs, an additional cue, such as gradations of color from a pale pink (on the "No pain" side) to a dark red (on the "Unbearable pain" side) (Grossi et al., 1983), is provided. The reverse side of the mechanical VAS usually indicates (numerically), usually in millimeters, how far the patient has slid the marker from the "No pain" end toward the "Unbearable pain" end. After the patient rates his or her pain, all the researcher or clinician need do is examine the other side of the scale to obtain the intensity score. Mechanical VASs have been shown to be strongly associated with classic paper-and-pencil VASs (Choinière & Amsel, 1996; Grossi et al., 1983; Grossman et al., 1992; Thomas & Griffiths, 1982) and have been shown to have good test–retest reliability over a 2-hour period (Gaston-Johansson, 1996). In addition, like paper-and-pencil VASs, mechanical VASs appear to have ratio-like qualities (Price et al., 1994).

One drawback to both the paper-and-pencil and mechanical or computer VASs is that they require the respondent to have a minimum level of motor abilities to use the scale. Any study that uses these measures must therefore exclude persons with significant motor disabilities. Also, and perhaps of greater concern, research consistently shows that VAS scales are more difficult to understand than other measures of pain intensity, especially among persons at risk for cognitive difficulties, such as some older adult individuals or persons on high doses of opioid analgesics (Jensen et al., 1986; Kremer et al., 1981; Paice & Cohen, 1997; Walsh, 1984). This may explain why patients prefer to use the more straightforward NRSs or VRSs (Choinière & Amsel, 1996). Therefore, unless a clinician or researcher has a strong rationale for using the VAS (e.g., he or she may require a scale more likely to have ratio-like qualities), and the population being studied is limited to persons who are unlikely to have cognitive difficulties, we do not recommend the VAS as a primary (or sole) measure of pain intensity. If an investigator plans to use VAS measures, careful explanation and patient practice with the scale may decrease the failure rate (Scott & Huskisson, 1976), although high failure rates can still occur despite careful explanations (Walsh, 1984).

Numerical Rating Scales

An NRS involves asking patients to rate their pain from 0 to 10 (an 11-point scale), 0 to 20 (a 21-point scale), or 0 to 100 (a 101-point scale), with the understanding that the 0 represents one end of the pain intensity continuum (i.e., "No pain"), while the 10 or 100 represents the other extreme of pain intensity (e.g., "Pain as bad as it can be"). Verbal NRSs do not require paper and pencil. The patient is simply asked to state verbally his or her pain intensity on a 0- to 10-point (or 0–20, or 0–100) scale. Nonetheless, a number of paper-and-pencil NRSs exist. One simply asks patients to record the number that best represents their pain intensity (e.g., Jensen et al., 1986, 1989). Another presents the numbers in ascending order, with the endpoint descriptors near the 0 and the highest number of the scale, and asks patients to circle the number that best represents their pain intensity (cf. the pain intensity scales of the Brief Pain Inventory; Cleeland & Ryan, 1994). Yet another version of the NRS is the Box Scale, which consists of 11 numbers (0–10) presented in ascending order and surrounded by boxes (Downie et al., 1978). For the Box Scale, patients are asked to place an "X" through the number that represents their pain. In some ways, the NRSs that display all of the numbers in ascending order, from left to right, might be considered a kind of "combined" VAS and NRS, since these measures provide both numerical and visual cues for rating pain. Interestingly, in the single study that examined preferences between a VAS, an NRS, and combined VAS and NRS, the combined scale was preferred over the individual scales (Price et al., 2008). For all of these scales, the patient's pain intensity score is simply the number he or she has indicated.

The validity of NRSs has been well documented. They demonstrate positive and significant correlations with other measures of pain intensity (Jensen et al., 1986, 1989; Kremer et al., 1981; Seymour, 1982; Wilkie, Lovejoy, Dodd, & Tesler, 1990). They have also demonstrated sensitivity to treatments expected to impact pain intensity (Chesney & Shelton, 1976; Keefe, Schapira, Williams, Brown, & Surwit, 1981; Paice & Cohen, 1997; Stenn, Mothersill, & Brooke, 1979). NRSs are likewise extremely easy to administer and score, so they can be used with a greater variety of patients (e.g., geriatric patients, patients with marked motor difficulties) than is possible with the VAS. Because verbal NRSs do not require special materials (e.g., a pencil, printed cards, or paper), they can also be administered conveniently over the phone. The simplicity of the measure may be one reason for the high rate of comparative compliance with the measurement task. Moreover, older people do not appear to have as much difficulty with NRSs as they do with the traditional VAS (Jensen et al., 1986; Paice & Cohen, 1997). Also, if an investigator wishes to maximize the number of response categories, he or she may use a 101-point NRS.

The primary weakness is that NRSs may not have ratio scale qualities (Price et al., 1994), especially when compared to VASs, which do appear to have ratio qualities in groups of patients (although not necessarily in individual patients). Although this possibility may not impact the reliability, validity, or sensitivity of NRSs to treatment outcome, an evaluator cannot necessarily conclude that a change in perceived pain from 9.0 to 6.0 as measured by a NRS represents a 33% decrease in perceived pain. On the other hand, the only scale that has been shown to have ratio qualities (VAS) has other weaknesses not shared by NRSs. Taking all these issues into consideration, we choose 0- to 10-point NRSs over other measures because they work with a diversity of patients.

Picture or Faces Scales

Picture or face scales employ photographs or line drawings that illustrate facial expressions of persons experiencing different levels of pain severity (e.g., Beyer & Knott, 1998; Frank, Moll, & Hort, 1982; Keck, Gerkensmeyer, Joyce, & Schade, 1996; Wong & Baker, 1988). These scales are described in detail in Ruskin, Amaria, Warnock, and

McGrath, Chapter 11, and Hadjistavropoulos, Breau, and Craig, Chapter 13, this volume, and are only briefly mentioned here.

Although picture and face scales were developed primarily to provide an option for assessing pain in individuals who have difficulty with written language or are at risk for having cognitive difficulties (i.e., the very young or the very old), there is evidence these measures are valid in literate populations and in those not at risk for cognitive difficulties, as demonstrated by their association with other measures of pain intensity (see Frank et al., 1982; Stuppy, 1998; Wilson, Cason, & Grissom, 1995). These measures may also useful when assessing pain in samples that cover a large age range (e.g., 8 to 100 years old) or in those whose individuals vary with respect to cognitive function, and comparisons across the sample are needed.

Summary and Recommendations Regarding Pain Intensity Measures

A summary of the strengths and weaknesses of the four primary measures of pain intensity is presented in Table 2.1. Because pain intensity is a relatively easy dimension of pain experience for patients to report, most self-report measures of pain intensity are strongly related to one another; therefore, most of these measures can be used in most situations. However, each procedure has its particular strengths and weaknesses that merit consideration when choosing among measures.

ASSESSING PAIN AFFECT

Evidence suggests that although the affective component of pain is conceptually and empirically distinct from pain intensity (Gracely et al., 1978a, 1978b; Huber et al., 2007; Jensen et al., 1989; Tursky, 1976), it is not a completely independent dimension (Fernandez & Turk, 1992; Gracely, 1992). Whereas *pain intensity* is defined as how much a person hurts, *pain affect* is defined as the emotional arousal and discomfort engendered by the pain experience. Because people's feelings about events can be mixed, it is likely that the domain of pain affect consists of multiple, coactivated dimensions that may be closely related to one another (Morley, 1989; Morley & Pallin, 1995). However, it

TABLE 2.1. The Strengths and Weaknesses of Four Measures of Pain Intensity

Scale	Strengths	Weaknesses
Verbal rating scale	• Easy to administer. • Easy to score. • Good evidence for construct validity. • Compliance with measurement task is high. • May approximate ratio scaling if cross-modality matching (CMM) methods (or scores developed from CMM methods) are used.	• Can be difficult for persons with limited vocabulary. • Relatively few response categories compared to the VAS or NRS-101. • If scored using the ranking method, the scores do not necessarily have ratio qualities. • People are forced to choose one word, even if no word on the scale adequately describes their pain intensity.
Visual analogue scale	• Easy to administer. • Many ("infinite") response categories. • Scores can be treated as ratio data. • Some people, especially older people, have difficulty using VASs. • Good evidence for construct validity.	• Extra step in scoring the paper-and-pencil version can take more time and adds an additional source of error.
Numerical rating scale	• Easy to administer. • Many response categories if NRS-101 is chosen. • Easy to score. • Good evidence for construct validity.	• Limited number of response categories if the NRS-11 is used. • Compliance with measurement task is high. • Scores cannot necessarily be treated as ratio data.
Picture or faces scales	• Easy to administer. • Easy to score.	• No evidence regarding relative compliance rates. • Limited number of response categories. • Scores cannot necessarily be treated as ratio data.

remains unclear whether it is most useful to assess pain affect as a single global response to sensory arousal or as multiple responses, or whether affect may be reliably assessed as both a global construct and a set of related affect dimensions (Cacioppo & Berntson, 1999).

By far the most widely used measure of pain affect is the Affective subscale of the McGill Pain Questionnaire (Melzack, 1975a, 1975b; see also Dworkin et al., 2009). This subscale, along with the other subscales of the McGill Pain Questionnaire, is described in detail by Katz and Melzack (Chapter 3, this volume) and is not discussed in detail here. Pain affect can also be assessed with single-item VRSs or VASs.

Verbal Rating Scales

The two VRSs developed to assess the suffering component of pain are illustrated in Table 2.2. Similar to VRSs for pain inten-

sity, VRSs for pain affect consist of adjectives that describe increasing amounts of discomfort and suffering. Respondents select from the list a single word that best describes the degree of unpleasantness of their pain. Like VRS intensity measures, VRS affect scales may be scored in three ways: (1) the ranking method, (2) the cross-modality matching method, or (3) the standardized score method (using scores developed from cross-modality matching procedures with a standardization group). The advantages and disadvantages of these methods have already been discussed with respect to VRSs of pain intensity; therefore, we offer the same cautions here; that is, we recommend the simpler ranking method if the investigator wishes to examine the relation between pain intensity and other constructs, and the standardized scores method developed from cross-modality matching procedures if the investigator requires a measure more likely to have ratio scale properties.

TABLE 2.2. Verbal Rating Scales of Pain Affect

12-point scale (from Tursky, Jamner, & Friedman, 1982)	15-point scale (from Gracely, McGrath, & Dubner, 1978a)
• Not unpleasant	• Bearable
• Bearable	• Distracting
• Tolerable	• Unpleasant
• Uncomfortable	• Uncomfortable
• Distracting	• Distressing
• Unpleasant	• Oppressive
• Distressing	• Miserable
• Miserable	• Bearable
• Unbearable	• Tolerable
• Intolerable	• Uncomfortable
• Agonizing	• Distracting
	• Unpleasant
	• Distressing
	• Miserable
	• Awful
	• Frightful
	• Dreadful
	• Horrible
	• Agonizing
	• Unbearable
	• Intolerable
	• Excruciating

Evidence for the validity of VRSs of pain affect is mixed. On the positive side, VRSs of pain affect appear to be more sensitive than measures of pain intensity in treatments designed to impact the emotional component of pain (Fernandez & Turk, 1994; Gracely, Dubner, & McGrath, 1979; Gracely et al., 1978a, 1978b; Heft, Gracely, & Dubner, 1984). On the other hand, factor-analytic and correlational investigations among chronic pain patients, postoperative pain patients, and laboratory volunteers indicate that VRSs designed to measure pain affect are not always distinct from measures of pain intensity (Jensen et al., 1989; Jensen & Karoly, 1987; Levine & De Simone, 1991). This pattern of overlap may have something to do with the relatively low level of reliability of single-item measures. Alternatively, a lack of independence among measures of pain intensity versus pain affect may reflect the simple fact that some degree of pain intensity is necessary for there to be pain affect and, presumably, pain affect should increase as pain intensity increases. Thus, pain intensity and pain affect may be related to one another in the same way that height and weight are distinct but closely associated with each other (Gracely, 1992). Another drawback is that VRS measures of pain affect force respondents to choose only one descriptor, even when none of the available descriptors (or more than one of the available descriptors) captures their affective response to pain.

Visual Analogue Scales

VASs for pain affect are very similar to VASs for pain intensity. Only the endpoint descriptors are different. Examples of the extremes used in VAS affect scales are "Not bad at all" and "The most unpleasant feeling possible for me" (Price, Harkins, & Baker, 1987). A great deal of evidence supports the validity of VAS affect measures. They are more sensitive than VAS intensity measures to treatments that impact pain affect and intensity (Price, Barrell, & Gracely, 1980; Price et al., 1987). They appear to have the qualities of ratio scales (Price & Harkins, 1987; Price et al., 1983). Finally, they are sensitive to general treatment effects (Price & Barber, 1987; Price, Harkins, Rafii, & Price, 1986; Price, Von der Gruen, Miller, Rafii, & Price, 1985).

The weaknesses of VAS affect measures are likely to be similar to those of VAS intensity measures. Most research using these measures has been conducted with young or middle-aged subjects. The utility of such measures in geriatric populations has not yet been examined, and it may be that older people have the same difficulty with VAS affect scales as with VAS intensity scales. Because VAS affect measures are single-item scales, they may be less reliable and less valid for examining the full spectrum of affective responses relative to multiple-item measures, such as the Affective subscales of the McGill Pain Questionnaire. Also, there is limited research comparing VAS affect measures to other measures of pain affect. A single experiment suggests that VAS affect measures may be less able than VRS affect measures to discriminate between pain intensity and pain affect (Duncan, Bushnell, & Lavigne, 1989), perhaps because words are so often used to describe emotional reaction, whereas VASs (and NRSs for that matter) may pull for more of the intensity (magnitude) component of the pain experience.

Summary and Recommendations for Assessing Pain Affect

Pain affect is more complex than pain intensity, and there are fewer measures available to assess this construct. In addition, unresolved questions linger regarding the psychometrics and meaning of pain affect. In view of the multidimensional nature of pain affect, is it reasonable to use a global measure of the distress associated with pain, or is there a need for separate indices that tap distinct affective dimensions of pain? Are single-item measures of pain affect less reliable than multiple-item measures, as would be suggested by the complexity of pain affect? These and other basic questions need to be addressed in future research.

In the meantime, investigators have several options for the assessment of pain affect. Among the single-item measures are VRS affect and VAS affect scales. Both procedures have demonstrated discriminant validity (from pain intensity) in some treatment outcome studies. However, both also appear closely related to single-item measures of pain intensity in other situations. Additional research is also needed to clarify the specific dimensions of pain affect (Morley & Pallin, 1995) in order to then develop pain affect measures that best capture these dimensions. Until additional research is performed, clinicians and researchers may wish to use both single- and multiple-item measures, then perform psychometric analyses to determine which measure(s) are most useful in their particular situation.

ASSESSING PAIN QUALITY

A large number of measures of pain quality have been developed. The two primary purposes of such measures are (1) to help diagnose the pain problem and (2) to describe more thoroughly the pain experience and determine the effects of pain treatments on that experience. The use of pain quality measures as diagnostic aides, in particular, as instruments to distinguish neuropathic from non-neuropathic pain conditions, is covered in another chapter in this volume (see Gilron, Attal, Bouhassira, & Dworkin, Chapter 17) and is not addressed in detail here.

To date, six measures have been developed as outcome measures in clinical trials. They include the original McGill Pain Questionnaire (MPQ; Melzack, 1975b), the Short-Form McGill Pain Questionnaire (SF-MPQ; Melzack, 1987), the Revised Version of the Short-Form McGill Pain Questionnaire (SF-MPQ-2; Dworkin et al., 2009), the Neuropathic Pain Symptom Inventory (NPSI; Bouhassira et al., 2004), the Neuropathic Pain Scale (NPS; Galer & Jensen, 1997), and the Pain Quality Assessment Scale (PQAS; Jensen, Gammaitoni, et al., 2006). The three versions of the MPQ are described and discussed in detail in Katz and Melzack, Chapter 3, this volume; this section focuses on the three additional measures of pain quality.

Neuropathic Pain Symptom Inventory

The NPSI (Bouhassira et al., 2004) includes 12 items selected to assess four global domains of neuropathic pain (spontaneous ongoing pain, spontaneous paroxysmal pain, evoked pain, and paraesthesia/dysesthesia). Respondents rate the severity or intensity of each descriptor item on 0- to 10-point NRSs. Two additional items assess the temporal qualities of pain (number of hours of spontaneous pain in the past 24 hours, number of paroxysms during the past 24 hours).

As reported in the initial development study, short-term (3 hours) and long-term (1 month) test–retest stability of NPSI items was very high, as measured by intraclass correlation coefficients (short-term: range .87–.98; long-term: .78–.98). Also, validity for the evoked pain items was evidenced through their significant associations (r's range .66–.73) with related clinician scores of pain evoked by brushing, pressure, and cold stimuli. Changes in the NPSI total score were also found to be associated significantly with patient and provider ratings of global improvement over a 1-month period.

An exploratory factor analysis of the NPSI items in 482 patients with a variety of neuropathic pain conditions yielded five factors: (1) evoked pain (pain evoked by brushing, pressure, and cold stimuli), (2) paraesthesia/dysesthesia (pins and needles, tingling), (3) deep pain (pressure, squeezing), (4) paroxysmal pain (electric shocks, stabbing), and (5) burning pain (burning) (Attal et al., 2008). In addition, and consistent with the original developmental sample, the three NPSI evoked pain items were strongly associated with allodynia/hyperalgesia assessed by quantitative sensory testing (Attal et al., 2008). Attal and colleagues (2008) also examined the ability of the NPSI items to distinguish among presumed etiology of the pain (postherpetic neuralgia, stroke, etc.), pain site (e.g., trunk, face and/or neck), and site of injury (e.g., peripheral, central). The primary finding from these analyses was that patients with postherpetic neuralgia, trigeminal neuralgia, and pain localized to the face and/or neck were not likely to described their pain using the terms "tingling" or "pins and needles." Otherwise, no clear association emerged between NPSI items and pain type, suggesting that neuropathic pain problems across etiologies are more similar than they are different (Attal et al., 2008). On the negative side, a qualitative study of neuropathic pain sensations has identified a large number of pain descriptors commonly used by patients with neuropathic pain that are not included on the NPSI (Crawford, Bouhassira, Wong, & Dukes, 2008). These included, for example, "numb," "itchy," "sharp," and "shooting pain," among others.

Neuropathic Pain Scale

The NPS was developed as measure of neuropathic pain both to (1) describe neuropathic pain qualities in different pain populations, and (2) document the impact of pain treatments on pain qualities in clinical trials (Galer & Jensen, 1997). The NPS includes 10 items, two that assess global pain intensity and unpleasantness, and eight that reflect specific pain domains (six pain qualities and two spatial characteristics) likely to be reported by patients with neuropathic pain syndromes. Respondents rate each item on 0- to 10-point NPSs. An 11th item allows patients to report the temporal pattern of their pain ("Constant with intermittent increases," "Intermittent," or "Constant with fluctuation"). The NPS items were intended primarily to assess distinct pain qualities, which could then be used to create a profile of a person's pain quality experience. A substantial body of research supports the validity of the NPS for describing neuropathic pain conditions (Carter et al., 1998; Galer, Gianas, & Jensen, 2000; Galer, Henderson,

Perander, & Jensen, 2000; Torrance, Smith, Bennett, & Lee, 2006), distinguishing between pain diagnoses (Bennett, Smith, Torrance, & Potter, 2005; Carter et al., 1998; Galer & Jensen, 1997), predicting treatment outcome (Fishbain et al., 2005, 2006), and detecting treatment effects (Fishbain et al., 2006; Galer & Jensen, 1997; Galer, Jensen, Ma, Davies, & Rowbotham, 2002; Gammaitoni, Galer, Lacouture, Domingos, & Schlagheck, 2003; Geha et al., 2007; Jensen, Chiang, & Wu, 2009; Jensen, Dworkin, et al., 2005; Levendoglu, Ogün, Ozerbil, Ogün, & Ugurlu, 2004; Lynch, Clark, & Sawynok, 2002; Moseley, 2004; Semenchuk & Sherman, 2000; Tai et al., 2002; Weintraub & Cole, 2008).

The NPS is also useful for identifying the pain qualities affected by different pain treatments. For example, one study examined the effectiveness of the NPS for assessing changes in pain qualities in three groups (peripheral neuropathic pain, low back pain, and osteoarthritis) of patients treated with an open-label lidocaine 5% patch (Jensen, Hoffman, & Cardenas, 2005). Although significant changes in almost all NPS pain qualities were found, significantly larger changes were seen for NPS items measuring sharp and deep pain than for items measuring cold, sensitive, or itching pain (Jensen, Hoffman, & Cardenas, 2005). In another study, controlled-release oxycodone was found to be associated with decreases in sharp, dull, deep, and surface pain, but had little impact on hot, cold, itchy, or sensitive pain in patients with painful diabetic neuropathy (Jensen, Friedman, Bonzo, & Richards, 2006). In a sample of patients with mixed neuropathic pain conditions, intravenous lidocaine and phentolamine were found to have similar effects on 8 of 10 NPS items, although lidocaine had a greater effect on global pain unpleasantness and deep pain (Galer & Jensen, 1997). Another study showed that tizanidine for neuropathic pain impacted the hot, cold, and sensitive NPS items (as well as global intensity and unpleasantness) after 2 weeks of treatment, then impacted sharp, dull, and deep pain NPS items after 8 weeks, indicating that the NPS may show how treatments impact various pain qualities over time (Semenchuk & Sherman, 2000). Finally, a recent study examining the effects of an extended-release gabapentin formulation had more effects on sharp, dull, sensitive, and itchy pain than on other pain qualities, such as hot, cold, deep, or surface pain (Jensen et al., 2009). An additional strength of the NPS is its brevity, which makes it potentially useful in survey research and in settings where assessment burden may be a significant issue. Also, the NPS has been translated into 24 languages, so it may be useful for cross-cultural research comparing neuropathic pain conditions and treatments across cultures.

Although the NPS was originally designed to be scored to create a "profile" of sensation severity across different pain qualities, it is possible to combine the items into composite scores. Galer, Henderson, Perander, and Jensen (2002), for example, created four different NPS composite scores when examining the effects of a lidocaine 5% patch in a sample of patients with postherpetic neuralgia: an average of all 10 items (NPS 10); an average of the eight specific descriptors, excluding the global ratings of pain intensity and unpleasantness (NPS 8); an average of the eight items that do not reflect allodynia (i.e., excluding the "sensitive" and "surface" items; NPS NA); and an average of four items thought to reflect nonperipheral pain mechanisms ("dull," "deep," "sharp," and "burning" items; NPS 4).

The primary limitation of the NPS is associated with one of its strengths—its brevity. The NPS does not assess a number of pain qualities commonly reported by patients with some neuropathic pain conditions, such as shooting, electrical, and tingling pain. Also, the NPS does not assess some pain qualities experienced by individuals with non-neuropathic pain, limiting its utility in populations with musculoskeletal problems, such as individuals with low back pain or arthritis.

Pain Quality Assessment Scale

The PQAS (Jensen, 2008; Jensen, Gammaitoni, et al., 2006; see Appendix 2.1) was developed to make available a measure with the strengths of the NPS, but without its primary limitation. In addition to the original NPS items, the PQAS includes the following pain qualities that make it possible to assess additional common neuropathic and nociceptive pain qualities: tender, shooting,

numb, electrical, tingling, cramping, radiating, throbbing, aching, and heavy. Like the NPS, the PQAS includes an additional item to differentiate among three primary temporal patterns of pain: intermittent (i.e., variable pain with some pain free periods), variable (variable pain without pain-free periods), and stable (i.e., constant pain with little variation). Thus, the final 21-item PQAS was intended to be comprehensive enough to capture the majority of a patient's pain experience, yet brief enough to minimize assessment burden.

A factor analysis of the PQAS pain descriptors in a sample of 823 patients with low back pain or osteoarthritis of the knee yielded three clear pain quality factors that appeared to represent (1) paroxysmal pain sensations (PQAS descriptors: shooting, sharp, electric, hot, radiating), (2) superficial pain (itchy, cold, numb, sensitive, tingling), and (3) deep pain (aching, heavy, dull, cramping, throbbing) (Victor et al., 2008). These three factors are similar to three of the five factors identified in the first factor analysis of the NPSI items in a sample of patients with a variety of neuropathic pain conditions (Attal et al., 2008). Specifically, the NPSI paraesthesia/dysaesthesia factor is similar to the PQAS superficial factor, the NPSI deep factor is similar to the PQAS deep factor, and the NPSI paroxysmal factor is similar to the PQAS paroxysmal factor. The two additional factors of the NPSI were hot (the hot item loaded on the PQAS paroxysmal factor) and evoked pain (the PQAS does not include any evoked pain items). The three-factor PQAS solution that Victor and colleagues (2008) identified in the low back pain and osteoarthritis sample was confirmed in a sample of patients with carpal tunnel syndrome. Overall, the findings from both the PQAS and NPSI factor-analytic studies support the hypothesis that pain qualities cluster into distinct groups, and raise the interesting possibility of the development and use of pain quality subscales that may represent these factors.

All of the data that support the validity of the NPS also support the validity of the PQAS, since NPS items are contained in the PQAS. In addition, in the first published report using the PQAS items, all 10 of the new PQAS items (i.e., the non-NPS items) were responsive to the effects of both lidocaine patch 5% and a corticosteroid injection in a sample of patients with carpal tunnel syndrome (Jensen, Gammaitoni, et al., 2006). Further support for the validity of the PQAS items for detecting changes in pain quality comes from a study showing significant effects of an extended-release formula of oxymorphone in 19 of the 20 PQAS items and all three of the PQAS subscales based on the factor-analytic findings of Victor and colleagues (2008), relative to placebo in a sample of patients with low back pain. In addition, in support of the ability of PQAS items to identify a "treatment response profile," larger effects were found for the PQAS intense, unpleasant, deep, aching and sharp items, and the PQAS Paroxysmal and Deep scales, relative to the other PQAS items and scales in the oxymorphone study.

A described in Katz and Melzack, Chapter 3, this volume, the SF-MPQ-2 was developed to address the same need that the PQAS addresses, that is, to have available a measure broad enough to assess both neuropathic and nonneuropathic pain conditions and key pain quality domains, yet brief enough to limit assessment burden. The end result of this effort, the SF-MPQ-2, is much like the PQAS. Both measures allow respondents to rate individual pain qualities on 0- to 10-point NPSs, and there is a great deal of overlap in the pain qualities assessed. The only nonoverlapping pain quality items are "gnawing pain" and "spitting pain," assessed by the SF-MPQ-2, and "radiating" and "dull" pain assessed by the PQAS. Also, the SF-MPQ-2 includes four items that assess pain affect that are not included in the PQAS, whereas the PQAS includes two items that assess pain location (deep and surface pain), two global ratings (that assess overall pain intensity and pain unpleasantness), and an item that assesses pain's temporal characteristics (e.g., intermittent vs. constant). Thus, although there is significant overlap, some components of the SF-MPQ-2 and the PQAS are unique to each measure. Interestingly, factor analyses of the SF-MPQ-2 and PQAS pain quality items have yielded similar factor solutions, with many of SF-MPQ-2 intermittent factor items showing overlap with the PQAS paroxysmal factor items (i.e., "shooting," "sharp/stabbing/piercing"), many of the SF-MPQ-2 continuous items showing overlap with PQAS deep items (i.e., "aching," "heavy," "cramping," "throbbing"), and many of the SF-MPQ-2 predominantly neuropathic items showing overlap with the PQAS superficial items ("itchy," "cold," "numb," "sensitive/caused by light touch").

Summary and Recommendations for Assessing Pain Quality

At this point in time, the NPS has the most empirical evidence supporting its validity as a measure of the distinct pain qualities impacted by pain treatments. However, given its brevity, the NPS has limited content validity. This limitation inspired development of the PQAS, which includes pain qualities common to patients with neuropathic and nonneuropathic pain conditions. Preliminary evidence supports the utility of the PQAS for identifying the effects of pain treatment on multiple pain qualities. The PQAS also shares many items with the revised SF-MPQ (SF-MPQ-2). When a thorough assessment of pain qualities is indicated, therefore, either the SF-MPQ-2 or the PQAS would appear to be measures of choice. Perhaps the SF-MPQ-2 would be chosen over the PQAS if a multiple-item measure of pain affect is needed, and the PQAS over the SF-MPQ-2 if the study would benefit from inclusion of global measures of pain intensity and pain unpleasantness, as well as measures of pain's spatial (deep vs. surface) and temporal qualities.

ASSESSING PAIN LOCATION

A fourth dimension of subjective experience is the location of pain. The instrument most commonly used to assess pain location is the pain drawing. This procedure usually involves a line drawing of the front and back of the human body. Sometimes, line drawings of the face, head, and neck are also presented for patients experiencing localized pain. Patients are asked to indicate the location of their pain on the surface of the drawings. It is possible to vary the instructions regarding how patients are to indicate their pain to suit the purposes of the investigator. Patients may be asked to distinguish between various sensations of their pain experience, and to indicate the location of these sensations by means of different symbols. For example, the letters "E" and "I" have been used for external (surface) and internal (deep somatic) pain, respectively (Melzack, 1975b). Similarly, "—" has been used for numbness; "oo," for pins and needles; "xx," for burning; and "//," for stabbing pain (Ransford, Cairns, & Mooney, 1976). The most common procedure is to ask patients simply to shade in the areas of the body that are "in pain."

Pain drawings are included in a number of standard pain questionnaires, such as the MPQ (Melzack, 1975b), the Leeds Assessment of Neuropathic Symptoms and Signs (LANSS; Bennett, 2001), and the original (non-short-form) Brief Pain Inventory (Cleeland & Ryan, 1994). Toomey, Gover, and Jones (1983) divided line drawings of the human body into 32 regions, and gave their patients with chronic pain a score equal to the number of regions that were shaded. This score was found to be related to many important, pain-related constructs, such as dimensions of the MPQ (Number of Words Chosen, MPQ Sensory and MPQ Total subscale scores); self-report of time spent reclining; interference of pain with basic activities, such as walking, working, socializing, and recreation; number of health care professionals consulted; and medication use. Interestingly, the number of pain sites shaded was unrelated to duration of the pain problem (Toomey et al., 1983).

Other investigators have similarly found the percentage of body surface in pain to show moderate associations with disability, pain severity, and tendency to focus on and report physical symptoms (Öhlund, Eek, Palmblad, Areskoug, & Nachemson, 1996; Staud, Price, Robinson, & Vierck, 2004; Staud, Vierck, Robinson, & Price, 2006; Tait, Chibnall, & Margolis, 1990; Toomey, Mann, Abashian, & Thompson-Pope, 1991). Pain extent scores derived from pain drawings among patients with recent-onset low back pain have also predicted return to work (Öhlund et al., 1996). Evidence for the predictive validity of specific pain site was found by Toomey, Gover, and Jones (1984), who demonstrated that patients with low back pain (or low back pain plus head and neck pain) were more likely than other patients to report interference of pain with life's activities.

The reliability of pain drawing data has also been established. Test–retest stability is high and does not appear to decrease even after 3 months (Margolis, Chibnall, & Tait, 1988). Scoring for "inappropriate" drawings (see below) as well as for total body area in pain, appears to be extremely reliable from person to person (Chan, Goldman, Ilstrup, Kunselman, & O'Neil, 1993; Margolis, Tait, & Krause, 1986; Parker, Wood, & Main, 1995; Udén, Åström, & Bergenudd, 1988).

Some clinicians have suggested that information regarding psychopathology may be extracted from the manner in which patients complete pain drawings. To examine this hypothesis, Ransford and colleagues (1976) developed a system for rating the normality versus abnormality of pain drawings. These investigators found patients with abnormal drawings to have higher Hysteria (Hs) and Hypochondriasis (Hy) scale scores on the Minnesota Multiphasic Personality Inventory, suggesting that exaggerated pain drawing may reflect a tendency toward somatic preoccupation. Similarly, Gil, Phillips, Abrams, and Williams (1990) found that pain drawing responses of persons with sickle cell disease that were rated as "inconsistent" with sickle cell disease had significantly higher somatization scores on the revised Symptom Checklist–90 (SCL-90-R; Derogatis, 1983). High scores on the SCL-90-R reflect a tendency to focus on somatic symptoms. Although the relationship between abnormal pain drawings and various measures of psychopathology has continued to be positive in subsequent research, the magnitude of the relationship has generally been weak (Ginzburg, Merskey, & Lau, 1988; Hildebrandt, Franz, Choroba-Mehnen, & Temme, 1988; Parker et al., 1995; Schwartz & DeGood, 1984; Von Baeyer, Bergstrom, Brodwin, & Brodwin, 1983).

A second measure of pain location commonly used in pain research is the pain site checklist. A pain site checklist is a simple list of possible sites for pain. The respondent is asked to indicate which site(s) are currently painful (cf. Jensen, Hoffman, et al., 2005). Like pain drawings, site checklists can be scored for both the specific site(s) chosen and "pain extent" (total number of sites chosen). One can also have patients indicate the relative depth of pain (as an indication of pain location) by asking them to indicate the relative severity of "deep" and "surface" pain (see the PQAS reflecting these in Appendix 2.1).

Summary and Recommendations for Assessing Pain Location

The assessment of pain location is a necessary part of any thorough pain evaluation. Although research suggests that pain extent scores predict, in some patients, disability, pain interference, medication use, return to work, and psychological functioning, this same body of research indicates that these associations are typically inconsistent and weak. Therefore, we do not recommend that pain drawings be relied upon as a proxy measure of psychopathology or disability. Although drawings that appear overly detailed or exaggerated may raise questions about possible hypochondriacal tendencies or disability, it is possible that a detailed drawing may reflect a person's wish to be extremely thorough in providing data. Caution should be applied in any attempt to overinterpret pain drawing data. Many researchers choose to assess pain location using pain site checklists instead of pain drawings, since the latter require additional scoring steps that can take additional time and be a source of additional measurement error. However, there is no direct evidence comparing the psychometric properties of pain drawings and pain site checklists. Thus, there are no strong grounds to justify one method over the other.

GENERAL SUMMARY AND CONCLUSION

The assessment of pain intensity, pain affect, pain quality, and pain location continues to be important to clinicians and researchers, and self-report is the most direct way to access these pain domains. Although additional research is needed to answer important questions regarding the nature and dimensionality of pain experience, most of the measures now available have demonstrated adequate to excellent reliability and validity. Clinicians and researchers should have full knowledge of the psychometric strengths and weaknesses of selected measures, and choose measures in keeping with their explicit conceptual model(s) of pain. In this chapter, we

have attempted to provide investigators with some of the information necessary to make informed decisions regarding the use of self-report measures of pain in adults.

NOTE

1. There is probably an upper limit to the number of response categories necessary to characterize fully different levels of perceived pain intensity. For example, 1,000,001 response categories (i.e., "choose a number between 0 and 1,000,000 that best represents your pain intensity") is unlikely to be more sensitive than 101 response categories. Laboratory research indicates that people are unable to identify more than 21 noticeable differences between weak and intolerable experimental pain (Hardy, Wolff, & Goodell, 1952; see also Vierck, Cannon, Fry, Maixner, & Whitsel, 1997). Based on these findings, scale sensitivity is likely to be maximal if a measure has at least 22 levels.

REFERENCES

Aaron, L. A., Mancl, L., Turner, J. A., Sawchuk, C. N., & Klein, K. M. (2004). Reasons for missing interviews in the daily electronic assessment of pain, mood, and stress. *Pain, 109,* 389–398.

Ahles, T. A., Ruckdeschel, J. C., & Blanchard, E. B. (1984). Cancer-related pain: II. Assessment with visual analogue scales. *Journal of Psychosomatic Research, 28,* 121–124.

Andrasik, F., & Holroyd, K. A. (1980). Reliability and concurrent validity of headache questionnaire data. *Headache, 20,* 44–46.

Attal, N., Fermanian, C., Fermanian, J., Lanteri-Minet, M., Alchaar, H., & Bouhassira, D. (2008). Neuropathic pain: Are there distinct subtypes depending on the aetiology or anatomical lesion? *Pain, 31,* 343–353.

Baker, B. O., Hardyck, C. D., & Petrinovich, L. F. (1966). Weak measurement vs strong statistics: An empirical critique of S. S. Stevens' prescriptions on statistics. *Educational and Psychological Measurement, 26,* 291–309.

Bennett, M. (2001). The LANSS pain scale: The Leeds Assessment of Neuropathic Symptoms and Signs. *Pain, 92,* 147–157.

Bennett, M. I., Smith, B. H., Torrance, N., & Potter, J. (2005). The S-LANSS score for identifying pain of predominantly neuropathic origin: Validation for use in clinical and postal research. *Journal of Pain, 6,* 149–158.

Beyer, J. E., & Knott, C. B. (1998). Construct

validity estimation for the African-American and Hispanic versions of the Oucher Scale. *Journal of Pediatric Nursing, 13*, 20–31.

Bolger, N., Davis, A., & Rafaeli, E. (2003). Diary methods: Capturing life as it is lived. *Annual Review of Psychology, 54*, 579–616.

Bolton, J. E. (1999). Accuracy of recall of usual pain intensity in back pain patients. *Pain, 83*, 533–539.

Bolton, J. E., & Wilkinson, R. C. (1998). Responsiveness of pain scales: A comparison of three pain intensity measures in chiropractic patients. *Journal of Manipulative and Physiological Therapeutics, 21*, 1–7.

Bouhassira, D., Attal, N., Fermanian, J., Alchaar, H., Gautron, M., Masquelier, E., et al. (2004). Development and validation of the Neuropathic Pain Symptom Inventory. *Pain, 108*, 248–257.

Burton, C., Weller, D., & Sharpe, M. (2007). Are electronic diaries useful for symptoms research?: A systematic review. *Journal of Psychosomatic Research, 62*, 553–561.

Cacioppo, J. T., & Berntson, G. G. (1999). The affect system: Architecture and operating characteristics. *Current Directions in Psychological Science, 8*, 133–137.

Carter, G. T., Jensen, M. P., Galer, B. S., Kraft, G. H., Crabtree, L. D., Beardsley, R. M., et al. (1998). Neuropathic pain in Charcot–Marie–Tooth disease. *Archives of Physical Medicine and Rehabilitation, 79*, 1560–1564.

Chan, C. W., Goldman, S., Ilstrup, D. M., Kunselman, A. R., & O'Neil, P. I. (1993). The pain drawing and Waddell's nonorganic physical signs in chronic low-back pain. *Spine, 18*, 1717–1722.

Chesney, M. A., & Shelton, J. L. (1976). A comparison of muscle relaxation and electromyogram biofeedback treatments for muscle contraction headache. *Journal of Behavior Therapy and Experimental Psychiatry, 7*, 221–225.

Choinière, M., & Amsel, R. (1996). A visual analogue thermometer for measuring pain intensity. *Journal of Pain and Symptom Management, 11*, 299–311.

Christensen, T. C., Feldman Barrett, L., Bliss-Moreau, E., Lebo, K., & Kaschub, C. (2003). A practical guide to experience sampling procedures. *Journal of Happiness Studies, 4*, 53–78.

Cicchetti, D. V., Showalter, D., & Tyrer, P. J. (1985). The effect of number of rating scale categories on levels of interrater reliability: A Monte Carlo investigation. *Applied Psychological Measurement, 9*, 31–36.

Clark, W. C., Kuhl, J. P., Keohan, M. L., Knotkova, H., Winer, R. T., & Griswold, G. A. (2003). Factor analysis validates the cluster structure of the dendrogram underlying the Multidimensional Affect and Pain Survey (MAPS) and challenges the a priori classification of the descriptors in the McGill Pain Questionnaire (MPQ). *Pain, 106*, 357–363.

Cleeland, C. S., & Ryan, K. M. (1994). Pain assessment: Global use of the Brief Pain Inventory. *Annals of the Academy of Medicine, 23*, 129–138.

Craig, K. D., & Weiss, S. M. (1971). Vicarious influences on pain-threshold determinations. *Journal of Personality and Social Psychology, 19*, 53–59.

Dar, R., Ariely, D., & Frank, H. (1995). The effect of past-injury on pain threshold and tolerance. *Pain, 60*, 189–193.

Derogatis, L. R. (1983). *SCL-90-R: Administration, scoring and procedures manual II.* Towson, MD: Clinical Psychometric Research.

Downie, W. W., Leatham, P. A., Rhind, V. M., Wright, V., Branco, J. A., & Anderson, J. A. (1978). Studies with pain rating scales. *Annals of the Rheumatic Diseases, 37*, 378–381.

Duncan, G. H., Bushnell, M. C., & Lavigne, G. J. (1989). Comparison of verbal and visual analogue scales for measuring the intensity and unpleasantness of experimental pain. *Pain, 37*, 295–303.

Dworkin, R. H., Turk, D. C., Revicki, D. A., Harding, G., Coyne, K. S., Peirce-Sandner, S., et al. (2009). Development and initial validation of an expanded and revised version of the Short-Form McGill Pain Questionnaire (SF-MPQ-2). *Pain, 144*, 35–42.

Dworkin, S. F., & Chen, A. C. N. (1982). Pain in clinical and laboratory contexts. *Journal of Dental Research, 6*, 772–774.

Evans, S. R., Simpson, D. M., Kitch, D. W., King, A., Clifford, D. B., Cohen, B. A., et al. (2007). A randomized trial evaluating Prosaptide for HIV-associated sensory neuropathies: Use of an electronic diary to record neuropathic pain. *PLoS ONE, 25*, e551.

Fernandez, E., & Turk, D. C. (1992). Sensory and affective components of pain: Separation and synthesis. *Psychological Bulletin, 112*, 205–217.

Ferraz, M. B., Quaresma, M. R., Aquino, L. R. L., Atra, E., Tugwell, P., & Goldsmith, C. H. (1990). Reliability of pain scales in the assessment of literate and illiterate patients with rheumatoid arthritis. *Journal of Rheumatology, 17*, 1022–1024.

Fishbain, D. A., Lewis, J., Cole, B., Cutler, B., Smets, E., Rosomoff, H., et al. (2005). Multidisciplinary pain facility treatment outcome for pain-associated fatigue. *Pain Medicine, 6*, 299–304.

Fishbain, D. A., Lewis, J. E., Cole, B., Cutler, B., Rosomoff, H. L., & Rosomoff, R. S. (2006).

Lidocaine 5% patch: An open-label naturalistic chronic pain treatment trial and prediction of response. *Pain Medicine, 7,* 135–142.

Fox, E. J., & Melzack, R. (1976). Transcutaneous electrical stimulation and acupuncture: Comparison of treatment for low-back pain, *Pain, 2,* 141–148.

Frank, A. J. M., Moll, J. M. H., & Hort, J. F. (1982). A comparison of three ways of measuring pain. *Rheumatology and Rehabilitation, 21,* 211–217.

Gaertner, J., Elsner, F., Pollmann-Dahmen, K., Radbruch, L., & Sabatowski, R. (2004). Electronic pain diary: A randomized crossover study. *Journal of Pain and Symptom Management, 28,* 259–267.

Galer, B. S., Gianas, A., & Jensen, M. P. (2000). Painful diabetic polyneuropathy: Epidemiology, pain description, and quality of life. *Diabetes Research and Clinical Practice, 47,* 123–128.

Galer, B. S., Henderson, J., Perander, J., & Jensen, M. P. (2000). Course of symptoms and quality of life measurement in complex regional pain syndrome: A pilot survey. *Journal of Pain and Symptom Management, 20,* 286–292.

Galer, B. S., & Jensen, M. P. (1997). Development and preliminary validation of a pain measure specific to neuropathic pain: The Neuropathic Pain Scale. *Neurology, 48,* 332–338.

Galer, B. S., Jensen, M. P., Ma, T., Davies, P. S., & Rowbotham, M. C. (2002). The lidocaine patch 5% effectively treats all neuropathic pain qualities: Results of a randomized, double-blind, vehicle-controlled, 3-week efficacy study with use of the Neuropathic Pain Scale. *Clinical Journal of Pain, 18,* 297–301.

Gammaitoni, A. R., Galer, B. S., Lacouture, P., Domingos, J., & Schlagheck, T. (2003). Effectiveness and safety of new oxycodone/acetaminophen formulations with reduced acetaminophen for the treatment of low back pain. *Pain Medicine, 4,* 21–30.

Gaston-Johansson, F. (1996). Measurement of pain: The psychometric properties of the Pain-O-Meter, a simple, inexpensive pain assessment tool that could change health care practices. *Journal of Pain and Symptom Management, 12,* 172–181.

Geha, P. Y., Baliki, M. N., Chialvo, D. R., Harden, R. N., Paice, J. A., & Apkarian, A. V. (2007). Brain activity for spontaneous pain of postherpetic neuralgia and its modulation by lidocaine patch therapy. *Pain, 128,* 88–100.

Gil, K. M., Phillips, G., Abrams, M. R., & Williams, D. A. (1990). Pain drawings and sickle cell disease pain. *Clinical Journal of Pain, 6,* 105–109.

Ginzburg, B. M., Merskey, H., & Lau, C. L. (1988). The relationship between pain drawings and the psychological state. *Pain, 35,* 141–146.

Gracely, R. H. (1992). Evaluation of multidimensional pain scales. *Pain, 48,* 297–300.

Gracely, R. H., Dubner, R., & McGrath, P. A. (1979). Narcotic analgesia: Fentanyl reduces the intensity but not the unpleasantness of painful tooth pulp sensations. *Science, 203,* 1261–1263.

Gracely, R. H., McGrath, P., & Dubner, R. (1978a). Ratio scales of sensory and affective verbal pain descriptors. *Pain, 5,* 5–18.

Gracely, R. H., McGrath, P., & Dubner, R. (1978b). Validity and sensitivity of ratio scales of sensory and affective verbal pain descriptors: Manipulation of affect by diazepam. *Pain, 5,* 19–29.

Gramling, S. E., & Elliot, T. R. (1992). Efficient pain assessment in clinical settings. *Behaviour Research and Therapy, 30,* 71–73.

Grossi, E., Borghi, C., Cerchiari, E. L., Della Puppa, T., & Francucci, B. (1983). Analogue Chromatic Continuous Scale (ACCS): A new method for pain assessment. *Clinical and Experimental Rheumatology, 4,* 337–340.

Grossman, S. A., Sheidler, V. R., McGuire, D. B., Geer, C., Santor, D., & Piantadosi, S. (1992). A comparison of the Hopkins Pain Rating Instrument with standard visual analogue and verbal descriptor scales in patients with cancer pain. *Journal of Pain and Symptom Management, 7,* 196–203.

Hall, W. (1981). On "ratio scales of sensory and affective verbal pain descriptors." *Pain, 4,* 101–107.

Hardy, J. D., Wolff, H. G., & Goodell, H. (1952). *Pain sensations and reactions.* Baltimore: Williams & Wilkins.

Heft, M. W., Gracely, R. H., & Dubner, R. (1984). Nitrous oxide analgesia: A psychophysical evaluation using verbal descriptor scaling. *Journal of Dental Research, 63,* 129–132.

Heiberg, T., Kvien, T. K., Dale, Ø., Mowinckel, P., Aanerud, G. J., Songe-Møller, A. B., et al. (2007). Daily health status registration (patient diary) in patients with rheumatoid arthritis: A comparison between personal digital assistant and paper–pencil format. *Arthritis and Rheumatism, 57,* 454–460.

Hildebrandt, J., Franz, C. E., Choroba-Mehnen, B., & Temme, M. (1988). The use of pain drawings in screening for psychological involvement in complaints of low-back pain. *Spine, 13,* 681–685.

Huber, A., Suman, A. L., Rendo, C. A., Biasi, G., Marcolongo, R., & Carli, G. (2007). Dimensions of "unidimensional" ratings of pain and emotions in patients with chronic musculoskeletal pain. *Pain, 130,* 216–224.

Jamison, R. N., Raymond, S. A., Slawsby, E. A.,

McHugo, G. J., & Baird, J. C. (2006). Pain assessment in patients with low back pain: Comparison of weekly recall and momentary electronic data. *Journal of Pain, 7*, 192–199.

Jamison, R. N., Sbrocco, T., & Parris, W. C. (1989). The influence of physical and psychosocial factors on accuracy of memory for pain in chronic pain patients. *Pain, 37*, 289–294.

Jensen, M. P. (2008). Pain assessment in clinical trials. In H. Wittink & D. Carr (Eds.), *Pain management: evidence, outcomes, and quality of life in pain treatment* (pp. 57–88). Amsterdam: Elsevier.

Jensen, M. P. (2010). Measurement of pain. In J. D. Loeser, D. C. Turk, C. R. Chapman, & S. Butler (Eds.), *Bonica's management of pain* (4th ed., pp. 251–270). Media, PA: Williams & Wilkins.

Jensen, M. P., Chiang, Y., & Wu, J. (2009). Assessment of pain quality in a clinical trial of gabapentin extended release for postherpetic neuralgia. *Clinical Journal of Pain, 25*, 286–292.

Jensen, M. P., Dworkin, R. H., Gammaitoni, A. R., Olaleye, D. O., Oleka, N., & Galer, B. S. (2005). Assessment of pain quality in chronic neuropathic and nociceptive pain clinical trials with the Neuropathic Pain Scale. *Journal of Pain, 6*, 98–106.

Jensen, M. P., Friedman, M., Bonzo, D., & Richards, P. (2006). The validity of the Neuropathic Pain Scale for assessing diabetic neuropathic pain in a clinical trial. *Clinical Journal of Pain, 22*, 97–103.

Jensen, M. P., Gammaitoni, A. R., Olaleye, D. O., Oleka, N., Nalamachu, S. R., & Galer, B. S. (2006). The Pain Quality Assessment Scale: Assessment of pain quality in carpal tunnel syndrome. *Journal of Pain, 7*, 823–832.

Jensen, M. P., Hoffman, A. J., & Cardenas, D. D. (2005). Chronic pain in individuals with spinal cord injury: A survey and longitudinal study. *Spinal Cord, 43*, 704–712.

Jensen, M. P., & Karoly, P. (1987). *Assessing the subjective experience of pain: What do the scale scores of the McGill Pain Questionnaire measure?* Poster presented at the Eighth Annual Scientific Sessions of the Society of Behavioral Medicine, Washington, DC.

Jensen, M. P., Karoly, P., & Braver, S. (1986). The measurement of clinical pain intensity: A comparison of six methods. *Pain, 27*, 117–126.

Jensen, M. P., Karoly, P., O'Riordan, E. F., Bland, F., Jr., & Burns, R. S. (1989). The subjective experience of acute pain: An assessment of the utility of 10 indices. *Clinical Journal of Pain, 5*, 153–159.

Jensen, M. P., Mardekian, J., Lakshminarayanan, M., & Boye, M. E. (2008). Validity of 24-hour recall ratings of pain severity: Biasing effects of "peak" and "end" pain. *Pain, 137*, 422–427.

Jensen, M. P., & McFarland, C. A. (1993). Increasing the reliability and validity of pain intensity measurement in chronic pain patients. *Pain, 55*, 195–203.

Jensen, M. P., Turner, J. A., Romano, J. M., & Fisher, L. (1999). Comparative reliability and validity of chronic pain intensity measures. *Pain, 83*, 157–162.

Jensen, M. P., Turner, L. R., Turner, J. A., & Romano, J. M. (1996). The use of multiple-item scales for pain intensity measurement in chronic pain patients. *Pain, 67*, 35–40.

Joyce, C. R. B., Zutshi, D. W., Hrubes, V., & Mason, R. M. (1975). Comparison of fixed interval and visual analogue scales for rating chronic pain. *European Journal of Clinical Pharmacology, 8*, 415–420.

Kállai, I., Barke, A., & Voss, U. (2004). The effects of experimenter characteristics on pain reports in women and men. *Pain, 112*, 142–147.

Karoly, P. (1985). The assessment of pain: Concepts and issues. In P. Karoly (Ed.), *Measurement strategies in health psychology* (pp. 1–43). New York: Wiley.

Karoly, P. (1991). Assessment of pediatric pain. In J. P. Bush & S. W. Harkins (Eds.), *Children in pain: Clinical and research issues from a developmental perspective* (pp. 59–82). New York: Springer-Verlag.

Karoly, P., & Jensen, M. P. (1987). *Multimethod assessment of chronic pain*. New York: Pergamon.

Keck, J. F., Gerkensmeyer, J. E., Joyce, B. A., & Schade, J. G. (1996). Reliability and validity of the faces and word descriptor scales to measure procedural pain. *Journal of Pediatric Nursing, 11*, 368–374.

Keefe, F. J., Schapira, B., Williams, R. B., Brown, C., & Surwit, R. S. (1981). EMG-assisted relaxation training in the management of chronic low back pain. *American Journal of Clinical Biofeedback, 4*, 93–103.

Kikuchi, H., Yoshiuchi, K., Miyasaka, N., Ohashi, K., Yamamoto, Y., Kumano, H., et al. (2006). Reliability of recalled self-report on headache intensity: Investigation using ecological momentary assessment technique. *Cephalalgia, 26*, 1335–1343.

Kremer, E., Atkinson, J. H., & Ignelzi, R. J. (1981). Measurement of pain: Patient preference does not confound pain measurement. *Pain, 10*, 241–248.

Levendoglu, F., Ogün, C. O., Ozerbil, O., Ogün, T. C., & Ugurlu, H. (2004). Gabapentin is a first line drug for the treatment of neuropathic pain in spinal cord injury. *Spine, 28*, 743–751.

Levine, F. M., & De Simone, L. L. (1991). The effects of experimenter gender on pain report in male and female subjects. *Pain*, *44*, 69–72.

Litcher-Kelly, L., Kellerman, Q., Hanauer, S. B., & Stone, A. A. (2007). Feasibility and utility of an electronic diary to assess self-report symptoms in patients with inflammatory bowel disease. *Annals of Behavioral Medicine*, *33*, 207–212.

Lynch, M. E., Clark, A. J., & Sawynok, J. (2003). Intravenous adenosine alleviates neuropathic pain: A double blind placebo controlled crossover trial using an enriched enrollment design. *Pain*, *103*, 111–117.

Margolis, R. B., Chibnall, J. T., & Tait, R. C. (1988). Test–retest reliability of the pain drawing instrument. *Pain*, *33*, 49–51.

Margolis, R. B., Tait, R. C., & Krause, S. J. (1986). A rating system for use with patient pain drawings. *Pain*, *24*, 57–65.

Max, M. B. (1991). Neuropathic pain syndromes. In M. Max, R. Portenoy, & E. Laska (Eds.), *Advances in pain research and therapy* (Vol. 18, pp. 193–219). New York: Springer.

Max, M. B., Schafer, S. C., Culnane, M., Dubner, R., & Gracely, R. H. (1987). Association of pain relief with drug side effects in postherpetic neuralgia: A single-dose study of clonidine, codeine, ibuprofen, and placebo. *Clinical Pharmacology and Therapeutics*, *43*, 363–371.

Melzack, R. (1975a). The McGill Pain Questionnaire. In R. Melzack (Ed.), *Pain measurement and assessment* (pp. 41–47). New York: Raven Press.

Melzack, R. (1975b). The McGill Pain Questionnaire: Major properties and scoring methods. *Pain*, *1*, 277–299.

Melzack, R. (1987). The Short-Form McGill Questionnaire. *Pain*, *30*, 191–197.

Morley, S. (1989). The dimensionality of verbal descriptors in Tursky's Pain Perception Profile. *Pain*, *37*, 41–49.

Morley, S., & Pallin, V. (1995). Scaling the affective domain of pain: A study of the dimensionality of verbal descriptors. *Pain*, *63*, 39–49.

Moseley, G. L. (2004). Graded motor imagery is effective for long-standing complex regional pain syndrome: A randomised controlled trial. *Pain*, *108*, 192–198.

Myles, P. S., Troedel, S., Boquest, M., & Reeves, M. (1999). The pain visual analog scale: Is it linear or nonlinear? *Anesthesia and Analgesia*, *91*, 248–291.

Myles, P. S., & Urquhart, N. (2005). The linearity of the visual analogue scale in patients with severe acute pain. *Anaesthesia and Intensive Care*, *33*, 54–58.

Öhlund, C., Eek, C., Palmblad, S., Areskoug, B., & Nachemson, A. (1996). Quantified pain drawing in subacute low back pain. *Spine*, *21*, 1021–1031.

Ohnhaus, E. E., & Adler, R. (1975). Methodological problems in the measurement of pain: A comparison between the verbal rating scale and the visual analogue scale. *Pain*, *1*, 379–384.

Paice, J. A., & Cohen, F. L. (1997). Validity of a verbally administered numeric rating scale to measure cancer pain intensity. *Cancer Nursing*, *20*, 88–93.

Palermo, T. M., Valenzuela, D., & Stork, P. P. (2004). A randomized trial of electronic versus paper pain diaries in children: Impact on compliance, accuracy, and acceptability. *Pain*, *107*, 213–219.

Parker, H., Wood, P. L. R., & Main, C. J. (1995). The use of the pain drawing as a screening measure to predict psychological distress in chronic low back pain. *Spine*, *20*, 236–243.

Peters, M. L., Sorbi, M. J., Kruise, D. A., Kerssens, J. J., Verhaak, P. F., & Bensing, J. M. (2000). Electronic diary assessment of pain, disability and psychological adaptation in patients differing in duration of pain. *Pain*, *84*, 181–192.

Philip, B. K. (1990). Parametric statistics for evaluation of the visual analog scale. *Anesthesia and Analgesia*, *71*, 710.

Piasecki, T., Hufford, M. R., Solhan, M., & Trull, T. J. (2007). Assessing clients in their natural environments with electronic diaries: Rationale, benefits, limitations, and barriers. *Psychological Assessment*, *19*, 25–43.

Price, D. D., & Barber, J. (1987). An analysis of factors that contribute to the efficacy of hypnotic analgesia. *Journal of Abnormal Psychology*, *96*, 46–51.

Price, D. D., Barrell, J. J., & Gracely, R. H. (1980). A psychophysical analysis of experiential factors that selectively influence the affective dimension of pain. *Pain*, *8*, 137–149.

Price, D. D., Bush, F. M., Long, S., & Harkins, S. W. (1994). A comparison of pain measurement characteristics of mechanical visual analogue and simple numerical rating scales. *Pain*, *56*, 217–226.

Price, D. D., & Harkins, S. W. (1987). Combined use of experimental pain and visual analogue scales in providing standardized measurement of clinical pain. *Clinical Journal of Pain*, *3*, 1–8.

Price, D. D., Harkins, S. W., & Baker, C. (1987). Sensory–affective relationships among different types of clinical and experimental pain. *Pain*, *28*, 297–307.

Price, D. D., Harkins, S. W., Rafii, A., & Price, C. (1986). A simultaneous comparison of fentanyl's analgesic effects on experimental and clinical pain. *Pain*, *24*, 197–203.

Price, D. D., McGrath, P. A., Rafii, A., & Buckingham, B. (1983). The validation of visual analogue scales as ratio scale measures for chronic and experimental pain. *Pain*, *17*, 45–56.

Price, D. D., Patel, R., Robinson, M. E., & Staud, R. (2008). Characteristics of electronic visual analogue and numerical scales for ratings of experimental pain in healthy subjects and fibromyalgia patients. *Pain*, *140*, 158–166.

Price, D. D., Von der Gruen, A., Miller, J., Rafii, A., & Price, C. (1985). A psychophysical analysis of morphine analgesia. *Pain*, *22*, 261–269.

Ransford, A. O., Cairns, D., & Mooney, V. (1976). The pain drawing as an aid to the psychologic evaluation of patients with low-back pain. *Spine*, *1*, 127–134.

Rasmussen, J. L. (1989). Analysis of Likert-scale data: A reinterpretation of Gregoire and Driver. *Psychological Bulletin*, *105*, 167–170.

Roelofs, J., Peters, M. L., Patijn, J., Schouten, E. G., & Vlaeyen, J. W. (2006). An electronic diary assessment of the effects of distraction and attentional focusing on pain intensity in chronic low back pain patients. *British Journal of Health Psychology*, *11*, 595–606.

Rybstein-Blinchik, E. (1979). Effects of different cognitive strategies on chronic pain experience. *Journal of Behavioral Medicine*, *2*, 93–101.

Salovey, P., Smith, A. F., Turk, D. C., Jobe, J. B., & Willis, G. B. (1993). The accuracy of memory for pain: Not so bad most of the time. *American Pain Society Journal*, *2*, 184–191.

Schwartz, D. P., & DeGood, D. E. (1984). Global appropriateness of pain drawings: Blind ratings predict patterns of psychological distress and litigation status. *Pain*, *19*, 383–388.

Scott, J., & Huskisson, E. C. (1976). Graphic representation of pain. *Pain*, *2*, 175–184.

Semenchuk, M. R., & Sherman, S. (2000). Effectiveness of tizanidine in neuropathic pain: An open-label study. *Journal of Pain*, *1*, 285–292.

Seymour, R. A. (1982). The use of pain scales in assessing the efficacy of analgesics in postoperative dental pain. *European Journal of Clinical Pharmacology*, *23*, 441–444.

Shiffman, S., Stone, A. A., & Hufford, M. R. (2008). Ecological momentary assessment. *Annual Review of Clinical Psychology*, *4*, 1–32.

Sriwatanakul, K., Kelvie, W., Lasagna, L., Calimlim, J. F., Weis, O. F., & Mehta, G. (1983). Studies with different types of visual analog scales for measurement of pain. *Clinical Pharmacology and Therapeutics*, *34*, 235–239.

Staud, R., Price, D. D., Robinson, M. E., & Vierck, C. J., Jr. (2004). Body pain area and pain-related negative affect predict clinical pain intensity in patients with fibromyalgia. *Journal of Pain*, *5*, 338–343.

Staud, R., Vierck, C. J., Robinson, M. E., & Price, D. D. (2006). Overall fibromyalgia pain is predicted by ratings of local pain and pain-related negative affect—possible role of peripheral tissues. *Rheumatology*, *45*, 1409–1415.

Stenn, P. G., Mothersill, K. J., & Brooke, R. I. (1979). Biofeedback and a cognitive behavioral approach to treatment of myofascial pain dysfunction syndrome. *Behavior Therapy*, *10*, 29–36.

Stinson, J. N., Stevens, B. J., Feldman, B. M., Streiner, D., McGrath, P. J., Dupuis, A., et al. (2008). Construct validity of a multidimensional electronic pain diary for adolescents with arthritis. *Pain*, *136*, 281–292.

Stone, A. A., Broderick, J. E., Kaell, A. T., DelesPaul, P. A., & Porter, L. E. (2000). Does the peak-end phenomenon observed in laboratory pain studies apply to real-world pain in rheumatoid arthritics? *Journal of Pain*, *1*, 212–217.

Stone, A. A., Broderick, J. E., Schwartz, J. E., Shiffman, S., Litcher-Kelly, L., & Calvanese, P. (2003). Intensive momentary reporting of pain with an electronic diary: Reactivity, compliance, and patient satisfaction. *Pain*, *104*, 343–351.

Stone, A. A., Broderick, J. E., Shiffman, S. S., & Schwartz, J. E. (2004). Understanding recall of weekly pain from a momentary assessment perspective: Absolute agreement, between- and within-person consistency, and judged change in weekly pain. *Pain*, *107*, 61–69.

Stuppy, D. J. (1998). The Faces Pain Scale: Reliability and validity with mature adults. *Applied Nursing Research*, *11*, 84–89.

Tai, Q., Kirshblum, S., Chen, B., Millis, S., Johnston, M., & DeLisa, J. A. (2002). Gabapentin in the treatment of neuropathic pain after spinal cord injury: A prospective, randomized, double-blind, crossover trial. *Journal of Spinal Cord Medicine*, *25*, 100–105.

Tait, R. C., Chibnall, J. T., & Margolis, R. B. (1990). Pain extent: Relations with psychological state, pain severity, pain history, and disability. *Pain*, *41*, 295–301.

Teske, K., Daut, R. L., & Cleeland, C. S. (1983). Relationships between nurses' observations and patients' self-reports of pain. *Pain*, *16*, 289–296.

Thomas, T. A., & Griffiths, M. J. (1982). A pain slide rule. *Anaesthesia*, *37*, 960–961.

Toomey, T. C., Gover, V. F., & Jones, B. N. (1983). Spatial distribution of pain: A descriptive characteristic of chronic pain. *Pain*, *17*, 289–300.

Toomey, T. C., Gover, V. F., & Jones, B. N. (1984). Site of pain: Relationship to measures of pain description, behavior and personality. *Pain*, *19*, 389–397.

Toomey, T. C., Mann, J. D., Abashian, S., & Thompson-Pope, S. (1991). Relationship of pain drawing scores to ratings of pain description and function. *Clinical Journal of Pain, 7,* 269–274.

Torrance, N., Smith, B. H., Bennett, M. I., & Lee, A. J. (2006). The epidemiology of chronic pain of predominantly neuropathic origin: Results from a general population survey. *Journal of Pain, 7,* 281–289.

Turner, J. A. (1982). Comparison of group progressive-relaxation training and cognitive-behavioral group therapy for chronic low back pain. *Journal of Consulting and Clinical Psychology, 50,* 757–765.

Tursky, B. (1976). The development of a pain perception profile: A psychophysical approach. In M. Weisenberg & B. Tursky (Eds.), *Pain: New perspectives in therapy and research* (pp. 171–194). New York: Plenum Press.

Tursky, B., Jamner, L. D., & Friedman, R. (1982). The pain Perception Profile: A psychophysical approach to the assessment of pain report. *Behavior Therapy, 13,* 376–394.

Udén, A., Åström, M., & Bergenudd, H. (1988). Pain drawings in chronic back pain. *Spine, 13,* 389–392.

Urban, B. J., Keefe, F. J., & France, R. D. (1984). A study of psychophysical scaling in chronic pain patients. *Pain, 20,* 157–168.

Victor, T. W., Jensen, M. P., Gammaitoni, A. R., Gould, E. M., White, R. E., & Galer, B. S. (2008). The dimensions of pain quality: Factor analysis of the Pain Quality Assessment Scale. *Clinical Journal of Pain, 24,* 550–555.

Vierck, C. J., Cannon, R. L., Fry, G., Maixner, W., & Whitsel, B. L. (1997). Characteristics of temporal summation of second pain sensations elicited by brief contact of glabrous skin by a preheated thermode. *Journal of Neurophysiology, 78,* 992–1002.

Von Baeyer, C. L., Bergstrom, K. J., Brodwin, M. G., & Brodwin, S. K. (1983). Invalid use of pain drawings in psychological screening of back pain patients. *Pain, 16,* 103–107.

Wallenstein, S. L., Heidrich, G., III, Kaiko, R., & Houde, R. W. (1980). Clinical evaluation of mild analgesics: The measurement of clinical pain. *British Journal of Clinical Pharmacology, 10,* 319S–327S.

Walsh, T. D. (1984). Practical problems in pain measurement. *Pain, 19,* 96–98.

Weintraub, M. I., & Cole, S. P. (2008). A randomized controlled trial of the effects of a combination of static and dynamic magnetic fields on carpal tunnel syndrome. *Pain Medicine, 9,* 493–504.

Wilkie, D., Lovejoy, N., Dodd, M., & Tesler, M. (1990). Cancer pain intensity measurement: Concurrent validity of three tools—finger dynamometer, pain intensity number scale, visual analogue scale. *Hospice Journal, 6,* 1–13.

Wilson, J. S., Cason, C. L., & Grissom, N. L. (1995). Distraction: An effective intervention for alleviating pain during venipuncture. *Journal of Emergency Nursing, 21,* 87.

Wong, D., & Baker, C. (1988). Pain in children: Comparison of assessment scales. *Pediatric Nursing, 14,* 9–17.

APPENDIX 2.1. The Pain Quality Assessment Scale

Instructions: There are different aspects and types of pain that patients experience and that we are interested in measuring. Pain can feel sharp, hot, cold, dull, and achy. Some pains may feel like they are very superficial (at skin level), or they may feel like they are from deep inside your body. Pain can also be described as unpleasant. The Pain Quality Assessment Scale helps us measure these and other different aspects of your pain. For one patient, a pain might feel extremely hot and burning but not at all dull, while another patient may not experience any burning pain but feel very dull and achy pain. Therefore, we expect you to rate very high on some of the scales below and very low on others.

Please use the 19 rating scales below to rate how much of each different pain quality and type you may or may not have felt *OVER THE PAST WEEK, ON AVERAGE.*

Place an "X" through the number that best describes your pain. For example:

0   1   2   3   4   X   6   7   8   9   10

1. Please use the scale below to tell us how **intense** your pain has been over the past week, on average.

   No pain   0   1   2   3   4   5   6   7   8   9   10   The most **intense** pain sensation imaginable

2. Please use the scale below to tell us how sharp your pain has felt over the past week. Words used to describe sharp feelings include **"like a knife,"** **"like a spike,"** or **"piercing."**

   Not sharp   0   1   2   3   4   5   6   7   8   9   10   The most **sharp** sensation imaginable ("like a knife")

3. Please use the scale below to tell us how **hot** your pain has felt over the past week. Words used to describe very hot pain include **"burning"** and **"on fire."**

   Not hot   0   1   2   3   4   5   6   7   8   9   10   The most **hot** sensation imaginable ("burning")

4. Please use the scale below to tell us how **dull** your pain has felt over the past week.

   Not dull   0   1   2   3   4   5   6   7   8   9   10   The most **dull** sensation imaginable

5. Please use the scale below to tell us how **cold** your pain has felt over the past week. Words used to describe very cold pain include **"like ice"** and **"freezing."**

   Not cold   0   1   2   3   4   5   6   7   8   9   10   The most **cold** sensation imaginable ("freezing")

6. Please use the scale below to tell us how **sensitive** your skin has been to light touch or clothing rubbing against it over the past week. Words used to describe sensitive skin include **"like sunburned skin"** and **"raw skin."**

   Not sensitive   0   1   2   3   4   5   6   7   8   9   10   The most **sensitive** sensation imaginable ("raw skin")

7. Please use the scale below to tell us how **tender** your pain is when something has pressed against it over the past week. A phrase that can be used to describe tender pain is "**like a bruise**."

Not tender   0 1 2 3 4 5 6 7 8 9 10   The most **tender** sensation imaginable ("like a bruise")

8. Please use the scale below to tell us how **itchy** your pain has felt over the past week. Words used to describe itchy pain include "**like poison ivy**" and "**like a mosquito bite**."

Not itchy   0 1 2 3 4 5 6 7 8 9 10   The most **itchy** sensation imaginable ("like poison ivy")

9. Please use the scale below to tell us how much your pain has felt like it has been **shooting** over the past week. Another word used to describe shooting pain is "**zapping**."

Not shooting   0 1 2 3 4 5 6 7 8 9 10   The most **shooting** sensation imaginable ("zapping")

10. Please use the scale below to tell us how **numb** your pain has felt over the past week. A phrase that can be used to describe numb pain is "like it is **asleep**."

Not numb   0 1 2 3 4 5 6 7 8 9 10   The most **numb** sensation imaginable ("asleep")

11. Please use the scale below to tell us how much your pain sensations have felt **electrical** over the past week. Words used to describe electrical pain include "**shocks**," "**lightning**," and "**sparking**."

Not electrical   0 1 2 3 4 5 6 7 8 9 10   The most **electrical** sensation imaginable ("shocks")

12. Please use the scale below to tell us how **tingling** your pain has felt over the past week. Words used to describe tingling pain include "**like pins and needles**" and "**prickling**."

Not tingling   0 1 2 3 4 5 6 7 8 9 10   The most **tingling** sensation imaginable ("pins and needles")

13. Please use the scale below to tell us how **cramping** your pain has felt over the past week. Words used to describe cramping pain include "**squeezing**" and "**tight**."

Not cramping   0 1 2 3 4 5 6 7 8 9 10   The most **cramping** sensation imaginable ("squeezing")

14. Please use the scale below to tell us how **radiating** your pain has felt over the past week. Another word used to describe radiating pain is "**spreading**."

Not radiating   0 1 2 3 4 5 6 7 8 9 10   The most **radiating** sensation imaginable ("spreading")

15. Please use the scale below to tell us how **throbbing** your pain has felt over the past week. Another word used to describe throbbing pain is "**pounding**."

Not throbbing   0 1 2 3 4 5 6 7 8 9 10   The most **throbbing** sensation imaginable ("pounding")

16. Please use the scale below to tell us how **aching** your pain has felt over the past week. A phrase that can be used to describe aching pain is "**like a toothache.**"

    Not aching   0   1   2   3   4   5   6   7   8   9   10   The most **aching** sensation imaginable ("like a toothache")

17. Please use the scale below to tell us how **heavy** your pain has felt over the past week. Other words used to describe heavy pain are "**pressure**" and "**weighted down.**"

    Not heavy   0   1   2   3   4   5   6   7   8   9   10   The most **heavy** sensation imaginable ("weighted down")

18. Now that you have told us the different types of pain sensations you have felt, we want you to tell us overall how **unpleasant** your pain has been to you over the past week. Words used to describe very unpleasant pain include "**annoying,**" "**bothersome,**" "**miserable,**" and "**intolerable.**" Remember, pain can have a low intensity but still feel extremely unpleasant, and some kinds of pain can have a high intensity but be very tolerable. With this scale, please tell us how **unpleasant** your pain feels.

    Not unpleasant   0   1   2   3   4   5   6   7   8   9   10   The most **unpleasant** sensation imaginable ("intolerable")

19. Finally, we want you to give us an estimate of the severity of your **deep** versus **surface** pain over the past week. We want you to rate each location of pain separately. We realize that it can be difficult to make these estimates, and most likely it will be a "best guess," but please give us your best estimate.

    HOW INTENSE IS YOUR *DEEP* PAIN?

    No deep pain   0   1   2   3   4   5   6   7   8   9   10   The most **intense deep** pain sensation imaginable

    HOW INTENSE IS YOUR *SURFACE* PAIN?

    No surface pain   0   1   2   3   4   5   6   7   8   9   10   The most **intense surface** pain sensation imaginable

20. Pain can also have different time qualities. For some people, the pain comes and goes, and so they have some moments that are completely without pain; in other words, the pain "comes and goes." This is called **intermittent** pain. Others are never pain-free, but their pain types and pain severity can vary from one moment to the next. This is called **variable** pain. For these people, the increases can be severe, so that they feel they have moments of very intense pain ("breakthrough" pain), but at other times they can feel lower levels of pain ("background" pain). Still, they are never pain-free. Other people have pain that really does not change that much from one moment to another. This is called **stable** pain. Which of these best describes the time pattern of your pain (please select only one):

    ( ) I have **intermittent** pain (I feel pain sometimes but I am pain-free at other times).

    ( ) I have **variable** pain ("background" pain all the time, but also moments of more pain, or even severe "breakthrough pain or varying types of pain).

    ( ) I have **stable** pain (constant pain that does not change very much from one moment to another, and no pain-free periods).

CHAPTER 3

The McGill Pain Questionnaire

Development, Psychometric Properties, and Usefulness
of the Long Form, Short Form, and Short Form–2

JOEL KATZ
RONALD MELZACK

People with acute or chronic pain provide valuable opportunities to study the mechanisms of pain and analgesia. The measurement of pain is therefore essential to determine the intensity, perceptual qualities, and time course of the pain, so that the differences among pain syndromes can be ascertained and investigated. Furthermore, measurement of these variables provides valuable clues that help in the differential diagnosis of the underlying causes of the pain. They also help determine the most effective treatment, such as the types of analgesic drugs, or other therapies, necessary to control the pain, and are essential to evaluate the relative effectiveness of different therapies. The measurement of pain, then, is important (1) to determine pain intensity, quality, and duration; (2) to aid in diagnosis; (3) to help decide the choice of therapy; and (4) to evaluate the relative effectiveness of different therapies.

DIMENSIONS OF PAIN EXPERIENCE

Research on pain, since the beginning of the 1900s, has been dominated by the concept that pain is purely a sensory experience. Yet pain also has a distinctly unpleasant, affective quality. It becomes overwhelming, demands immediate attention, and disrupts ongoing behavior and thought. It motivates or drives the organism into activity aimed at stopping the pain as quickly as possible. To consider only the sensory features of pain and ignore its motivational–affective properties is to look at only part of the problem. Even the concept of pain as a perception, with full recognition of past experience, attention, and other cognitive influences, still neglects the crucial motivational dimension.

These considerations led Melzack and Casey (1968) to suggest that there are three major psychological dimensions of pain: sensory–discriminative, motivational–affective, and cognitive–evaluative. They proposed, moreover, that these dimensions of pain experience are subserved by physiologically specialized systems in the brain: the sensory–discriminative dimension of pain is influenced primarily by the rapidly conducting spinal systems; the powerful motivational drive and unpleasant affect characteristic of pain are subserved by activities in reticular and limbic structures that are influenced primarily by the slowly conducting spinal systems; neocortical or higher central

45

nervous system processes, such as evaluation of the input in terms of past experience, exert control over activity in both the discriminative and motivational systems.

It is assumed that these three categories of activity interact with one another to provide perceptual information on the location, magnitude, and spatiotemporal properties of the noxious stimuli, motivational tendency toward escape or attack, and cognitive information based on past experience and probability of outcome of different response strategies (Melzack & Casey, 1968). All three forms of activity could then influence motor mechanisms responsible for the complex pattern of overt responses that characterize pain.

THE LANGUAGE OF PAIN

Clinical investigators have long recognized the varieties of pain experience. Descriptions of the burning qualities of pain after peripheral nerve injury, or the stabbing, cramping qualities of visceral pains frequently provide the key to diagnosis and may even suggest the course of therapy. Despite the frequency of such descriptions, and the seemingly high agreement that they are valid descriptive words, studies of their use and meaning are relatively recent.

Anyone who has suffered severe pain and tried to describe the experience to a friend or to the doctor often finds him- or herself at a loss for words. The reason for this difficulty in expressing pain experience, actually, is not because the words do not exist. As we shall soon see, there is an abundance of appropriate words. Rather, the main reason is that, fortunately, they are not words we have occasion to use often. Another reason is that the words may seem absurd. We may use descriptors such as splitting, shooting, gnawing, wrenching, or stinging as useful metaphors, but there are no external objective references for these words in relation to pain. If we talk about a blue pen or a yellow pencil we can point to an object and say "That is what I mean by yellow," or "The color of the pen is blue." But what can we point to in telling another person precisely what we mean by smarting, tingling, or rasping? A person who suffers terrible pain may say that the pain is burning and add

that "it feels as if someone is shoving a red-hot poker through my toes and slowly twisting it around." These "as if" statements are often essential to convey the qualities of the experience.

If the study of pain in people is to have a scientific foundation, it is essential to measure it. If we want to know how effective a new drug is, we need numbers to say that the pain decreased by some amount. Yet, whereas overall intensity is important information, we also want to know whether the drug specifically decreased the burning quality of the pain, or whether the especially miserable, tight, cramping feeling is gone.

TRADITIONAL MEASURES OF PAIN INTENSITY

Traditional methods of pain measurement treat pain as though it were a single unique quality that varies only in intensity (Beecher, 1959). These methods include the use of verbal rating scales (VRSs), numerical rating scales (NRSs), and visual analogue scales (VASs) (Jensen & Karoly, 2001). These simple methods have all been used effectively in hospital clinics, and have provided valuable information about pain and analgesia. VRSs, NRSs, and VASs provide simple, efficient, and minimally intrusive measures of pain intensity that have been used widely in clinical and research settings that require a quick index of pain intensity to which a numerical value can be assigned (Katz & Melzack, 1999). The main disadvantage of VASs, NRSs, and VRSs is the assumption that pain is a unidimensional experience that can be measured with a single item scale (Melzack, 1975). Although intensity is, without a doubt, a salient dimension of pain, it is clear that the word "pain" refers to an endless variety of qualities categorized under a single linguistic label, not to a specific, single sensation that varies only in intensity or affect. The development of rating scales to measure pain affect or pain unpleasantness (Price, Harkins, & Baker, 1987) has partially addressed the problem, but the same shortcoming applies within the affective domain. Each pain has unique qualities. Unpleasantness is only one such quality. The pain of a toothache is obviously different from that of a pinprick, just as the pain of a coronary occlusion is uniquely different from the pain of a broken leg. To describe pain solely in terms of intensity or affect is like specifying the visual world only in terms of light flux, without regard to pattern, color, texture, and the many other dimensions of visual experience.

THE McGILL PAIN QUESTIONNAIRE

Development and Description

Melzack and Torgerson (1971) developed the procedures to specify the qualities of pain. In the first part of their study, physicians and other university graduates were asked to classify 102 words, obtained from the clinical literature, into small groups that describe distinctly different aspects of the experience of pain. On the basis of the data, the words were categorized into three major classes and 16 subclasses. The classes are (1) words that describe the sensory qualities of the experience in terms of temporal, spatial, pressure, thermal, and other properties; (2) words that describe affective qualities in terms of tension, fear, and autonomic properties that are part of the pain experience; and (3) evaluative words that describe the subjective overall intensity of the total pain experience. Each subclass was given a descriptive label and consists of a group of words considered by most subjects to be qualitatively similar, but whereas some of these words are undoubtedly synonyms, others seem to be synonymous yet vary in intensity, and still others provide subtle differences or nuances (despite their similarities) that may be of importance to a patient trying desperately to communicate to a physician.

The second part of the Melzack and Torgerson (1971) study was an attempt to determine the pain intensities implied by the words within each subclass. Groups of physicians, patients, and students were asked to assign an intensity value to each word, using a numerical scale ranging from least (or mild) pain to worst (or excruciating) pain. When this was done, it was apparent that several words within each subclass had the same relative intensity relationships in all three sets. For example, in the spatial subclass, "shooting" was found to represent more pain than "flashing," which in turn implied more pain than "jumping." Although the precise intensity scale values differed for the groups, all three agreed on the positions of the words relative to each other.

Because of the high degree of agreement on the intensity relationships among pain descriptors by subjects who have different cultural, socioeconomic, and educational backgrounds, a pain questionnaire (Figure 3.1) was developed as an experimental tool for studies of the effects of various methods of pain management. In addition to the list of pain descriptors, the questionnaire contains line drawings of the body to show the spatial distribution of the pain, words that describe temporal properties of pain, and descriptors of the overall present pain intensity (PPI). The PPI is recorded as a number from 1 to 5, in which each number is associated with the following words: 1, "mild"; 2, "discomforting"; 3, "distressing"; 4, "horrible"; and 5, "excruciating." The mean scale values of these words, which were chosen from the evaluative category, are approximately equally far apart, so that they represent equal scale intervals and thereby provide "anchors" for the specification of the overall pain intensity (Melzack & Torgerson, 1971).

In a preliminary study, the pain questionnaire consisted of the 16 subclasses of descriptors shown in Figure 3.1, as well as the additional information deemed necessary for the evaluation of pain. It soon became clear, however, that many of the patients found certain key words to be absent. These words were then selected from the original word list used by Melzack and Torgerson (1971), categorized appropriately, and ranked according to their mean scale values. A further set of words—"cool," "cold," "freezing"— was used by patients on rare occasions but was indicated to be essential for an adequate description of some types of pain. Thus, four supplementary—or "miscellaneous"— subclasses were added to the word lists of the questionnaire (Figure 3.1). The final classification, then, appeared to represent the most parsimonious and meaningful set of subclasses without at the same time losing subclasses that represent important qualitative properties. The questionnaire, which is known as the McGill Pain Questionnaire (MPQ; Melzack, 1975), has become a widely used clinical and research tool (Melzack, 1983; Wilkie, Savedra, Holzemier, Tesler, & Paul, 1990).

McGill Pain Questionnaire

Patient's Name ______________ **Date** __________ **Time** ________ **am/pm**

PRI: S ______ **A** ______ **E** ______ **M** ______ **PRI(T)** ______ **PPI** ______
(1-10) **(11-15)** **(16)** **(17-20)** **(1-20)**

1 FLICKERING ___
QUIVERING ___
PULSING ___
THROBBING ___
BEATING ___
POUNDING ___

2 JUMPING ___
FLASHING ___
SHOOTING ___

3 PRICKING ___
BORING ___
DRILLING ___
STABBING ___
LANCINATING ___

4 SHARP ___
CUTTING ___
LACERATING ___

5 PINCHING ___
PRESSING ___
GNAWING ___
CRAMPING ___
CRUSHING ___

6 TUGGING ___
PULLING ___
WRENCHING ___

7 HOT ___
BURNING ___
SCALDING ___
SEARING ___

8 TINGLING ___
ITCHY ___
SMARTING ___
STINGING ___

9 DULL ___
SORE ___
HURTING ___
ACHING ___
HEAVY ___

10 TENDER ___
TAUT ___
RASPING ___
SPLITTING ___

11 TIRING ___
EXHAUSTING ___

12 SICKENING ___
SUFFOCATING ___

13 FEARFUL ___
FRIGHTFUL ___
TERRIFYING ___

14 PUNISHING ___
GRUELING ___
CRUEL ___
VICIOUS ___
KILLING ___

15 WRETCHED ___
BLINDING ___

16 ANNOYING ___
TROUBLESOME ___
MISERABLE ___
INTENSE ___
UNBEARABLE ___

17 SPREADING ___
RADIATING ___
PENETRATING ___
PIERCING ___

18 TIGHT ___
NUMB ___
DRAWING ___
SQUEEZING ___
TEARING ___

19 COOL ___
COLD ___
FREEZING ___

20 NAGGING ___
NAUSEATING ___
AGONIZING ___
DREADFUL ___
TORTURING ___

PPI

0 NO PAIN ___
1 MILD ___
2 DISCOMFORTING ___
3 DISTRESSING ___
4 HORRIBLE ___
5 EXCRUCIATING ___

BRIEF ___	RHYTHMIC ___	CONTINUOUS ___
MOMENTARY ___	PERIODIC ___	STEADY ___
TRANSIENT ___	INTERMITTENT ___	CONSTANT ___

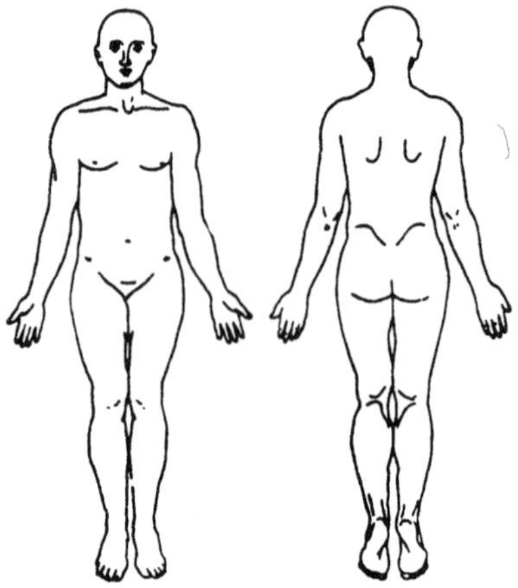

E = EXTERNAL
I = INTERNAL

COMMENTS:

FIGURE 3.1. The McGill Pain Questionnaire (MPQ). The descriptors fall into four major groups: Sensory, 1–10; Affective, 11–15; Evaluative, 16; and Miscellaneous, 17–20. The rank value for each descriptor is based on its position in the word set. The sum of the rank values is the pain rating index (PRI). The present pain intensity (PPI) is based on a scale of 0 to 5. Copyright 1996 by Ronald Melzack. Reprinted by permission.

Measures of Pain Experience

The descriptor lists of the MPQ are read to a patient with the explicit instruction that he or she choose only those words that describe his or her feelings and sensations at that moment. Three major indices are obtained:

1. The pain rating index (PRI) based on the rank values of the words. In this scoring system, the word in each subclass implying the least pain is given a value of 1, the next word is given a value of 2, and so forth. The rank values of the words chosen by a patient are summed to obtain separate scores for the sensory (subclasses 1–10), affective (subclasses 11–15), evaluative (subclass 16), and miscellaneous (subclasses 17–20) words, in

addition to providing a total score (subclasses 1–20). Figure 3.2 shows MPQ scores (total score from subclasses 1–20) obtained by patients with a variety of acute and chronic pains.
2. The number of words chosen (NWC).
3. The present pain intensity (PPI), the number–word combination chosen as the indicator of overall pain intensity at the time of administration of the questionnaire.

Usefulness

The most important requirements are that a measure be valid, reliable, consistent, and above all, useful. The MPQ appears to meet all of these requirements (Chapman et al., 1985; Melzack, 1983; Wilkie et al., 1990)

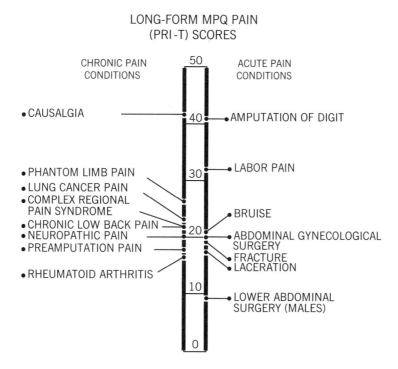

FIGURE 3.2. Comparison of pain scores, using the MPQ, obtained from women during labor (Melzack et al., 1981), patients in a general hospital pain clinic (Melzack, 1975), and an emergency department (Melzack et al., 1982). The pain score for causalgic pain is reported by Tahmoush (1981). Other pain ratings come from studies of patients with chronic pain conditions, including lung cancer pain (Wilkie et al., 2001), low back pain (Scrimshaw & Maher, 2001), complex regional pain syndromes (Birklein, Riedl, Sieweke, Weber, & Neundorfer, 2000), neuropathic pain (Lynch et al., 2003), preamputation pain (Nikolajsen, Ilkjaer, Kroner, Christensen, & Jensen, 1997), and rheumatoid arthritis (Roche et al., 2003), as well patients with acute pain after abdominal gynecological surgery (Katz, Cohen, Schmid, Chan, & Wowk, 2003) and lower abdominal surgery (Katz et al., 1994).

and provides a relatively rapid way of measuring subjective pain experience (Melzack, 1975). When administered to a patient by reading each subclass, it can be completed in about 5 minutes. It can also be filled out by the patient in a more leisurely way as a paper-and-pencil test, though the scores are somewhat different (Klepac, Dowling, Rokke, Dodge, & Schafer, 1981).

Since its introduction in 1975, the MPQ has been used in more than 500 studies of acute, chronic, and laboratory-produced pains. It has been translated into several languages and has also spawned the development of similar pain questionnaires in other languages (Table 3.1).

TABLE 3.1. Pain Questionnaires in Different Languages Based on the McGill Pain Questionnaire

Language	Authors
Amharic (Ethiopia)	Aboud et al. (2003)
Arabic	Harrison (1988)
Chinese	Hui & Chen (1989)
Danish	Drewes et al. (1993)
Dutch (Flemish)	Vanderiet et al. (1987); Verkes et al. (1989); van Lankveld et al. (1992); van der Kloot et al. (1995)
Finnish	Ketovuori & Pöntinen (1981)
French	Boureau et al. (1984, 1992)
German	Kiss et al. (1987); Radvila et al. (1987); Stein & Mendl (1988)
Greek	Georgoudis et al. (2000, 2001b); Mystakidou et al. (2002)
Italian	De Benedittis et al. (1988); Ferracuti et al. (1990); Maiani & Sanavio (1985)
Japanese	Satow et al. (1990); Hobara et al. (2003); Hasegawa et al. (2001)
Norwegian	Strand & Wisnes (1991); Kim et al. (1995)
Polish	Sedlak (1990)
Portuguese	Pimenta & Teixeiro (1996)
Slovak	Bartko et al. (1984)
Spanish	Laheurta et al. (1982); Bejarano et al. (1985); Lázaro et al. (1994); Escalante et al. (1996); Masedo & Esteve (2000)

Because pain is a private, personal experience, it is impossible for us to know precisely what someone else's pain feels like. No man can possibly know what it is like to have menstrual cramps or labor pain. Nor can psychologically healthy persons know what psychotic patients are feeling when they say they have excruciating pain (Veilleux & Melzack, 1976). But the MPQ provides us with an insight into the qualities that are experienced. Studies indicate that each kind of pain is characterized by a distinctive constellation of words. There is a remarkable consistency in the choice of words by patients experiencing the same or similar pain syndromes (Graham, Bond, Gerkovitch, & Cook, 1980; Grushka & Sessle, 1984; Katz, 1992; Katz & Melzack, 1991; Melzack, Taenzer, Feldman, & Kinch, 1981; Van Buren & Kleinknecht, 1979). For example, in a study of amputees with phantom limb pain (Group PLP) or nonpainful phantom limb sensations (Group PLS), every MPQ descriptor chosen by 33% or more participants in Group PLS was also chosen by 33% or more participants in Group PLP, although there were other descriptors the latter group endorsed with greater frequency (Katz & Melzack, 1991). These data indicated that the phantom limb experiences of the two groups have in common a paresthetic quality (e.g., tingling, numb), although painful phantoms consist of more than this shared component.

Reliability and Validity

Reading, Everitt, and Sledmere (1982) investigated the reliability of the groupings of adjectives in the MPQ by using different methodological and statistical approaches. Subjects sorted each of the 78 words of the MPQ into groups that described similar pain qualities. The mean number of groups was 19 (with a range of 7 to 31), which is remarkably close to the MPQ's 20 groups. Moreover, there were distinct subgroups for sensory and affective–evaluative words. Since the cultural backgrounds of subjects in this study and in that of Melzack and Torgerson (1971) were different, and the methodology and data analysis were dissimilar, the degree of correspondence is impressive. Gaston-Johansson, Albert, Fagan, and Zimmerman (1990) reported that subjects with diverse ethnic–cultural and educational backgrounds use similar MPQ adjectives to describe commonly used words such as "pain," "hurt," and "ache." Nevertheless, interesting differences were found between the studies, which suggest alternative approaches for future revisions of the MPQ.

Evidence for the stability of pain measures can be difficult to obtain, since many pains fluctuate over time, resolve spontaneously, or improve as a function of a treatment. In cases such as these, repeated administration of the same pain instrument would not be expected to yield similar estimates. Chronic pain conditions that remain relatively constant over time offer the opportunity to evaluate the stability of pain measures. Evidence of the stability the MPQ comes from a study of patients with chronic low back pain who completed the MPQ on two occasions separated by several days (Love, Leboeuf, & Crisp, 1989). The results showed very strong test–retest reliability coefficients for the MPQ PRIs, as well as for some of the 20 categories. The lower coefficients for the 20 categories may be explained by the suggestion that clinical pains show fluctuations in quality over time yet still represent the "same" pain to the person who experiences it. More recently, a study of patients with rheumatoid arthritis showed a stable pattern of MPQ scores across three pain assessments over a 6-year period (Roche, Klestov, & Heim, 2003). The pain remained moderate over the 6-year period in the presence of ongoing disease activity, and the MPQ revealed a consistent choice of descriptors, with no significant change in MPQ ratings over time.

There are many validity studies of the three-dimensional framework of the MPQ. Generally, the distinction between sensory and affective dimensions has held up extremely well, but there is still considerable debate on the separation of the affective and evaluative dimensions. Nevertheless, several excellent studies (Holroyd et al., 1992; McCreary, Turner, & Dawson, 1981; Prieto et al., 1980; Reading, 1979) have reported a discrete evaluative factor. The different factor-analytic procedures that were used undoubtedly account for the reports of four factors (Holroyd et al., 1992; Reading, 1979), five factors (Crockett, Prkachin, & Craig, 1977), six factors (Burckhardt, 1984),

or seven factors (Leavitt, Garron, Whisler, & Sheinkop, 1978). The major source of disagreement, however, seems to be the different patient populations used to obtain data for factor analyses. The range includes brief laboratory-induced pains, dysmenorrhea, back pain, and cancer pain. In some studies, relatively few words are chosen, while large numbers are selected in others. It is not surprising, then, that factor-analytic studies based on such diverse populations have confused rather than clarified some of the issues.

Turk, Rudy, and Salovey (1985) examined the internal structure of the MPQ using techniques that avoided the problems of most earlier studies and confirmed the three (sensory, affective, and evaluative) dimensions. Lowe, Walker, and McCallum (1991) also confirmed the three-factor structure of the MPQ, using elegant statistical procedures and a large number of subjects. Finally, a paper by Chen, Dworkin, Haug, and Gehrig (1989) presented data on the remarkable consistency of the MPQ across five studies using the cold pressor task, and Pearce and Morley (1989) provided further confirmation of the construct validity of the MPQ using the Stroop color-naming task with patients with chronic pain.

Sensitivity

Recent studies show that the MPQ is sensitive to interventions designed to reduce pain of neuropathic origin (Lynch, Clark, & Sawynok, 2003), including phantom limb pain (Nikolajsen et al., 1996), spinal cord injury pain (Defrin, Grunhaus, Zamir, & Zeilig, 2007), and postherpetic neuralgia (Dworkin et al., 2003). The relative sensitivity of the MPQ to change in postoperative pain following administration of oral analgesics was evaluated by comparing it with VAS and VRS measures of pain intensity (Jenkinson et al., 1995). While all three measures of pain revealed the same pattern of change over time, effect sizes for the MPQ were consistently related to self-reported, directly assessed change in pain using a VRS. These findings probably underestimate the MPQ's sensitivity to change, since the benchmark for change was a VRS. In support of this, the MPQ appears to provide a more sensitive measure of mild postoperative pain than does a simple VAS that assesses pain intensity, only because patients can be more precise in describing their experience by selecting appropriate descriptors (Katz et al., 1994). This increased ability of the MPQ to detect differences in pain at the low end of the pain continuum most likely is a function of the multidimensional nature of the MPQ and the large number of descriptors from which to choose.

Discriminative Capacity

One of the most exciting features of the MPQ is its potential value as an aid in the differential diagnosis among various pain syndromes. The first study to demonstrate the discriminative capacity of the MPQ was carried out by Dubuisson and Melzack (1976), who administered the questionnaire to patients with eight different pain syndromes: postherpetic neuralgia, phantom limb pain, metastatic carcinoma, toothache, degenerative disc disease, rheumatoid arthritis or osteoarthritis, labor pain, and menstrual pain. Discriminant analysis revealed that each type of pain is characterized by a distinctive constellation of verbal descriptors. Furthermore, when the descriptor set for each patient was classified into one of the eight diagnostic categories, a correct classification was made in 77% of cases. Table 3.2 shows the pain descriptors that are most characteristic of the eight clinical pain syndromes in the Dubuisson and Melzack (1976) study.

Descriptor patterns can also provide the basis for discriminating between two major types of low back pain. Some patients have clear physical causes, such as degenerative disc disease, while others suffer low back pain even though no physical causes can be found. Using a modified version of the MPQ, Leavitt and Garron (1980) found that patients with physical ("organic") causes use distinctly different patterns of words from patients whose pain has no detectable cause and is labeled as "functional." A concordance of 87% was found between established medical diagnosis and classification based on the patients' choice of word patterns from the MPQ. Along similar lines, Perry, Heller, and Levine (1988, 1991) reported differences in the pattern of MPQ subscale correlations in patients with and without demonstrable organic pathology.

Further evidence of the discriminative capacity of the MPQ was furnished by Melzack, Terrence, Fromm, and Amsel (1986), who correctly classified patients with trigeminal neuralgia or atypical facial pain with 91% accuracy based on seven key descriptors. The authors then used a second, independent validation sample of patients with trigeminal neuralgia or atypical facial pain and showed a correct prediction for 90% of the patients. Specific verbal descriptors of the MPQ have also been shown to discriminate between reversible and irreversible damage of the nerve fibers in a tooth (Grushka & Sessle, 1984), among various facial pain disorders (Mongini & Italiano, 2001; Mongini, Italiano, Raviola, & Mossolov, 2000), and between leg pain caused by diabetic neuropathy and leg pain arising from other causes (Masson, Hunt, Gem, & Boulton, 1989). Mongini, Deregibus, Raviola, and Mongini (2003) further showed that the MPQ consistently discriminates between migraine and tension-type headache, confirming an earlier report (Jerome et al., 1988) that cluster headache pain is more intense and distressing than other vascular (migraine and mixed) headache pain, and is characterized by a distinct constellation of descriptors. Wilkie, Huang, Reilly, and Cain (2001) compared MPQ descriptors chosen by patients with previously classified nociceptive and neuropathic pain sites due to lung cancer. They found that four descriptors (i.e., "lacerating," "stinging," "heavy," "suffocating") were used significantly more frequently to describe nociceptive pain sites than neuropathic pain sites, and that 11 other descriptors were used more often to describe the latter than the former pain sites. Using a multivariate regression equation, they showed that 78% of the pain sites were accurately identified using 10 MPQ descriptors as nociceptive (81% sensitivity) or neuropathic (59% sensitivity).

It is evident, however, that the discriminative capacity of the MPQ has limits. High levels of anxiety and other psychological disturbance, which may produce high affective scores, may obscure the discriminative capacity (Kremer & Atkinson, 1983). Moreover, certain key words that discriminate among specific syndromes may be absent (Reading, 1982). Nevertheless, it is clear that there are appreciable and quantifiable

TABLE 3.2. Descriptions Characteristic of Clinical Pain Syndromes

Menstrual pain (n = 25)	Arthritic pain (n = 16)	Labor pain (n = 11)	Disc disease pain (n = 10)	Toothache (n = 10)	Cancer pain (n = 8)	Phantom limb pain (n = 8)	Postherpetic pain (n = 6)
			Sensory				
Cramping (44%) Aching (44%)	Gnawing (38%) Aching (50%)	Pounding (37%) Shooting (46%) Stabbing (37%) Sharp (64%) Cramping (82%) Aching (46%)	Throbbing (40%) Shooting (50%) Stabbing (40%) Sharp (60%) Cramping (40%) Aching (40%)	Throbbing (50%) Boring (40%) Sharp (50%)	Shooting (50%) Sharp (50%) Gnawing (50%) Burning (50%) Heavy (50%)	Throbbing (38%) Stabbing (50%) Sharp (38%) Cramping (50%) Burning (50%) Aching (38%)	Sharp (84%) Pulling (67%) Aching (50%) Tender (83%) Heavy (40%) Tender (50%)
			Affective				
Tiring (44%) Sickening (56%)	Exhausting (50%)	Tiring (37%) Exhausting (46%) Fearful (36%)	Tiring (46%) Exhausting (40%)	Sickening (40%)	Exhausting (50%)	Tiring (50%) Exhausting (38%) Cruel (38%)	Exhausting (50%)
			Evaluative				
	Annoying (38%)	Intense (46%)	Unbearable (40%)	Annoying (50%)	Unbearable (50%)		
			Temporal				
Constant (56%)	Constant (44%) Rhythmic (56%)	Rhythmic (91%)	Constant (80%) Rhythmic (70%)	Constant (60%) Rhythmic (40%)	Constant (100%) Rhythmic (88%)	Constant (88%) Rhythmic (63%)	Constant (50%) Rhythmic (50%)

Note. Only those words chosen by more than one-third of the patients are listed, and the percentage of patients who chose each word is shown below the word.

differences in the way various types of pain are described, and that patients with the same disease or pain syndrome tend to use remarkably similar words to communicate what they feel.

Multidimensional Pain Experience

Several groups of researchers have evaluated the theoretical structure of the MPQ using factor-analytic methods (Holroyd et al., 1992; Turk et al., 1985). Turk and colleagues (1985) concluded that the three-factor structure of the MPQ—sensory, affective, and evaluative—is strongly supported by the analyses; Holroyd's "most clearly interpretable structure" was provided by a four-factor solution obtained by oblique rotation in which two sensory factors were identified in addition to an affective and an evaluative factor.

Like most others who have used the MPQ, Turk and colleagues (1985) and Holroyd and colleagues (1992) find high intercorrelations among the factors. However, significant intercorrelations among identified factors should not be taken as evidence for the lack of discriminative capacity and clinical utility of the MPQ. There is, in fact, considerable evidence that the MPQ is effective in discriminating among the three factors despite the high intercorrelations. First, Gracely (1992) has convincingly argued that factor-analytic methods may be inappropriate for assessing the factor structure of the MPQ, although they provide useful information about patient characteristics. Torgerson (1988) distinguished between semantic meaning (how the MPQ descriptors are arranged) and associate meaning (how patients arrange the MPQ descriptors) to emphasize that factor analysis provides a context-dependent structure of the latter; that is, the outcome depends on how specific patient samples make use of the MPQ descriptors. Gracely (1992) elaborated further on the difference between semantic and associative meaning and concluded that factor-analytic techniques do not "directly evaluate the semantic structure of the questionnaire" (p. 297).

Second, a high correlation among variables does not necessarily imply a lack of discriminant capacity. Traditional psychophysics has shown repeatedly that, in the case of vision, increasing the intensity of light produces increased capacity to discriminate color, contours, texture, and distance (Kling & Riggs, 1971). Similarly, in the case of hearing, increases in volume lead to increased discrimination of timbre, pitch, and spatial location (Kling & Riggs, 1971). In these cases, there are clearly very high intercorrelations among the variables in each modality. But this does not mean that we should forget about the differences between color and texture, or between timbre and pitch, just because they intercorrelate highly. This approach would lead to the loss of valuable, meaningful data (Gracely, 1992).

Third, many papers have demonstrated the discriminant validity of the MPQ (Melzack, Kinch, Dobkin, Lebrun, & Taenzer, 1984; Melzack & Perry, 1975; Melzack et al., 1981; Reading, 1982; Reading & Newton, 1977). In studies on labor pain, Melzack and colleagues (1981, 1984) found that distinctly different variables correlate with the sensory, affective, and evaluative dimensions. Prepared childbirth training, for example, correlates significantly with the sensory and affective dimensions but not the evaluative one. Menstrual difficulties correlate with the affective but neither the sensory nor evaluative dimensions. Physical factors, such as mother's and infant's weight, also correlate selectively with one or another dimension.

Similarly, a study of acute pain in emergency ward patients (Melzack, Wall, & Ty, 1982, p. 33) has "revealed a normal distribution of sensory scores but very low affective scores compared to patients with chronic pain." Finally, Chen and colleagues (1989) have consistently identified a group of pain-sensitive and pain-tolerant subjects in five laboratory studies of *tonic* (prolonged) pain. Compared with pain-tolerant subjects, pain-sensitive subjects show significantly higher scores on all PRIs except the sensory dimension. Atkinson, Kremer, and Ignelzi (1982) are undoubtedly right that high affect scores tend to diminish the discriminant capacity of the MPQ, so that, at high levels of anxiety and depression, some discriminant capacity is lost. However, the MPQ still retains good discriminant function even at high levels of anxiety.

In summary, (1) high intercorrelations among psychological variables do not mean that they are all alike and can therefore be lumped into a single variable, such as intensity; rather, certain biological and psychological variables can covary to a high degree yet represent distinct, discriminable entities; and (2) the MPQ has been shown in many studies to be capable of discriminating among the three component factors.

THE SHORT-FORM MPQ

The Short-Form MPQ (SF-MPQ; Melzack, 1987; Figure 3.3) was developed for use in specific research settings in which the time to obtain information from patients is limited and more information is desired than that provided by intensity measures such as the VAS or PPI. The SF-MPQ consists of 15 representative words from the sensory (n = 11) and affective (n = 4) categories of the standard, Long-Form MPQ (LF-MPQ). The PPI and a VAS are included to provide indices of overall pain intensity. The 15 descriptors making up the SF-MPQ were selected on the basis of their frequency of endorsement by patients with a variety of acute, intermittent, and chronic pains. An additional word— "splitting"—was added because it was reported to be a key discriminative word for

SHORT-FORM McGILL PAIN QUESTIONNAIRE

RONALD MELZACK

PATIENT'S NAME: _____   DATE: _____

	NONE	MILD	MODERATE	SEVERE
THROBBING	0) _____	1) _____	2) _____	3) _____
SHOOTING	0) _____	1) _____	2) _____	3) _____
STABBING	0) _____	1) _____	2) _____	3) _____
SHARP	0) _____	1) _____	2) _____	3) _____
CRAMPING	0) _____	1) _____	2) _____	3) _____
GNAWING	0) _____	1) _____	2) _____	3) _____
HOT-BURNING	0) _____	1) _____	2) _____	3) _____
ACHING	0) _____	1) _____	2) _____	3) _____
HEAVY	0) _____	1) _____	2) _____	3) _____
TENDER	0) _____	1) _____	2) _____	3) _____
SPLITTING	0) _____	1) _____	2) _____	3) _____
TIRING-EXHAUSTING	0) _____	1) _____	2) _____	3) _____
SICKENING	0) _____	1) _____	2) _____	3) _____
FEARFUL	0) _____	1) _____	2) _____	3) _____
PUNISHING-CRUEL	0) _____	1) _____	2) _____	3) _____

NO PAIN |————————————————————————————| WORST POSSIBLE PAIN

PPI

0	NO PAIN	_____
1	MILD	_____
2	DISCOMFORTING	_____
3	DISTRESSING	_____
4	HORRIBLE	_____
5	EXCRUCIATING	_____

FIGURE 3.3. The Short-Form McGill Pain Questionnaire (SF-MPQ). Descriptors 1–11 represent the sensory dimension of pain experience, and descriptors 12–15 represent the affective dimension. Each descriptor is ranked on an intensity scale of 0 = "none," 1 = "mild," 2 = "moderate," 3 = "severe." The PPI of the standard Long-Form McGill Pain Questionnaire (LF-MPQ) and the VAS are also included to provide overall pain intensity scores. Copyright 1987 by Ronald Melzack. Reprinted by permission.

dental pain (Grushka & Sessle, 1984). Each descriptor is ranked by the patient on an intensity scale of 0 = "none," 1 = "mild," 2 = "moderate," 3 = "severe." The SF-MPQ exists in both Canadian English and French versions (Melzack, 1987).

Psychometric Properties

The SF-MPQ correlates very highly with the major PRI indices (Sensory (S), Affective (A), and Total (T)) of the LF-MPQ (Dudgeon, Ranbertas, & Rosenthal, 1993; Melzack, 1987). Concurrent validity and test–retest reliability of the SF-MPQ were reported in a study of patients with chronic pain due to cancer (Dudgeon et al., 1993). On each of three occasions separated by at least a 3-week period, the PRI-S, PRI-A, and PRI-T scores correlated highly with corresponding scores on the LF-MPQ. Other studies also have demonstrated the SF-MPQ to have good to excellent test–retest reliability (Strand, Ljunggren, Bogen, Ask, & Johnsen, 2008), with lower intraclass correlation coefficients (ICCs) associated with longer intervals between testings (Burckhardt & Bjelle, 1994) and higher ICCs reported when the interval between test occasions is short and not confounded by treatment (Georgoudis, Oldham, & Watson, 2001a; Grafton, Foster, & Wright, 2005; Yakut, Yakut, Bayar, & Uygur, 2007).

Factor-analytic studies of the SF-MPQ have generally supported the two-factor structure proposed by Melzack (1987). The presence of sensory and affective factors has been confirmed using both confirmatory and exploratory analyses and in varied patient populations, including patients with burn injuries (Mason et al., 2008), chronic low back pain (Beattie, Dowda, & Feuerstein, 2004; Wright, Asmundson, & McCreary, 2001), and fibromyalgia or rheumatoid arthritis (Burckhardt & Bjelle, 1994). The most methodologically sound study was conducted by Beattie and colleagues (2004), who cross-validated the two-factor solution obtained using exploratory factor analysis with a subsequent confirmatory factor analysis in a large sample of patients with chronic low back pain. Factor solutions suggesting a structure other than that proposed by Melzack are still consistent with the general distinction between sensory and affective dimensions. For example, Burckhardt and Bjelle (1994) reported a three-factor solution that comprised two sensory factors and one affective factor. As reviewed by Mason and colleagues (2008), two studies have evaluated the cross-cultural validity of the SF-MPQ in African American and European American patients with upper and lower back pain (Cassisi et al., 2004) and in Asian American cancer patients (Shin, Kim, Young Hee, Chee, & Im, 2008). Both studies used exploratory factor-analytic methods and both failed to find a two-factor solution consistent with the sensory and affective dimensions proposed by Melzack (1987). In one study (Cassisi et al., 2004) a four- and five-factor solution emerged, and in the other (Shin et al., 2008) a two-factor solution was found in which both factors contained sensory and affective descriptors. Methodological limitations associated with these studies may, in part, explain the inconsistent findings.

The SF-MPQ is sensitive to change brought about by various therapies—analgesic drugs (Rice & Maton, 2001; Ruoff, Rosenthal, Jordan, Karim, & Kamin, 2003), epidurally or spinally administered agents (Harden, Carter, Gilman, Gross, & Peters, 1991; Melzack, 1987; Serrao, Marks, Morley, & Goodchild, 1992), transcutaneous electrical nerve stimulation (TENS) (Melzack, 1987), acupuncture (Birch & Jamison, 1998), low-power light therapy (Stelian et al., 1992), and an intensive 3½-week multidisciplinary treatment program (Strand et al., 2008). It is notable that the SF-MPQ is also capable of detecting clinically significant reductions in various neuropathic pain conditions associated with pharmacological interventions administered in the context of randomized, placebo-controlled trials (Backonja et al., 1998; Gilron et al., 2005; Lesser, Sharma, LaMoreaux, & Poole, 2004; Lyrica Study Group, 2006).

Voorhies, Jiang, and Thomas (2007) reported the SF-MPQ to be useful in predicting outcome in response to surgical intervention for lumbar radiculopathy. Patients with preoperative SF-MPQ Sensory and Affective scores of 17 and 7 or more, respectively (i.e., 50% of the total possible SF-MPQ scores) had between a 42 and 50% chance of obtaining an excellent or good surgical outcome 12 months after surgery.

Figure 3.4 shows SF-MPQ scores obtained by patients with a variety of acute and chronic pains. As can be seen, the SF-MPQ has been used in studies of chronic pain (al Balawi, Tariq, & Feinmann, 1996; Bruehl, Chung, & Burns, 2003; Burckhardt, Clark, & Bennett, 1992; Dudgeon et al., 1993; Gagliese & Melzack, 1997; Grönblad, Lukinmaa, & Konttinen, 1990; Ruoff et al., 2003; Stelian et al., 1992; Turner, Cardenas, Warms, & McClellan, 2001) and acute pain (Hack, Cohen, Katz, Robson, & Goss, 1999; Harden et al., 1991; King, 1993; McGuire et al., 1993; Melzack, 1987; Thomas, Heath, Rose, & Flory, 1995; Watt-Watson, Stevens,

Costello, Katz, & Reid, 2000) of diverse etiology, and to evaluate pain and discomfort in response to medical interventions (Fowlow, Price, & Fung, 1995).

An important property of the LF-MPQ is that it is has been shown to distinguish between different pains. Initial data (Melzack, 1987) suggesting that the SF-MPQ may be capable of discriminating among different pain syndromes have been confirmed by Closs, Nelson, and Briggs (2008), who reported that venous leg ulcers were frequently described as "throbbing," "burning," and "itchy," whereas arterial ulcers were described as "sharp" and "hurting." Similarly, modest predictability was reported for distinguishing between pain of neuropathic and

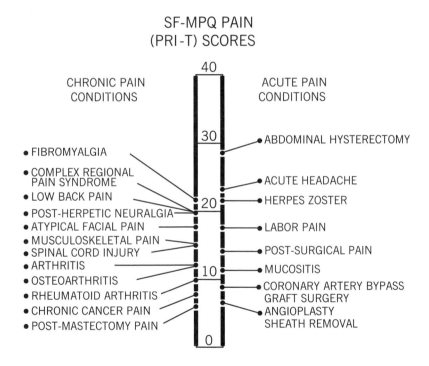

FIGURE 3.4. Comparison of total pain rating index (PRI-T) scores using the SF-MPQ for acute and chronic pain conditions. References for the various pain conditions are as follows: labor pain, musculoskeletal pain, and postsurgical pain (Melzack, 1987); abdominal hysterectomy (Thomas et al., 1995); acute headache (Harden et al., 1991); herpes zoster and postherpetic neuralgia (King, 1993); mucositis (McGuire et al., 1993); angioplasty sheath removal (Fowlow et al., 1995); fibromyalgia and rheumatoid arthritis (Burckhardt & Bjelle, 1994); atypical facial pain (al Balawi et al., 1996); arthritis (Gagliese & Melzack, 1997); osteoarthritis (Stelian et al., 1992); chronic cancer pain (Dudgeon et al., 1993); postmastectomy pain (Hack et al., 1999); spinal cord injury (Turner et al., 2001); complex regional pain syndrome (Bruehl et al., 2003); low back pain (Ruoff et al., 2003); and coronary artery bypass graft surgery (Watt-Watson et al., 2000).

musculoskeletal origin among patients with spinal cord injuries (Putzke et al., 2002). Czech (Solcová, Jacoubek, Sÿkora, & Hnïk, 1990) and Swedish (Burckhardt & Bjelle, 1994) versions of the SF-MPQ have been developed. In addition, an established translation institute (Mapi, 2003), using forward- and backward-translation techniques, has translated the SF-MPQ into 50 languages.

A study of patients with chronic arthritis suggests that the SF-MPQ may be appropriate for use with geriatric patients with pain (Gagliese & Melzack, 1997). In that study, the frequency of failing to complete the SF-MPQ appropriately did not differ among young, middle-aged, and older adult patients. In addition, the subscales showed high intercorrelations and consistency. Although older adult patients endorsed fewer adjectives than their younger counterparts, there was a consistency among the three age groups in the most frequently chosen pain descriptors. These results suggest that pain patients across the lifespan approach the SF-MPQ in a similar manner.

THE SF-MPQ-2

Recent advances in identifying the mechanisms of neuropathic pain (Treede et al., 2008) and in improving its management (Dworkin et al., 2007) have led to the development of new instruments (Jensen, 2006) designed to measure the unique aspects of pain initiated or caused by a primary lesion or dysfunction in the nervous system. While there are merits to a neuropathic pain-specific questionnaire, there are also disadvantages. For example, measurement of the various qualities of pain can aid in the process of diagnosis. Use of a neuropathic pain-specific questionnaire will clearly bias diagnosis in that direction and miss potentially important information that might suggest the presence of a non-neuropathic pain problem. As well, it is not uncommon for patients to present, clinically, with pains that comprise both neuropathic and non-neuropathic components (e.g., nociceptive, inflammatory, musculoskeletal). Neuropathic pain-specific questionnaires provide descriptions of the qualities and other features of neuropathic but not the non-neuropathic components.

Large-scale, population-based, epidemiological studies of chronic pain would be aided by a single, reliable, valid measure of the many qualities of pain. These factors argue for a single pain questionnaire designed to measure the qualities of neuropathic and non-neuropathic pain.

As described earlier, the SF-MPQ has been used successfully in treatment trials of neuropathic pain. However, it does not contain certain descriptors that have been shown to be reliably associated with neuropathic pain conditions. Dworkin and colleagues (2009) developed the SF-MPQ-2, an expanded and revised version of the SF-MPQ, designed to measure of the qualities of both neuropathic and non-neuropathic pain in research and clinical settings.

The following modifications were involved in the development of the SF-MPQ-2 (Figure 3.5): (1) inclusion of seven new descriptors relevant to neuropathic pain; (2) use of an 11-point NRS for each descriptor; (3) addition of the qualifier "pain" to 13 descriptors; and (4) expansion of the instructions to take into account "different qualities of pain and related symptoms" (Dworkin et al., 2009, p. 37).

The SF-MPQ-2 was administered, in a Web-based format, to 882 participants with diverse chronic pain conditions and to 226 patients with painful diabetic peripheral neuropathy enrolled in a randomized controlled trial. Exploratory and confirmatory factor analyses revealed the presence of the following four factors or subscales (Table 3.3); Continuous Pain descriptors, Intermittent Pain descriptors, Predominantly Neuropathic Pain descriptors, and Affective descriptors. Subscale scores are computed by calculating the mean NRS ratings associated with subscale descriptors. The total SF-MPQ-2 score is the mean of the four subscale scores.

Preliminary analyses indicate that the SF-MPQ-2 has very good to excellent psychometric properties, including adequate to high internal consistency reliability estimates for the subscale (.73–.87) and total scores (.91–.95), respectively. Construct validity was demonstrated by correlations with another well-validated measure of pain, the Brief Pain Inventory (Cleeland et al., 1996). Consistent with the goal of developing a questionnaire that is sensitive to both neu-

Short-Form McGill Pain Questionnaire–2 (SF-MPQ-2)

This questionnaire provides you with a list of words that describe some of the different qualities of pain and related symptoms. Please put an **X** through the numbers that best describe the intensity of each of the pain and related symptoms you felt during the past week. Use 0 if the word does not describe your pain or related symptoms.

1. Throbbing pain	none	0	1	2	3	4	5	6	7	8	9	10	worst possible
2. Shooting pain	none	0	1	2	3	4	5	6	7	8	9	10	worst possible
3. Stabbing pain	none	0	1	2	3	4	5	6	7	8	9	10	worst possible
4. Sharp pain	none	0	1	2	3	4	5	6	7	8	9	10	worst possible
5. Cramping pain	none	0	1	2	3	4	5	6	7	8	9	10	worst possible
6. Gnawing pain	none	0	1	2	3	4	5	6	7	8	9	10	worst possible
7. Hot-burning pain	none	0	1	2	3	4	5	6	7	8	9	10	worst possible
8. Aching pain	none	0	1	2	3	4	5	6	7	8	9	10	worst possible
9. Heavy pain	none	0	1	2	3	4	5	6	7	8	9	10	worst possible
10. Tender	none	0	1	2	3	4	5	6	7	8	9	10	worst possible
11. Splitting pain	none	0	1	2	3	4	5	6	7	8	9	10	worst possible
12. Tiring-exhausting	none	0	1	2	3	4	5	6	7	8	9	10	worst possible
13. Sickening	none	0	1	2	3	4	5	6	7	8	9	10	worst possible
14. Fearful	none	0	1	2	3	4	5	6	7	8	9	10	worst possible
15. Punishing-cruel	none	0	1	2	3	4	5	6	7	8	9	10	worst possible
16. Electro-shock pain	none	0	1	2	3	4	5	6	7	8	9	10	worst possible
17. Cold-freezing pain	none	0	1	2	3	4	5	6	7	8	9	10	worst possible
18. Piercing	none	0	1	2	3	4	5	6	7	8	9	10	worst possible
19. Pain caused by light touch	none	0	1	2	3	4	5	6	7	8	9	10	worst possible
20. Itching	none	0	1	2	3	4	5	6	7	8	9	10	worst possible
21. Tingling or "pins and needles"	none	0	1	2	3	4	5	6	7	8	9	10	worst possible
22. Numbness	none	0	1	2	3	4	5	6	7	8	9	10	worst possible

FIGURE 3.5. The Short-Form McGill Pain Questionnaire–2 (SF-MPG-2). The 22 descriptors comprise the following four subscales: Continuous Pain (Items 1, 5, 6, 8–10); Intermittent Pain (Items 2–4, 11, 16, 18); Neuropathic Pain (Items 7, 17, 19–22); and Affective descriptors (Items 12–15). Each descriptor is rated on an 11-point NRS ranging from 0 = "none" to 10 = "worst possible." Subscale scores are computed by calculating the mean ratings for subscale descriptors. Total score is the mean of the four subscale scores. Copyright by Ronald Melzack and the Initiative on Methods, Measurement, and Pain Assessment in Clinical Trials (IMMPACT). Reprinted by permission. Information regarding permission to reproduce the SF-MPQ-2 can be obtained at *www.immpact.org.*

TABLE 3.3. SF-MPQ-2 Subscales

Subscale	Item
1. Continuous Pain	1. Throbbing pain 5. Cramping pain 6. Gnawing pain 8. Aching pain 9. Heavy pain 10. Tender
2. Intermittent Pain	2. Shooting pain 3. Stabbing pain 4. Sharp pain 11. Splitting pain 16. Electric-shock pain 18. Piercing
3. Predominantly Neuropathic Pain	7. Hot-burning pain 17. Cold-freezing pain 19. Pain caused by light touch 20. Itching 21. Tingling or "pins and needles" 22. Numbness
4. Affective	12. Tiring-exhausting 13. Sickening 14. Fearful 15. Punishing-cruel

ropathic and non-neuropathic pain, the SF-MPQ-2 total score and scores on the Intermittent Pain and Neuropathic Pain subscales were significantly higher for the Web-based participants with neuropathic pain than for participants with non-neuropathic pain. In contrast, subscale scores for Continuous Pain and Affective descriptors did not differ significantly between the participants with neuropathic and non-neuropathic pain. Finally, the SF-MPQ-2 subscale and total scores showed sensitivity to change in the context of a randomized controlled treatment trial. Taken together, the results of the study by Dworkin and colleagues (2009) suggest that the SF-MPQ-2 is a reliable, valid, and sensitive measure of chronic pain that is capable of discriminating between neuropathic and non-neuropathic pain. Further psychometric evaluation of the SF-MPQ-2 is required to address some of the shortcomings involved in using a Web-based sample of participants to validate the questionnaire and to confirm the scale's ability to discriminate between pains of neuropathic and non-neuropathic origin (Bouhassira & Attal, 2009).

CONCLUSION

Accurate, valid, and reliable measurement of pain is essential to progress in (1) better understanding the factors that determine pain intensity, quality, and duration; (2) diagnosis and treatment of pain; and (3) evaluation of the relative effectiveness of different therapies. The MPQ and SF-MPQ have become "gold standards" in the measurement of the various qualities of acute and chronic pain. Both forms have been shown to be psychometrically sound, valid, and reliable instruments with good discriminative capacity. The newly developed SF-MPQ-2 has improved some of the shortcomings of the SF-MPQ and has made available, in one questionnaire, the measurement of both neuropathic and non-neuropathic pain. Further research is needed to determine the psychometric properties of the SF-MPQ-2 in acute pain contexts (e.g., after surgery, work injuries, accidents) and across the lifespan (from adolescents to older adults). Application of powerful statistical techniques, such as item response theory, will permit a more precise evaluation of the psychometric properties of the SF-MPS-2 across a range of pain levels.

ACKNOWLEDGMENT

This work was supported by a Canadian Institutes of Health Research Canada Research Chair in Health Psychology to Joel Katz.

REFERENCES

Aboud, F. E., Hiwot, M. G., Arega, A., Molla, M., Samson, S., Seyoum, N., et al. (2003). The McGill Pain Questionnaire in Amharic: Zwai Health Center patients' reports on the experience of pain. *Ethiopian Medical Journal*, 41(1), 45–61.

al Balawi, S., Tariq, M., & Feinmann, C. (1996). A double-blind, placebo-controlled, crossover, study to evaluate the efficacy of subcutaneous sumatriptan in the treatment of atypical facial pain. *International Journal of Neuroscience*, 86(3–4), 301–309.

Atkinson, J. H., Kremer, E. F., & Ignelzi, R. J. (1982). Diffusion of pain language with affective disturbance confounds differential diagnosis. *Pain*, 12, 375–384.

Backonja, M., Beydoun, A., Edwards, K. R.,

Schwartz, S. L., Fonseca, V., Hes, M., et al. (1998). Gabapentin for the symptomatic treatment of painful neuropathy in patients with diabetes mellitus: A randomized controlled trial. *Journal of the American Medical Association*, *280*(21), 1831–1836.

Bartko, D., Kondos, M., & Jansco, S. (1984). Slovak version of the McGill–Melzack's Questionnaire on pain. *Ceskoslovenska Neurologie a Neurochirurgie*, *47*, 113–121.

Beattie, P. F., Dowda, M., & Feuerstein, M. (2004). Differentiating sensory and affective-sensory pain descriptions in patients undergoing magnetic resonance imaging for persistent low back pain. *Pain*, *110*(1–2), 189–196.

Beecher, H. K. (1959). *Measurement of subjective responses*. New York: Oxford University Press.

Bejarano, P. F., Noriego, R. D., Rodriguez, M. L., & Berrio, G. M. (1985). Evaluación del dolor: Adaptatión del cuestionario del McGill [Evaluation of pain: Adaptation of the McGill Pain Questionniare]. *Revista Columbia Anesesia*, *13*, 321–351.

Birch, S., & Jamison, R. N. (1998). Controlled trial of Japanese acupuncture for chronic myofascial neck pain: Assessment of specific and nonspecific effects of treatment. *Clinical Journal of Pain*, *14*(3), 248–255.

Birklein, F., Riedl, B., Sieweke, N., Weber, M., & Neundorfer, B. (2000). Neurological findings in complex regional pain syndromes—analysis of 145 cases. *Acta Neurologica Scandanavica*, *101*(4), 262–269.

Bouhassira, D., & Attal, N. (2009). All in one: Is it possible to assess all dimensions of any pain with a simple questionnaire? *Pain*, *144*(1–2), 7–8.

Boureau, F., Luu, M., & Doubrère, J. F. (1992). Comparative study of the validity of four French McGill Pain Questionnaire (MPQ) versions. *Pain*, *50*, 59–65.

Boureau, F., Luu, M., Doubrère, J. F., & Gay, C. (1984). Elaboration d'un questionnaire d'auto-évaluation de la douleur par liste de qualicatifs [Development of a self-evaluation questionnaire comprising pain descriptors.]. *Thérapie*, *39*, 119–129.

Bruehl, S., Chung, O. Y., & Burns, J. W. (2003). Differential effects of expressive anger regulation on chronic pain intensity in CRPS and non-CRPS limb pain patients. *Pain*, *104*(3), 647–654.

Burckhardt, C. S. (1984). The use of the McGill Pain Questionnaire in assessing arthritis pain. *Pain*, *19*(3), 305–314.

Burckhardt, C. S., & Bjelle, A. (1994). A Swedish version of the Short-Form McGill Pain Questionnaire. *Scandinavian Journal of Rheumatology*, *23*(2), 77–81.

Burckhardt, C. S., Clark, S. R., & Bennett, R. M. (1992). A comparison of pain perceptions in women with fibromyalgia and rheumatoid arthritis: Relationship to depression and pain extent. *Arthritis Care and Research*, *5*(4), 216–222.

Cassisi, J. E., Umeda, M., Deisinger, J. A., Sheffer, C., Lofland, K. R., & Jackson, C. (2004). Patterns of pain descriptor usage in African Americans and European Americans with chronic pain. *Cultural Diversity and Ethnic Minority Psychology*, *10*(1), 81–89.

Chapman, C. R., Casey, K. L., Dubner, R., Foley, K. M., Gracely, R. H., & Reading, A. E. (1985). Pain measurement: An overview. *Pain*, *22*, 1–31.

Chen, A. C. N., Dworkin, S. F., Haug, J., & Gehrig, J. (1989). Human pain responsivity in a tonic pain model: Psychological determinants. *Pain*, *37*, 143–160.

Cleeland, C. S., Nakamura, Y., Mendoza, T. R., Edwards, K. R., Douglas, J., & Serlin, R. C. (1996). Dimensions of the impact of cancer pain in a four country sample: New information from multidimensional scaling. *Pain*, *67*(2–3), 267–273.

Closs, S. J., Nelson, E. A., & Briggs, M. (2008). Can venous and arterial leg ulcers be differentiated by the characteristics of the pain they produce? *Journal of Clinical Nursing*, *17*(5), 637–645.

Crockett, D. J., Prkachin, K. M., & Craig, K. D. (1977). Factors of the language of pain in patients and normal volunteer groups. *Pain*, *4*, 175–182.

De Benedittis, G., Massei, R., Nobili, R., & Pieri, A. (1988). The Italian Pain Questionnaire. *Pain*, *33*, 53–62.

Defrin, R., Grunhaus, L., Zamir, D., & Zeilig, G. (2007). The effect of a series of repetitive transcranial magnetic stimulations of the motor cortex on central pain after spinal cord injury. *Archives of Physical Medicine and Rehabilitation*, *88*(12), 1574–1580.

Drewes, A. M., Helweg-Larsen, S., Petersen, P., Brennum, J., Andreasen, A., Poulsen, L. H., et al. (1993). McGill Pain Questionnaire translated into Danish: Experimental and clinical findings. *Clinical Journal of Pain*, *9*(2), 80–87.

Dubuisson, D., & Melzack, R. (1976). Classification of clinical pain descriptors by multiple group discriminant analysis. *Experimental Neurology*, *51*, 480–487.

Dudgeon, D., Ranbertas, R. F., & Rosenthal, S. (1993). The Short-Form McGill Pain Questionnaire in chronic cancer pain. *Journal of Pain and Symptom Management*, *8*, 191–195.

Dworkin, R. H., Corbin, A. E., Young, J. P., Jr., Sharma, U., LaMoreaux, L., Bockbrader,

H., et al. (2003). Pregabalin for the treatment of postherpetic neuralgia: A randomized, placebo-controlled trial. *Neurology*, 60(8), 1274–1283.

Dworkin, R. H., O'Connor, A. B., Backonja, M., Farrar, J. T., Finnerup, N. B., Jensen, T. S., et al. (2007). Pharmacologic management of neuropathic pain: Evidence-based recommendations. *Pain*, 132(3), 237–251.

Dworkin, R. H., Turk, D. C., Revicki, D. A., Harding, G., Coyne, K. S., Peirce-Sandner, S., et al. (2009). Development and initial validation of an expanded and revised version of the Short-Form McGill Pain Questionnaire (SF-MPQ-2). *Pain*, 144(1–2), 35–42.

Escalante, A., Lichtenstein, M. J., Rios, N., & Hazuda, H. P. (1996). Measuring chronic rheumatic pain in Mexican Americans: Cross-cultural adaptation of the McGill Pain Questionnaire. *Journal of Clinical Epidemiology*, 49(12), 1389–1399.

Ferracuti, S., Romeo, G., Leardi, M. G., Cruccu, G., & Lazzari, R. (1990). New Italian adaptation and standardization of the McGill Pain Questionnaire. *Pain* (Suppl. 1), S300.

Fowlow, B., Price, P., & Fung, T. (1995). Ambulation after sheath removal: A comparison of 6 and 8 hours of bedrest after sheath removal in patients following a PTCA procedure. *Heart and Lung*, 24(1), 28–37.

Gagliese, L., & Melzack, R. (1997). Age differences in the quality of chronic pain: A preliminary study. *Pain Research and Management*, 2, 157–162.

Gaston-Johansson, F., Albert, M., Fagan, E., & Zimmerman, L. (1990). Similarities in pain descriptors of four different ethnic–culture groups. *Journal of Pain and Symptom Management*, 5, 94–100.

Georgoudis, G., Oldham, J. A., & Watson, P. J. (2001a). Reliability and sensitivity measures of the Greek version of the short form of the McGill Pain Questionnaire. *European Journal of Pain*, 5(2), 109–118.

Georgoudis, G., Oldham, J. A., & Watson, P. J. (2001b). Reliability and sensitivity measures of the Greek version of the short form of the McGill Pain Questionnaire. *European Journal of Pain*, 5(2), 109–118.

Georgoudis, G., Watson, P. J., & Oldham, J. A. (2000). The development and validation of a Greek version of the Short-Form McGill Pain Questionnaire. *European Journal of Pain*, 4(3), 275–281.

Gilron, I., Bailey, J. M., Tu, D., Holden, R. R., Weaver, D. F., & Houlden, R. L. (2005). Morphine, gabapentin, or their combination for neuropathic pain. *New England Journal of Medicine*, 352(13), 1324–1334.

Gracely, R. H. (1992). Evaluation of multidimensional pain scales. *Pain*, 48, 297–300.

Grafton, K. V., Foster, N. E., & Wright, C. C. (2005). Test–retest reliability of the Short-Form McGill Pain Questionnaire: Assessment of intraclass correlation coefficients and limits of agreement in patients with osteoarthritis. *Clinical Journal of Pain*, 21(1), 73–82.

Graham, C., Bond, S. S., Gerkovitch, M. M., & Cook, M. R. (1980). Use of the McGill Pain Questionnaire in the assessment of cancer pain: Replicability and consistency. *Pain*, 8, 377–387.

Grönblad, M., Lukinmaa, A., & Konttinen, Y. T. (1990). Chronic low-back pain: Intercorrelation of repeated measures for pain and disability. *Scandinavian Journal of Rehabilitation Medicine*, 22, 73–77.

Grushka, M., & Sessle, B. J. (1984). Applicability of the McGill Pain Questionnaire to the differentiation of "toothache" pain. *Pain*, 19, 49–57.

Hack, T. F., Cohen, L., Katz, J., Robson, L. S., & Goss, P. (1999). Physical and psychological morbidity after axillary lymph node dissection for breast cancer. *Journal of Clinical Oncology*, 17(1), 143–149.

Harden, R. N., Carter, T. D., Gilman, C. S., Gross, A. J., & Peters, J. R. (1991). Ketorolac in acute headache management. *Headache*, 31, 463–464.

Harrison, A. (1988). Arabic pain words. *Pain*, 32, 239–250.

Hasegawa, M., Hattori, S., Mishima, M., Matsumoto, I., Kimura, T., Baba, Y., et al. (2001). The McGill Pain Questionnaire, Japanese version, reconsidered: Confirming the theoretical structure. *Pain Research and Management*, 6(4), 173–180.

Hobara, M., Fujiwara, H., Clark, W. C., & Wharton, R. N. (2003). A translation of the Multidimensional Affect and Pain Survey (MAPS) from English to Japanese. *Gan To Kagaku Ryoho*, 30(5), 721–729.

Holroyd, K. A., Holm, J. E., Keefe, F. J., Turner, J. A., Bradley, L. A., Murphy, W. D., et al. (1992). A multi-center evaluation of the McGill Pain Questionnaire: Results from more than 1,700 chronic pain patients. *Pain*, 48, 301–311.

Hui, Y. L., & Chen, A. C. (1989). Analysis of headache in a Chinese patient population. *Ma Tsui Hsueh Tsa Chi*, 27, 13–18.

Jenkinson, C., Carroll, D., Egerton, M., Frankland, T., McQuay, H., & Nagle, C. (1995). Comparison of the sensitivity to change of long and short form pain measures. *Quality of Life Research*, 4(4), 353–357.

Jensen, M. P. (2006). Review of measures of neuropathic pain. *Current Pain and Headache Reports, 10*(3), 159–166.

Jensen, M. P., & Karoly, P. (2001). Self-report scales and procedures for assessing pain in adults. In D. C. Turk & R. Melzack (Eds.), *Handbook of pain assessment* (2nd ed., pp. 15–34). New York: Guilford Press.

Jerome, A., Holroyd, K. A., Theofanous, A. G., Pingel, J. D., Lake, A. E., & Saper, J. R. (1988). Cluster headache pain vs. other vascular headache pain: Differences revealed with two approaches to the McGill Pain Questionnaire. *Pain, 34*, 35–42.

Katz, J. (1992). Psychophysical correlates of phantom limb experience. *Journal of Neurology, Neurosurgery, and Psychiatry, 55*, 811–821.

Katz, J., Clairoux, M., Kavanagh, B. P., Roger, S., Nierenberg, H., Redahan, C., et al. (1994). Pre-emptive lumbar epidural anaesthesia reduces postoperative pain and patient-controlled morphine consumption after lower abdominal surgery. *Pain, 59*, 395–403.

Katz, J., Cohen, L., Schmid, R., Chan, V. W., & Wowk, A. (2003). Postoperative morphine use and hyperalgesia are reduced by preoperative but not intraoperative epidural analgesia: Implications for preemptive analgesia and the prevention of central sensitization. *Anesthesiology, 98*(6), 1449–1460.

Katz, J., & Melzack, R. (1991). Auricular TENS reduces phantom limb pain. *Journal of Pain and Symptom Management, 6*, 73–83.

Katz, J., & Melzack, R. (1999). Measurement of pain. *Surgical Clinics of North America, 79*(2), 231–252.

Ketovuori, H., & Pöntinen, P. J. (1981). A pain vocabulary in Finnish—the Finnish Pain Questionnaire. *Pain, 11*, 247–253.

Kim, H. S., Schwartz-Barcott, D., Holter, I. M., & Lorensen, M. (1995). Developing a translation of the McGill pain questionnaire for cross-cultural comparison: An example from Norway. *Journal of Advanced Nursing, 21*(3), 421–426.

King, R. B. (1993). Topical aspirin in chloroform and the relief of pain due to herpes zoster and postherpetic neuralgia. *Archives of Neurology, 50*(10), 1046–1053.

Kiss, I., Müller, H., & Abel, M. (1987). The McGill Pain Questionnaire—German version: A study on cancer pain. *Pain, 29*, 195–207.

Klepac, R. K., Dowling, J., Rokke, P., Dodge, L., & Schafer, L. (1981). Interview vs. paper-and-pencil administration of the McGill Pain Questionnaire. *Pain, 11*, 241–246.

Kling, J. W., & Riggs, L. A. (1971). *Experimental psychology.* New York: Holt, Rinehart & Winston.

Kremer, E., & Atkinson, J. H. (1983). Pain language as a measure of effect in chronic pain patients. In R. Melzack (Ed.), *Pain measurement and assessment* (pp. 119–127). New York: Raven Press.

Lahuerta, J., Smith, B. A., & Martinez-Lage, J. L. (1982). An adaptation of the McGill Pain Questionnaire to the Spanish Language. *Schmerz, 3*, 132–134.

Lázaro, C., Bosch, F., Torrubia, R., & Baños, J. E. (1994). The development of a Spanish questionnaire for assessing pain: Preliminary data concerning reliability and validity. *European Journal of Psychological Assessment, 10*, 145–151.

Leavitt, F., & Garron, D. C. (1980). Validity of a back pain classification scale for detecting psychological disturbance as measured by the MMPI. *Journal of Clinical Psychology, 36*, 186–189.

Leavitt, F., Garron, D. C., Whisler, W. W., & Sheinkop, M. B. (1978). Affective and sensory dimensions of pain. *Pain, 4*, 273–281.

Lesser, H., Sharma, U., LaMoreaux, L., & Poole, R. M. (2004). Pregabalin relieves symptoms of painful diabetic neuropathy: A randomized controlled trial. *Neurology, 63*(11), 2104–2110.

Love, A., Leboeuf, D. C., & Crisp, T. C. (1989). Chiropractic chronic low back pain sufferers and self-report assessment methods: Part I. A reliability study of the Visual Analogue Scale, the pain drawing and the McGill Pain Questionnaire. *Journal of Manipulative and Physiological Therapeutics, 12*, 21–25.

Lowe, N. K., Walker, S. N., & McCallum, R. C. (1991). Confirming the theoretical structure of the McGill Pain Questionnaire in acute clinical pain. *Pain, 46*, 53–60.

Lynch, M. E., Clark, A. J., & Sawynok, J. (2003). Intravenous adenosine alleviates neuropathic pain: A double blind placebo controlled crossover trial using an enriched enrolment design. *Pain, 103*(1–2), 111–117.

Lyrica Study Group. (2006). Pregabalin for peripheral neuropathic pain: Results of a multicenter, non-comparative, open-label study in Indian patients. *International Journal of Clinical Practice, 60*(9), 1060–1067.

Maiani, G., & Sanavio, E. (1985). Semantics of pain in Italy: The Italian version of the McGill Pain Questionnaire. *Pain, 22*, 399–405. Retrieved May 18, 2009 from .

Mapi, R. I. (2003). Quality of life instruments data base. *www.qolid.org*.

Masedo, A. I., & Esteve, R. (2000). Some empirical evidence regarding the validity of the Spanish version of the McGill Pain Questionnaire (MPQ-SV). *Pain, 85*(3), 451–456.

Mason, S. T., Arceneaux, L. L., Abouhassan, W., Lauterbach, D., Seebach, C., & Fauerbach, J. A. (2008). Confirmatory factor analysis of the Short Form McGill Pain Questionnaire with burn patients. *Eplasty, 8*, e54.

Masson, E. A., Hunt, L., Gem, J. M., & Boulton, A. J. M. (1989). A novel approach to the diagnosis and assessment of symptomatic diabetic neuropathy. *Pain, 38*, 25–28.

McCreary, C., Turner, J., & Dawson, E. (1981). Principal dimensions of the pain experience and psychological disturbance in chronic low back pain patients. *Pain, 11*, 85–92.

McGuire, D. B., Altomonte, V., Peterson, D. E., Wingard, J. R., Jones, R. J., & Grochow, L. B. (1993). Patterns of mucositis and pain in patients receiving preparative chemotherapy and bone marrow transplantation. *Oncology Nursing Forum, 20*(10), 1493–1502.

Melzack, R. (1975). The McGill Pain Questionnaire: Major properties and scoring methods. *Pain, 1*(3), 277–299.

Melzack, R. (1983). *Pain measurement and assessment.* New York: Raven Press.

Melzack, R. (1987). The Short-Form McGill Pain Questionnaire. *Pain, 30*, 191–197.

Melzack, R., & Casey, K. L. (1968). Sensory, motivational, and central control determinants of pain: A new conceptual model. In D. Kenshalo (Ed.), *The skin senses* (pp. 423–443). Springfield, IL: Thomas.

Melzack, R., Kinch, R., Dobkin, P., Lebrun, M., & Taenzer, P. (1984). Severity of labour pain: Influence of physical as well as psychologic variables. *Canadian Medical Association Journal, 130*, 579–584.

Melzack, R., & Perry, C. (1975). Self-regulation of pain: The use of alpha-feedback and hypnotic training for the control of chronic pain. *Experimental Neurology, 46*, 452–469.

Melzack, R., Taenzer, P., Feldman, P., & Kinch, R. A. (1981). Labour is still painful after prepared childbirth training. *Canadian Medical Association Journal, 125*, 357–363.

Melzack, R., Terrence, C., Fromm, G., & Amsel, R. (1986). Trigeminal neuralgia and atypical facial pain: Use of the McGill Pain Questionnaire for discrimination and diagnosis. *Pain, 27*, 297–302.

Melzack, R., & Torgerson, W. S. (1971). On the language of pain. *Anesthesiology, 34*, 50–59.

Melzack, R., Wall, P. D., & Ty, T. C. (1982). Acute pain in an emergency clinic: Latency of onset and description patterns related to different injuries. *Pain, 14*, 33–43.

Mongini, F., Deregibus, A., Raviola, F., & Mongini, T. (2003). Confirmation of the distinction between chronic migraine and chronic tension-type headache by the McGill Pain Questionnaire. *Headache, 43*(8), 867–877.

Mongini, F., & Italiano, M. (2001). TMJ disorders and myogenic facial pain: A discriminative analysis using the McGill Pain Questionnaire. *Pain, 91*(3), 323–330.

Mongini, F., Italiano, M., Raviola, F., & Mossolov, A. (2000). The McGill Pain Questionnaire in patients with TMJ pain and with facial pain as a somatoform disorder. *Cranio, 18*(4), 249–256.

Mystakidou, K., Parpa, E., Tsilika, E., Kalaidopoulou, O., Georgaki, S., Galanos, A., et al. (2002). Greek McGill Pain Questionnaire: Validation and utility in cancer patients. *Journal of Pain and Symptom Management, 24*(4), 379–387.

Nikolajsen, L., Hansen, C. L., Nielsen, J., Keller, J., Arendt-Nielsen, L., & Jensen, T. S. (1996). The effect of ketamine on phantom pain: A central neuropathic disorder maintained by peripheral input. *Pain, 67*(1), 69–77.

Nikolajsen, L., Ilkjaer, S., Kroner, K., Christensen, J. H., & Jensen, T. S. (1997). The influence of preamputation pain on postamputation stump and phantom pain. *Pain, 72*(3), 393–405.

Pearce, J., & Morley, S. (1989). An experimental investigation of the construct validity of the McGill Pain Questionnaire. *Pain, 39*, 115–121.

Perry, F., Heller, P. H., & Levine, J. D. (1988). Differing correlations between pain measures in syndromes with or without explicable organic pathology. *Pain, 34*, 185–189.

Perry, F., Heller, P. H., & Levine, J. D. (1991). A possible indicator of functional pain: Poor pain scale correlation. *Pain, 46*, 191–193.

Pimenta, C. A., & Teixeiro, M. J. (1996). [Proposal to adapt the McGill Pain Questionnaire into Portuguese]. *Revista Da Escola de Enfermagem Da USP, 30*(3), 473–483.

Price, D. D., Harkins, S. W., & Baker, C. (1987). Sensory–affective relationships among different types of clinical and experimental pain. *Pain, 28*(3), 297–307.

Prieto, E. J., Hopson, L., Bradley, L. A., Byrne, M., Geisinger, K. F., Midax, D., et al. (1980). The language of low back pain: Factor structure of the McGill Pain Questionnaire. *Pain, 8*, 11–19.

Putzke, J. D., Richards, J. S., Hicken, B. L., Ness, T. J., Kezar, L., & DeVivo, M. (2002). Pain classification following spinal cord injury: The utility of verbal descriptors. *Spinal Cord, 40*(3), 118–127.

Radvila, A., Adler, R. H., Galeazzi, R. L., & Vorkauf, H. (1987). The development of a German language (Berne) pain questionnaire and its application in a situation causing acute pain. *Pain, 28*, 185–195.

Reading, A. E. (1979). The internal structure of

the McGill Pain Questionnaire in dysmenorrhea patients. *Pain*, 7, 353–358.

Reading, A. E. (1982). An analysis of the language of pain in chronic and acute patient groups. *Pain*, 13, 185–192.

Reading, A. E., Everitt, B. S., & Sledmere, C. M. (1982). The McGill Pain Questionnaire: A replication of its construction. *British Journal of Clinical Psychology*, 21, 339–349.

Reading, A. E., & Newton, J. R. (1977). On a comparison of dysmenorrhea and intrauterine device related pain. *Pain*, 3, 265–276.

Rice, A. S., & Maton, S. (2001). Gabapentin in postherpetic neuralgia: A randomised, double blind, placebo controlled study. *Pain*, 94(2), 215–224.

Roche, P. A., Klestov, A. C., & Heim, H. M. (2003). Description of stable pain in rheumatoid arthritis: A 6 year study. *Journal of Rheumatology*, 30(8), 1733–1738.

Ruoff, G. E., Rosenthal, N., Jordan, D., Karim, R., & Kamin, M. (2003). Tramadol/acetaminophen combination tablets for the treatment of chronic lower back pain: A multicenter, randomized, double-blind, placebo-controlled outpatient study. *Clinical Therapeutics*, 25(4), 1123–1141.

Satow, A., Nakatani, K., Taniguchi, S., & Higashiyama, A. (1990). Perceptual characteristics of electrocutaneous pain estimated by the 30-word list and Visual Analog Scale. *Japanese Psychological Review*, 32, 155–164.

Scrimshaw, S. V., & Maher, C. G. (2001). Randomized controlled trial of neural mobilization after spinal surgery. *Spine*, 26(24), 2647–2652.

Sedlak, K. (1990). A Polish version of the McGill Pain Questionnaire. *Pain* (Suppl. 1), S308.

Serrao, J. M., Marks, R. L., Morley, S. J., & Goodchild, C. S. (1992). Intrathecal midazolam for the treatment of chronic mechanical low back pain: A controlled comparison with epidural steroid in a pilot study. *Pain*, 48, 5–12.

Shin, H., Kim, K., Young Hee, K., Chee, W., & Im, E. O. (2008). A comparison of two pain measures for Asian American cancer patients. *Western Journal of Nursing Research*, 30(2), 181–196.

Solcová, I., Jacoubek, B., Sýkora, J., & Hník, P. (1990). Characterization of vertebrogenic pain using the short form of the McGill Pain Questionnaire. *Casopis Lekaru Ceskych*, 129, 1611–1614.

Stein, C., & Mendl, G. (1988). The German counterpart to McGill Pain Questionnaire. *Pain*, 32, 251–255.

Stelian, J., Gil, I., Habot, B., Rosenthal, M., Abramovici, I., Kutok, N., et al. (1992). Improvement of pain and disability in elderly patients with degenerative osteoarthritis of the knee treated with narrow-band light therapy. *Journal of the American Geriatrics Society*, 40, 23–26.

Strand, L. I., Ljunggren, A. E., Bogen, B., Ask, T., & Johnsen, T. B. (2008). The Short-Form McGill Pain Questionnaire as an outcome measure: Test–retest reliability and responsiveness to change. *European Journal of Pain*, 12(7), 917–925.

Strand, L. I., & Wisnes, A. R. (1991). The development of a Norwegian pain questionnaire. *Pain*, 46, 61–66.

Tahmoush, A. J. (1981). Causalgia: Redefinition as a clinical pain syndrome. *Pain*, 10, 187–197.

Thomas, V., Heath, M., Rose, D., & Flory, P. (1995). Psychological characteristics and the effectiveness of patient-controlled analgesia. *British Journal of Anaesthesia*, 74(3), 271–276.

Torgerson, W. S. (1988). *Critical issues in verbal pain assessment: Multidimensional and multivariate issues*. Washington, DC: American Pain Society Abstracts.

Treede, R. D., Jensen, T. S., Campbell, J. N., Cruccu, G., Dostrovsky, J. O., Griffin, J. W., et al. (2008). Neuropathic pain: Redefinition and a grading system for clinical and research purposes. *Neurology*, 70(18), 1630–1635.

Turk, D. C., Rudy, T. E., & Salovey, P. (1985). The McGill Pain Questionnaire reconsidered: Confirming the factor structures and examining appropriate uses. *Pain*, 21, 385–397.

Turner, J. A., Cardenas, D. D., Warms, C. A., & McClellan, C. B. (2001). Chronic pain associated with spinal cord injuries: A community survey. *Archives of Physical Medicine and Rehabilitation*, 82(4), 501–509.

Van Buren, J., & Kleinknecht, R. (1979). An evaluation of the McGill Pain Questionnaire for use in dental pain assessment. *Pain*, 6, 23–33.

van der Kloot, W. A., Oostendorp, R. A., van der Meij, J., & van den Heuvel, J. (1995). [The Dutch version of the McGill pain questionnaire: A reliable pain questionnaire]. *Nederlands Tijdschrift voor Geneeskunde*, 139(13), 669–673.

van Lankveld, W., van 't Pad Bosch, P., van de Putte, L., van der Staak, C., & Naring, G. (1992). [Pain in rheumatoid arthritis measured with the visual analogue scale and the Dutch version of the McGill Pain Questionnaire]. *Nederlands Tijdschrift voor Geneeskunde*, 136(24), 1166–1170.

Vanderiet, K., Adriaensen, H., Carton, H., & Vertommen, H. (1987). The McGill Pain Questionnaire constructed for the Dutch language (MPQ-DV): Preliminary data concerning reliability and validity. *Pain*, 30, 395–408.

Veilleux, S., & Melzack, R. (1976). Pain in psychotic patients. *Experimental Neurology, 52,* 535–563.

Verkes, R. J., Van der Kloot, W. A., & Van der Meij, J. (1989). The perceived structure of 176 pain descriptive words. *Pain, 38,* 219–229.

Voorhies, R. M., Jiang, X., & Thomas, N. (2007). Predicting outcome in the surgical treatment of lumbar radiculopathy using the Pain Drawing Score, McGill Short Form Pain Questionnaire, and risk factors including psychosocial issues and axial joint pain. *Spine Journal, 7*(5), 516–524.

Watt-Watson, J., Stevens, B., Costello, J., Katz, J., & Reid, G. (2000). Impact of preoperative education on pain management outcomes after coronary artery bypass graft surgery: A pilot. *Canadian Journal of Nursing Research, 31*(4), 41–56.

Wilkie, D. J., Huang, H. Y., Reilly, N., & Cain, K. C. (2001). Nociceptive and neuropathic pain in patients with lung cancer: A comparison of pain quality descriptors. *Journal of Pain and Symptom Management, 22*(5), 899–910.

Wilkie, D. J., Savedra, M. C., Holzemier, W. L., Tesler, M. D., & Paul, S. M. (1990). Use of the McGill Pain Questionnaire to measure pain: A meta-analysis. *Nursing Research, 39,* 36–41.

Wright, K. D., Asmundson, G. J., & McCreary, D. R. (2001). Factorial validity of the short-form McGill Pain Questionnaire (SF-MPQ). *European Journal of Pain, 5*(3), 279–284.

Yakut, Y., Yakut, E., Bayar, K., & Uygur, F. (2007). Reliability and validity of the Turkish version Short-Form McGill Pain Questionnaire in patients with rheumatoid arthritis. *Clinical Rheumatology, 26*(7), 1083–1087.

CHAPTER 4

Psychosocial Assessment

Comprehensive Measures
and Measures Specific to Pain Beliefs and Coping

DOUGLAS E. DeGOOD
ANDREW J. COOK

The purpose of this chapter is to describe and evaluate selected psychometric assessment tools available to clinicians and researchers to assess critical psychosocial variables impacting on the experience of chronic pain. The chapter contains descriptions of several comprehensive self-report measures intended to capture multiple psychosocial dimensions within a single questionnaire, as well as examples of specialized instruments designed to measure the specific dimensions of beliefs about pain and strategies for coping with pain.

A psychosocial evaluation of a patient with chronic pain can take several forms. Undoubtedly, the most commonly used process for collecting such information is via the clinical interview, using standardized self-report questionnaires supplement the interview. However, coverage in this chapter is limited to the self-report questionnaires only. Questionnaire-based psychosocial assessment is by no means limited to the measures described in this chapter. Not covered here are the traditional psychiatric symptom measures employed by many clinicians, for example, the Minnesota Multiphasic Personality Inventory (MMPI; Hathaway et al., 1989); Symptom Checklist–90 (SCL-90;

Derogatis, 1983); and Profile of Mood States (POMS; McNair, Lorr, & Droppleman, 1992). Likewise excluded here are many specialized measures that target specific psychosocial concerns, such as couple/family variables, fear of pain, pain avoidance, or measures that target a specific type of pain condition, such as cancer, low back pain, or arthritis. Some of these targeted measures are reviewed in other chapters of this *Handbook*.

HISTORICAL AND THEORETICAL BACKGROUND

Generalized Psychosocial Considerations

It is universally recognized that the experience of pain is affected by psychological and social factors. Because pain is simultaneously a sensory, an emotional, and a behavioral event, whenever the pain experience is prolonged, the emotional and behavioral components have increasing opportunity to interact with the social environment. Frustration and fear regarding the pain and its consequences are commonplace for people with chronic pain and for others that fall under the shadow of its plight. Overt psychological distress in the form of depression and anxiety disorders is a frequent result (e.g., Banks & Kerns, 1996). Accompanying such pain-generated emotional upset, one often observes financial stress from unemployment or underemployment, marital and family dysfunction, substance abuse and dependence, and a general decline in social and recreational functioning (Jacob & Kerns, 2001). Thus, combined with biomedical considerations, attention to psychosocial components of pain is an essential part of current multidimensional and multimodal clinical pain management programs. Replacing discipline-specific or one-dimensional treatment approaches, such broad-based programs are considered state of the art in chronic pain management.

The *gate control theory* of pain (Melzack & Wall, 1965), *operant pain behavior* (Fordyce, 1976), and general *cognitive-behavioral* formulations of the pain experience (Turk, Meichenbaum, & Genest, 1983) have played a key role in focusing attention on the importance of psychological and interpersonal/environmental variables in the development, maintenance, and treatment of chronic pain. These psychosocial factors have become integrated into the now widely accepted *biopsychosocial model of chronic pain* (Gatchel, Peng, Peters, Fuchs, & Turk, 2007). This perspective views coping with pain as a dynamic process wherein patients' understanding, beliefs, and thinking styles mediate emotional and behavioral responses to their pain. In turn, such cognitive variables can directly influence effectiveness at coping with pain.

Pain Beliefs and Coping Considerations

In our clinical practices of chronic pain management, we have consistently encountered patients with persistent maladaptive beliefs about the diagnosis and treatment of pain. Despite multiple diagnostic studies and failed, invasive treatments, it is not uncommon for patients to expect, if not demand, more of the same. Also, beliefs regarding the origin and meaning of pain, physical functioning, fault, and compensation may often feature prominently in patients' progress during treatment.

In multidisciplinary clinics, pain beliefs significantly and independently predict both physical disability and depression, even after researchers control for age, sex, pain intensity, catastrophizing, and coping (Turner, Jensen, & Romano, 2000). Negative pain beliefs have been identified as significant predictors of pain and related disability in the transition from acute to chronic pain (Young Casey, Greenberg, Nicassio, Harpin, & Hubbard, 2008). Changes in pain beliefs have been shown to predict or mediate the therapeutic outcomes (e.g., reductions in pain, disability and physical limitations) of cognitive-behavioral therapy (CBT) and multidisciplinary management for chronic pain (Turner, Holtzman, & Mancl, 2007; Walsh & Radcliffe, 2002). Changes in pain beliefs following treatment completion may be equally important. Increases in beliefs regarding disability in the year following a multidisciplinary pain program are associated with worsening disability and depression during this time (Jensen, Turner, & Romano, 2007). The significance of pain beliefs to disability, health care utilization, and treatment delivery has been reflected in public media campaigns designed to alter pain beliefs in several countries, with varying degrees of success (Buchbinder & Jolley, 2007; Werner, Gross, Atle Lie, & Ihlebaek, 2008).

The origin of such dysfunctional pain beliefs is a separate though interesting topic. There is some evidence that level of educational achievement is relevant: Persons with less education have stronger beliefs that pain signals harm, is unrelated to emotional experience, is disabling and uncontrollable, while they also report more passive and maladaptive coping strategies (Roth & Geisser, 2002).

Closely aligned with beliefs regarding pain is the topic of pain coping skills. In fact, the psychology of pain management is mostly about how people cope with pain. Coping, whether adaptive or maladaptive, represents an individual's attempts to resolve pain-related problems and is strongly influenced by psychosocial variables, including one's beliefs about the pain and its appropriate treatment. If beliefs directly influence coping, beliefs about pain should not be viewed simply as an artifact of the chronic pain experience that will disappear once a correct diagnosis is made and corresponding treatment is initiated. Rather, maladaptive cognitions, and corresponding poor coping, can lie at the heart of the chronic pain problem. Recognizing that beliefs compatible with treatment must exist if patients are to cope effectively with pain, the New Zealand National Advisory Committee on Health and Disability (1997) has identified "maladaptive attitudes and beliefs about back pain" as a significant risk factor (a psychosocial "yellow flag") for developing long-term disability from low back pain. Likewise, Gatchel and Epker (1999) list "maladaptive attitudes and beliefs about pain" as one of the prime risk factors in identifying patients likely to move from acute pain into chronic pain and disability. The Orebro Musculoskeletal Pain Questionnaire (OMPQ; Hockings, McAuley, & Maher, 2008; Linton & Hallden, 1998), a validated screening measure for identifying chronicity risk in patients with acute or subacute spinal pain, includes questions to assess basic beliefs about the meaning of pain.

COMPREHENSIVE MEASURES OF PSYCHOSOCIAL VARIABLES

History

As mentioned previously, the collection of psychosocial information usually begins with a clinical interview. As the multidisciplinary pain movement began to emerge in the 1960s and 1970s, interviews were often supplemented by standardized psychological tests of psychiatric symptoms, especially indicators of mood state. Since these tests had been standardized almost exclusively with psychiatric patients; there was a considerable initial effort to revalidate traditional symptom inventories, such as the MMPI and SCL-90, for use with pain patients. But as the discipline of behavioral medicine continued to grow, there was also a significant effort toward development of scales and inventories that were more specific to cognitive-behavioral dimensions of medical illness.

Comprehensive Generic (Not Specific to Pain) Psychosocial Measures

A plethora of self-report measures for quantifying psychosocial variables associated with medical problems have been used in pain research and treatment settings. How-

ever, many of these measures are generic instruments, not specific to the symptoms of a particular medical condition such as chronic pain. Only a few of the more commonly used generic measures are mentioned here.

The Illness Behavior Questionnaire (IBQ; Pilowsky & Spence, 1983) and the Illness Behavior Inventory (IBI; Turkat & Pettegrew, 1983) are seldom used today, but we mentioned them here due to their historical importance. Expanding on concepts borrowed from the sociology of illness, as formulated by Parsons (1951) and Mechanic and Volkart (1960), Pilowsky began to apply these ideas directly to clinical patient samples with hypochondrias and other manifestations of abnormal illness behavior (e.g., Pilowsky, 1969). This effort grew into the development of the IBQ, one of the first questionnaires containing questions about patients' attitudes toward their illnesses, perceived reactions of others, and other psychosocial variables. The IBI, one of the first self-report inventories developed from a behavioral perspective, in contrast to the IBQ, placed a greater focus on scales of overt behavior. Both of these measures, used in several early pain studies, were covered in more detail in prior editions of this *Handbook*.

Sickness Impact Profile

Of the generic psychosocial health inventories, the instrument that has been most extensively used in pain studies is probably the Sickness Impact Profile (SIP). A version of the SIP appeared as early as 1972, although the current, most widely used version first appeared in 1981 (Bergner, Bobbitt, Carter, & Gilson, 1981). The authors' stated goal was to develop a psychometrically sound measure that could be used to evaluate the impact of disease on both physical and emotional functioning.

The SIP is a 136-item questionnaire with "yes" or "no" responses. Scales with the labels Sleep and Rest, Eating, Work, Management, and Recreation and Pastimes are labeled Independent scales. The scales Ambulation, Mobility, Body Care, and Movement are called Physical scales, and Social Interaction, Alertness Behavior, Emotional Behavior, and Communication are considered Psychosocial scales. A 24-item short form of the SIP, worded especially for patients with back pain, was developed by Roland and Morris (1983). However, it is limited to the assessment of physical disability due to pain. A more comprehensive, but still abbreviated, 68-item version has more recently become available (Naurda, McLendon, Andresen, & Armbrecht, 2003).

Psychometric data presented in the Bergner and colleagues (1981) publication suggest good reliability and validity for the SIP. The data are collected from group general medical practice enrollees, as well as patients with specialty treatment for hyperthyroidism, rheumatoid arthritis, and hip replacement surgery. Test–retest reliability ($r = .92$) and internal consistency ($r = .94$) were both very high. Convergent and discriminant validity, assessed via the multitrait–multimethod technique, were also good. Clinical validity, determined by the relationship between SIP scores and clinical measures of disease, was also reported to be high.

The value of the SIP has been well established through dozens of published studies. However, from our unsystematic perusal of the literature, it seems to have received less use in recent pain studies. This may be due to its length, binary response choice, and more importantly, the growing number of options available to the pain clinician and researcher.

Short Form–36 Health Survey

The Short Form–36 Health Survey (SF-36; Ware, Kosinski, & Keller, 1994) is a 36-item questionnaire intended to assess both physical and emotional dimensions of health. Documented in over 4,000 publications, it has been judged, according to Garratt, Schmidt, Mackintosh, and Fitzpatrick (2002), to be the most extensively used of all generic patient health outcome measures. The 36 items yield an eight-scale profile of functional health and well-being scores, as well as psychometrically based physical and mental health summary measures. These two higher-order clusters have been confirmed by factor analysis (Ware et al., 1994). The four Physical Health scales are named: Physical Functioning, Role–Physical, Bodily Pain, and General Health. The Mental Scales are called Vitality, Social Functioning, Role–Emotional, and Mental Health.

Most SF-36 items have their roots in instruments that have been in use since the 1970s and 1980s. The eight scales included in the SF-36 were chosen to represent the most frequently measured concepts in widely used health surveys and those most likely to be affected by disease and treatment (Ware, Snow, Kosinski, & Gandek, 1993). Version 1 became available in a developmental form in 1988 and in a "standard" form in 1990. Several years later, version 2 (SF-36v2) was released, with improvements in layout, wording, and increases in five-level response format (Ware, Kosinski, & Dewey, 2000). Norms are available for the newer v2 format.

Due to its sheer bulk, the extensive psychometric developmental work supporting the reliability and validity of this inventory can only be briefly summarized here. According to Ware and colleagues (1993), median test–retest reliability across 15 studies has been at least .80 for seven of the eight scales, with .76 for the Social Functioning scale. Dozens of studies give indication of adequate content, concurrent, criterion, construct, and predictive validity. However, the validity of its Physical (PCS) and Mental Component scores (MCS) has been questioned by some research showing that these scores can have significant overlap (Taft, Karlsson, & Sullivan, 2001). Significant correlations ($r = -.74 - .67$) between PCS and MCS were found at their upper scoring intervals, with indication that substantial variance in each component score (greater than 50%) was accounted for by subscales classified under the other component. It was suggested that component scores be interpreted with caution, and only in combination with profile scores (Taft et al., 2001). Other limitations of the SF-36 in the pain context include lack of specificity for assessing established pain constructs and cost.

Although, the SF-36 is a generic instrument, not targeting a specific disease, it has found it way into many pain studies (e.g., Krousael-Wood, McCune, Abdoh, & Re, 1994; Osterhaus, Townsend, Gandek, & Ware, 1994). An advantage of the SF-36 is the ability to compare directly and connect results from any given study with a huge literature. The questionnaire can be self-administered, computer-administered, or administered by a trained interviewer in person or by telephone. In addition to individual use for clinical or research purposes, it has been widely used in general population surveys in the United States and other countries. Although it can now be considered an "older" instrument, it remains widely used in current medical survey research, but less so as an individual-patient clinical assessment tool.

Millon Behavioral Medicine Diagnostic

The Millon Behavioral Medicine Diagnostic (MBMD; Millon, Antoni, Millon, Meagher, & Grossman, 2000) is a self-report instrument that has largely replaced the Millon Behavioral Health Inventory (MBHI; Millon, Green, & Meagher, 1983) described in prior editions of this volume. Like its predecessor, the MBMD was developed by Millon and colleagues to evaluate the psychosocial functioning of medical patients. According to its authors, the newer MBHD places relatively more emphasis on psychosocial assets that may support response to treatment. This reflects an increasing assessment trend toward assessment of dimensions that contribute to positive coping rather than a focus solely on identification of psychosocial pathologies that may interfere with response to treatment.

The test contains 165 dichotomous response items, grouped into 32 clinical scales in seven categories entitled Response Patterns, Negative Health Habits, Psychiatric Indicators, Coping Styles, Stress Moderators, Treatment Prognostics, and Management Guide. Commercially handled computer scoring and profiling is available for a fee.

Current norms are based on 700 patients with a wide variety of medical conditions, including chronic pain. Reliability appears to be adequate, with a median internal consistency coefficient of .79 for all scales and median test–retest coefficient for all scales of .83 (Millon et al., 2000). Scale development went through the standard procedures of internal consistency refinement followed by correlations with related scales for construct and concurrent validity, which appear to be quite adequate. The authors report (Millon et al., 2000) that the MDMD De-pression score correlated .87 with the Beck Depression Inventory and .58 with the Brief Symptom Inventory–Depression scale. Medical professionals rated 100 patients on targeted attitudes and behaviors thought to be important to treatment outcome (e.g., compliance, medication problems, and utilization problems). The MBMD Pain Sensitivity scale correlated .62 with a rating of Pain Reports, and the Adjustment Difficulties scale correlated .61 with a rating of Utilization Problems. Two recent reports suggest that the MBMD can predict adherence to highly active antiretroviral therapy (Cruess, Minor, Antoni, & Millon, 2007). However, the data on discriminate and predictive validity remain very limited, and there has been recent debate about the reliability and validity of the test when used for screening of bariatric surgery candidates (Strack, 2008; Walfish, Wise, & Streiner, 2008). To date, most of the empirical effort has gone into internal test construction efforts and generation of norms. We are unaware of studies specific to pain. Despite its youth, we feel that this test deserves consideration because of its convenience and the fact it was created by a group with a long history of successful test development for psychosocial assessment of medical patients.

Comprehensive Psychosocial Measures Specific to Pain

McGill Pain Questionnaire

The first of the comprehensive assessment tools specific to pain, and still the most widely recognized, is the McGill Pain Questionnaire (MPQ; Melzack, 1975). This questionnaire is described in detail elsewhere in this *Handbook*.

While the value of the MPQ as a research tool is unquestioned, it has been relatively less popular with clinicians, many of whom feel that too much time is focused on gathering sensory information, a dimension that may be relatively independent of overall cognitive-behavioral functioning. The two comprehensive psychosocial instruments described below tend to place relatively greater emphasis on dimensions such as activity level, personal and family reactions to pain, and current employment issues.

West Haven–Yale Multidimensional Pain Inventory

For the past two decades, in both research and clinical pain settings, the most widely used comprehensive measure of psychosocial variables has been the West Haven–Yale Multidimensional Pain Inventory (MPI; Kerns, Turk, & Rudy, 1985). The origin of the instrument is closely linked to a cognitive-behavioral perspective on chronic pain (Turk, Meichenbaum, & Genest, 1983).

The original version of MPI is a 52-item, 12-scale questionnaire divided into three parts. Section 1 contains five scales designed to evaluate important dimensions of the pain experience: Perceived Interference of pain in vocational, social/recreational, and family and marital/couple functioning; Support and Concern from significant others; Pain Severity; Life Control with regard to activities of daily living and daily problems; and Affective Distress. Section 2 is intended for the assessment of patients' perceptions of the responses of others to their pain. Its three scales measure the perceived frequencies of Negative, Solicitous, and Distracting responses. Section 3 assesses patients' participation in four types of common daily activities: Household Chores, Outdoor Work, Activities Away from Home, and Social Activities. Several of the scales can also be combined to produce composite scores for General Activity and Affective Distress. A 60-item version with modified instructions is also available (Okifuji, Turk, & Everleigh, 1999).

Psychometric procedures for developing the MPI are thoroughly documented elsewhere (Jacob & Kerns, 2001; Kerns et al., 1985; Turk & Kerns, 1985). Internal consistency of scales is adequate, and factorial structure of items has been consistent across several studies (e.g., see Riley, Zawacki, Robinson, & Geisser, 1999). Also, interscale correlations were all found to be lower than each scale's internal consistency, suggesting that each scale contributes some unique variance to the overall inventory. Concurrent validity was evidenced by the fact that a scale-level factor analysis of the 12 scales, along with several other standardized measures of pain-relevant constructs, revealed that the MPI scales loaded significantly on conceptually related factors found in other standardized measures.

Since it first publication nearly 25 years ago, the MPI has demonstrated considerable heuristic value by its adaptation in numerous research and clinical settings. Rudy, Turk, and colleagues, in a series of studies (Rudy, Turk, Zaki, & Curtin, 1989; Turk & Rudy, 1988, 1990), have identified three reliable categories of pain patients from cluster analyses of MPI scale scores: Dysfunctional, Interpersonally Distressed, and Adaptive Copers. Recently, it has been argued (Hopwood, Creech, Clark, Meagher, & Morey, 2008) that the addition of a fourth cluster, labeled Repressors, can further improve treatment outcome prediction. Whether with three or four clusters, this type of classification system can provide useful information to the clinician who must plan interventions tailored to the particular patient's unique cognitive-behavioral profile. In summary, the enduring strength of the MPI lies in the fact that it is a psychometrically sound instrument that despite its relative brevity provides comprehensive psychosocial information that is useful in both clinical and research settings.

Profile of Chronic Pain: Extended Assessment and Profile of Chronic Pain: Screen

The Profile of Chronic Pain: Extended Assessment (PCP:EA; Ruehlman, Karoly, Newton, & Aiken, 2005b) and the PCP: Screen (PCP:S; Ruehlman, Karoly, Newton, & Aiken, 2005a) reflect a recent ambitious effort to develop a new instrument for the assessment of multiple psychosocial aspects of chronic pain adaptation. The PCP:EA provides information on the qualitative features of pain experience, pain location, pain severity, health care status, pain medication use, pain coping, catastrophizing, pain attitudes and beliefs, social responses to pain, and functional limitations across 10 areas of everyday life. Seemingly, the goals are quite similar to those of the authors' of the SF-36, but in this case focus on the symptom of chronic pain.

The PCP:EA consists of 33 ordinally scored items evaluating Pain Location and Severity, Pain Characteristics (e.g., worst daily pain, medication use, health care status, identification of the most important person in the patient's life), and Functional Limitations in 10 areas of daily living. Also, the instrument includes 13 multi-item subscales addressing dimensions of Coping (guarding, ignoring, task persistence, and positive self-talk), Catastrophizing, Pain Attitudes and Beliefs, and Positive (behavioral and emotional) and Negative (insensitivity and impatience) Social Responses.

Supportive data were drawn from two large (approximately 4,800 subjects) national samples, stratified by age, via telephone interview. These two samples provide (1) confirmation of the factor structure of the scales, (2) support for internal consistency of the scales, (3) evidence of adequate concurrent and predictive validity for most of the scales, and (4) data for development of norms for the scales. Specific to predictive validity, it was determined that many of the PCP:EA scales were significant predictors of adjustment indices collected after a 3-month interval. The adjustment indices included measures of depression, anxiety, and disability indicators. However, the predictive utility of PCP:EA Coping scales need more psychometric work before their validity can be established. This may be due to the lack of item-content conformity among differing comparative measures of coping and catastrophizing.

The 15-item screening version of the PCP (PCP:S) was developed simultaneously with the longer 86-item extended version. It is designed to gauge Pain Severity, Interference with Daily Activity, and Emotional Burden. In addition to the national sample data, a secondary cross-validation of the PCP:S has been completed with 244 patients from primary care settings (Karoly, Ruehlman, Aiken, Todd, & Newton, 2006).

A significant effort has gone into the development of this new comprehensive psychosocial measure. To date, with its application restricted primarily to large-scale survey research, its use mirrors the use of the SF-36. But the PCP, unlike the SF-36, is designed specifically for use with chronic pain assessment. Seemingly, the instrument captures information that should be useful for individual clinical assessment, as well as survey research. Time will determine how this measure compares to the MPI. It seems likely that the brief screening form will be the more popular version in time-pressed clinical settings.

ASSESSMENT OF PAIN BELIEFS

The reader who is particularly interested in the history of pain beliefs and measurement of coping strategies is encouraged to refer to the prior editions of this *Handbook*. Many of the earlier measures mentioned in those volumes, although making important contributions to the evolution of beliefs assessment, due to space limitations are not included here.

Definitions and Relationships among Beliefs and Coping Constructs

Research into cognitive-behavioral constructs is often hampered by poorly defined terms, and terms used in different ways by different investigators. Thus, we feel that an effort to review definitions of terms found in pain beliefs and coping research is important.

Beliefs have been defined as personally formed or culturally shared cognitive configurations (Wrubel, Benner, & Lazarus, 1981). They differ from *attitudes*, defined as our feelings about events, because beliefs refer to our understanding of events (Fishbein & Ajzen, 1975). Thus, beliefs are preexisting notions about the nature of reality that mold our perception of our environment and ourselves, and shape its meaning (Lazarus & Folkman, 1984). (*Note.* By this definition, many of the belief questionnaires discussed here are actually both *belief* and *attitude* measures). Beliefs may be so generalized, or wide-ranging, as to qualify as a stable personality disposition, or they may be highly specific to a particular context (Lazarus & Folkman, 1984).

Although *expectancy* is often considered to be synonymous with beliefs, it refers more specifically to beliefs about the future, especially relationships between a set of events and future consequences. Most relevant to pain management are so-called *self-efficacy expectancies* that refer to beliefs about one's capacity to execute the behavior required to produce a certain outcome (Bandura, 1977).

Self-efficacy beliefs differ from *outcome expectancy beliefs*. The latter refers to beliefs that a behavior will lead to a specific outcome, regardless of whether the person can execute the behavior. By comparison, self-efficacy beliefs are based on behaviors within a person's repertoire, thus representing appraisals of personal control. These self-efficacy beliefs have strong clinical relevance; in an investigation of mediators, moderators, and predictors of therapeutic change in CBT for chronic pain, change in perceived pain control (self-efficacy) was the mediator that explained the greatest proportion of the total treatment effect on each measured outcome (Turner et al., 2007).

Pain beliefs differ in significant ways from *coping responses*. Whereas pain beliefs refer to mental appraisals of a situation, coping involves the set of responses an individual produces. Hence, a pain belief is always a cognition, whereas a coping response may be a cognition or an overt behavior. Moreover, patients readily acknowledge their beliefs about pain and its treatment, whereas self-reports regarding their coping responses to pain may or may not be the ones that are actually employed (DeGood, 2000). Finally, coping responses may be either adaptive or maladaptive, depending on variables such as the internal and external resources available to the individual and the demands posed by the stressor (Lazarus & Folkman, 1984).

An example may clarify the meaning of the preceding terms and illustrate how beliefs can interact with actual coping behavior. Picture a patient with musculoskeletal back pain who has been told that a set of stretching exercises will be helpful for managing pain. The patient may or may not believe this information to be accurate (a treatment *outcome expectancy belief*). Even if the recommendation is believed to be valid, the patient may doubt his or her own ability to perform the exercises (*self-efficacy belief*). For either or both of these reasons, the patient may not engage in the *coping response* of performing the exercises. If he or she does perform the exercises and encounters an increase in pain, the patient may or may not continue with the exercise regimen. Therefore, if the exercise routine is to become a stable coping response, four steps must occur: (1) The therapeutic benefit of

the prescribed exercise must be believed; (2) the capability to perform the exercise must exist; (3) the exercise must actually be performed: and (4) the outcome must contribute to a perception of pain mastery. Although exercising might be viewed as the critical (coping) behavior, the beliefs regarding this behavior may be more critical in determining whether the coping response occurs or is maintained. If the coping response were a cognitive rather than overt behavior, a similar analysis would apply.

Several other psychological constructs in chronic pain are closely linked to pain beliefs. *Acceptance* is now a well-established construct in chronic pain research and treatments (McCracken, Carson, Eccleston, & Keefe, 2004). Measures of acceptance have been shown to capture unique variance in pain adjustment relative to traditional coping measures (McCracken & Eccleston, 2003, 2006). Acceptance is understood to be based on beliefs about the nature and permanence of chronic pain, and measures for chronic pain acceptance rely heavily on assessment of these beliefs. The relationship between acceptance beliefs and traditional domains of pain beliefs remains unclear, though there is some evidence of divergence (Rankin & Holttum, 2003). We describe tools for measurement of acceptance below.

Fear–avoidance has also been established as an important mediator of pain coping and adjustment (Leeuw et al., 2007). The emotional and behavioral aspects of fear avoidance are understood to be rooted in beliefs about pain, underlying disease, and pain as a signal of (re)injury. Therefore, most psychometric tools for fear avoidance assess these types of beliefs.

Another growing specialty area of beliefs assessment involves *readiness to change*. The stages of change, part of the transtheoretical model of behavior change, have been applied successfully to predict response to treatment for a number of health risk behaviors (Prochaska & DiClemente, 1984). The transtheoretical model has been integrated with other models of health behavior to identify approaches to increase patient motivation for self-management of pain (Jensen, Nielson, & Kerns, 2003). However, clinical pain applications of the model are still in their infancy (Dijkstra, 2005). The application of the stages of change construct to chronic pain management involves assessment of beliefs about the value of engaging in components of treatment, and perceived benefits of changing the current management approach. Below we describe measures designed to assess readiness to change and associated beliefs.

Domains of Pain Beliefs

Most beliefs relevant to pain can be categorized into three domains: (1) basic philosophical assumptions about the nature of the self and the world; (2) beliefs sufficiently generalized and stable to be considered personality traits; and (3) beliefs specific to the experience of pain. The first category of beliefs has to do with loosely organized but deep-seated ethical and philosophical assumptions about values such as justice, fairness, suffering, and personal responsibility. If one believes that life should be free of pain, that belief can intensify suffering associated with the experience of chronic pain. Because beliefs in this category are often highly personalized, inconsistent, and at times contradictory, they are difficult to assess.

Beliefs falling into the second category tend to be more organized and rooted in everyday life. Because they are stable across time and situations, such beliefs are often conceptualized as personality traits. Considering beliefs that translate into negative traits, Lazarus (1991) suggests that "people carry around with them private and recurrent personal meanings that lead them to react inappropriately to an encounter with a sense of betrayal, victimization, rejection, abandonment, inadequacy, or whatever" (p. 363). Of course, other such beliefs may contribute to positive adaptation, including popular psychological constructs such as "hardiness" (Kobasa, 1979; Pollock & Duffy, 1990), "locus of control" (Rotter, 1966; Wallston, Wallston, & DeVellis, 1978), "attributional style" (Abramson, Seligman, & Teasdale, 1978), and "self-efficacy" (Bandura, 1977).

Certainly, beliefs falling into the first and second domains can be studied in patients with pain (e.g., Weisberg & Gatchel, 2000); nevertheless, the most productive beliefs research has focused on the third category:

specific patient beliefs about pain. These pain-specific beliefs have to do with the "nuts and bolts" of what patients believe should be done to diagnose and control pain.

Pain Beliefs Instruments Currently Recommended for Research and Clinical Applications

Survey of Pain Attitudes

The pain beliefs instrument that has been most extensively studied and has gained the widest use is the Survey of Pain Attitudes (SOPA). The initial published version (Jensen, Karoly, & Huger, 1987) had 24 items, each rated on a 5-point scale. These items were designed to assess five dimensions related to patient beliefs: (1) Pain Control, (2) Pain-Related Disability, (3) Medical Cures for Pain, (4) Solicitude from Others, and (5) Medication for Pain. A sixth dimension, Emotionality (i.e., beliefs about the influence of emotions on pain), was added in a subsequent 35-item version (Jensen & Karoly, 1989). Initial psychometric analyses revealed the 35-item SOPA to have high internal consistency within subscales and to be stable over time (Jensen & Karoly, 1989). Subsequent analyses revealed the SOPA to be associated with patient reports of pain behavior and coping responses, as well as sensitive to belief changes following conservative pain treatment (Jensen & Karoly, 1991; Jensen, Turner, & Romano, 1991).

In a third revision of the SOPA (Jensen, Turner, Romano, & Lawler, 1994), the scale was increased to 57 items (SOPA-57). Additional items were added to the Medication and Disability subscales, and a seventh dimension was added, assessing beliefs that pain is evidence of physical harm. Subscale scores with this version continued to demonstrate acceptable internal consistency, test–retest reliability, and convergent/discriminant validity (Jensen et al., 1994). Scale scores derived from this version have been related to treatment outcomes: Changes in beliefs from pre- to posttreatment correlated with changes in measures of physical and emotional functioning. Translations and validation of the SOPA into Portuguese (Pimenta & da Cruz, 2006) and Quebec-French (Duquette, McKinley, & Litowski, 2005) languages have been reported.

Tait and Chibnall (1997), who found through factor analysis that the SOPA-57 did not contain seven unique dimensions, developed a briefer, 30-item version (SOPA-30) that exhibited a seven-dimension factor structure. All but the three-item Medication scale had good internal consistency. Correlations between subscales in the brief and standard versions of the SOPA ranged from .79 to .90. The SOPA-30 also demonstrated other desirable psychometric properties, including convergent/discriminative validity with other pain variables that appear similar to the lengthier version. Unfortunately, the SOPA-30 has seen limited use in clinical research. Subsequently, Jensen, Turner, and Romano (2000) developed a 35-item short form of the SOPA (SOPA-35), with the goal of more closely reflecting the subscale content of the SOPA-57. They compared the SOPA-30, SOPA-35, and SOPA-57 in a longitudinal study of multidisciplinary pain rehabilitation program participants. Internal consistencies of all scales were adequate to good, except for the SOPA-30 Disability (alpha = .53) and SOPA-35 Harm (alpha = .66) scales. The SOPA-30 Disability and Medication scales were found to have marginal test–retest stabilities, though this dimension was assessed posttreatment, which, as previously described, is a time when belief changes are known to occur. Jensen and colleagues provide reasonable advice on selecting a version of the SOPA: The SOPA-57 is most appropriate when reliability is a prominent concern (e.g., longitudinal testing); the SOPA-35 is the most appropriate short form when similarity to the original SOPA scale content is desired (e.g., comparing scores with prior SOPA-57 research); and the SOPA-30 can be selected when brevity is a primary concern.

The SOPA has now undergone three major revisions and is available in two abbreviated versions. Since its inception, it has consistently demonstrated strong psychometric qualities and good clinical utility involving patient responses to multidisciplinary pain management. Its demonstrated relationship to treatment outcome makes it especially appealing both to clinicians and researchers interested in the assessment of pain cognition. The choice of long and short versions provides flexibility for different applications. However, recommended normative standards for interpreting individual response profiles are lacking. Nonetheless, it is a useful and psychometrically sound instrument for both research and clinical applications.

Pain Beliefs and Perceptions Inventory

The Pain Beliefs and Perceptions Inventory (PBAPI; Williams & Thorn, 1989), a 16-item questionnaire, originally measured three dimensions of patient beliefs derived from factor analysis: (1) self-blame for pain, (2) perception of pain as mysterious, and (3) beliefs about the stability/permanence of pain over time. The initial study (Williams & Thorn, 1989) showed that the three scales are face valid and possess high internal consistency. The belief that pain is permanent and likely to persist despite treatment was positively associated with pain intensity ratings and decreased compliance with conservative treatment. In addition, the belief that "pain is mysterious" (i.e., that pain has no explanation) was inversely associated with posttreatment ratings of psychological distress and somatization. Finally, both "pain stability" and "pain as mystery" beliefs were associated with negative self-perceptions and decreased control over pain. A study by Williams and Keefe (1991) also supported the validity of the PBAPI. A cluster analysis of PBAPI responses revealed three patient subgroups that differed in patterns of coping strategies. For example, patients who believed that their pain was mysterious and permanent reported a greater tendency to catastrophize about pain and employed fewer cognitive coping strategies compared to patients who believed their pain was of short duration and understandable.

Subsequent factor analyses (Herda, Siegeris, & Basler, 1994; Strong, Ashton, & Chant, 1992) indicated a four-factor structure in which the Stability scale subdivides into two subscales: beliefs that pain is a constant and enduring experience (Constancy) and beliefs about the chronicity of pain (Acceptance). Constancy showed higher correlations with self-reported symptoms (anxiety, general physical troubles, and pain intensity) than did Acceptance, Self-Blame, or Pain as a Mystery.

Clearly this measure has strong psychometric grounding and taps dimensions that have proven relevance to patient behavior. These properties have contributed to its broad use, including German (Herda et al., 1994) and Spanish (Gonzalez, Soler, & Ferrer, 2002) translations. Several caveats should be noted, however. First, the limited scope (content) of the PBAPI may restrict its clinical utility. Furthermore, high levels of self-blame are uncommonly reported, potentially reducing the utility of this scale. Finally, Pain as a Mystery seems to measure something very akin to catastrophizing, so that its added value for assessment is unclear. Nonetheless, these are empirical questions requiring further attention. Other dimensions of the PBAPI (Constancy, Acceptance) have shown considerable clinical utility.

Cognitive Risk Profile for Pain

After initial research with the Pain Information and Beliefs Questionnaire (Shutty & DeGood, 1990), based on a videotaped format, DeGood and colleagues began development of a wider-ranging pain beliefs instrument. This instrument, the *Cognitive Risk Profile for Pain* (CRPP; Cook & DeGood, 2006) has now gone through several iterations and is a clinically based self-report instrument with a primary focus on clinical risk assessment for treatment planning. It measures several belief dimensions identified through prior research as potential roadblocks to successful pain management. The most recent version of the CRPP consists of 53 items, each rated on a 6-point scale. Each item asks patients to rate their level of agreement–disagreement with a statement about pain that has been judged to be either adaptive or maladaptive, and thus potentially related to treatment response. The CRPP produces a total risk score, as well as nine subscale scores: (1) Philosophic Beliefs about Pain (PB), (2a) Denial that Mood Affects Pain (MP), (2b) Denial that Pain Affects Mood (PM), (3) Perception of Blame (BL), (4) Inadequate Support (IS), (5) Disability Entitlement (DE), (6) Desire for Medical Breakthrough (MB), (7) Skepticism of Multidisciplinary Approach (SM), and (8) Conviction of Hopelessness (CH). Confirmatory factor analysis indicated an improved fit of the nine-factor model in comparison to the previous 68-item version (Cook & DeGood, 2006). Internal consistency/reliability was found to be excellent for the total score (.82)

and acceptable (> .70) to excellent (> .80) for seven of the nine scales, with marginal levels for scales BL (.64) and MB (.65). Consistent with the design and intent of the scales, low to moderate intercorrelations were reported. Construct and criterion validation were demonstrated through associations of CRPP scores with concurrent measures of pain and psychosocial functioning, and with longitudinal treatment outcomes. Further evaluation of the MP, BL, and MB scales was recommended. A comparative study of pain beliefs across three age groups (< 40, 41–59, 60–90) using the CRPP-68 found significant differences for seven of the nine CRPP scales. Older adults were found to have lower risk scores than young and/or middle-aged patients for four of the scales, though patterns varied across belief domains (Cook, DeGood, & Chastain, 1999).

We believe that the intent of the CRPP, to identify factors that put patients at risk for poor treatment outcomes, enhances clinical utility. In addition, many of the scales assess belief dimensions that are very familiar and of interest to clinicians, thus providing face validity. We have suggested that the CRPP may be useful in some clinical settings for identifying specific domains of pain beliefs that can interfere with an individual patient's treatment progress. These in turn can be used to target interventions addressing these beliefs and to facilitate general treatment planning. To date, the CRPP has been used in a variety of clinical settings in at least seven countries, and translations for French and German versions are in process. The primary current limitation of the CRPP in clinical practice is its length, and work on a short-form version is underway. Clinical use of the CRPP will be assisted by additional studies of its role in treatment planning and publication of normative data from different clinical settings.

New Beliefs Measures

Several new measures of pain-related cognitions have been developed. Inadequate data or other limitations keep us from recommending their use at this time, and/or they provide a specialized scope of assessment. However, initial data suggest that they offer potential to expand the scope of pain beliefs assessment.

Cognitive Appraisal Inventory for Chronic Pain Patients

Based on the transactional theory of stress and coping (Lazarus & Folkman, 1984), the Cognitive Appraisal Inventory for Chronic Pain Patients (CAI; Ramirez-Maestre, Esteve, & Lopez, 2008) assesses appraisals in three categories: harm or loss, threat, and challenge. Good initial psychometrics were reported for the Spanish version, though the published English translation requires validation.

Revised Cognitive Evaluation Questionnaire

The Cognitive Evaluation Questionnaire (Philips, 1989) was designed to assess the types of cognitions provoked by the onset of a painful episode. The Revised Cognitive Evaluation Questionnaire (R-CEQ; Helmes & Goburdhun, 2007) maintains a focus on cognitive reactions to chronic pain, with addition of new items and expansion to eight scales: Positive Coping, Desire to Withdraw, Disappointment with Self, Causal Rumination, Helplessness, Concern with Effects of Pain, Endogenous Emotion, and Reactive Emotion. Further validation is needed to address psychometric concerns from initial testing.

Pain Attitudes Questionnaire

The Pain Attitudes Questionnaire (PAQ; Yong, Bell, Workman, & Gibson, 2003; Yong, Gibson, de L. Horne, & Helms, 2001) was developed to assess stoicism and cautiousness beliefs, and to provide a basis for age group comparisons. An initial version was evaluated in a sample of community-dwelling healthy adults (Yong et al., 2001), and subsequently revised and tested with a clinical sample of patients with chronic pain (Yong et al., 2003). The *Pain Attitudes Questionnaire—Revised (PAQ-R)* includes 24 items that load on three Stoicism factors (Fortitude, Concealment, Superiority) and two Cautiousness factors (Self-Doubt, Reluctance). A different pattern of age group differences was reported across the two studies. In follow-up analyses with the clinical sample, PAQ-R scores were found to mediate the relationships between age and measures of pain, mood, and functional interference (Yong, 2006). The PAQ-R has

introduced important dimensions of beliefs assessment with possible age cohort differences. We hope that there will be continued research in this area.

Readiness to Change Measures

Pain Stages of Change Questionnaire

The Pain Stages of Change Questionnaire (PSOCQ; Kerns, Rosenberg, Jamison, Caudill, & Haythornwaite, 1997) measures cognitions that are relevant to a patient's readiness for change, based on the stages of change in the transtheoretical model (Prochaska & DiClemente, 1984). The PSOCQ is a 30-item self-report instrument designed to assesses attitudes and beliefs connected to four of the stages of change, as applied to self-management of chronic pain: Precontemplation, Contemplation, Action, and Maintenance.

The initial study of 241 patients supported the factor structure of the scales, as well as their discriminant and criterion validities (Kerns et al., 1997). Moreover, each of the four scales was found to be internally consistent and stable over time. A subsequent study (Kerns & Rosenberg, 1999) of 109 chronic pain patients participating in cognitive-behavioral treatment found that, relative to patients that completed treatment, 50 patient dropouts had significantly higher Precontemplation scores and lower Contemplation scores prior to treatment. Overall, it was found that pre- to posttreatment changes in the PSOCQ scales were associated with improved outcomes. Studies by Jensen, Nielson, Turner, Romano, and Hill (2003, 2004) have demonstrated that PSOCQ scores are associated with concurrent coping measures in expected patterns, but variably associated with measures of depression and disability, and that changes in PSOCQ scores predict improvement in multidisciplinary pain treatment and pain coping.

The PSOCQ is easily administered and has evident face validity. Continued research has established a good base of support for its psychometric properties. It fits nicely within the tradition of cognitive assessment of pain beliefs, and adds a conceptual framework that is appealing to clinicians interested in gauging potential treatment response.

Multidimensional Pain Readiness to Change Questionnaire

The Multidimensional Pain Readiness to Change Questionnaire (MPRCQ; Nielson, Jensen, & Kerns, 2003) was developed to advance the assessment of readiness to change by focusing on specific skills taught in multidisciplinary pain programs rather than overall readiness beliefs about self-management. As such, it is more of a coping than beliefs measure. It comprises 46 items loading on nine scales: Exercise, Task Persistence, Relaxation, Cognitive Control, Pacing, Avoid Contingent Rest, Avoid Asking for Assistance, Assertive Communication, and Proper Body Mechanics. Factor analyses in two samples suggested two higher-order factors, labeled Active Coping and Perseverance. Internal consistency reliabilities were found to be acceptable for all but two scales (Pacing, Relaxation), and test–retest reliability was adequate. There was a lack of association with a measure of social desirability, an important finding given expected demand characteristics of clinical settings where the measure is intended for use. The MPRCQ scales were associated with PSOCQ scores in predicted directions, though patterns of correlations were different in two clinical samples.

A recent revision (MPRCQ2) incorporated several modifications to enhance the questionnaire's psychometric properties and provide additional validation (Nielson, Jensen, Ehde, Kerns, & Molton, 2008). The MPRCQ2 items are divided into two sections, separating items describing Adaptive Coping behaviors from those reflecting Maladaptive Coping. The resulting measure contains 69 items. Initial validation suggests good psychometric properties. However, its length may limit its use in clinical settings, and cross-validation in other samples will be important for interpretation. In response to these issues, the authors have recently published two short-form versions: the MPRCQ2-13 and the MPRCQ2-26, based on one- and two-item versions of the subscales (Nielson, Armstrong, Jensen, & Kerns, 2009). Initial psychometric analyses, though based on a single sample of patients with rheumatic disease, are promising, with nine of the 10 subscales showing responsiveness to change following multidisciplinary

treatment. These shortened versions are likely to increase the utility of the MPRCQ2 in both clinical and research applications. Additional studies will help to establish the psychometrics of the brief versions.

Concluding Comment on Pain Beliefs

Maladaptive beliefs continue to be recognized as a major risk factor for poor response to treatment for chronic pain. Change in beliefs has become clearly linked to treatment outcomes. However, beliefs about pain are still most likely to be clinically assessed by interview rather than with psychometric assessment tools. There has been an increase in the choice of beliefs measures available to clinicians and researchers. Of the measures that have been described, the SOPA and its short forms (SOPA-35 and SOPA-30) have the strongest combination of psychometric support and clinical utility. Other options with high clinical appeal are described in a later section of this chapter on brief versions of beliefs and coping measures, including versions of the SOPA and PBAPI. For applications in which readiness to change is of interest, the PSOCQ provides reliable beliefs assessment, while the MPRCQ2 and its shortened versions show promise as measures emphasizing coping strategies. Many of the other measures we have described will benefit from further development, especially for clinical applications.

Several problems relevant to assessment of pain beliefs remain. First, there is ongoing conceptual confusion between pain beliefs and pain coping. Similarly, the relationship between pain beliefs and coping behaviors is confusing and difficult to sort out in the literature. Likewise, the process by which pain beliefs translate into attempts at coping is often unclear. Clearer conceptual models, such as an adaptation of the Lazarus and Folkman transactional model of stress, as proposed by Thorn, Rich, and Boothby (1999), may be helpful.

There also are problems associated with research design. In many studies, beliefs, coping, and even outcome measures are intertwined in a manner that leads to conceptual confusion. One solution to this problem might be to restrict beliefs to the realm of cognition, and coping to the realm of overt behavior (Jensen, Turner, Romano, & Strom,

1995). At a less radical level and at the very least, further attention to conceptual issues is needed as researchers design studies of these challenging constructs.

There is also an issue involving measurement and scaling. Belief measures have emphasized the assessment of maladaptive beliefs. It is not clear, however, that a low score on a negative beliefs scale is the equivalent of a positive belief. More research is needed on relations between adaptive and maladaptive pain beliefs, as well as the relative contribution of each to coping and treatment outcome.

Another ongoing question concerns the origin of beliefs relevant to pain. Are pain beliefs a product of misinformation, idiosyncratic medical experiences, or the psychosocial environment? To what degree do they precede or follow the onset of pain? What are the effects of general and health-specific education on these beliefs? Such information is critical in terms of prevention and modification of maladaptive beliefs. In light of information that mere exposure to new (and more accurate) information is not always sufficient to change pain beliefs (Shutty, DeGood, & Tuttle, 1990), it is important to explore sources from which maladaptive beliefs are derived. Little research has considered the impact of beliefs, particularly on response to treatment, in interaction with moderator variables such as age, gender, employment, and economic circumstances. Similarly, little attention has been paid to the interface between beliefs and recent developments in the field of pain management. While beliefs have been heavily studied in the context of cognitive-behavioral interventions, they have been less studied as they apply to the interventional strategies frequently employed in current pain management practice (e.g., implantable spinal cord stimulators and drug pumps).

COPING WITH PAIN

Any discussion of coping should begin with the transactional model of stress (Lazarus & Folkman, 1984), a theory that continues to guide research on coping with pain. Accordingly, the first part of this section addresses that model and very briefly measures directly associated with it, followed by a review of several established and newer measures of pain coping, and provides conclusions on clinical applications and directions for further study.

Conceptual Basis of Coping

The transactional model of stress defines *coping* as "constantly changing cognitive and behavioral efforts to manage specific external and/or internal demands that are appraised as taxing, or exceeding the resources of the person" (Lazarus & Folkman, 1984, p. 141). This definition recognizes that coping is a fluid process, subject to change across situations and over time. Similarly, it represents coping as a process that comprises appraisals, responses, and reappraisals. Appraisals and responses are both colored by individual differences, including differences in beliefs, expectancies, personality and biological characteristics, and social roles. Faced with similar stressors (e.g., pain), individuals are likely to respond differently: One may appraise pain as a threat, while another may appraise it as a challenge.

The Ways of Coping Checklist (WCCL; Folkman & Lazarus, 1980) was developed to assess coping responses to a broad range of emotion-focused (internal) and problem-focused (external) demands, dimensions intrinsic to the transactional model. Both the WCCL and a modified version (Vitaliano, Russo, Carr, Maiuro, & Becker, 1985) were used extensively in early research on pain patients (DeGood & Shutty, 1992; Jensen, Turner, Romano, & Karoly, 1991). They have seen relatively little recent use, possibly because the factor structure of the instruments has not held up with medical patients (Wineman, Durand, & McCulloch, 1994), and because they were not designed for specific health conditions such as chronic pain (Endler, Parker, & Summerfeldt, 1993).

Established Measures

Vanderbilt Pain Management Inventory

The Vanderbilt Pain Management Inventory (VPMI; Brown & Nicassio, 1987) is a 19-item questionnaire that assesses active and passive coping strategies specifically relevant to chronic pain. The VPMI defines *active strategies* as attempts by the patient to deal with pain through his or her own resources, and *passive strategies* as helplessness or relying on others (Nicholas, Wilson, & Goyen, 1992). The VPMI was significantly revised with the introduction of the 49-item, 11-subscale Vanderbilt Multidimensional Pain Coping Inventory (VMPCI; Smith, Wallston, Dwyer, & Dowdy, 1997). Research with the VPMI and VMPCI is described in the previous edition of this *Handbook*. Both measures appear infrequently in the recent pain literature, having been displaced by alternative pain coping measures.

Coping Strategies Questionnaire

The Coping Strategies Questionnaire (CSQ; Rosenstiel & Keefe, 1983) has for many years formed the backbone of research on coping and adjustment to pain. Unlike the VPMI, the CSQ was designed to assess relatively specific coping strategies: six cognitive and one behavioral coping strategy. Items for each coping strategy subscale are rated as to the frequency with which they are used. Cognitive coping strategies include Diverting Attention, Reinterpreting Pain Sensations, Coping Self-Statements, Ignoring Pain Sensations, Praying or Hoping, and Catastrophizing. The behavioral coping strategy subscale is Increasing Activity. In addition, there are two self-efficacy items reflecting "perceived control over pain" and "ability to decrease pain." Although the CSQ has been studied extensively as an assessment measure, a study on its use as an outcome measure in chronic pain rehabilitation suggests low responsiveness for most of the subscales (Angst, Verra, Lehmann, & Aeschlimann, 2008), with the Catastrophizing scale, and Control and Decrease Pain items showing the greatest responsiveness to interdisciplinary treatment. The CSQ has been translated into several languages, including French (Irachabal, Koleck, Rascle, & Bruchon-Schweitzer, 2008) and German (Verra, Angst, Lehmann, & Aeschlemann, 2006), and has been used in two major lines of research: (1) factor-analytic studies aimed at identifying superordinate constructs relevant to coping, and (2) studies of individual scales aimed at identifying specific coping strategies associated with good or poor adjustment.

CSQ COMPOSITE MEASURES

Numerous composites derived from the CSQ since 1992 include following:

• *Coping Attempts*, a construct that subsumes Coping Self-Statements, Reinterpreting Pain, Ignoring Pain, Increasing Activity, and Diverting Attention (all of the cognitive coping strategies except Catastrophizing) (Gil et al., 1993; Jensen, Turner, & Romano, 1992; Martin et al., 1996; Nicassio, Schoenfeld-Smith, Radojevic, & Schuman, 1995; Thompson, Gil, Abrams, & Phillips, 1992).

• *Pain Control and Rational Thinking*, which has typically included the Catastrophizing subscale (loading negatively) and the two control ratings (loading positively), and has been found to be associated with a variety of desirable pain characteristics (Beckham, Keefe, Caldwell, & Roodman, 1991; Dozois, Dobson, Wong, Hughes, & Long, 1996; Keefe et al., 1991; Schanberg, Lefebvre, Keefe, Kredich, & Gil, 1997; Tota-Faucette, Gil, Williams, Keefe, & Goli, 1993).

• *Active Coping*, composed of items such as "I pretend it's not part of me," has correlated with higher levels of activity and lower levels of psychological distress (e.g., Snow-Turek, Norris, & Tan, 1996). Longitudinal research has shown that Active Coping predicts positive functional gains (Spinhoven & Linssen, 1991; Turner, Whitney, Dworkin, Massoth, & Wilson, 1995).

• *Coping Flexibility* (Haythornthwaite, Menefee, Heinberg, & Clark, 1998), defined as the number of strategies (excluding Catastrophizing) frequently employed to cope with pain. Patients describing a high number of frequently used coping strategies have reported higher levels of perceived control over pain, suggesting that flexibility contributes to effective coping. This finding is consistent with research suggesting that coping flexibility is important for effective pain management (Blalock, DeVellis, & Giorgino, 1995; McCracken & Vowles, 2007; Vowles, McCracken, McLeod, & Eccleston, 2008).

• Several CSQ composites associated with poor adjustment to pain and/or poor outcomes: Negative Thinking/Passive Adherence (Gil, Abrams, Phillips, & Williams, 1992; Gil et al., 1993; Thompson et al., 1992), and Pain Avoidance (Geisser, Robinson, & Henson, 1994).

Although research on composite measures has identified several constructs of clinical significance, several problems characterize this line of study. Because most composites were empirically derived, their composition typically varies somewhat across samples (Boothby, Thorn, Stroud, & Jensen, 1999). Furthermore, because the superordinate constructs reflected in the composites include items from multiple CSQ subscales, the subscales within these constructs may be differentially associated with criterion variables (e.g., Geisser, Robinson, & Henson, 1994). Thus, theoretically and clinically important information can be lost.

DIVERTING ATTENTION

Research regarding the use of attention diversion (e.g., "I try to think of something pleasant") as a coping strategy has been inconclusive. When diverting attention has been associated with positive adjustment to pain, the association generally has been moderated by another variable, such as low levels of pain intensity (Affleck, Urrows, Tennen, & Higgins, 1992), flexible goal setting (Schmitz, Saile, & Nilges, 1996), or pain acuity (Stevens, 1992).

REINTERPRETING SENSATIONS

There is some evidence supporting the efficacy of reinterpretation strategies (e.g., "I tell myself it doesn't hurt") in reducing pain of patients undergoing painful procedures (e.g., Buckelew et al., 1992). Research results with chronic pain, however, have been mixed. The best support has come from longitudinal studies, although these have yielded mixed results (Affleck et al., 1992; Keefe, Affleck, et al., 1997).

COPING SELF-STATEMENTS

Despite the fact that coping self-statements (e.g., "I tell myself that I can overcome the pain") often are taught in multidisciplinary treatment settings, research findings on their efficacy have been sufficiently mixed that some argue that further study of this coping strategy is not warranted (Boothby et al., 1999). It may be, however, that coping self-statements are efficacious only under certain conditions, such as relatively low levels of

pain intensity (Jensen et al., 1992). Similarly, coping self-statements may be mediated by beliefs, such as self-efficacy (Haythornthwaite et al., 1998; Keefe, Kashikar-Zuck, et al., 1997; Large & Strong, 1997). Research that provides a better understanding of mediating and moderating variables appears important to the understanding of coping self-statements in adjustment to pain.

IGNORING PAIN SENSATIONS

The strategy of ignoring pain (e.g., "I don't think about the pain") also has generated mixed results, even in studies where its efficacy is likely to be greatest, such as painful procedures (e.g., Chaves & Brown, 1987; Kashikar-Zuck et al., 1997). Because the preponderance of studies shows no relations between ignoring pain as a coping strategy and adjustment to chronic pain, Boothby and colleagues (1999) have concluded that further research on this strategy does not appear promising.

PRAYING OR HOPING

The use of praying and hoping (e.g., "I have faith in doctors that someday there will be a cure for my pain") as coping strategies generally has been associated with poor adjustment to pain (e.g., Ashby & Lenhart, 1994). Inconsistencies in the research (e.g., Jensen et al., 1992) have been explained several ways. In a factor analysis of the CSQ, praying and hoping items loaded on distinct factors (Robinson et al., 1997), suggesting that inconsistencies may have been the product of psychometric properties of the CSQ. From a more clinical perspective, Boothby and colleagues (1999) suggest that the findings may reflect people's tendency to hope and pray more often when they are doing badly, rather than to do badly because of praying/hoping. The value of this set of coping strategies for clinical practice is not clear.

INCREASING ACTIVITIES

Unlike routine physical exercise, the strategy of increasing activities to distract from pain (e.g., "I do something active, like household chores or projects") has demonstrated little utility as a means of coping with pain (Boothby et al., 1999). It may be, as with other coping strategies, that other variables (e.g., pain intensity, pain acuity) moderate the effects of increased activity on chronic pain adjustment.

MODIFIED VERSIONS OF THE CSQ

The CSQ has been in use for more than two decades and has been studied extensively. Several revisions have been proposed. In a factor analysis of 965 patients with chronic pain, Robinson and colleagues (1997) identified five factors that were generally consistent with CSQ subscales, and four other factors that differed from the CSQ (Hoping, Praying, Increasing Activity, and Distancing from Pain). The factor solution was reduced to six factors due to poor internal reliability of three of the factors. The resulting questionnaire, with 21 of the original CSQ items eliminated, was later named the *Coping Strategies Questionnaire—Revised (CSQ-R)*. A follow-up study of 472 patients with chronic pain (Riley & Robinson, 1997) that employed confirmatory factor analyses to compare available factor solutions found that the 27-item, six-factor model of the CSQ-R provided the best fit: Distraction, Catastrophizing, Ignoring Pain, Distancing from Pain, Coping Self-Statements, and Praying. The CSQ-R factor structure was subsequently replicated in samples of healthy young adults, including both European American and African American subsamples (Hastie, Riley, & Fillingim, 2004). Though the CSQ-R has been used in some studies, it does not appear to have been widely adopted.

Another revision of the CSQ that has gained some clinical interest is the Coping Strategies Questionnaire–24 (CSQ-24; Harland & Georgieff, 2003). A principal components analysis of CSQ data from 214 British patients with back pain revealed a four-factor solution: Catastrophising, Diversion, Cognitive Coping (encompassing items from prior Ignoring Pain and Coping Self-Statements scales), and Reinterpreting. A Praying and Hoping factor was dropped due to low internal consistency reliability. The similarity of this factor solution to past solutions, including the CSQ-R model, was argued as evidence in support of the model's stability. The strengths of the CSQ-24 include brevity; ease of scoring; construct validity per correlations with measures of pain, physical disability, and anxiety/depression; and good internal consistencies (alpha = .75 to .85). A limitation is the need to adjust the Cognitive Coping score (+20%) to allow direct comparison with the other scale scores. Because the development work involved a single sample, cross-validation and additional normative data for the CSQ-24 are needed.

Methodological Developments and More Recently Developed Coping Measures

Moderating Variables

Because coping is a fluid phenomenon (Lazarus & Folkman, 1984), it is important that situation-specific, changeable elements of the coping process be better understood. Research on variables that may moderate relations between coping and adjustment has clarified some of the conditions that influence coping effectiveness. For example, several studies have shown that level of pain intensity moderates relations between coping strategies and adjustment. Affleck and colleagues (1992) found that high levels of coping activity are associated with improved mood for patients reporting low levels of pain, but with worsened mood for patients reporting high levels of pain. Similarly, Jensen and Karoly (1991) found that diverting attention, ignoring pain, and using coping self-statements were positively associated with levels of activity for patients with lower levels of pain, but not for patients with high levels of pain. Associations that hold only for high levels of pain also have been found: Frequent use of coping self-statements has been linked to poor adjustment to pain in patients reporting high (but not low) levels of pain intensity (Jensen et al., 1992). These and other studies underscore the importance of pain intensity as a moderating factor that differentially affects relations between coping and adjustment.

Demographic variables also moderate relations between coping and adjustment. A study of patients with rheumatoid arthritis showed that older patients were more likely than younger patients to use maladaptive coping strategies in response to mild pain, but not severe pain (Watkins, Shifren, Park, & Morrell, 1999). On the other hand, adults across the age range used more active coping strategies in response to mild pain and more maladaptive strategies in response to severe pain. Other studies (e.g., Sullivan, Bishop, & Pivik, 1995) have suggested that gender may be another demographic variable that moderates coping and pain.

Whereas pain intensity and demographic variables have been studied as moderator variables, psychological moderators are relatively understudied. One variable that has been examined involves flexibility of goal setting. In a study of expectations regarding goal setting among patients with chronic pain, patients who were flexible in setting goals reported less depression and disability than did inflexible patients (Schmitz et al., 1996). These data suggest that flexible goal setting may moderate the efficacy of specific coping strategies used with pain, a finding that is consistent with other studies of patients who have adapted successfully to pain (e.g., Large & Strong, 1997; Strong & Large, 1995). It is likely that flexibility in goal setting represents only one of a larger set of beliefs and expectancies that moderate coping efficacy. Other pain-specific beliefs and/or attitudes that deserve further attention as potential moderators include acceptance (McCracken, Carson, et al., 2004), readiness to change (Kerns et al., 1997), and catastrophizing (DeGood, 2000; Geisser, Robinson, & Riley, 1999).

Chronic Pain Coping Inventory

In contrast to the many instruments that have focused on cognitive strategies, the Chronic Pain Coping Inventory (CPCI; Jensen et al., 1995) was developed in both a self-report and significant other format to assess behavioral coping. The item pool for the CPCI was derived from a list of coping responses incorporated into pain treatment programs and/or emphasized in the literature. Factor analysis (based on 176 patients with chronic pain) of 65 total items yielded eight factors, reflecting illness- and wellness-focused strategies. The eight subscales included Guarding, Resting, Asking for Assistance, Relaxation, Task Persistence, Exercising/Stretching, Coping Self-Statements, and Seeking Social Support. Initial results showed that Guarding, Resting, and Asking for Assistance (illness-focused strategies) were associated with poor adjust-

ment to pain. Task Persistence was the only wellness-focused strategy associated with a good adjustment.

A follow-up study of the CPCI (Hadjistavropoulos, MacLeod, & Asmundson, 1999) examined its psychometric properties in a group of 210 patients with chronic pain, all of whom were involved in workers' compensation cases. Factor analysis revealed a similar eight-factor solution. Regression analyses showed that several CPCI subscales discussed in the previous study (Asking for Assistance, Guarding, and Task Persistence) accounted for significant variance in a measure of adjustment. A subsequent study with a sample of 564 veterans with chronic pain validated the eight-factor structure of the CPCI via confirmatory factor analysis, and supported predictive validity of its scales for measures of patient adjustment (Tan, Nguyen, Anderson, Jensen, & Thornby, 2005). In a longitudinal study of subacute low back pain, the Guarding scale of the CPCI and the CSQ Catastrophizing scale were found to have good predictive validity for measures of patient adjustment over a 6-month study period (Truchon & Côté, 2005).

Nielson, Jensen, and Hill (2001) proposed and tested a six-item Pacing scale addition for the CPCI. They noted that this commonly recommended coping strategy in chronic pain programs has no available measures to assess its use. In their sample of 110 fibromyalgia patients, they found evidence for high internal consistency, moderate test–retest reliability and predictive validity of the Pacing scale. Unfortunately, addition of this scale increases the CPCI to 71 items, compromising clinical utility in many settings. However, this shortcoming of the CPCI was addressed by Romano, Jensen, and Turner (2003) through development of a shortened version, the CPCI-42. Their validation study with 154 patients with chronic pain found comparable internal consistency, test–retest stability, and criterion validity correlations for the CPCI-65 and CPCI-42, with high correlations between scales of the two versions. Though further validation is needed for the CPCI-42, it appears to gaining use as a briefer alternative to the assessment of behavioral coping.

Preliminary validation and normative data for the CPCI-65 and CPCI-42 with older adults in retirement communities have been published (Ersek, Turner, & Kemp, 2006). The scales appear to have adequate reliability and construct validity within this subpopulation of persistent pain sufferers. Several translations of the CPCI measures have been reported: a Spanish version of the CPCI-42 (Garcia-Campayo, Pascual, Alda, & Ramirez, 2007) and a French version of the CPCI-65 (Truchon, Côté, & Irachabal, 2006).

Brief Pain Coping Inventory

Another approach to pain coping assessment seeks to incorporate coping responses involving both control and acceptance. Mc-Cracken, Eccleston, and Bell (2005) developed the Brief Pain Coping Inventory (BPCI) in support of an acceptance-based approach to pain coping. The BPCI is an 18-item questionnaire that asks respondents to rate the frequency of engaging in various coping responses on a 0- to 7-point Likert scale. It includes five items designed to measure acceptance coping responses (two reverse scored), with the remaining items querying common cognitive and behavioral coping strategies. Initial results in a sample of 200 patients assessed for interdisciplinary treatment suggested moderate test–retest stability and adequate construct and predictive validities. The authors reported that the BPCI was sensitive to treatment effects. In a follow-up study, 11 items were added to form the Brief Pain Coping Inventory–2 (BPCI-2), which incorporates two scales (Pain Management Strategies, Psychological Flexibility; McCracken & Vowles, 2007). The former includes common cognitive-behavioral strategies as per existing coping inventories, whereas Psychological Flexibility assesses responses associated with mindfulness, acceptance, values-based action, and cognitive diffusion. Initial analyses resulted in elimination of 10 items, resulting in a 19-item measure. The two-factor structure of the BPCI-2 was supported, with evidence of adequate reliability for each scale and moderate construct validity. Psychological Flexibility scores had stronger and broader correlations than Pain Management Strategies with measures of patient functioning, and accounted for significant variance in these measures after researchers controlled for pain and demographic variables. The

BPCI-2 shows promise as a brief measure assessing a broad range of coping strategies. Replication of results in other samples and other clinical settings will help to establish its validity and clinical utility.

Catastrophizing

Catastrophizing, defined as "an exaggerated negative orientation toward pain stimuli and pain experience" (Sullivan, Stanish, Waite, Sullivan, & Tripp, 1998, p. 253), is the single construct from the coping literature that has received the most attention since the early 1990s. Catastrophizing has been associated with many variables reflecting poor adjustment to pain: psychological distress (Geisser, Robinson, Keefe, & Weiner, 1994; Hill, Niven, & Knussen, 1995; Jensen et al., 1992; Ulmer, 1997), disability (Lester, Lefebvre, & Keefe, 1996; Lin & Ward, 1996; Martin et al., 1996; Robinson et al., 1997), and levels of pain intensity (Geisser, Robinson, Keefe, & Weiner, 1994; Harkapaa, 1991; Hill, 1993; Wilkie & Keefe, 1991). There have been discrepant findings, such as those regarding catastrophizing and disability (e.g., Jensen et al., 1992; Pfingsten, Hildebrandt, Leibing, Franz, & Saur, 1997).

Several important practical and theoretical questions about catastrophizing have been raised. For example, Sullivan and D'Eon (1990) found that clinical psychologists viewed catastrophizing and depression as virtually synonymous. Evidence shows, however, that they are not synonymous: Catastrophizing has been associated with self-reports of pain intensity independent of depression (Flor, Behle, & Birbaumer, 1993; Geisser, Robinson, Keefe, & Weiner, 1994; Sullivan et al., 1995). Similarly, Geisser and Roth (1998), after controlling for negative affect, still found a significant relationship between catastrophizing and disability. Recently, Hirsh, George, Riley, and Robinson (2007) studied this relationship with the CSQ-Catastrophizing (CAT) scale in a varied sample of 152 patients with chronic pain. They found that the CSQ-CAT was highly related to measures of negative mood, and added little to the prediction of pain after they controlled for measures of depression, anxiety and anger. Though the acknowledged limitations of the cross-sectional, correlational study design restrict the conclusions that can be drawn, the use of the CSQ-CAT as a catastrophizing measure warrants further investigation.

There also is considerable disagreement regarding the category to which the concept belongs. By dint of its inclusion in the CSQ, it was judged initially to represent a way of coping with pain. Because the CSQ-CAT reflects automatic, irrational cognitions rather than purposeful responses, it has been suggested that catastrophizing is better considered as an appraisal (Jensen, Turner, et al., 1991). Noting that catastrophizing can "increase distress and can mobilize the individual for action" (Keefe, Kashikar-Zuck, et al., 1997, p. 197), others have contended that catastrophizing does represent a coping strategy.

While most research using the CSQ has included catastrophizing as a measure of coping, the view that that catastrophizing represents a belief rather than a coping response gained increasing acceptance over time (Boothby et al., 1999; Geisser et al., 1999; Haythornthwaite et al., 1998). Regardless of its category, the weight of research evidence clearly underscores the importance of catastrophizing in coping research. Geisser and colleagues (1999), in fact, have argued that it should receive increased attention, perhaps, as a variable that moderates the likelihood of coping adaptively to pain. Although this stance has not been universally embraced (Haythornthwaite & Heinberg, 1999; Keefe, Lefebvre, & Smith, 1999; Thorn et al., 1999), the debate has served to stimulate further research aimed at clarifying its theoretical and clinical role.

Pain Catastrophizing Scale

The Pain Catastrophizing Scale (PCS; Sullivan et al., 1995) is a brief, 12-item instrument that examines three components of catastrophizing: Rumination ("I can't stop thinking about how much it hurts"), Magnification ("I worry that something serious may happen"), and Helplessness ("There is nothing I can do to reduce the intensity of the pain"). Initial studies of the PCS with undergraduates showed that catastrophizing predicts levels of pain and distress reported in response to pain inductions. In a more applied setting, PCS scores predicted

levels of pain and distress among clinical patients undergoing electromyographic (EMG) procedures (Sullivan et al., 1995). PCS scores also have been associated with thought intrusions among patients awaiting painful dental procedures (Sullivan & Neish, 1997), and with pain, disability, and employment status among patients with intractable musculoskeletal pain (Sullivan et al., 1998). The latter study also showed PCS scores, especially the Ruminative subscale, to predict disability after controlling for variance associated with levels of pain intensity, depression, and anxiety. Osman and colleagues (1997) provided additional psychometric support for the PCS in undergraduate samples, and in adult community and outpatient pain samples (Osman et al., 2000).

In recent years, additional research has provided information on the psychometrics of the PCS in demographic subgroups, and has expanded its utility through significant other and child versions. Support for the PCS model representing catastrophizing as a single construct with three underlying dimensions (factors) was found in a large undergraduate Canadian sample, with invariance of the model across gender (D'Eon, Harris, & Ellis, 2004). In a racially diverse sample of workers' compensation claimants with low back injuries, Chibnall and Tait (2005) found support for a two-factor model of the PCS: Rumination and Powerlessness. This fit of this model was superior in the African American subsample. Because comparative data on the PCS in an occupational injury sample have not been reported, confirmation of these findings is needed. Cano, Leonard, and Franz (2005) developed the Significant Other Version of the PCS (PCS-S) to assess individuals' catastrophizing about their significant other's pain. A similar three-factor model (with two cross-loadings) was identified in undergraduate samples, with invariance across gender and racial groups. This factor structure was then replicated, and content validity of the scale supported, in a clinical sample of pain patients and their spouses. Preliminary validation of a Child Version of the PCS (PCS-C) has also been reported (Crombez et al., 2003). The growing body of psychometric and normative data in clinical samples has increased the utility of the PCS, and the PCS-S will provide additional benefit in some clinic and research applications.

The utility of the PCS has also been enhanced by multiple translations in recent years. These include Dutch (Van Damme, Crombez, Bijttebier, Goubert, & Van Houdenhove, 2002), Catalan (Miro, Nieto, & Huguet, 2008), German (Meyer, Sprott, & Mannion, 2008), and Chinese (Yap et al., 2008) versions.

Acceptance Measures

Though space limitations preclude a full review, measures of chronic pain acceptance warrant mention as valuable tools in the assessment of pain beliefs and coping. The most widely used measure of acceptance has been the Chronic Pain Acceptance Questionnaire (CPAQ; McCracken, Vowles, & Eccleston, 2004). It comprises 20 items loading on two factors: Activities Engagement and Pain Willingness. Adequate psychometric properties have been reported, along with three subgroups from cluster analysis: high scores on both subscales, low scores on both subscales, and high Activities Engagement with low Pain Willingness (McCracken, Vowles, & Eccleston, 2004; Vowles et al., 2008). These subgroupings were found to be predictive of other aspects of chronic pain adjustment.

A promising newer measure is the Pain Solutions Questionnaire (PaSol), designed to assess several dimensions of assimilative and accommodative coping responses to pain (De Vlieger, Van den Bussche, Eccleston, & Crombez, 2006). It contains 14 items with a four-factor structure: Solving Pain, Meaningfulness of Life Despite Pain, Acceptance of Insolubility of Pain, and Belief in a Solution. In a follow-up validation study, a combined assimilative coping score was generated, based on three of the subscale scores (Crombez, Eccleston, Van Hamme, & De Vlieger, 2008). In construct validity analyses, expected patterns of correlations with the CPAQ scales were demonstrated (De Vlieger et al., 2006). The PaSol was developed and evaluated in Dutch. An English version was published (De Vlieger et al., 2006) but we are not aware of a published evaluation of its psychometrics.

Brief Versions of Beliefs and Coping Measures

Length of beliefs and coping assessment measures, and the associated time demands and patient burden have long been recognized as barriers to use of these tools in many clinical and research contexts. This is especially true when a multidimensional assessment is desired, requiring use of longer composite measures or concurrent multiple tools. Jensen, Keefe, Lefebvre, Romano, and Turner (2003) have directly tackled this problem through the development and testing of one- and two-item measures of pain beliefs and coping. The very brief measures were developed in two clinical chronic pain samples (n's = 141 and 87). The authors used correlations of each item with the Parent subscale and with other measures of pain and functioning, and pre- to posttreatment item t-test comparisons, combined with expert agreement, to identify the items from common beliefs and coping measures (including the CPCI, SOPA, PBAPI, and CSQ) that best represented the respective subscales and their constructs.

Once the primary item was identified, hierarchical regression was used to identify the second item accounting for the most incremental variance in predicting the relevant subscale. Validity and treatment sensitivity analyses were then conducted for each one- and two-item scale.

Though the one-item measures were found to be reasonable representations of their parent subscales, the two-item versions showed consistently higher associations (median R at pretreatment = .88, median R posttreatment = .87), and were more sensitive to treatment changes. The authors concluded that use of both one- and two-item versions was supported, with the two-item versions providing a psychometric advantage. The total length of the resulting one- and two-item per scale versions of the measures were CPCI, 8 and 16 items; CSQ, 7 and 14 items; SOPA, 7 and 14 items; and PBAPI, 4 and 8 items.

In a follow-up study, the utility of the two-item per scale versions of several of these measures (CPCI-16, CSQ-14, and SOPA-14) was tested in a sample of 563 veterans referred to an outpatient pain program (Tan, Nguyen, Cardin, & Jensen, 2006). Strong associations of the two-item versions with the respective subscales were found (R = .70–.91). Construct validity of the brief scales was supported by their ability to predict concurrent measures of depression, functional activities and interference, and pain. Though Jensen, Keefe, and colleagues (2003) acknowledged the reduction in reliability for the brief versions, they suggested several suitable applications: epidemiological research; research with individuals having cognitive or communication difficulties; exploratory studies; clinical screening and monitoring when longer measures are not feasible; and, for diary and ecological momentary assessment study designs, where repeated assessments are required. Since practical considerations preclude the use of longer measures in most of these circumstances, these brief measures provide reasonable alternatives with acceptable validity. Given the necessary reductions in reliability, examination of test–retest stability in future studies will be beneficial.

Concluding Comments on Coping

Coping continues to be a highly studied construct in the field of pain management. Since 2001, this continued research has helped to clarify our understanding of coping processes in pain, while highlighting its complexity. The CSQ remains the most widely studied and used measure of coping. Its clinical utility has been enhanced by the development of shortened versions and language translations. The original version continues to have the strongest base of supporting research and normative data. The CSQ-R and the CSQ-24 appear to have good potential, particularly in clinical settings, though recommendations regarding their use await further study. We recommend the CPCI for applications in which a focus on behavioral strategies is appropriate, particularly in the context of interdisciplinary pain rehabilitation programs. Length, even in its shortened form, is a barrier to use in some settings. The BPCI-2 may help to fill the need for a brief, clinically oriented coping measure in settings where an expanded view that incorporates acceptance-based approaches is desired. It is our hope that further research will support its use in varied clinical settings.

Catastrophizing and acceptance are now well-established constructs in the psychology of pain. The availability of several well-studied measures to assess these important domains is encouraging. We recommend the PCS and CPAQ for applications in which reliable assessment of these constructs is desired. Further development of newer measures will likely broaden the choices of clinicians and researchers in future years.

Several general comments about research on coping are warranted. Although existing tools allow assessment of a broader range of coping strategies than was available in the past, they still do not exhaust the coping strategies that can be assessed. For example, research has suggested that problem solving, a construct for which there is no established measure in the pain literature, is a skill relevant to adjustment to pain (Kole-Snijders et al., 1999). Pacing, a poorly studied but widely taught coping skill in many self-management programs, has only recently been incorporated into a coping measure (Nielson et al., 2001). For adjustment to chronic pain, the comparative value of traditional cognitive-behavioral coping strategies versus those based on acceptance and psychological flexibility has recently been explored (McCracken & Eccleston, 2006; Vowles & McCracken, 2010). We expect further elaboration of the role of specific coping skills and approaches to coping in adjusting to pain.

Longitudinal studies have begun to clarify processes relevant to coping and pain adjustment. The daily tracking strategy used in longitudinal research, while laborious, holds considerable promise for a better understanding of causal mechanisms linking coping and adjustment. Clearly, further attention to this area is needed. Attention also is needed to assess coping in outcome research. Outcome instruments keyed to treatment interventions (e.g., CPCI; Jensen et al., 1995) hold promise for outcome research, especially if treatment interventions are linked to coping variables. In addition, the daily tracking methodology holds promise for tracking the course of treatment-related change in outcome research.

Finally, a methodological issue that continues to deserve more study is the role of moderating variables. Several descriptive variables have been shown to moderate relations between coping and adjustment, including levels of pain intensity, age, gender, and pain duration. Other variables that might influence relations between coping and adjustment have received less attention. There is a particular need for research that examines attitudes/beliefs that moderate or mediate coping efficacy, such as readiness for change, flexibility in goal setting, and self-efficacy. More attention to these and other variables is likely to give us a better theoretical understanding of the fluid processes that influence the efficacy of coping efforts. At least as important, a better understanding of moderating and mediating influences will help us to identify for whom and under what conditions coping strategies are most likely to help and/or hinder adjustment to pain.

CONCLUDING COMMENTS

Pain research has become internationalized. A shortcoming in our chapter coverage may be an insufficient awareness of the many measures used outside of North America, especially in non-English-speaking countries. Also, we have ignored many of the controversial issues in test construction theory. Some measures are developed via internal consistency models, whereas others are much more concerned with face validity and external criterion validation. Based on test construction philosophy and goals, measures attempting to capture multiple dimensions of a behavioral construct may or may not contain factorially pure scales. Furthermore, measures developed via traditional classical test theory methodology are significantly limited in interpretation of scores. Variance attributable to characteristics of the test cannot be separated, and differential functioning of test items at varying levels of the measured construct is not taken into account. Newer health measures developed through item response theory methods provide an alternative (Hays, Morales, & Reise, 2000).

There are several current general needs and trends in psychosocial assessment that we expect to continue into the next decade. First of all, we expect there to be a continuing shift toward the assessment of psychosocial factors contributing to positive coping and positive treatment outcome, rather than a focus on primarily psychosocial risk factors.

We expect the trend toward use of brief self-report forms to continue, especially in applied clinical settings where administrative costs and efficiency are primary. This is particularly important in light of the fact that most pain management services are outpatient settings. There is increasing need for forms that can readily be computer-administered and -scored by the clinician or a commercial scoring service. Psychometric equivalence of pain self-report measures, when administered by computer, is an often neglected but important assessment consideration (Cook, Roberts, Henderson, Van Winkle, Chastain, & Hamill-Ruth, 2004).

Additional attention to pain beliefs and coping across the lifespan is needed. In the previous edition of this volume, we commented on the development of the Pain Coping Questionnaire (Reid, Gilbert, & McGrath, 1998), an instrument showing good potential for coping assessment among children and adolescents. The adaptation and testing of an established measure such as the PCS for children represents another positive advance for coping assessment across the lifespan. Since 2001, there have also been several positive developments relating to beliefs and coping assessment across adult age groups. These include the publication of psychometrics and norms of the CPCI with older adults (Ersek et al., 2006) and the development of the revised PAQ (PAQ-R; Yong et al., 2003). Parmalee (2005) has reviewed measures of mood and psychosocial function, including beliefs and coping, and known research supporting use with older adults. With continued shifting of age demographics, the assessment of pain in older adults has gained increasing attention (Hadjistavropoulos et al., 2007), but assessment of beliefs and coping in this age group remains an underdeveloped area (see Gauthier & Gagliese, Chapter 12, this volume).

Finally, although use of comprehensive psychosocial measures may remain the standard in treatment settings, much of the assessment research for the past two decades has focused on the more specialized aspects of psychosocial adjustment and functioning, as reflected in all the work on beliefs and coping measurement. This trend may have peaked in the past few years, which makes it difficult to speculate on future trends. Practical clinical and market dictates continue to pose a barrier between pain assessment activities in research-oriented settings and strictly applied settings.

REFERENCES

Abramson, L. Y., Seligman, M. E. P., & Teasdale, J. D. (1978). Learned helplessness in humans: Critique and reformulations. *Journal of Abnormal Psychology, 87*, 49–74.

Affleck, G., Urrows, S., Tennen, H., & Higgins, P. (1992). Daily coping with pain from rheumatoid arthritis: Patterns and correlates. *Pain, 51*, 221–229.

Angst, F., Verra, M. L., Lehmann, S., & Aeschlimann, A. (2008). Responsiveness of five condition-specific and generic outcome assessment instruments for chronic pain. *BMC Medical Research Methodology, 8*, 26.

Ashby, J. S., & Lenhart, R. S. (1994). Prayer as a coping strategy for chronic pain patients. *Rehabilitation Psychology, 39*, 205–209.

Bandura, A. (1977). Self-efficacy: Toward a unifying theory of behavioral change. *Psychological Review, 84*, 191–215.

Banks, S. M., & Kerns, R. D. (1996). Explaining high rates of depression in chronic pain: A diathesis–stress framework. *Psychological Bulletin, 119*, 95–100.

Beckham, J. C., Keefe, F. J., Caldwell, D. S., & Roodman, A. A. (1991). Pain coping strategies in rheumatoid arthritis: Relationships to pain, disability, depression, and daily hassles. *Behavior Therapy, 22*, 113–124.

Bergner, M., Bobbitt, R. A., Carter, W. B., & Gilson, B. S. (1981). The Sickness Impact Profile: Development and final revision of a health status measure. *Medical Care, 19*, 787–805.

Blalock, S. J., DeVellis, B. M., & Giorgino, K. B. (1995). The relationship between coping and psychological well-being among people with osteoarthritis: A problem-specific approach. *Annals of Behavioral Medicine, 17*, 107–115.

Boothby, J. L., Thorn, B. E., Stroud, M. W., & Jensen, M. P. (1999). Coping with pain. In R. J. Gatchel & D. C. Turk (Eds.), *Psychosocial factors in pain: Critical perspectives* (pp. 343–359). New York: Guilford Press.

Brown, G. K., & Nicassio, P. M. (1987). Development of a questionnaire for the assessment of active and passive coping strategies in chronic pain patients. *Pain, 31*, 53–63.

Buchbinder, R., & Jolley, D. (2007). Improvements in general practitioner beliefs and stated management of back pain persist 4.5 years after the cessation of a public media campaign. *Spine, 32*, 156–162.

Buckelew, S. P., Conway, R. C., Shutty, M. S., Lawrence, J. A., Grafing, M. R., Anderson, S. K., et al. (1992). Spontaneous coping strategies to manage acute pain and anxiety during electrodiagnostic studies. *Archives of Physical Medicine and Rehabilitation, 73*, 594–598.

Cano, A., Leonard, M. T., & Franz, A. (2005). The Significant Other Version of the Pain Catastrophizing Scale (PCS-S): Preliminary validation. *Pain, 119*, 26–37.

Chaves, J. F., & Brown, J. M. (1987). Spontaneous cognitive strategies for the control of clinical pain and stress. *Journal of Behavioral Medicine, 10*, 263–276.

Chibnall, J. T., & Tait, R. C. (2005). Confirmatory factor analysis of the Pain Catastrophizing Scale in African American and Caucasian Workers' Compensation claimants with low back injuries. *Pain, 113*, 369–375.

Cook, A. J., & DeGood, D. E. (2006). The Cognitive Risk Profile for Pain: Development of a self-report inventory for identifying beliefs and attitudes that interfere with pain management. *Clinical Journal of Pain, 22*, 332–345.

Cook, A. J., DeGood, D. E., & Chastain, D. C. (1999, August). *Age differences in pain beliefs*. Poster presented at 9th World Congress on Pain, Vienna, Austria.

Cook, A. J., Roberts, D. A., Henderson, M. D., Van Winkle, L. C., Chastain, D. C., & Hamill-Ruth, R. J. (2004). Electronic pain questionnaires: A randomized, crossover comparison with paper questionnaires for chronic pain assessment. *Pain, 110*, 310–317.

Crombez, G., Bijttebier, P., Eccleston, C., Mascagni, T., Mertens, G., Goubert, L., et al. (2003). The Child Version of the Pain Catastrophizing Scale (PCS-C): A preliminary validation. *Pain, 104*, 639–646.

Crombez, G., Eccleston, C., Van Hamme, G., & De Vlieger, P. (2008). Attempting to solve the problem of pain: A questionnaire study in acute and chronic pain patients. *Pain, 137*, 556–563.

Cruess, D. G., Minor, S., Antoni, M. H., & Millon, T. (2007). Utility of the MBMD to predict adherence to highly active antiretroviral therapy (HAART) medication regimens among HIV-positive men and women. *Journal of Personality Assessment, 89*, 277–290.

DeGood, D. E. (2000). The relationship of pain coping strategies to adjustment and functioning. In J. N. Weisburg & R. J. Gatchel (Eds.), *Personality characteristics of pain patients: Recent advances and future directions* (pp. 129–164). Washington, DC: American Psychological Association.

DeGood, D. E., & Shutty, M. S. (1992). Assessment of pain beliefs, coping, and self-efficacy.

In D. C. Turk & R. Melzack (Eds.), *Handbook of pain assessment* (pp. 214–234). New York: Guilford Press.

D'Eon, J. L., Harris, C. A., & Ellis, J. A. (2004). Testing factorial validity and gender invariance of the Pain Catastrophizing Scale. *Journal of Behavioral Medicine, 27*, 361–372.

Derogatis, L. R. (1983). *SCL-90R: Administration, scoring and procedures manual-II for the revised version.* Towson, MD: Clinical Psychometric Research.

De Vlieger, P., Van den Bussche, E., Eccleston, C., & Crombez, G. (2006). Finding a solution to the problem of pain: Conceptual formulation and the development of the Pain Solutions Questionnaire (PaSol). *Pain, 123*, 285–293.

Dijkstra, A. (2005). The validity of the stages of change model in the adoption of the self-management approach in chronic pain. *Clinical Journal of Pain, 21*, 27–37.

Dozois, D. J. A., Dobson, K. S., Wong, M., Hughes, D., & Long, A. (1996). Predictive utility of the CSQ in low back pain: Individual vs. composite measures. *Pain, 66*, 171–180.

Duquette, J., McKinley, P. A., & Litowski, J. (2005). Test–retest reliability and internal consistency of the Quebec-French version of the Survey of Pain Attitudes. *Archives of Physical Medicine and Rehabilitation, 86*, 782–288.

Endler, N. S., Parker, J. D. A., & Summerfeldt, L. J. (1993). Coping with health problems: Conceptual and methodological issues. *Canadian Journal of Behavioral Science, 25*, 384–399.

Ersek, M., Turner, J. A., & Kemp, C. A. (2006). Use of the Chronic Pain Coping Inventory to assess older adults' pain coping strategies. *Journal of Pain, 7*, 833–842.

Fishbein, M., & Ajzen, I. (1975). *Belief, attitude, intention and behavior: An introduction to theory and research.* Reading, MA: Addison-Wesley.

Flor, H., Behle, D. J., & Birbaumer, N. (1993). Assessment of pain-related cognitions in chronic pain patients. *Behaviour Research and Therapy, 31*, 63–73.

Folkman, S., & Lazarus, R. S. (1980). An analysis of coping in a middle-aged community sample. *Journal Health and Social Behavior, 21*, 219–239.

Fordyce, W. E. (1976). *Behavioral methods for chronic pain and illness.* St Louis, MO: Mosby.

Garcia-Campayo, J., Pascual, A., Alda, M., & Ramirez, M. T. G. (2007). Coping with fibromyalgia: Usefulness of the Chronic Pain Coping Inventory–42. *Pain, 132*, S68–S76.

Garratt, A. M., Schmidt, L., Mackintosh, A., & Fitzpatrick, R. (2002). Quality of life measurement: Bibliographic study of patient assessed health outcome measures. *British Medical Journal, 324*, 1417–1421.

Gatchel, R. J., & Epker, J. (1999). Psychosocial predictors of chronic pain and response to treatment. In R. J. Gatchel & D. C. Turk (Eds.), *Psychosocial factors in pain: Critical perspectives* (pp. 412–434). New York: Guilford Press.

Gatchel, R. J., Peng, Y. B., Peters, M. L., Fuchs, P. N., & Turk, D. C. (2007). The biopsychosocial approach to chronic pain: Scientific advances and future directions. *Psychological Bulletin, 33*, 581–624.

Geisser, M. E., Robinson, M. E., & Henson, C. D. (1994). The Coping Strategies Questionnaire and chronic pain adjustment: A conceptual and empirical reanalysis. *Clinical Journal of Pain, 10*, 98–106.

Geisser, M. E., Robinson, M. E., Keefe, F. J., & Weiner, M. L. (1994). Catastrophizing, depression and the sensory, affective and evaluative aspects of chronic pain. *Pain, 59*, 79–83.

Geisser, M. E., Robinson, M. E., & Riley, J. L. (1999). Pain beliefs, coping, and adjustment to chronic pain: Let's focus more on the negative. *Pain Forum, 8*, 161–168.

Geisser, M. E., & Roth, R. S. (1998). Knowledge of and agreement with pain diagnosis: Relation to pain beliefs, pain severity, disability, and psychological distress. *Journal of Occupational Rehabilitation, 8*, 73–88.

Gil, K. M., Abrams, M. R., Phillips, G., & Williams, D. A. (1992). Sickle cell disease pain: 2. Predicting health care use and activity level at 9-month follow-up. *Journal of Consulting and Clinical Psychology, 60*, 267–273.

Gil, K. M., Thompson, R. J., Keith, B. R., Tota-Faucette, M., Noll, S., & Kinney, T. R. (1993). Sickle cell disease pain in children and adolescents: Change in pain frequency and coping strategies over time. *Journal of Pediatric Psychology, 18*, 621–637.

Gonzalez, R., Soler, E., & Ferrer, V. A. (2002). Pain Beliefs and Perceptions Inventory: Confirmatory factor analysis [Spanish]. *Revista Iberoamericana de Diagnostico y Evaluacion Psicologica, 14*, 135–148.

Hadjistavropoulos, H. D., MacLeod, F. K., & Asmundson, G. J. G. (1999). Validation of the Chronic Pain Coping Inventory. *Pain, 80*, 471–481.

Hadjistavropoulos, T., Herr, K., Turk, D. C., Fine, P. G., Dworkin, R. H., Helme, R., et al. (2007). An interdisciplinary expert consensus statement on assessment of pain in older persons. *Clinical Journal of Pain, 23*, S1–S43.

Harkapaa, K. (1991). Relationships of psychological distress and health locus of control beliefs with the use of cognitive and behavioral coping strategies in low back pain patients. *Clinical Journal of Pain, 7*, 275–282.

Harland, N. J., & Georgieff, K. (2003). Development of the Coping Strategies Questionnaire 24, a clinically utilitarian version of the Coping Strategies Questionnaire. *Rehabilitation Psychology, 48*, 296–300.

Hastie, B. A., Riley, J. L., & Fillingim, R. B. (2004). Ethnic differences in pain coping: Factor structure of the Coping Strategies Questionnaire and Coping Strategies Questionnaire—Revised. *Journal of Pain, 5*, 304–316.

Hathaway, S. R., McKinley, J. C., Butcher, J. N., Dahlstrom, W. G., Graham, J. R., Tellegen, A., et al. (1989). *Minnesota Multiphasic Personality Inventory-2: Manual for administration.* Minneapolis: University of Minnesota Press.

Hays, R., Morales, L., & Reise, S. (2000). Item response theory and health outcomes measurement in the 21st century. *Medical Care, 38*(Suppl. 2), 28–42.

Haythornthwaite, J. A., & Heinberg, L. J. (1999). Coping with pain: What works, under what circumstances, and in what ways? *Pain Forum, 8*, 172–175.

Haythornthwaite, J. A., Menefee, L. A., Heinberg, L. J., & Clark, M. R. (1998). Pain coping strategies predict perceived control over pain. *Pain, 77*, 33–39.

Helmes, E., & Goburdhun, A. (2007). Cognitions related to chronic pain: Revision and extension of the Cognitive Evaluation Questionnaire. *Clinical Journal of Pain, 23*, 53–61.

Herda, C. A., Siegeris, K., & Basler, H. D. (1994). The Pain Beliefs and Perceptions Inventory: Further evidence for a 4-factor structure. *Pain, 57*, 85–90.

Hill, A. (1993). The use of pain coping strategies by patients with phantom limb pain. *Pain, 55*, 347–353.

Hill, A., Niven, C. A., & Knussen, C. (1995). The role of coping in adjustment to phantom limb pain. *Pain, 62*, 79–86.

Hirsh, A. T., George, S. A., Riley, J. L., & Robinson, M. E. (2007). An evaluation of the measurement of pain catastrophizing by the Coping Strategies Questionnaire. *European Journal of Pain, 11*, 75–81.

Hockings, R. L., McAuley, J. H., & Maher, C. G. (2008). A systematic review of the predictive ability of the Orebro Musculoskeletal Pain Questionnaire. *Spine, 33*, E494–E500.

Hopwood, C. J., Creech, S. K., Clark, T. S., Meagher, M. W., & Morey, L. C. (2008). Optimal scoring of the Multidimensional Pain Inventory in a chronic pain sample. *Journal of Clinical Psychology in Medical Settings, 15*, 301–307.

Irachabal, S., Koleck, M., Rascle, N., & Bruchon-Schweitzer, M. (2008). Pain coping strategies:

French adaptation of the Coping Strategies Questionnaire (CSQ-F) [French]. *Encéphale, 34*, 47–53.

Jacob, M. C., & Kerns, R. D. (2001). Assessment of the psychosocial context of the experience of chronic pain. In D. C. Turk & R. Melzack (Eds.), *Handbook of pain assessment* (2nd ed., pp. 362–384). New York: Guilford Press.

Jensen, M. P., & Karoly, P. (1989, March). *Revision and cross-validation of the Survey of Pain Attitudes (SOPA).* Poster presented at the annual meeting of the Society of Behavioral Medicine, San Francisco.

Jensen, M. P., & Karoly, P. (1991). Control beliefs, coping efforts, and adjustment to chronic pain. *Journal of Consulting and Clinical Psychology, 59*, 431–438.

Jensen, M. P., Karoly, P., & Huger, R. (1987). The development and preliminary validation of an instrument to assess patients' attitudes toward pain. *Journal of Psychosomatic Research, 31*, 393–400.

Jensen, M. P., Keefe, F. J., Lefebvre, J. C., Romano, J. M., & Turner, J. A. (2003). One- and two-item measures of pain beliefs and coping strategies. *Pain, 104*, 453–469.

Jensen, M. P., Nielson, W. R., & Kerns, R. D. (2003). Toward the development of a motivational model of pain self-management. *Journal of Pain, 4*, 477–492.

Jensen, M. P., Nielson, W. R., Turner, J. A., Romano, J. M., & Hill, M. L. (2003). Readiness to self-manage pain is associated with coping and with psychological and physical functioning among patients with chronic pain. *Pain, 104*, 529–537.

Jensen, M. P., Nielson, W. R., Turner, J. A., Romano, J. M., & Hill, M. L. (2004). Changes in readiness to self-manage pain are associated with improvement in multidisciplinary pain treatment and pain coping. *Pain, 111*, 84–95.

Jensen, M. P., Turner, J. A., & Romano, J. M. (1991). Self-efficacy and outcome expectancies: Relationship to chronic pain coping strategies and adjustment. *Pain, 44*, 263–269.

Jensen, M. P., Turner, J. A., & Romano, J. M. (1992). Chronic pain coping measures: Individual vs. composite scores. *Pain, 51*, 273–280.

Jensen, M. P., Turner, J. A., & Romano, J. M. (2000). Pain belief assessment: A comparison of the short and long versions of the Survey of Pain Attitudes. *Journal of Pain, 1*, 138–150.

Jensen, M. P., Turner, J. A., & Romano, J. M. (2007). Changes after multidisciplinary pain treatment in patient pain beliefs and coping are associated with concurrent changes in patient functioning. *Pain, 131*, 38–47.

Jensen, M. P., Turner, J. A., Romano, J. M., & Karoly, P. (1991). Coping with chronic pain:

A critical review of the literature. *Pain*, *47*, 249–283.

Jensen, M. P., Turner, J. A., Romano, J. M., & Lawler, B. K. (1994). Relationship of pain-specific beliefs to chronic pain adjustment. *Pain*, *57*, 301–309.

Jensen, M. P., Turner, J. A., Romano, J. M., & Strom, S. E. (1995). The Chronic Pain Coping Inventory: Development and preliminary validation. *Pain*, *60*, 203–216.

Karoly, P., Ruehlman, L. S., Aiken, L. S., Todd, M., & Newton, C. (2006). Evaluating chronic pain impact among patients in primary care: Further validation of a brief assessment instrument. *Pain Medicine*, *7*, 289–298.

Kashikar-Zuck, S., Keefe, F. J., Kornguth, P., Beaupre, P., Holzberg, A., & Delong, D. (1997). Pain coping and the pain experience during mammography: A preliminary study. *Pain*, *73*, 165–172.

Keefe, F. J., Affleck, G., Lefebvre, J. C., Starr, K., Caldwell, D. S., & Tennen, H. (1997). Pain coping strategies and coping efficacy in rheumatoid arthritis: A daily process analysis. *Pain*, *69*, 35–42.

Keefe, F. J., Caldwell, D. S., Martinez, S., Nunley, J., Beckham, J., & Williams, D. A. (1991). Analyzing pain in rheumatoid arthritis patients: Pain coping strategies in patients who have had knee replacement surgery. *Pain*, *46*, 153–160.

Keefe, F. J., Kashikar-Zuck, S., Robinson, E., Salley, A., Beaupre, P., Caldwell, D., et al. (1997). Pain coping strategies that predict patients' and spouses' ratings of patients' self-efficacy. *Pain*, *73*, 191–199.

Keefe, F. J., Lefebvre, J. C., & Smith, S. J. (1999). Catastrophizing research: Avoiding conceptual errors and maintaining a balanced perspective. *Pain Forum*, *8*, 176–180.

Kerns, R. D., & Rosenberg, R. (1999). Predicting responses to self-management treatments for chronic pain: Application of the pain stages of change model. *Pain*, *82*, 1–7.

Kerns, R. D., Rosenberg, R., Jamison, R. N., Caudill, M. A., & Haythornthwaite, J. (1997). Readiness to adopt a self-management approach to chronic pain: The Pain Stages of Change Questionnaire (PSOCQ). *Pain*, *72*, 227–234.

Kerns, R. D., Turk, D. C., & Rudy, T. E. (1985). The West Haven–Yale Multidimensional Pain Inventory (WHYMPI). *Pain*, *23*, 345–356.

Kobasa, S. C. (1979). Stressful life events, personality, and health: An inquiry into hardiness. *Journal of Personality and Social Psychology*, *37*, 1–11.

Kole-Snijders, A. M., Vlaeyen, J. W., Goossens, M. E., Ruten-van Molken, M. P., Heuts, P. H., van Breukelen, G., et al. (1999). Chronic low-

back pain: What does cognitive coping skills training add to operant behavioral treatment?: Results of a randomized clinical trial. *Journal of Consulting and Clinical Psychology*, *67*, 931–944.

Krousael-Wood, M. A., McCune, T. W., Abdoh, A., & Re, R. N. (1994). Predicting work status for patients in an occupational medicine setting who report back pain. *Archives of Family Medicine*, *3*, 349–355.

Large, R. G., & Strong, J. (1997). The personal constructs of coping with chronic low back pain: Is coping a necessary evil? *Pain*, *73*, 245–252.

Lazarus, R. A. (1991). Cognition and motivation in emotion. *American Psychologist*, *46*, 353–367.

Lazarus, R. S., & Folkman, S. (1984). *Stress, appraisal, and coping*. New York: Springer.

Leeuw, M., Goossens, M. E., Linton, S. J., Crombez, G., Boersma, K., & Vlaeyen, J. W. S. (2007). The fear–avoidance model of musculoskeletal pain: Current state of scientific evidence. *Journal of Behavioral Medicine*, *30*, 77–94.

Lester, N., Lefebvre, J. C., & Keefe, F. J. (1996). Pain in young adults: III. Relationships of three pain-coping measures to pain and activity interference. *Clinical Journal of Pain*, *12*, 291–300.

Lin, C., & Ward, S. E. (1996). Perceived self-efficacy and outcome expectancies in coping with chronic low back pain. *Research in Nursing and Health*, *19*, 299–310.

Linton, S. J., & Hallden, K. B. A. (1998). Can we screen for problematic back pain?: A screening questionnaire for predicting outcome in acute and subacute back pain. *Clinical Journal of Pain*, *14*, 209–215.

Martin, M. Y., Bradley, L. A., Alexander, R. W., Alarcon, G. S., Triana-Alexander, M., Aaron, L. A., et al. (1996). Coping strategies predict disability in patients with primary fibromyalgia. *Pain*, *68*, 45–53.

McCracken, L. M., Carson, J. W., Eccleston, C., & Keefe, F. J. (2004). Acceptance and change in the context of chronic pain. *Pain*, *109*, 4–7.

McCracken, L. M., & Eccleston, C. (2003). Coping or acceptance: What to do about chronic pain? *Pain*, *105*, 197–204.

McCracken, L. M., & Eccleston, C. (2006). A comparison of the relative utility of coping and acceptance-based measures in a sample of chronic pain sufferers. *European Journal of Pain*, *10*, 23–29.

McCracken, L. M., Eccleston, C., & Bell, L. (2005). Clinical assessment of behavioral coping responses: Preliminary results from a brief inventory. *European Journal of Pain*, *9*, 69–78.

McCracken, L. M., & Vowles, K. E. (2007). Psychological flexibility and traditional pain management strategies in relation to patient functioning with chronic pain: An examination of a revised instrument. *Journal of Pain, 8,* 700–707.

McCracken, L. M., Vowles, K. E., & Eccleston, C. (2004). Acceptance of chronic pain: Component analysis and a revised assessment tool. *Pain, 107,* 159–166.

McNair, D. M., Lorr, M., & Droppleman, L. F. (1992). *Manual for the Profile of Mood States (POMS): Revised.* San Diego, CA: Educational and Industrial Testing Service.

Mechanic, D., & Volkart, E. H. (1960). Illness behavior and medical diagnosis. *Journal of Health and Human Behavior, 1,* 86–96.

Melzack, R. (1975). The McGill Pain Questionnaire: Major properties and scoring methods. *Pain, 1,* 277–299.

Melzack, R., & Wall, P. D. (1965). Pain mechanisms: A new theory. *Science, 150,* 971–979.

Meyer, K., Sprott, H., & Mannion, A. F. (2008). Cross-cultural adaptation, reliability, and validity of the German version of the Pain Catastrophizing Scale. *Journal of Psychosomatic Research, 64,* 469–478.

Millon, T., Antoni, M., Millon, C., Meagher, S., & Grossman, S. (2000). *Millon Behavioral Medicine Diagnostic (MBMD) manual.* Minneapolis, MN: National Computer Systems.

Millon, T., Green, C., & Meagher, R. (1983). *Millon Behavioral Health Inventory manual* (3rd ed.). Minneapolis, MN: National Computer Systems.

Miro, J., Nieto, R., & Huguet, A. (2008). The Catalan version of the Pain Catastrophizing Scale: A useful instrument to assess catastrophic thinking in whiplash patients. *Journal of Pain, 9,* 397–406.

National Advisory Committee on Health and Disability. (1997). *Guide to assessing yellow flags in acute low back pain.* Wellington, New Zealand: Ministry of Health.

Naurda, U., McLendon, P. M., Andresen, E. M., & Armbrecht, E. (2003). The SIP68: An abbreviated sickness impact profile for disability. *Quality of Life Research, 12,* 583–595.

Nicassio, P. M., Schoenfeld-Smith, K., Radojevic, V., & Schuman, C. (1995). Pain coping mechanisms in fibromyalgia: Relationship to pain and functional outcomes. *Journal of Rheumatology, 22,* 1552–1558.

Nicholas, M. K., Wilson, P. H., & Goyen, J. (1992). Comparison of cognitive-behavioral group treatment and an alternative nonpsychological treatment for chronic low back pain. *Pain, 48,* 339–347.

Nielson, W. R., Armstrong, J. M., Jensen, M. P., & Kerns, R. D. (2009). Two brief versions of the Multidimensional Pain Readiness to Change Questionnaire, Version 2 (MPRCQ2). *Clinical Journal of Pain, 25,* 48–57.

Nielson, W. R., Jensen, M. P., Ehde, D. M., Kerns, R. D., & Molton, I. R. (2008). Further development of the Multidimensional Pain Readiness to Change Questionnaire: The MPRCQ2. *Journal of Pain, 9,* 552–565.

Nielson, W. R., Jensen, M. P., & Hill, M. L. (2001). An activity pacing scale for the Chronic Pain Coping Inventory: Development in a sample of patients with fibromyalgia syndrome. *Pain, 89,* 111–115.

Nielson, W. R., Jensen, M. P., & Kerns, R. D. (2003). Initial development and validation of a Multidimensional Pain Readiness to Change Questionnaire. *Journal of Pain, 4,* 148–158.

Okifuji, A., Turk, D. C., & Everleigh, D. J. (1999). Improving the rate of classification of patients with the Multidimensional Pain Inventory (MPI): Clarifying the meaning of "significant other." *Clinical Journal of Pain, 15,* 290–296.

Osman, A., Barrios, F. X., Guttierez, P. M., Kopper, B. A., Merrifield, T., & Grittman, L. (2000). The Pain Catastrophizing Scale: Further psychometric evaluation with adult samples. *Journal of Behavioral Medicine, 23,* 351–365.

Osman, A., Barrios, F. X., Kopper, B. A., Hauptmann, W., Jones, J., & O'Neill, E. (1997). Factor structure, reliability and validity of the Pain Catastrophizing Scale. *Journal of Behavioral Medicine, 20,* 589–605.

Osterhaus, J. T., Townsend, R. J., Gandek, B., & Ware, J. E. (1994). Measuring the functional status and well-being of patients with migraine headaches. *Headache, 34,* 337–343.

Parmalee, P. A. (2005). Measuring mood and psychosocial function associated with pain in late life. In S. J. Gibson & D. K. Weiner (Eds.), *Pain in older persons: Progress in pain research and management* (Vol. 35). Seattle, WA: IASP Press.

Parsons, T. (1951). *The social system.* New York: Free Press.

Pfingsten, M., Hildebrandt, J., Leibing, E., Franz, C., & Saur, P. (1997). Effectiveness of a multimodal treatment program for chronic low-back pain. *Pain, 73,* 77–85.

Philips, H. C. (1989). Thoughts provoked by pain. *Behaviour Research and Therapy, 27,* 469–473.

Pilowsky, I. (1969). Abnormal illness behavior. *British Journal of Medical Psychology, 42,* 347–351.

Pilowsky, I., & Spence, N. D. (1983). *Manual for the Illness Behavior Questionnaire (IBQ)* (2nd ed.). Adelaide, Australia: University of Adelaide, Department of Psychiatry.

Pimenta, C. A., & da Cruz, D. de A. (2006). Chronic pain beliefs: Validation of the Survey of Pain Attitudes for the Portugese language. [Portugese]. *Revista Da Escola de Enfermagem Da Usp, 40,* 365–373.

Pollock, S. E., & Duffy, M. E. (1990). The Health-Related Hardiness Scale: Development and psychometric analysis. *Nursing Research, 39,* 218–222.

Prochaska, J. O., & DiClemente, C. C. (1984). *The transtheoretical approach: Crossing traditional boundaries of change.* Homewood, IL: Dow Jones/Irwin.

Ramirez-Maestre, C., Esteve, R., & Lopez, A. E. (2008). Cognitive appraisal and coping in chronic pain patients. *European Journal of Pain, 12,* 749–756.

Rankin, H., & Holttum, S. E. (2003). The relationship between acceptance and cognitive representations of pain in participants of a pain management programme. *Psychology, Health and Medicine, 8,* 329–334.

Reid, G. J., Gilbert, C. A., & McGrath, P. J. (1998). The Pain Coping Questionnaire: Preliminary validation. *Pain, 76,* 83–96.

Riley, J. L., & Robinson, M. E. (1997). CSQ: Five factors or fiction? *Clinical Journal of Pain, 13,* 156–162.

Riley, J. L., Zawacki, T. M., Robinson, M. E., & Geisser, M. E. (1999). Empirical test of the factor structure of the West Haven–Yale Multidimensional Pain Inventory. *Pain, 15,* 24–30.

Robinson, M. E., Riley, J. L., Myers, C. D., Sadler, I. J., Kvaal, S. A., Geisser, M. E., et al. (1997). The Coping Strategies Questionnaire: A large sample, item level factor analysis. *Clinical Journal of Pain, 13,* 43–49.

Roland, M., & Morris, R. (1983). A study of the natural history of back pain: Part I. Development of a reliable and sensitive measure of disability in low back pain. *Spine, 8,* 141–144.

Romano, J. M., Jensen, M. P., & Turner, J. A. (2003). The Chronic Pain Coping Inventory–42: Reliability and validity. *Pain, 104,* 65–73.

Rosenstiel, A. K., & Keefe, F. J. (1983). The use of coping strategies in chronic low back pain patients: Relationship to patient characteristics and current adjustment. *Pain, 17,* 33–44.

Roth, R. S., & Geisser, M. E. (2002). Educational achievement and chronic pain disability: Mediating role of pain-related cognitions. *Clinical Journal of Pain, 18,* 286–296.

Rotter, J. B. (1966). Generalized expectancies for internal versus external control of reinforcement. *Psychological Monographs: General and Applied, 80*(Whole No. 609).

Rudy, T. E., Turk, D. C., Zaki, H. S., & Curtin, H. D. (1989). An empirical taxometric alternative to traditional classification of temporomandibular disorders. *Pain, 36,* 311–320.

Ruelman, L. S., Karoly, P., Newton, C., & Aiken, L. S. (2005a). The development and preliminary validation of a brief measure of chronic pain impact for use in the general population. *Pain, 113,* 82–90.

Ruelman, L. S., Karoly, P., Newton, C., & Aiken, L. S. (2005b). The development and preliminary validation of the Profile of Chronic Pain: Extended assessment battery. *Pain, 118,* 380–389.

Schanberg, L. E., Lefebvre, J. C., Keefe, F. J., Kredich, D. W., & Gil, K. M. (1997). Pain coping and the pain experience in children with juvenile chronic arthritis. *Pain, 73,* 181–189.

Schmitz, U., Saile, H., & Nilges, P. (1996). Coping with chronic pain: Flexible goal adjustment as an interactive buffer against pain-related distress. *Pain, 67,* 41–51.

Shutty, M. S., & DeGood, D. E. (1990). Patient knowledge and beliefs about pain and its treatment. *Rehabilitation Psychology, 35,* 43–54.

Shutty, M. S., DeGood, D. E., & Tuttle, D. H. (1990). Chronic pain patients' beliefs about their pain and treatment outcomes. *Archives of Physical Medicine and Rehabilitation, 71,* 128–132.

Smith, C. A., Wallston, K. A., Dwyer, K. A., & Dowdy, S. W. (1997). Beyond good and bad coping: A multidimensional examination of coping with pain in persons with rheumatoid arthritis. *Annals of Behavioral Medicine, 19,* 11–21.

Snow-Turek, A. L., Norris, M. P., & Tan, G. (1996). Active and passive coping strategies in chronic pain patients. *Pain, 64,* 455–462.

Spinhoven, P., & Linssen, A. C. G. (1991). Behavioral treatment of chronic low back pain: I. Relation of coping strategy use to outcome. *Pain, 45,* 29–34.

Stevens, J. J. (1992). Interaction of coping style and cognitive strategies in the management of acute pain. *Imagination, Cognition, and Personality, 11,* 225–232.

Strack, S. (2008). The Millon Behavioral Medicine Diagnostic (MBMD) is a valid, reliable, and relevant choice for bariatric surgery candidates. *Obesity Surgery, 18,* 1657–1659.

Strong, J., Ashton, R., & Chant, D. (1992). The measurement of attitudes towards and beliefs about pain. *Pain, 48,* 227–236.

Strong, J., & Large, R. G. (1995). Coping with chronic pain: An idiographic exploration through focus groups. *International Journal of Psychiatry in Medicine, 25,* 361–377.

Sullivan, M. J. L., Bishop, S., & Pivik, J. (1995). The Pain Catastrophizing Scale: Development and validation. *Psychological Assessment, 7,* 524–532.

Sullivan, M. J. L., & D'Eon, J. (1990). Relation between catastrophizing and depression in chronic pain patients. *Journal of Abnormal Psychology, 99,* 260–263.

Sullivan, M. J. L., & Neish, N. (1997). Psychological predictors of pain during dental hygiene treatment. *Probe, 31,* 123–127.

Sullivan, M. J. L., Stanish, W., Waite, H., Sullivan, M., & Tripp, D. A. (1998). Catastrophizing, pain, and disability in patients with soft-tissue injuries. *Pain, 77,* 253–260.

Taft, C., Karlsson, J., & Sullivan, M. (2001). Do SF-36 summary component scores accurately summarize subscale scores? *Quality of Life Research, 10,* 395–404.

Tait, R. C., & Chibnall, J. T. (1997). Development of a brief version of the Survey of Pain Attitudes. *Pain, 70,* 229–235.

Tan, G., Nguyen, Q., Anderson, K. O., Jensen, M., & Thornby, J. (2005). Further validation of the Chronic Pain Coping Inventory. *Journal of Pain, 6,* 29–40.

Tan, G., Nguyen, Q., Cardin, S. A., & Jensen, M. P. (2006). Validating the use of two-item measures of pain beliefs and coping strategies for a veteran population. *Journal of Pain, 7,* 252–260.

Thompson, R. J., Gil, K. M., Abrams, M. R., & Phillips, G. (1992). Stress, coping, and psychological adjustment of adults with sickle cell disease. *Journal of Consulting and Clinical Psychology, 60,* 433–440.

Thorn, B. E., Rich, M. A., & Boothby, J. L. (1999). Pain beliefs and coping attempts: Conceptual model building. *Pain Forum, 8,* 169–171.

Tota-Faucette, M. E., Gil, K. M., Williams, D. A., Keefe, F. J., & Goli, V. (1993). Predictors of response to pain management treatment. *Clinical Journal of Pain, 9,* 115–123.

Truchon, M., & Côté, D. (2005). Predictive validity of the Chronic Pain Coping Inventory in subacute low back pain. *Pain, 116,* 205–212.

Truchon, M., Côté, D., & Irachabal, S. (2006). The Chronic Pain Coping Inventory: Confirmatory factor analysis of the French version. *BMC Musculoskeletal Disorders, 7,* 13.

Turk, D. C., & Kerns, R. D. (1985). Assessment in health psychology: A cognitive-behavioral perspective. In P. Karoly (Ed.), *Measurement strategies in health psychology* (pp. 335–372). New York: Wiley.

Turk, D. C., Meichenbaum, D., & Genest, M. (1983). *Pain and behavioral medicine: A cognitive-behavioral perspective.* New York: Guilford Press.

Turk, D. C., & Rudy, T. E. (1988). Toward an empirically derived taxonomy of chronic pain patients: Integration of psychological assessment data. *Journal of Consulting and Clinical Psychology, 56,* 233–238.

Turk, D. C., & Rudy, T. E. (1990). The robustness of an empirically derived taxonomy of chronic pain patients. *Pain, 43,* 27–36.

Turkat, I. D., & Pettegrew, L. S. (1983). Development and validation of the Illness Behavior Inventory. *Journal of Behavioral Assessment, 5,* 35–47.

Turner, J. A., Holtzman, S., & Mancl, L. (2007). Mediators, moderators, and predictors of therapeutic change in cognitive-behavioral therapy for chronic pain. *Pain, 127,* 276–286.

Turner, J. A., Jensen, M. P., & Romano, J. M. (2000). Do beliefs, coping and catastrophizing independently predict functioning in patients with chronic pain? *Pain, 85,* 115–125.

Turner, J. A., Whitney, C., Dworkin, S. F., Massoth, D., & Wilson, L. (1995). Do changes in patient beliefs and coping strategies predict temporomandibular disorder treatment outcomes? *Clinical Journal of Pain, 11,* 177–188.

Ulmer, J. F. (1997). An exploratory study of pain, coping, and depressed mood following burn injury. *Journal of Pain and Symptom Management, 13,* 148–157.

Van Damme, S., Crombez, G., Bijttebier, P., Goubert, L., & Van Houdenhove, B. (2002). A confirmatory factor analysis of the Pain Catastrophizing Scale: Invariant factor structure across clinical and non-clinical populations. *Pain, 96,* 319–324.

Verra, M. L., Angst, F., Lehmann, S., & Aeschlimann, A. (2006). Translation, cross-cultural adaptation, reliability and validity of the German version of the Coping Strategies Questionnaire (CSQ-D). *Journal of Pain, 7,* 327–336.

Vitaliano, P. P., Russo, J., Carr, J. E., Maiuro, R. D., & Becker, J. (1985). The Ways of Coping Checklist: revision and psychometric properties. *Multivariate Behavioral Research, 20,* 3–26.

Vowles, K. E., & McCracken, L. M. (2010). Comparing the role of psychological flexibility and traditional pain management coping strategies in chronic pain treatment outcomes. *Behaviour Research and Therapy, 48,* 141–146.

Vowles, K. E., McCracken, L. M., McLeod, C., & Eccleston, C. (2008). The Chronic Pain Acceptance Questionnaire: Confirmatory factor analysis and identification of patient subgroups. *Pain, 140,* 284–291.

Walfish, S., Wise, E. A., & Streiner, D. L. (2008). Limitations of the Millon Behavioral Diagnostic (MBMD) with bariatric surgery candidates. *Obesity Surgery, 18,* 1318–1322.

Wallston, K. A., Wallston, B. S., & DeVellis, R. (1978). Development of the Multidimensional Health Locus of Control (MHLC) scales. *Health Education Monographs, 6,* 160–170.

Walsh, D. A., & Radcliffe, J. C. (2002). Pain beliefs and perceived physical disability of patients with chronic low back pain. *Pain*, *97*, 23–31.

Ware, J. E., Kosinski, M., & Dewey, J. E. (2000). *How to score version two of the SF-36 Health Survey*. Lincoln, RI: QualityMetric.

Ware, J. E., Kosinski, M., & Keller, S. D. (1994). *SF-36 Physical and Mental Health summary scales: A user's manual*. Boston: Health Institute.

Ware, J. E., Snow, K. K., Kosinski, M., & Gandek, B. (1993). *SF-36 Health Survey manual and interpretation guide*. Boston: Health Institute.

Watkins, K. W., Shifren, K., Park, D. C., & Morrell, R. W. (1999). Age, pain, and coping with rheumatoid arthritis. *Pain*, *82*, 217–228.

Weisberg, J. N., & Gatchel, R. J. (Eds.). (2000). *Personality characteristics of pain patients: Recent advances and future directions*. Washington, DC: American Psychological Association.

Werner, E. L., Gross, D. P., Atle Lie, S., & Ihlebaek, C. (2008). Healthcare provider back pain beliefs unaffected by a media campaign. *Scandanavian Journal of Primary Health Care*, *26*, 50–56.

Wilkie, D. J., & Keefe, F. J. (1991). Coping strategies of patients with lung cancer-related pain. *Clinical Journal of Pain*, *7*, 292–299.

Williams, D. A., & Keefe, F. J. (1991). Pain beliefs and the use of cognitive-behavioral coping strategies. *Pain*, *46*, 185–358.

Williams, D. A., & Thorn, B. E. (1989). An empirical assessment of pain beliefs. *Pain*, *36*, 351–358.

Wineman, N. M., Durand, E. J., & McCulloch, B. J. (1994). Examination of the factor structure of the Ways of Coping Questionnaire with clinical populations. *Nursing Research*, *43*, 268–273.

Wrubel, J., Benner, P., & Lazarus, R. S. (1981). Social competence from the perspective of stress and coping. In J. Wine & M. Syme (Eds.), *Social competence* (pp. 61–99). New York: Guilford Press.

Yap, J. C., Lau, J., Chen, P. P., Gin, T., Wong, T., Chan, I., et al. (2008). Validation of the Chinese Pain Catastrophizing Scale (HK-PCS) in patients with chronic pain. *Pain Medicine*, *9*, 186–195.

Yong, H.-H. (2006). Can attitudes of stoicism and cautiousness explain observed age-related variation in levels of self-rated pain, mood disturbance and functional interference in chronic pain patients? *European Journal of Pain*, *10*, 399–407.

Yong, H.-H., Bell, R., Workman, B., & Gibson, S. J. (2003). Psychometric properties of the Pain Attitudes Questionnaire (revised) in adult patients with chronic pain. *Pain*, *104*, 673–681.

Yong, H.-H., Gibson, S. J., de L. Horne, D. J., & Helms, R. D. (2001). Development of a pain attitudes questionnaire to assess stoicism and cautiousness for possible age differences. *Journals of Gerontology B: Psychological Sciences*, *56*, 279–284.

Young Casey, C., Greenberg, M. A., Nicassio, P. M., Harpin, R. E., & Hubbard, D. (2008). Transition from acute to chronic pain and disability: A model including cognitive, affective, and trauma factors. *Pain*, *134*, 69–79.

CHAPTER 5

Assessment of Couples and Families with Chronic Pain

JOAN M. ROMANO
ANNMARIE CANO
KAREN B. SCHMALING

Any attempt to understand the patient suffering from chronic pain must include an assessment of the psychosocial context in which the patient functions. The primary examples of such a context are, of course, the couple and family. As we noted in the previous edition of this book, the family arguably provides the most important social influence on the development of concepts of health and illness, and on responses to acute and chronic health care problems (Kerns, 1995). Families provide the context in which early experiences of illness and caretaking occur, and in which beliefs about the meanings of symptoms and the appropriate individual and family response to them are formed. Current approaches to chronic pain recognize that adjustment and functioning are multidimensional and involve an ongoing dynamic interplay between the patient and his or her social environment. The patient and his or her partner affect each other in how they appraise, cope with, and respond to the challenges of living with chronic pain, as well as other life stresses. Since the previous edition of this book was published, there have been a number of developments in conceptualization and assessment of the social context of the patient with chronic pain. In this chapter, we provide an updated selective review of this area.

We have chosen to focus primarily on the couple given that most of the research literature pertaining to the families of patients with chronic pain is based on the study of couples. The partner also is more likely than other family members to be available to the clinician during assessment and treatment of adults with chronic pain. We first provide an overview of major theoretical models that have been applied to the study of couples and family systems in which one member has chronic pain. We then describe and review the most commonly used methods and measures for assessing couple and family functioning, including recently developed measures and advances in the use of behavioral observation and electronic momentary assessment. Finally, we discuss areas in need of further research and suggest directions for future studies.

MODELS OF THE ROLE OF THE FAMILY IN CHRONIC PAIN

Behavioral Models

Arguably, the most influential description of the role of the social environment and its impact on chronic pain was provided by Wilbert Fordyce in his seminal work *Behavioral Methods in Chronic Pain and Illness* (1976).

Fordyce made the conceptual breakthrough of considering "pain behaviors" (behaviors that would be commonly construed as indicating pain) as not simply responses to a nociceptive stimulus, but as operant behaviors that could come under the control of social and environmental contingencies of reinforcement. According to this model, persistent pain behaviors and disability could be perpetuated, at least in part, by reinforcers, such as solicitous responses by significant others, or by avoidance of painful or otherwise aversive stimuli. This conceptualization was particularly pertinent to the patient with chronic pain, in that Fordyce hypothesized that the longer pain persists, the more opportunity exists for pain behaviors to be shaped by their environmental consequences, contributing to ongoing dysfunction.

Such a conceptualization, of course, does not imply that chronic pain is not "real" or that patients are not suffering, nor does it diminish the importance of other potential influences on pain behaviors, including physiological factors (e.g., deconditioning) and psychological disorders (e.g., depression). It does highlight, however, that the dysfunction associated with chronic pain is embedded in a psychosocial context and that the responses of partners and others close to the patient must be examined to provide a comprehensive picture of factors affecting function.

Although the operant behavioral model has been highly influential, it has been criticized for an overly restrictive conceptualization of chronic pain and insufficient attention to the role of cognitive factors (e.g., beliefs and attributions about pain or the responses of others) (Hadjistavropoulos & Craig, 2002; Novy, Nelson, Francis, & Turk, 1995; Turk & Flor, 1987). Newton-John and Williams (2006) have advocated the assessment of a wider array of responses by partners than has been commonly examined in the behavioral literature.

Cognitive-Behavioral Models

Cognitive-behavioral approaches to the assessment and treatment of chronic pain have become widely used over the last 25 years, with a growing body of evidence supporting their efficacy and applicability (Compas, Haaga, Keefe, Leitenberg, & Wil-liams, 1998; National Institutes of Health (NIH) Technology Assessment Panel, 1996). Cognitive-behavioral therapy (CBT) is based on a theoretical model in which patient affect and behavior are strongly influenced by how patients view and interpret their experiences. This model implies that patients' beliefs and attributions about pain impact their emotional and behavioral responses to it. However, this model also implies that the effect of the social environment on patients' pain behaviors and dysfunction is influenced by patients' cognitions, for example, the beliefs that patients hold regarding the meaning of others' responses to pain behaviors. In addition, the model implies that the responses of patients' partners may be strongly influenced by the beliefs they hold regarding the nature of patients' pain and disability, and the appropriateness of different responses to pain behaviors (Cano, Miller, & Loree, 2009; Turk, Kerns, & Rosenberg, 1992). An expanded version of the cognitive-behavioral model, termed the cognitive-behavioral transactional model (Kerns & Weiss, 1994), integrates concepts of family adjustment and adaptation, as well as stress and coping into a cognitive-behavioral perspective. This model supports assessment at multiple levels (individual, dyadic, and family) of behavior, cognition, mood, and global functioning.

More recently, Michael Sullivan and colleagues (2001) proposed the communal coping model (CCM), in which *catastrophizing* (a style of cognitive appraisal in which events are seen as threatening and beyond one's ability to cope) is hypothesized to function as a type of coping that mobilizes social support. Catastrophizing in patients with pain has been shown to be associated with greater reported pain, psychological distress, and disability (cf. Turner, Jensen, & Romano, 2000; Turner, Jensen, Warms, & Cardenas, 2002; Sullivan & D'Eon, 1990) but its relationship to partner responses is less clear, with some researchers finding a positive association (Cano, 2004; Giardino, Jensen, Turner, Ehde, & Cardenas, 2003) and others finding no significant association (Boothby, Thorn, Overduin, & Ward, 2004). Furthermore, the mechanism through which catastrophizing might relate to partners' awareness of distress, as well as their social responses to pain, has not been made explicit. Overt patient pain behavior would appear to be a necessary link between catastrophizing (a cognitive process within patients) and the responses of others in the environment. In a critique of the CCM, Severeijns, Vlaeyen, and van den Hout (2004) argue that catastrophizing is a cognitive construct rather than a coping behavior, and the communal coping formulation is conceptually confusing. Additionally, an appraisal model of catastrophizing provides a more parsimonious explanation than does the CCM of the empirical evidence regarding the relationship of catastrophizing to pain coping. Despite these concerns, the CCM has value in calling attention to the social context in which patients' appraisal processes occur. These cognitive processes can in turn influence patient pain behavior and subsequent responses from the social environment.

Acceptance and commitment therapy (Hayes, Strosahl, & Wilson, 1999), another cognitive-behavioral model that has been applied to patients with chronic pain (McCracken, 2005) evaluates cognitions for their functional value in influencing behavior, with a core concept that acceptance of the reality of pain is an important factor in improving adaptation to chronic pain. Pain-related cognitions may support avoidance of pain-related activities, whereas acceptance and lack of avoidance have been associated with better functioning (McCracken, 1998; McCracken & Eccleston, 2003). McCracken (2005) demonstrated that solicitous and punishing responses by partners are negatively correlated with patients' acceptance, suggesting another pathway by which partner responses may influence patient adjustment and function. Later generation cognitive-behavioral models such as this provide new and interesting directions for examining the role that social context may play to influence patient cognitive appraisals and provide social feedback in response to pain behavior.

Social Control Model

Social control processes form another lens through which to view the interactions between patients and partners in the context of chronic illness (Lewis & Rook, 1999). *Social control* refers to attempts to influence or change the behaviors of others. In the context of chronic pain, behaviors of the partner directed at helping the patient manage or change health-related behaviors, or that encourage reliance on others, have been examined as forms of control behaviors (Reich & Olmsted, 2007). In particular, behaviors that encourage reliance on others may have some overlap with behaviors considered solicitous in a cognitive-behavioral framework. Recent research has examined how such control behaviors may be related to relationships between patients with pain and their partners. When examined in conjunction with level of pain and uncertainty regarding illness among 51 patients with fibromyalgia and their partners, encouraging reliance on others was associated with greater relationship satisfaction when level of pain and illness uncertainty were high (Reich & Olmstead, 2007). Reich and Zautra (1995a, 1995b) also have found that encouraging reliance on others may be positively or negatively associated with patient outcomes depending on factors such as control beliefs, age, and patient health status. This application of social models provides a different perspective on the function that so-called "illness role" behaviors may play depending on the nature of the health problem and other factors within the relationship. Further research applying this model to the relationship between social control processes and patient functioning and health outcomes, as well as relationship satisfaction and psychological well-being, will be of interest.

THE IMPACT OF CHRONIC PAIN ON THE PARTNER

Given the enormous impact of chronic pain on patients' physical and psychosocial functioning, it is difficult to imagine that partner and family functioning also would not be affected by the experience of living with someone in chronic pain, as predicted by the models reviewed earlier. Previous research demonstrated that partners of patients with chronic pain experience increased psychological distress (cf. Ahern, Adams, & Follick, 1985; Kerns & Turk, 1984; Schwartz, Slater, Birchler, & Atkinson, 1991; Taylor, Lorentzen, & Blank, 1990). Relationship dissatisfaction also has been reported in patients with chronic pain (Flor, Turk, & Rudy, 1989; Kerns & Turk, 1984), and their partners (cf. Kerns, Haythornthwaite, Southwick, & Giller, 1990; Kerns & Turk, 1984;

Romano, Turner, & Clancy, 1989; Stampler, Wall, Cassisi, & Davis, 1997).

However, not all studies have reported relationship distress; some studies have reported relationship satisfaction in the normal range (cf. Flor, Breitenstein, Birbaumer, & Fürst, 1995; Hewitt, Flett, & Mikail, 1995; Romano et al., 1995; Stampler et al., 1997) using well-validated measures of relationship satisfaction and adjustment. Recent pain empathy work may offer an explanation for lower satisfaction in some partners. Goubert and colleagues (2005) suggest that partners' understanding of pain is based on patients' expressions of pain, as well as partners' experience with pain. In turn, understanding may promote personal distress (e.g., helplessness) or other-oriented distress (e.g., compassion). Differing patterns of relationship satisfaction findings may be due to the variety of distress responses of partners.

Other factors also may bear on the range of responses reported. First, patients with chronic pain are heterogeneous in their physical and psychological functioning, such that empirically derived subgroups can be identified (Jamison, Rudy, Penzien, & Mosley, 1994; Turk & Rudy, 1988, 1990). One such subgroup, labeled "interpersonally distressed," reported less perceived support and relationship satisfaction (Turk, Okifuji, Sinclair, & Starz, 1996; Turk & Rudy, 1988, 1990), suggesting that reliance on average group relationship satisfaction scores may obscure the presence of a significant subgroup of distressed couples. Second, self-selection bias may affect reports of relationship distress. Couples with significant relationship distress may not agree to participate in studies involving the relationship, perhaps resulting in an underrepresentation of distressed couples. In addition, patients and partners recruited from specialty pain clinics may not be representative of those seen in primary care settings, resulting in limited generalizability to the population of patients with chronic pain.

Research also has demonstrated that patients' pain may impact partners' cognitions. For instance, partners may catastrophize or feel helpless about patients' pain (Cano, Leonard, & Franz, 2005). In addition, patients' depressive symptoms were heightened when both partners endorsed high levels of pain catastrophizing. Furthermore, partner catastrophizing about the patient's pain was associated with partner depressive symptoms if the partner also reported chronic pain (Leonard & Cano, 2006).

In summary, a large subgroup of partners report significant relationship dissatisfaction and psychological distress. However, distress and dissatisfaction among partners of patients with chronic pain are not universal, and factors predictive of adjustment need further investigation. Continued research may be able to address the extent to which partners' cognitions impact distress and relationship satisfaction in the couple, as well as partners' responses to pain.

THE ROLE OF COUPLE AND FAMILY ASSESSMENT IN THE CLINICAL EVALUATION OF THE PATIENT WITH CHRONIC PAIN

An important part of the assessment process prior to and during treatment is the evaluation of patient–partner relationships, how partners and patients conceptualize and manage patients' pain and disability, and how partners respond to patients' pain behaviors. In this section, we describe some of the most commonly used methods to assess aspects of couple and family functioning, and review methods of clinical interviewing, questionnaires, and direct observational methods. Excellent reviews of couple and family assessment instruments are available, although they are not written with a focus on application to patients with chronic pain and their partners or families. Readers interested in self-report couple and family assessment instruments are referred to Fischer and Corcoran (2007). Good resources for readers interested in observational coding systems are the reviews of couple and family coding systems by Kerig and Baucom (2004) and Kerig and Lindahl (2000), respectively. Dyadic data-analytic techniques, which have not been used extensively in the pain literature, are described in a useful book by Kenny, Kashy, and Cook (2006).

The Clinical Interview

The clinical interview of the patient and partner is the primary source of information regarding the quality of interpersonal relationships in the family, and the patterns of partner and family responses to patient pain behaviors. Interviews may be supplemented by questionnaires or psychometric testing. Informal clinical observation of patient and partner behavior usually occurs in the course of the interview; more formal observational assessment of patient pain behaviors or of patient–partner interactions are more likely conducted in research rather than clinical settings.

Table 5.1 lists topics in the clinical interview of the patient and partner that are most pertinent to assessing couple and family functioning. It is important for the clinician first to establish rapport and to communicate empathically a desire to understand the nature of their experiences, and to help them and their physicians in formulating appropriate treatment options based on a thorough assessment.

It is helpful to hear from each partner separately his or her impressions of the severity and nature of the pain and its impact on the patient's functioning, as well as the couple's life together. Despite living with someone in pain for many years, partners typically are inaccurate in estimating the pain experienced by their partners (Cano, Johansen, & Franz, 2005; Cano, Johansen, & Geisser, 2004; Clipp & George, 1992; Cremeans-Smith et al., 2003; Miaskowski, Zimmer, Barrett, Dibble, & Wallhagen, 1997; Riemsma, Taal, & Rasker, 2000; Yeager, Miaskowski, Dibble, & Wallhagen, 1995). Patient depression appears to accentuate the incongruence within couples, such that partners underestimate the pain severity, interference, and disability of depressed patients to a greater degree than they do those of nondepressed patients (Cano, Johansen, & Franz, 2005; Cano, Johansen, & Geisser, 2004). Interestingly, partner distress was associated with higher patient pain and interference ratings than patients' self-ratings (Cano, Johansen, & Franz, 2005). Both partners may not feel comfortable discussing pain (Porter, Keefe, Wellington, & Williams, 2008), which may further complicate attempts to understand the extent of pain. Thus, clinicians should consider the factors that enter into couple incongruence in the family assessment of pain and interference.

The assessment of partners' responses to patient pain behaviors, including the behav-

TABLE 5.1. Couple and Family Issues to Assess in Interviewing Both Patient and Partner

Cognitive-behavioral analysis

1. Changes in patient and partner activity since pain onset and how these have affected the family.
2. Description of patient pain behaviors.
3. Responses of the partner/family to pain behaviors.
4. Responses of the partner/family to patient "well behaviors" and activity.
5. Beliefs of the patient and partner about the cause of the pain. Does either believe that pain is a signal of potential harm or damage?
6. Patient perceptions and interpretations of the partner's responses to his or her pain behaviors.
7. Partner perceptions and interpretations of the patient's pain behaviors.
8. Changes in roles and functions of the patient and partner since pain onset.
9. Partner observations concerning patient emotional distress and adjustment to chronic pain.

Relationship issues

1. Quality of relationship with partner.
2. Stresses and strains having an impact on the couple and family.
3. Changes in the relationship since pain onset.
4. Sexual adjustment and changes since pain onset; factors other than pain affecting sexual adjustment.
5. Strengths and resources of the couple.

Financial issues

1. Impact of pain on financial status of couple/ family.
2. Patient and partner perceptions of compensation/litigation issues.
3. Patient and partner views of vocational issues, return to work.

Social history and family of origin

1. Family relationships and attachment.
2. History of pain, disability, or chronic illness in family members.
3. Patient history of abuse or neglect.
4. Patient family psychiatric history: history of psychological disorders, alcohol or substance abuse.

ioral analysis of factors associated with increased or decreased pain and disability, continues to be an important part of the clinical interview when placed in the larger context of the psychosocial assessment. Both patients and partners should describe how the patient communicates pain (i.e., what pain behaviors the patient demonstrates) and how the partner and other family members respond to pain communications. The presence of frequent solicitous behaviors by partners, coupled with excessive patient disability and a relative absence of pathophysiology, raises the hypothesis that social contingencies may be playing a significant role in reinforcing pain behavior and dysfunction.

Patients' and partners' beliefs and attributions about patients' pain also should be assessed. Pain may be interpreted to mean that harm or damage is taking place, not only causing alarm and anxiety in the couple but also leading partners potentially to behave in an overprotective or solicitous manner. It is also important to inquire about how patients and partners interpret each others' behaviors. For example, apparently solicitous behaviors may occur frequently in response to pain behaviors, yet not be reinforcing if patients interpret partners' solicitousness as demeaning or as evidence of incapacity. Conversely, behaviors that appear to be negative or punishing, such as partners' withdrawal from patients when pain behaviors occur, may be positively reinforcing if they allow patients "time out" from stressful or conflictual interaction with partners. The responses of partners and families to activity and other *well behaviors* (behaviors incompatible with disability) also must be assessed. Partners may discourage activity for fear of injury to patients and may need help to overcome their fears, and learn to support and encourage activity as part of functional restoration.

In patient and partner interviews, assessment of the quality of the relationship is important to understand the context in which pain behaviors and partner responses occur. The possibility that pain behaviors and disability serve maintenance roles in the family must be considered; in some cases, couples may remain together primarily because of pain (e.g., "I couldn't leave him like this"). In other cases, caregiving may enhance feelings of closeness or intimacy, perhaps allowing emotional expression that was not otherwise possible (e.g., "The pain has brought us closer together"). These processes have important implications for treatment. If a pain problem has stabilized the relationship by providing additional closeness and intimacy, attempts to rehabilitate the patient to

work and to function more normally might threaten this homeostasis and meet with resistance if this pattern is not recognized and addressed during treatment. Likewise, if the only factor now holding the couple together is the pain problem, the patient may resist treatment for fear of losing the partner. Significant relationship conflict may form a major stressor in the patient's life that can contribute to depression and dysfunction. Conversely, a healthy partnership in which the relationship is not dependent on continuing patient dysfunction, and in which the partner can be a supportive ally of improved functioning, can bode well for treatment aimed at decreasing disability. Finally, couple and family strengths and resources should be assessed as well, including shared humor, mutual interests and activities outside of pain, strong commitments to children and work, capacity for caring and intimacy, and ability to support each other's problem-solving skills, among others.

Often chronic pain is associated with reductions in both the frequency and quality of couples' sexual activity, as well as sexual dysfunction (Kwan, Roberts, & Swalm, 2005; Maruta & Osborne, 1978; Maruta, Osborne, Swanson, & Halling, 1981), and it is important to assess sexual functioning before and after pain onset with patients and partners in a sensitive manner to determine how the pain problem has affected this aspect of the relationship. Patients may report that sexual activity provokes increased pain during and after the activity, which may lead to avoidance of sex. However, other factors, such as depression, relationship conflict, a history of abuse or trauma, or primary sexual dysfunction, may also result in decreased sexual interest or activity, with pain providing a more acceptable reason for reduced intimacy.

The financial implications of patients' pain problems for families are a difficult but important topic to address. When the patient is not working because of pain, there may be considerable anxiety on the part of the couple about the patient's ability to return to work and about the long-term financial stability of the family. Role changes can create stresses in relationships and contribute to depression. Although a full review of compensation and litigation issues and their implications for rehabilitation of patients with chronic pain is beyond the scope of this chapter (see review by Main, 1999), it is important to assess these areas because patient and partner concerns may need to be addressed if treatment aimed at improved functioning and work is to be successful.

Other important areas of query include basic information regarding patients' family of origin, including role models for chronic illness behavior and experiences patients or partners had earlier in life with their own or close family members' extended illness or disability. Family psychiatric history can provide important data about the presence of depression or other psychological disorders, alcohol, or other substance abuse in family members. Information about early developmental history may be important for treatment planning. Histories of abuse and neglect may be relevant to coping and adjustment to chronic pain.

Questionnaire Measurement

The use of reliable and valid questionnaires can provide valuable information to complement the clinical interviews of the patient and partner, and serves as a mainstay of research addressing questions of couple functioning and response to chronic pain. In this section, we review commonly used instruments for assessing general relationship satisfaction and their application to patients with chronic pain, and also questionnaire measures of partner responses to patient pain behavior.

Assessment of Relationship Satisfaction

An understanding of the intimate relationship and broader familial contexts in which chronic pain occurs is important for treatment planning and success, and because relationship satisfaction is associated with adjustment in patients and partners (Cano, Gillis, Heinz, Geisser, & Foran, 2004; Geisser, Cano, & Leonard, 2005). The two most frequently used such scales in the chronic pain literature are the Dyadic Adjustment Scale and the Locke–Wallace Marital Adjustment Test.

DYADIC ADJUSTMENT SCALE

The Dyadic Adjustment Scale (DAS; Spanier, 1976), a widely used relationship questionnaire, comprises 32 items designed to assess the quality of the relationship as perceived by each individual in a couple. Good internal consistency, test–retest reliability, and criterion-related validity have been reported (Spanier, 1976). The total score (range: 0–151) is used to measure global relationship satisfaction and has been shown to be sensitive to change in couples therapy (e.g., Jacobson et al., 1984). Adequate normative data exist, and reference ranges for scores that reflect normal and distressed relationships have been carefully developed (Eddy, Heyman, & Weiss, 1991; Jacobson, Follette, & Revenstorf, 1986; Jacobson & Truax, 1991). In addition to the total score, four component scores also can be derived for Dyadic Satisfaction, Cohesion, Consensus, and Affectional Expression. The DAS also includes items related to the individual's commitment to the relationship and willingness to work on improving the relationship; responses to these items may be useful for clinicians who consider initiating couples therapy.

Shorter versions of the DAS that have been developed have acceptable reliability and validity, including seven-item (Hunsley, Best, Lefebvre, & Vito, 2001; Sharpley & Rogers, 1984) and four-item (Sabourin, Valois, & Lussier, 2005) versions. Shorter versions may provide sufficient screening information to determine whether a more in-depth evaluation of relationship satisfaction is warranted.

The DAS is a useful instrument to quantify relationship satisfaction of couples dealing with pain. In addition to its positive psychometric qualities, DAS scores have potentially important relationships with pain-relevant variables. Another advantage of this measure is the ability to compare DAS scores in a couple, or sample of couples, with well-established normative data, and with other patient samples.

LOCKE–WALLACE MARITAL ADJUSTMENT TEST

The Marital Adjustment Test (MAT; Locke & Wallace, 1959) is a well-established, 15-item self-report instrument designed to assess intimate relationship quality. Items are scored with different weights, which are indicated on the instrument. The total score ranges between 2 and 158, with higher scores indicative of greater satisfaction. The MAT has been a useful instrument to characterize relationship satisfaction and has been a significant predictor of pain-relevant variables, both alone and in its interaction with partner responses to pain (Kerns et al., 1990).

COUPLE SATISFACTION INDEX

Newer indices of marital satisfaction also have been developed to address other measures' overreliance on communication items and problems relating to measurement precision. One of these indices, the Couples Satisfaction Index (CSI; Funk & Rogge, 2007), was created by subjecting items from the DAS, the MAT, and other freely available satisfaction measures to item response theory analyses. Funk and Rogge (2007) were able to develop 4-, 16-, and 32-item reliable and valid CSI versions that could be used for various research and clinical purposes. Although the CSI measures have not been used in pain research, they offer researchers additional options for assessing satisfaction with improved psychometric characteristics.

Assessment of Partner Responses to Patient Pain Behaviors and Disability

Assessment of partner responses to patients' pain behaviors and disability is important for both research and clinical purposes. It is facilitated by the use of questionnaire measures to assess these behavioral constructs.

MULTIDIMENSIONAL PAIN INVENTORY

The most commonly used measure of partner responses to patient pain behaviors is Part II of the West Haven–Yale Multidimensional Pain Inventory, also known as the Multidimensional Pain Inventory (MPI; Kerns, Turk, & Rudy, 1985). The MPI was developed as an assessment instrument for use in patients with chronic pain to provide a brief but comprehensive evaluation of salient dimensions of the experience of chronic pain. There are three parts to the inventory: Part I assesses pain severity and interference with activities and functioning; perceived life control; affective distress; and perceived support from family and partners. Part II evaluates patients' perceptions of the range and frequency of responses by partners to patients' pain and suffering behaviors and is most relevant

to this review. Fourteen specific responses are divided into three subscales: Solicitous, Punishing, and Distracting responses. Part III of the MPI assesses patient engagement in common domestic, household, social, and recreational activities.

The significant other version of Part II (MPI-SO), developed by Kerns and Rosenberg (1995), has the same scales as the patient version, described earlier, but is designed for the partner's self-report of his or her responses to the patient's pain behaviors. This measure has been demonstrated to have adequate internal consistency and criterion-related validity (Kerns & Rosenberg, 1995). A cluster analysis of MPI-SO items by Papas, Robinson, and Riley (2001) identified three subgroups that they term Positively Attentive, Negatively Attentive, and Inattentive.

Part II of the MPI has been used frequently in studies of the role of partner behavior in contributing to or maintaining chronic pain behavior. In general, studies have supported a positive relationship between solicitous partner responding and increased patient pain and dysfunction, although the correlational nature of these studies does not allow for conclusions about causation to be drawn. Solicitous responses by the partner to patient pain behaviors, as measured by the MPI, have been found to be related significantly to patient ratings of greater pain severity and lower patient activity (Flor, Kerns, & Turk, 1987; Flor et al., 1989; Stroud, Turner, Jensen, & Cardenas, 2006). These effects may differ by patient gender in terms of the specific negative outcomes associated with partner solicitous responses (Fillingim, Doleys, Edwards, & Lowery, 2003). The Solicitous Response scale of the MPI also has shown a significant association to more frequent patient pain behaviors (Kerns et al., 1991), as well as to observed solicitous behaviors in partners of patients with chronic pain (Romano et al., 1991; Romano, Jensen, Turner, Good, & Hops, 2000).

The relationship of the Punishing scale of the MPI to patient functioning has yielded less consistent findings. Flor and colleagues (1987) found a positive association between punishing responses and patient activity levels. However, other studies have not demonstrated significant relationships between punishing responses on the MPI and patient disability (Turk et al., 1992), pain intensity

(Kerns et al., 1990; Turk et al., 1992), or pain behavior (Turk et al., 1992). A more consistent finding has been that punishing responses are associated with poorer patient mood and psychological adjustment (Cano, Gillis, Heinz, Geisser, & Foran, 2004; Cano, Weisberg, & Gallagher, 2000; Kerns et al., 1990; Schwartz, Slater, & Birchler, 1996; Turk et al., 1992).

ADDITIONAL MEASURES

Other instruments have emerged more recently to assess partner responses to pain and well behavior in patients with chronic pain. Sharp and Nicholas (2000) examined the psychometric characteristics of the MPI-SO and designed significant other versions of three other measures of responses to and perceptions of patient pain: the Pain Self-Efficacy Questionnaire (PSEQ-SO; Patient Version developed by Nicholas, 1989; cited in Sharp & Nicholas, 2000); the Pain Responses Self-Statements (PRSS-SO; Patient Version developed by Flor, Behle, & Birbaumer, 1993); and the Pain Responses Coping Statements (PRCS-SO; Patient Version developed by Flor et al., 1993). Consistent with past research, they found that the MPI-SO demonstrated good internal consistency and convergent validity. Of these other scales, the PSEQ-SO had the strongest psychometric properties and demonstrated the most promise for future research in which the assessment of partner perceptions of patient self-efficacy may be clinically relevant.

SPOUSE RESPONSE INVENTORY

The Spouse Response Inventory (SRI; Schwartz, Jensen, & Romano, 2005) evaluates partner facilitative and negative responses to patient well behaviors and partner solicitous and negative responses to patient pain behaviors, thus providing a more comprehensive picture of responses to patient health-related behaviors. The SRI is a 39-item self-report instrument with strong internal consistency, test–retest stability, and predictive validity. Consistent with behavioral theory, negative partner responses to well behaviors, in addition to solicitous partner responses to pain behaviors, predicted more patient pain behavior, intensity,

and interference (Pence, Thorn, Jensen, & Romano, 2008; Schwartz et al., 2005).

Summary and Recommendations

Well-developed questionnaires assess relationship satisfaction and partner responses to patient pain behavior. Choosing from among multiple existing questionnaires requires a balanced consideration of factors such as questionnaire length and respondent burden, reliability and validity, and extant data applying the questionnaire to samples with chronic pain. Advanced statistical approaches may refine these instruments further. For example, item response theory has been used to pool items from the MAT, DAS, and other measures to create a more psychometrically sound measure of relationship satisfaction (Funk & Rogge, 2007).

For clinicians seeking to assess the interaction patterns of patients with chronic pain and their partners, the MPI (Kerns et al., 1985) has the greatest body of empirical support, but the SRI (Schwartz et al., 2005) additionally assesses the important dimension of partner responses to well behaviors.

Daily Interview and Electronic Momentary Assessment

In an effort to address limitations of self-report measures, such as potential inaccuracy of recall or the influence of current state on the reporting of past events, researchers may use daily interviews, diaries, or handheld electronic devices that sample patient experience in real time (Broderick et al., 2008; Peters et al., 2000; Turner, Mancl, & Aaron, 2004). More recently, these methods have been applied to the study of partner responses and their relationship to patient disability (Sorbi et al., 2006) and to patient pain, negative affect, and catastrophizing (Holtzman & DeLongis, 2007). Sorbi and colleagues (2006) utilized palm-top computers to prompt patients with chronic pain to respond four times daily to items assessing pain intensity, fear-avoidance responses, disability, and partner responses to patient pain. Partner responses were only assessed if the partner was actually present and the patient was in pain at the time of the prompt. While partner responses were found to be a weak predictor of pain intensity, partner discouragement of well behavior and activity was a stronger predictor (along with patient avoidance) of immobility due to pain.

Holtzman and DeLongis (2007) conducted 10-minute telephone interviews twice daily with patients with rheumatoid arthritis regarding pain intensity, pain catastrophizing, negative affect, and satisfaction with general partner support (not responses specific to pain). Satisfaction with partner responses reduced the likelihood of increased negative affect due to catastrophizing, as well as the likelihood of feeling overwhelmed and helpless in dealing with daily pain. Unfortunately, actual partner responses, as well as satisfaction with them, that would have provided a more comprehensive picture of the extent to which particular responses may be associated with both satisfaction and function were not assessed. However, both this study and the one by Sorbi and colleagues (2006) demonstrate the utility of simultaneously collecting data on the social context of pain, as well as patients' cognitions and behaviors related to pain and dysfunction, in examining the complex interrelationships among these variables.

Observational Measures

Observational methodology has continued to develop but it remains relatively infrequently used compared to self-report due to its cost and labor-intensive nature. Direct observation has unique strengths compared to questionnaire measurement, in that data may be more objective and less prone to reporting bias, and shared method variance is lessened when relationships with variables dependent on self-report are examined. In addition, the use of observational data allows for more precise measurement of dimensions of couple and family interaction that may have important theoretical and clinical implications. (See Heyman, 2001, for review, critique, and recommendations regarding couple observation methods.)

Early studies using observational techniques focused on measuring pain behaviors in patients in the presence versus absence of the partner (e.g., Keefe & Block, 1982). Presence of partners, especially those described as solicitous, was associated with more reported pain and more pain behaviors (Keefe & Block, 1982; Lousberg, Schmidt, & Groenman, 1992; Paulsen & Altmaier, 1995). A more complex coding scheme for measuring interactional patterns, the KPI (*Kategoriensystem für Partnerschaftliche Interaktion*; Hahlweg et al., 1984), was used by Flor and colleagues (1995) to examine the relationship of partner solicitousness to pain report and behaviors. The KPI, however, neither measures patient pain behavior nor captures directly the solicitous responses of the partner to patient pain behaviors.

In a series of studies Romano and her colleagues (1991, 1992, 1995, 2000) developed a methodology to observe directly and quantify patient pain behaviors and partner responses using the Living in Family Environments coding system (LIFE; Hops, Davis, & Longoria, 1995). The LIFE is a real-time, sequential coding system modified specifically to include affect and content codes reflecting verbal and nonverbal pain behaviors, as well as solicitous behaviors (see Romano et al., 1991, for a more detailed description of this methodology). Partner responses, especially those perceived as solicitous, accounted for significant variance in the pain behaviors and disability level of patients with chronic pain (Romano et al., 1995). Another study applying this methodology in a separate, larger sample of patients with pain and their partners replicated the finding that partner solicitous responses were associated with patient pain behaviors (Romano et al., 2000). More recently, this methodology was applied to the study of interactions between patients with chronic fatigue and their partners, with the finding of significant associations between observed and reported solicitous partner responses and patient illness behaviors (Romano, Jensen, Schmaling, Hops, & Buchwald, 2009).

Johansen and Cano (2007) examined affective interaction during a 15-minute marital problem-solving task. The Specific Affect Coding Scheme (SPAFF; Gottman & Levenson, 1992) was used to code each partner's utterances for humor, sadness, anger, and contempt. Patients' expressions of sadness were associated with greater pain and depressive symptoms only when patients, and not their partners, reported chronic pain. In contrast, sadness was inversely associated with pain and depression when both partners reported pain, which suggests that having a partner who also experiences pain may allow patients to express sadness in an empathic environment. However, the expression of anger and contempt by pain-free partners was associated with their own depression when patients also expressed anger and contempt. Thus, the assessment of anger may be particularly relevant for partners without personal experience of chronic pain.

Empathic interaction also has received interest because of the recent advancement of empathy models in the pain literature (Goubert et al., 2005). Cano, Barterian, and Heller (2008) used the Validating and Invalidating Behavior Coding System (VIBCS; Fruzetti, 2001) to code couples' discussions about the impact of pain on their lives. Validating responses included empathic responses, such as statements that convey an attempt to understand the feelings of patients. Invalidating responses included changing the subject, ignoring patients' emotional responses, and expressing disrespect or contempt for patients. In general, relationship satisfaction and perceived partner support were negatively correlated with invalidation and positively correlated with validation. To understand better the interrelatedness of partner empathic responses with the more traditional concepts of partner responses to pain, the data were subjected to an exploratory factor analysis that resulted in a two-factor solution, accounting for 57% of the variance in the data. Couples' reports of solicitous and distracting partner responses loaded on a Solicitous Responding factor. Couples' reports of punishing partner responses loaded with observations of partners' invalidation and validation on an Empathic Responding factor. The two factors were weakly related to one another ($r = -.17$). Although both factors correlated with relationship satisfaction and perceptions of support in both partners, the Empathic Responding factor was a significantly stronger correlate of patients' relationship satisfaction and partner support. A weakness of this study is that empathic interaction was observed, whereas partner responses to pain were self-reported. Nevertheless, this study suggests that validation and solicitousness are distinct concepts that should be further assessed in the interactions of patients and their partners.

Although observational research has advanced knowledge about the dynamics involved in patient–partner interaction, most studies in this area have been correlational, precluding conclusions regarding causation and direction of effects. In addition, there is likely a reciprocal and synergistic relationship between patient pain behaviors and responses from partners, such that over time each may shape the other's behavior. Longitudinal studies are needed to examine both the naturalistic course of patient–partner responses in the context of pain as well as studies in which partner responses to pain behavior and empathic expressions are systematically altered to provide information on possible causal pathways and more stringent tests of theoretical models.

SUMMARY AND FUTURE DIRECTIONS

The literature on assessment of the couple and family context of patients with chronic pain has grown in conceptual and methodological sophistication since the previous edition of this chapter was published. What has remained consistent, however, is empirical support for the importance of the couple and family to the adjustment of the patient with chronic pain. Conceptual advances include increasing incorporation of constructs such as acceptance, empathic communication, and validation into more traditional cognitive-behavioral formulations. Contributions from developmental perspectives, such as attachment theory, and from social psychological perspectives, such as social control theory, have the potential to enrich the conceptual background to research in this area. Methodologies such as electronic assessment and diary recording, and more sophisticated applications of observational technologies promise to increase the ecological validity of data on the psychosocial context and home environment of patients with pain.

However, many unresolved questions and issues remain. Research in this area remains descriptive and correlational, and more systematic tests of theoretical models are needed. Further development of well-validated instruments to assess cognitive, behavioral, contextual, and interactive variables are needed (Snyder, Heyman, & Haynes, 2005) to test complex models that posit synergistic effects among these classes of variables. Other developments in couple assessment that have not yet been applied to couples with chronic pain could be useful in this population. The Couple Attachment Interview (Alexandrov, Cowan, & Cowan, 2005) may elucidate the role that pain plays in couples with secure or insecure attachments. As another example, measures that characterize couple exchanges broadly, with the potential to apply specifically to pain behavior interaction, include the Communication Patterns Questionnaire (Christensen, 1988) and the Frequency and Acceptability of Partner Behavior Inventory (Doss & Christensen, 2006). Such information may assist clinicians who wish to pursue integrative behavioral couple therapy (Cano & Leonard, 2006). Longitudinal studies in which the beliefs and behavior of the patient and partner are assessed over time (ideally during the transition from acute to chronic pain) could potentially illuminate processes predictive of long-term functioning and adjustment in patients and family members.

Although this review has focused primarily on assessment of couples, the effects of parental chronic pain on children require additional research, as do the effects of parent–child interaction on the illness behaviors of children and adolescents with chronic pain (Walker, Levy, & Whitehead, 2006). Some studies have suggested that children of patients with chronic pain may be at increased risk for illness behaviors and maladjustment (Chun, Turner, & Romano, 1993; Jamison & Walker, 1992; Levy et al., 2004). While the mechanisms by which such increased risk may occur remain unclear, research has suggested an association between parent and child pain and dysfunction, and that this relationship may be mediated by processes such as catastrophizing (Schanberg et al., 2001).

Further research on the similarities and differences between solicitous behavior and social support in their topography, functional value, and perceptions by patients and partners is also needed. This issue has particular relevance for treatment given that these classes of partner responses may function to enhance patient psychosocial functioning and relationship satisfaction or contribute to ongoing pain behaviors and disability. Particular attention needs to be paid to determining optimal patterns of partner responses that support both physical and psychological functioning and relationship satisfaction. Moderating factors, such as gender or marital satisfaction, also require further investigation.

Although significant progress has been made, as noted earlier, concurrent multimodal assessment remains underutilized. Continued development, refinement, and application of combined behavioral, cognitive, and even physiological assessment instruments and methodologies to the evaluation of patients with chronic pain and their significant others will provide much-needed ability to test more complex models of the psychosocial context of chronic pain and their implications for treatment.

REFERENCES

Ahern, D. K., Adams, A. E., & Follick, M. J. (1985). Emotional and marital disturbance in spouses of chronic low back pain patients. *Clinical Journal of Pain, 1,* 69–74.

Alexandrov, E. O., Cowan, P. A., & Cowan, C. P. (2005). Couple attachment and the quality of marital relationship: Method and concept in the validation of the new Couple Attachment Interview and coding system. *Attachment and Human Development, 7,* 123–152.

Boothby, J. L., Thorn, B. E., Overduin, L. Y., & Ward, L. C. (2004). Catastrophizing and perceived partner responses to pain. *Pain, 109,* 500–506.

Broderick, J. E., Schwartz, J. E., Vikingstad, G., Pribbernow, M., Grossman, S., & Stone, A. A. (2008). The accuracy of pain and fatigue items across different reporting periods. *Pain, 139,* 146–157.

Cano, A. (2004). Pain catastrophizing and social support in married individuals with chronic pain: The moderating role of pain duration. *Pain, 110,* 656–664.

Cano, A., Barterian, J. A., & Heller, J. B. (2008). Empathic and nonempathic interaction in chronic pain couples. *Clinical Journal of Pain, 24,* 678–684.

Cano, A., Gillis, M., Heinz, W., Geisser, M., & Foran, H. (2004). Marital functioning, chronic pain, and psychological distress. *Pain, 107,* 99–106.

Cano, A., Johansen, A. B., & Franz, A. (2005). Multilevel analysis of spousal congruence on pain, interference, and disability. *Pain, 118,* 369–379.

Cano, A., Johansen, A. B., & Geisser, M. (2004).

Spousal congruence on disability, pain, and spouse responses to pain. *Pain, 109,* 258–265.

Cano, A., & Leonard, M. (2006). Integrative behavioral couple therapy for chronic pain: Promoting behavior change and emotional acceptance. *Journal of Clinical Psychology, 62,* 1409–1418.

Cano, A., Leonard, M. T., & Franz, A. (2005). The significant other version of the Pain Catastrophizing Scale (PCS-S): Preliminary validation. *Pain, 119,* 26–37.

Cano, A., Miller, L. R., & Loree, A. (2009). Spouse beliefs about partner chronic pain. *Journal of Pain, 10*(5), 486–492.

Cano, A., Weisberg, J., & Gallagher, M. (2000). Marital satisfaction and pain severity mediate the association between negative spouse responses to pain and depressive symptoms in a chronic pain patient sample. *Pain Medicine, 1,* 35–43.

Christensen, A. (1988). Dysfunctional interaction patterns in couples. In P. Noller & M. A. Fitzgerald (Eds.), *Perspectives on marital interaction* (pp. 31–52). Philadelphia: Multilingual Matters.

Chun, D. Y., Turner, J. A., & Romano, J. M. (1993). Children of chronic pain patients: Risk factors for maladjustment. *Pain, 52,* 311–317.

Clipp, E. C., & George, L. K. (1992). Patients with cancer and their spouse caregivers. Perceptions of the illness experience. *Cancer, 69,* 1074–1079.

Compas, B. E., Haaga, D. A., Keefe, F. J., Leitenberg, H., & Williams, D. A. (1998). Sampling of empirically supported psychological treatments from health psychology: Smoking, chronic pain, cancer, and bulimia nervosa. *Journal of Consulting and Clinical Psychology, 66,* 89–112.

Cremeans-Smith, J. K., Stephens, M. A., Franks, M. M., Martire, L. M., Druley, J. A., & Wojno, W. C. (2003). Spouses' and physicians' perceptions of pain severity in older women with osteoarthritis: Dyadic agreement and patients' well-being. *Pain, 106,* 27–34.

Doss, B. D., & Christensen, A. (2006). Acceptance in romantic relationships: The Frequency and Acceptability of Spouse Behavior Inventory. *Psychological Assessment, 18,* 289–302.

Eddy, J. M., Heyman, R. E., & Weiss, R. L. (1991). An empirical investigation of the Dyadic Adjustment Scale: Exploring the differences between marital "satisfaction" and "adjustment." *Behavioral Assessment, 13,* 199–220.

Fillingim, R. B., Doleys, D. M., Edwards, R. R., & Lowery, D. (2003). Spousal responses are differentially associated with clinical variables in women and men with chronic pain. *Clinical Journal of Pain, 19,* 217–224.

Fischer, J., & Corcoran, K. (2007). *Measures for clinical practice and research: A sourcebook: Vol. 1. Couples, families, and children.* New York: Oxford University Press.

Flor, H., Behle, D., & Birbaumer, N. (1993). Assessment of pain-related cognitions in chronic pain patients. *Journal of Psychosomatic Research, 31,* 251–259.

Flor, H., Breitenstein, C., Birbaumer, N., & Fürst, M. (1995). A psychophysiological analysis of spouse solicitousness towards pain behaviors, spouse interaction, and pain perception. *Behavior Therapy, 26,* 255–272.

Flor, H., Kerns, R. D., & Turk, D. C. (1987). The role of spouse reinforcement, perceived pain, and activity levels of chronic pain patients. *Journal of Psychosomatic Research, 31,* 251–259.

Flor, H., Turk, D. C., & Rudy, T. E. (1989). Relationship of pain impact and significant other reinforcement of pain behaviors: The mediating role of gender, marital status, and marital satisfaction. *Pain, 38,* 45–50.

Fordyce, W. E. (1976). *Behavioral methods in chronic pain and illness.* St. Louis, MO: Mosby.

Fruzetti, A. E. (2001). *Validation and invalidation coding system.* Unpublished manuscript, University of Nevada, Reno.

Funk, J. L., & Rogge, R. D. (2007). Testing the ruler with item response theory: Increasing the precision of measurement for relationship satisfaction with the Couples Satisfaction Index. *Journal of Family Psychology, 21,* 572–583.

Geisser, M. E., Cano, A., & Leonard, M. T. (2005). Factors associated with marital satisfaction and mood among spouses of persons with chronic back pain. *Journal of Pain, 6,* 518–525.

Giardino, N. D., Jensen, M. P., Turner, J. A., Ehde, D. M., & Cardenas, D. D. (2003). Social environment moderates the association between catastrophizing and pain among persons with a spinal cord injury. *Pain, 106,* 19–25.

Gottman, J. M., & Levenson, R. W. (1992). Toward a typology of marriage based on affective behavior: Preliminary differences in behavior, physiology, health, and risk for dissolution. *Journal of Personality and Social Psychology, 63,* 221–233.

Goubert, L., Craig, K. D., Vervoort, T., Morley, S., Sullivan, M. J. L., Williams, A., et al. (2005). Facing others in pain: The effects of empathy. *Pain, 118,* 285–288.

Hadjistavropoulos, T., & Craig, K. D. (2002). A theoretical framework for understanding self-report and observational measures of pain: A communications model. *Behaviour Research and Therapy, 440,* 551–570.

Hahlweg, K., Reisner, L., Kohli, G., Vollmer, M., Schindler, L., & Revenstorf, D. (1984). Development and validity of a new system to analyze interpersonal communication (KPI). In K. Hahlweg & N. Jacobson (Eds.), *Marital interaction: Analysis and modification* (pp. 182–198). New York: Guilford Press.

Hayes, S. C., Strosahl, K. D., & Wilson, K. G. (1999). *Acceptance and commitment therapy: An experiential approach to behavior change.* New York: Guilford Press.

Hewitt, P. L., Flett, G. L., & Mikail, S. F. (1995). Perfectionism and relationship adjustment in pain patients and their spouses. *Journal of Family Psychology, 9,* 335–347.

Heyman, R. E. (2001). Observation of couple conflicts: Clinical assessment applications, stubborn truths, and shaky foundation. *Psychological Assessment, 13,* 5–35.

Holtzman, S., & DeLongis, A. (2007). One day at a time: The impact of daily satisfaction with spouse responses on pain, negative affect and catastrophizing among individuals with rheumatoid arthritis. *Pain, 131,* 202–213.

Hops, H., Davis, B., & Longoria, N. (1995). Methodological issues in direct observation: Illustrations with the Living in Familial Environments (LIFE) coding system. *Journal of Clinical Child Psychology, 24,* 193–203.

Hunsley, J., Best, M., Lefebvre, M., & Vito, D. (2001). The seven-item short form of the Dyadic Adjustment Scale: Further evidence for construct validity. *American Journal of Family Therapy, 29,* 325–335.

Jacobson, N. S., Follette, W. C., & Revenstorf, D. (1986). Toward a standard definition of clinically significant change. *Behavior Therapy, 17,* 308–311.

Jacobson, N. S., Follette, W. C., Revenstorf, D., Baucom, D. H., Hahlweg, K., & Margolin, G. (1984). Variability in outcome and clinical significance of behavioral marital therapy: A reanalysis of outcome data. *Journal of Consulting and Clinical Psychology, 52,* 497–504.

Jacobson, N. S., & Truax, P. (1991). Clinical significance: A statistical approach to defining meaningful change in psychotherapy research. *Journal of Consulting and Clinical Psychology, 59,* 12–19.

Jamison, R. N., Rudy, T. E., Penzien, D. B., & Mosley, T. H. (1994). Cognitive-behavioral classification of chronic pain: Replication and extension of empirically derived patient profiles. *Pain, 57,* 277–292.

Jamison, R. N., & Walker, L. S. (1992). Illness behavior in children of chronic pain patients. *International Journal of Psychiatry in Medicine, 22,* 329–342.

Johansen, A., & Cano, A. (2007). A preliminary investigation of affective interaction in chronic pain couples. *Pain, 132,* S86–S95.

Keefe, F. J., & Block, A. R. (1982). Development of an observation method of assessing pain behavior in chronic low back pain patients. *Behavior Therapy, 13,* 363–375.

Kenny, D. A., Kashy, D. A., & Cook, W. L. (2006). *Dyadic data analysis.* New York: Guilford Press.

Kerig, P., & Baucom, D. H. (2004). *Couple observational coding systems.* Mahwah, NJ: Erlbaum.

Kerig, P., & Lindahl, K. (2000). *Family observational coding systems: Resources for systemic research.* Mahwah, NJ: Erlbaum.

Kerns, R. D. (1995). Family assessment and intervention. In P. M. Nicassio & T. W. Smith (Eds.), *Managing chronic illness: A biopsychosocial perspective* (pp. 207–244). Washington, DC: American Psychological Association.

Kerns, R. D., Haythornthwaite, J., Southwick, S., & Giller, E. L. (1990). The role of marital interaction in chronic pain and depressive symptom severity. *Journal of Psychosomatic Research, 34,* 401–408.

Kerns, R. D., & Rosenberg, R. (1995). Pain-relevant responses from significant others: Development of a significant other version of the WHYMPI scales. *Pain, 61,* 245–249.

Kerns, R. D., Southwick, S., Giller, E. L., Haythornthwaite, J. A., Jacob, M. C., & Rosenberg, R. (1991). The relationship between reports of pain-related social interactions and expressions of pain and affective distress. *Behavior Therapy, 22,* 101–111.

Kerns, R. D., & Turk, D. C. (1984). Depression and chronic pain: The mediating role of the spouse. *Journal of Marriage and the Family, 46,* 845–852.

Kerns, R. D., Turk, D. C., & Rudy, T. E. (1985). The West Haven–Yale Multidimensional Pain Inventory (WHYMPI). *Pain, 23,* 345–356.

Kerns, R. D., & Weiss, L. H. (1994). Family influences on the course of chronic illness: A cognitive-behavioral transactional model. *Annals of Behavioral Medicine, 16,* 116–121.

Kwan, K. S., Roberts, L. J., & Swalm, D. M. (2005). Sexual dysfunction and chronic pain: The role of psychological variables and impact on quality of life. *European Journal of Pain, 9,* 643–652.

Leonard, M. T., & Cano, A. (2006). Pain affects spouses too: Personal experience with pain and catastrophizing as correlates of spouse distress. *Pain, 126,* 139–146.

Levy, R. L., Whitehead, W. E., Walker, L. S., Von Korff, M., Feld, A. D., Garner, M., et al. (2004). Increased somatic complaints and health-care utilization in children: Effects of parent IBS status and parent response to gastrointestinal symptoms. *American Journal of Gastroenterology, 99,* 2442–2451.

Lewis, M. A., & Rook, K. S. (1999). Social control in personal relationships: Impact on health behaviors and psychological distress. *Health Psychology, 18,* 63–71.

Locke, H. J., & Wallace, K. M. (1959). Short marital adjustment and prediction tests: Their reliability and validity. *Marriage and Family Living, 21,* 251–255.

Lousberg, R., Schmidt, A. J., & Groenman, N. H. (1992). The relationship between spouse solicitousness and pain behavior: Searching for more experimental evidence. *Pain, 51,* 75–79.

Main, C. J. (1999). Medicolegal aspects of pain: The nature of psychological opinion in cases of personal injury. In R. J. Gatachel & D. C. Turk (Eds.), *Psychosocial factors in pain: Critical perspectives* (pp. 132–147). New York: Guilford Press.

Maruta, T., & Osborne, D. (1978). Sexual activity in chronic pain patients. *Psychosomatics, 19,* 531–537.

Maruta, T., Osborne, D., Swanson, D. W., & Halling, J. M. (1981). Chronic pain patients and spouses: Marital and sexual adjustment. *Mayo Clinic Proceedings, 56,* 307–310.

McCracken, L. M. (1998). Learning to live with the pain: Acceptance of pain predicts adjustment in persons with chronic pain. *Pain, 74,* 21–27.

McCracken, L. M. (2005). *Contextual cognitive-behavioral therapy for chronic pain: Progress in pain research and management* (Vol. 33). Seattle, WA: IASP Press.

McCracken, L. M., & Eccleston, C. (2003). Coping or acceptance: What to do about chronic pain? *Pain, 105,* 197–204.

Miaskowski, C., Zimmer, E. F., Barrett, K. M., Dibble, S. L., & Wallhagen, M. (1997). Differences in patients' and family caregivers' perceptions of the pain experience influence patient and caregiver outcomes. *Pain, 72,* 217–226.

Newton-John, T. R., & Williams, A. C. (2006). Chronic pain couples: Perceived marital interactions and pain behaviors. *Pain, 123,* 53–63.

NIH Technology Assessment Panel on Integration of Behavioral and Relaxation Approaches into the Treatment of Chronic Pain and Insomnia. (1996). Integration of behavioral and relaxation approaches into the treatment of chronic pain and insomnia. *Journal of the American Medical Association, 276,* 313–318.

Novy, D. M., Nelson, D. V., Francis, D. J., & Turk, D. C. (1995). Perspectives of chronic pain: An evaluative comparison of restrictive and comprehensive models. *Psychological Bulletin, 118,* 238–247.

Papas, R. K., Robinson, M. E., & Riley, J. L., III. (2001). Perceived spouse responsiveness to chronic pain: Three empirical subgroups. *Journal of Pain, 2,* 262–269.

Paulsen, J. S., & Altmaier, E. M. (1995). The effects of perceived versus enacted social support on the discriminative cue function of spouses for pain behaviors. *Pain, 60,* 103–110.

Pence, L. B., Thorn, B. E., Jensen, M. P., & Romano, J. M. (2008). Examination of perceived spouse responses to patient well and pain behavior in patients with headache. *Clinical Journal of Pain, 24,* 654–662.

Peters, M. L., Sorbi, M. J., Kruise, D. A., Kerssens, J. J., Verhaak, P. F., & Bensing, J. M. (2000). Electronic diary assessment of pain, disability and psychological adaptation in patients differing in duration of pain. *Pain, 84,* 181–192.

Porter, L. S., Keefe, F. J., Wellington, C., & Williams, A. C. (2008). Pain communication in the context of osteoarthritis: Patient and partner self-efficacy for pain communication and holding back from discussion of pain and arthritis-related concerns. *Clinical Journal of Pain, 24,* 662–668.

Reich, J. W., & Olmstead, M. (2007). Partner's social control effects on relationship satisfaction in fibromyalgia patients: Illness uncertainty and bodily pain as moderators. *Journal of Social and Clinical Psychology, 26,* 623–639.

Reich, J. W., & Zautra, A. J. (1995a). Other-reliance encouragement effects in female rheumatoid arthritis patients. *Journal of Social and Clinical Psychology, 14,* 119–133.

Reich, J. W., & Zautra, A. J. (1995b). Spouse encouragement of self-reliance and other-reliance in rheumatoid arthritis couples. *Journal of Behavioral Medicine, 18,* 249–260.

Riemsma, R. P., Taal, E., & Rasker, J. J. (2000). Perceptions about perceived functional disabilities and pain of people with rheumatoid arthritis: Differences between patients and their spouses and correlates with well-being. *Arthritis Care and Research, 13,* 255–261.

Romano, J. M., Jensen, M. P., Schmaling, K. B., Hops, H., & Buchwald, D. S. (2009). Illness behaviors in patients with unexplained chronic fatigue are associated with significant other responses. *Journal of Behavioral Medicine, 32,* 558–569.

Romano, J. M., Jensen, M. P., Turner, J. A., Good, A. B., & Hops, H. (2000). Chronic pain patient–partner interactions: Further support for a behavioral model of chronic pain. *Behavior Therapy, 31,* 415–440.

Romano, J. M., Turner, J. A., & Clancy, S. L. (1989). Sex differences in the relationship of pain patient dysfunction to spouse adjustment. *Pain, 39,* 289–295.

Romano, J. M., Turner, J. A., Friedman, L. S., Bulcroft, R. A., Jensen, M. P., & Hops, H. (1991). Observational assessment of chronic pain patient–spouse behavioral interactions. *Behavior Therapy, 11,* 549–567.

Romano, J. M., Turner, J. A., Friedman, L. S., Bulcroft, R. A., Jensen, M. P., Hops, H., et al. (1992). Sequential analysis of chronic pain behaviors and spouse responses. *Journal of Consulting and Clinical Psychology, 60,* 777–782.

Romano, J. M., Turner, J. A., Jensen, M. P., Friedman, L. S., Bulcroft, R. A., Hops, H., et al. (1995). Chronic pain patient–spouse behavioral interactions predict patient disability. *Pain, 63,* 353–360.

Sabourin, S., Valois, P., & Lussier, Y. (2005). Development and validation of a brief version of the Dyadic Adjustment Scale with a nonparametric item analysis model. *Psychological Assessment, 17,* 15–27.

Schanberg, L. E., Anthony, K. K., Gill, K. M., Lefebvre, J. C., Kredich, D. W., & Macharoni, L. M. (2001). Family pain history predicts child health status in children with chronic rheumatic disease. *Pediatrics, 108*(3), E47.

Schwartz, L., Jensen, M. P., & Romano, J. M. (2005). The development and psychometric evaluation of an instrument to assess spouse responses to pain and well behavior in patients with chronic pain: The Spouse Response Inventory. *Journal of Pain, 6,* 243–252.

Schwartz, L., Slater, M. A., & Birchler, G. R. (1996). The role of pain behaviors in the modulation of marital conflict in chronic pain couples. *Pain, 65,* 227–233.

Schwartz, L., Slater, M. A., Birchler, G. R., & Atkinson, J. H. (1991). Depression in spouses of chronic pain patients: The role of patient pain and anger, and marital satisfaction. *Pain, 44,* 61–67.

Severeijns, R., Vlaeyen, J. W., & van den Hout, M. A. (2004). Do we need a communal coping model of pain catastrophizing?: An alternative explanation. *Pain, 111,* 226–229.

Sharp, T. J., & Nicholas, M. K. (2000). Assessing the significant others of chronic pain patients: The psychometric properties of significant other questionnaires. *Pain, 88,* 135–144.

Sharpley, C. F., & Rogers, H. J. (1984). Preliminary validation of the Abbreviated Spanier Dyadic Adjustment Scale: Some psychometric data regarding a screening test of marital adjustment. *Educational and Psychological Measurement, 44,* 1045–1049.

Snyder, D. K., Heyman, R. E., & Haynes, S. N. (2005). Evidence-based approaches to assessing couple distress. *Psychological Assessment, 17,* 288–307.

Sorbi, M. J., Peters, M. L., Kruise, D. A., Maas, C. J., Kerssens, J. J., Verhaak, P. F., et al. (2006). Electronic momentary assessment in chronic pain II: Pain and psychological pain responses as predictors of pain disability. *Clinical Journal of Pain, 22,* 67–81.

Spanier, G. B. (1976). Measuring dyadic adjustment: New scales for assessing the quality of marriage and similar dyads. *Journal of Marriage and the Family, 38,* 15–28.

Stampler, D. B., Wall, J. R., Cassisi, J. E., & Davis, H. (1997). Marital satisfaction and psychophysiological responsiveness in spouses of patients with chronic pain. *International Journal of Rehabilitation and Health, 3,* 159–170.

Stroud, M. W., Turner, J. A., Jensen, M. P., & Cardenas, D. D. (2006). Partner responses to pain behaviors are associated with depression and activity interference among persons with chronic pain and spinal cord injury. *Journal of Pain, 7,* 91–99.

Sullivan, M. J., & D'Eon, J. L. (1990). Relation between catastrophizing and depression in chronic pain patients. *Journal of Abnormal Psychology, 99,* 260–263.

Sullivan, M. J., Thorn, B., Haythornthwaite, J. A., Keefe, F., Martin, M., Bradley, L. A., et al. (2001). Theoretical perspectives on the relation between catastrophizing and pain. *Clinical Journal of Pain, 17,* 52–64.

Taylor, A. G., Lorentzen, L. J., & Blank, M. B. (1990). Psychologic distress of chronic pain sufferers and their spouses. *Journal of Pain and Symptom Management, 5,* 6–10.

Turk, D. C., & Flor, H. (1987). Pain greater than pain behaviors: The utility and limitations of the pain behavior construct. *Pain, 31,* 277–295.

Turk, D. C., Kerns, R. D., & Rosenberg, R. (1992). Effects of marital interaction on chronic pain and disability: Examining the down side of social support. *Rehabilitation Psychology, 37,* 259–274.

Turk, D. C., Okifuji, A., Sinclair, J. D., & Starz, T. W. (1996). Pain, disability, and physical functioning in subgroups of patients with fibromyalgia. *Journal of Rheumatology, 23,* 1255–1262.

Turk, D. C., & Rudy, T. E. (1988). Toward an empirically derived taxonomy of chronic pain patients: Integration of psychological assessment data. *Journal of Consulting and Clinical Psychology, 56,* 233–238.

Turk, D. C., & Rudy, T. E. (1990). The robustness of an empirically derived taxonomy of chronic pain patients. *Pain, 43,* 27–35.

Turner, J. A., Jensen, M. P., & Romano, J. M. (2000). Do beliefs, coping, and catastrophizing independently predict functioning in patients with chronic pain? *Pain, 85,* 115–125.

Turner, J. A., Jensen, M. P., Warms, C. A., & Cardenas, D. D. (2002). Catastrophizing is associated with pain intensity, psychological distress, and pain-related disability among individuals with chronic pain after spinal cord injury. *Pain, 98,* 127–134.

Turner, J. A., Mancl, L., & Aaron, L. A. (2004). Pain-related catastrophizing: A daily process study. *Pain, 110,* 103–111.

Walker, L. S., Levy, R. L., & Whitehead, W. E. (2006). Validation of a measure of protective parent responses to children's pain. *Clinical Journal of Pain, 22,* 712–716.

Yeager, K. A., Miaskowski, C., Dibble, S. L., & Wallhagen, M. (1995). Differences in pain knowledge and perception of the pain experience between outpatients with cancer and their family caregivers. *Oncology Nursing Forum, 22,* 1235–1241.

PART II

MEASURES OF PAIN
NOT DEPENDENT ON SELF-REPORT

CHAPTER 6

The Facial Expression of Pain

KENNETH D. CRAIG
KENNETH M. PRKACHIN
RUTH E. GRUNAU

People in pain communicate their experience through a remarkable variety of actions, ranging from the use of language to diverse forms of nonverbal activity. The latter include (1) paralinguistic vocalizations, such as crying and moaning; (2) other nonverbal qualities of speech, such as amplitude, hesitancies, or timbre; (3) visible physiological activity, such as pallor or muscle tension; (4) bodily activity, including involuntary reflexes and purposeful action; and (5) facial expressions. Nonverbal expression adds context and meaning to verbal expression and tends to have greater credibility for observers because it is less subject to voluntary control. This chapter examines how facial expression allows clinicians, investigators, and others to formulate judgments about another person's pain, regardless of whether that person uses words to communicate.

A PRIMARY ROLE FOR FACIAL ACTIVITY IN SOCIAL COMMUNICATION

Facial expression is a powerful form of social communication (Ekman & Rosenberg, 2005). People attend carefully, if not continuously, to the facial activity of others and derive considerable information. People's facial expressions are readily accessible, available continuously, and highly plastic. They change rapidly to display a remarkable variety of patterns, revealing not only pain but a broad scope of emotions, motives, thoughts, attention, intentions, and social reactions. Utilizing facial cues enhances social effectiveness because this information is rarely entirely redundant with the content of speech. Personal safety, as well as the safety of others, may depend on accurate detection and interpretation of facial expressions. They have a primal capacity to warn others of personal threat and danger, thereby increasing the likelihood of escape or other preventive action. As well, these cues can instigate empathetic reactions and enhance caregiving (Goubert et al., 2005). The adaptive value of facial activity as a form of social communication reflects evolutionary dispositions to attend to others' actions and to communicate via this modality (Darwin (1872/1965; Fridlund, 1994; Langford et al., 2010; Williams, 2002).

Assessment of pain using facial expression relies on appreciating consistencies that differentiate pain from other subjective states. Genetic roots are evident in the anatomical structures, neurophysiological regulation, and behavioral organization of facial dis-

117

plays (Fridlund, 1994). In addition to this biological basis, children also become acculturated to family and ethnic environments in which they grow up, and people can modulate expression consistent with normative standards and the immediate social context.

SPECIFIC FACIAL ACTIONS ASSOCIATED WITH PAIN

Although most people intuitively recognize facial grimaces of pain, the speed and complexity of the response have led to diverse and sometimes inaccurate descriptions. Fortunately, objective, detailed coding of facial activity is possible, including fine-grained delineation of facial activity during all types of experiences. The Facial Action Coding System (FACS; Ekman & Friesen, 1978) provides objective, anatomically based descriptions of all possible facial actions, thereby avoiding inference as to underlying subjective states (see Cohn & Ekman, 2005, for a review of alternative measurement approaches). A comprehensive account of any facial display can be provided using 44 discrete facial actions and head movements. Each facial action represents the movement of a single facial muscle, or, in a few cases, a group of muscle strands that move as a unit.

Research applications of FACS typically use videotaped slow-motion or stop-frame feedback. Coders are trained to apply specific operational criteria to determine which actions are visible, and to identify their onset, offset, and (when possible) intensity during specified time intervals. Facial *expressions* (as opposed to specific movements) can be defined as two or more specific facial actions that have a common onset or overlap in time. Intercoder reliability for identifying pain-related actions has consistently been very good (LeResche & Dworkin, 1988; Prkachin & Mercer, 1989).

Numerous studies provide FACS-based accounts of facial activity during painful events. There is some variability in detail, but core actions tend to be consistent across different types of acute pain arising from clinical injury, persistent pain, and experimental pain stimulation. The core actions in adults described by Prkachin (1992) were brow lowering, orbit tightening, upper-lip raising/nose wrinkling, and eye narrowing

or closure, but there is variability with the severity, the source of distress, and personal and situational variables. Horizontal lip corner pull, oblique pull at the corner of the lips, and mouth open through vertical stretching of the mouth may also be observed. Anatomy of the facial muscles controlling facial actions associated with pain is shown in Figure 6.1. Figure 6.2 displays a patient with low back pain reacting to a painful range-of-motion exercise (Hadjistavropoulos & Craig, 1994), providing a composite of the facial actions commonly observed and some additional actions specific to the person or situation.

The distinct subset of facial actions is usually instigated by short, sharp acute pain, as demonstrated in clinical settings by examining reactions to invasive procedures, for example, injections (Lilley, Craig, & Grunau, 1997) or venipuncture (Grunau & Craig, 1987; Nader, Oberlander, Chambers, & Craig, 2004), and using instigated laboratory pain (e.g., Craig & Patrick, 1985; Prkachin, 1992). The reaction is also observed during acute exacerbation of persistent pain, such as temporomandibular joint disorder (LeResche & Dworkin, 1984), shoulder pathology (Prkachin & Mercer, 1989), chronic low back pain (Hadjistavropoulos & Craig, 1994), surgical repair (Hadjistavropoulos, LaChapelle, Hadjistavropoulos, Green, & Asmundson, 2002; Hadjistavropoulos, LaChapelle, MacLeod, Snider, & Craig, 2000), and muscle contraction headaches (Iezzi, Adams, Bugg, & Stokes, 1991). Reports of sex differences are variable, including differences (e.g., Sullivan, Tripp, & Santor, 2000) and no differences in adults (e.g., Kunz, Gruber, & Lautenbacher, 2006) and infants (Schiavenato et al., 2008).

Considerable evidence supports the position that facial activity represents pain:

1. This display pattern is observed as the response to acute clinical and experimental pain, as well as exacerbations of chronic pain, including the range of clinical conditions described earlier (Kunz, Mylius, Schepelmann, & Lautenbacher, 2008; Nader & Craig, 2008; Prkachin, 2009).
2. Facial displays diminish when analgesics are applied (Guinsburg et al., 1998; Scott et al., 1999; Taddio, Stevens, et al., 1997).

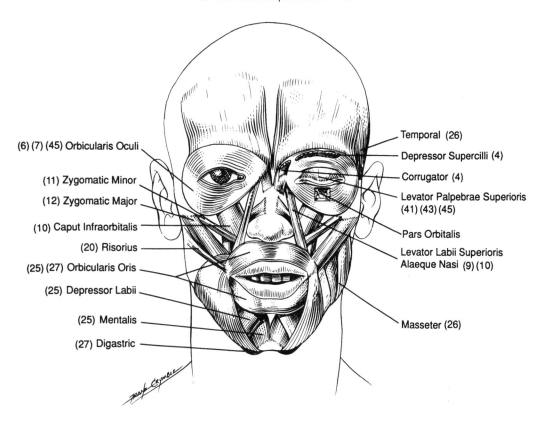

(6) (7) (45) Orbicularis Oculi

(11) Zygomatic Minor

(12) Zygomatic Major

(10) Caput Infraorbitalis

(20) Risorius

(25) (27) Orbicularis Oris

(25) Depressor Labii

(25) Mentalis

(27) Digastric

Temporal (26)

Depressor Supercilli (4)

Corrugator (4)

Levator Palpebrae Superioris
(41) (43) (45)

Pars Orbitalis

Levator Labii Superioris
Alaeque Nasi (9) (10)

Masseter (26)

FIGURE 6.1. Facial muscles controlling the various facial actions association with pain. Both core and ancillary actions are identified and labeled according to the Facial Action Coding System (FACS; Ekman & Friesen, 1978) as follows: (4) brow lowering, (6) cheek raising, (7) lids tight, (9) nose wrinkling, (11) nasolabial deepening, (10) raised upper lip, (12) lip corner pull, (20) lips stretching, (25) lips parting, (26) jaw dropping, (41) lids drooping, (43) eyes closing, (45) blinking.

3. The magnitude of the display covaries with verbal reports of pain severity, when circumstances are appropriate (Craig & Patrick, 1985; Kunz, Mylius, Schepelmann, & Lautenbaucher, 2004; Labus, Keefe, & Jensen, 2003). Social expectations or demand may result in decoupling of the measures, for example, leading to denial of pain when it is present (Hill & Craig, 2002). This is discussed in some detail below.

4. The facial display of pain can be differentiated from reactions to aversive, nonnoxious events (Hale & Hadjistavropoulos, 1997; Simon, Craig, Gosselin, Belin, & Rainville, 2008).

5. Untrained observers identify the facial display as indicative of pain (Pillai Riddell, Badali, & Craig, 2004; Xavier Balda et al., 2000) and are able to discriminate facial displays of pain from reactions to aversive but non-noxious emotional events (Kappesser & Williams, 2002; Simon et al., 2008).

6. Untrained observer judgments tend to be correlated with both the severity of the noxious insult applied (Patrick, Craig, & Prkachin, 1986; Prkachin & Mercer, 1989) and the objectively coded vigor of the facial display (Lints-Martindale, Hadjistavropoulos, Barber, & Gibson, 2007; Messmer, Nader, & Craig, 2008).

7. Witnessing others displaying facial expressions of pain instigates unique patterns of brain activity associated in part with the direct experience of pain (Botvinick et al., 2005), with the intensity of the observed pain encoded in observer brain activity (Saarela et al., 2007) and the pattern of brain activation differentia-

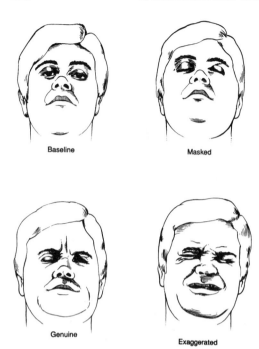

Baseline

Masked

Genuine

Exaggerated

FIGURE 6.2. Facial expressions of a patient with chronic low back pain during (top left) a neutral baseline period prior to onset of physical activity; (bottom left) straight-leg raising, provoking a sharp exacerbation of pain; (top right) repetition of the straight-leg raising, accompanied by instructions to mask the facial display; and (bottom right) repetition of this exercise, along with instructions to exaggerate the response. The video camera was placed above the patient's feet. See Hadjistavropoulos and Craig (1994) for details on the procedure.

ble from reactions to others' nonpainful but aversive emotional displays (Simon, Craig, Miltner, & Rainville, 2006).

In summary, the evidence provides support for the content, criterion, and construct validity of facial expression measures of pain. The facial expression displays both sensitivity and specificity as an index of acute pain and reflects the experience of chronic pain when it is exacerbated.

Judgment Study Approaches

Investigators or clinicians without resources to perform precise behavioral observation may consider judgment study approaches

(Rosenthal, 1993). Here, facial behavior during a potentially painful provocation, such as venipuncture or controlled heat, can be sampled using video recording technology. A behavioral rating scale, such as a pain unpleasantness scale, can then be applied to judge underlying dimensions of painful experience. Multiple judges are necessary to establish the reliability of judgments, with reliability indices (e.g., effective reliability or intraclass correlations) being commonly very high. Ratings of manageable (i.e., small) numbers of judges can be aggregated into overall scores (cf. Prkachin, Berzins, & Mercer, 1994). Judgment study approaches are relatively less resource-intensive than fine-grained behavioral coding procedures but have the advantage of enabling analysis of natural socioperceptive processes of observers. They have the disadvantage of not being able to provide insight into the specific behavioral determinants of judgments. Judges must be provided in advance, with the description of the facial display of pain appropriate to the age group, as summarized in the section "Essential Features in Clinical Coding of Facial Expressions of Pain" later in this chapter.

INDIVIDUAL DIFFERENCES

Although a distinctive and consistent pattern of facial activity is observed during painful events, variation has been observed across situations and within individuals.

Pain Severity

The intensity of acute pain experience appears to be encoded in the facial display, both in the vigor and the number of specific facial actions recruited. Facial reactions increase in frequency and intensity as a function of noxious stimulus intensity (Lints-Martindale et al., 2007). Lower levels of pain are manifest in brow lowering and narrowing of the eyes, with more severe experiences progressively recruiting more vigorous reactions in these actions and in the lower face. Some people begin to react at lower levels of noxious stimulation than others (Prkachin & Craig, 1995).

Facial expression can largely be characterized as a reflexive, automatic reaction to painful experience, whereas verbal report is representative of a deliberate, controlled, and goal-oriented response to the event (Hadjistavropoulos & Craig, 2002). While both indicators can be responsive to situational demands, the continuing stream of facial expression does not tend to be as carefully monitored (Craig, Versloot, Goubert, Vervoort, & Crombez, 2010). As well, discordance between the facial display and verbal report is most often observed during chronic pain, unless there is acute exacerbation.

Concurrent Emotional States

Pain often is accompanied by emotional distress, including fear, anxiety, anger, and depression (Hale & Hadjistavropoulos, 1997). Although the configuration displayed during pain shares components with facial displays during non-noxious but aversive emotional states (e.g., fear, anger, disgust), pain and other negative emotional states have unique patterns that can be distinguished when the detail and configurations of actions are examined (Kappesser & Williams, 2002; Kunz, Prkachin, & Lautenbacher, 2009; Prkachin & Solomon, 2008; Simon et al., 2008; Williams, 2002). For example, brow lowering is common to pain and fearful expressions, but fear is also associated with opening the eyes wide in contrast to narrowing of the eyes during pain.

Cognitive Functioning

Facial actions are important features of observational measures of pain for people with intellectual disabilities or declining cognitive functioning as a result of brain disease (see Chapter 13 by Hadjistavropoulos, Breau, & Craig, this volume). Contrary to widespread beliefs that people with intellectual disabilities or cognitive impairment are less sensitive or indifferent to pain, facial displays are often more vigorous among those with cognitive impairment (Hadjistavropoulos et al., 2000; Kunz, Scharmann, Hemmeter, Schepelmann, & Lautenbacher, 2007).

Other evidence indicates that the facial display of pain varies with the pattern of thinking and various coping styles. Adults and children who persistently engage in pain *catastrophizing* (Sullivan et al., 2001), characterized by magnifying severity of distress and its consequences, ruminating on the experience, and believing they cannot control the painful events, tend to display more vigorous facial activity (Sullivan, Adams, & Sullivan, 2004; Sullivan, Martel, Tripp, Savard, & Crombez, 2006; Vervoort et al., 2008; Vervoort, Goubert, & Crombez, 2009). When pain severity was controlled, this phenomenon was not observed (Kunz, Chatelle, Lautenbacher, & Rainville, 2008).

Context Influences

Variability in pain expression is associated with the pain setting (Sweet & McGrath, 1998), indicating that nonverbal expression is not exclusively an expression of internal states. Studies of audience effects suggest that people inhibit painful displays in the presence of strangers (Kleck et al., 1976; Sullivan et al., 2004; Vervoort et al., 2008), perhaps to avoid appearing vulnerable, or as not conforming to normative standards that encourage stoic forebearance of pain. This sensitivity to context is capable of being overridden: Children who catastrophize display more facial activity irrespective of the audience (Vervoort et al., 2008).

THE FACIAL EXPRESSION OF PAIN IN INFANTS AND YOUNG CHILDREN

Assessing pain in infants or young children who lack language is a particular challenge (see Ruskin, Amaria, Warnock, & McGrath, Chapter 11, this volume). A broad range of cues for pain is available, including crying, facial expression, body movement, and autonomic activity (Lehr et al., 2007). However, parents, clinicians, and other observers often find the cues ambiguous, because many are present during nonpainful states and stress. Facial expression has emerged as the most specific and consistent behavioral evidence for infant pain (e.g., Sharek, Powers, Koehn, & Anand, 2006; Slater, Cantarella, Franck, & Fitzgerald, 2008; Stevens et al., 2007). Johnston and Strada (1986) reported that the facial response to injection is more consistent across infants than cry patterns, heart rate, or body movement. Other studies demonstrate that facial activity contributes more to adult judgments of the severity of infant pain than do cry patterns and other contextual variables (Hadjistavropoulos, Craig, Grunau, & Whitfield, 1997).

The Neonatal Facial Coding System (NFCS) provides an objective, anatomically based, reliable, and detailed approach for studying the infant's facial reaction to pain (Grunau & Craig, 1987; Grunau, Johnston, & Craig, 1990). Numerous studies demonstrate content, empirical, and construct validity for this measure. Using the NFCS, a relatively stereotyped pattern of facial actions has emerged that is consistent throughout infancy in preterm neonates (Chimello, Gaspardo, Cugler, Martinez, & Linhares, 2009; Craig, Whitfield, Grunau, Linton, & Hadjistavropoulos, 1993; Grunau, Oberlander, Whitfield, Fitzgerald, & Lee, 2001; Grunau et al., 2005) or older infants (Grunau et al., 2001; Lilley et al., 1997; Oberlander et al., 2000). The facial display comprises lowered brow, eyes squeezed shut, deepened nasolabial furrow (a fold that extends down and out beyond the lip corners), and opened mouth. It is accompanied by a taut, cupped tongue in many infants. Figure 6.3 illustrates two infants' reactions to heel lancing, and the finding of Grunau and Craig (1987) that the severity of the infants' reactions is related to their sleep–wake behavioral state at the time of the lance. The display has striking similarities to the facial displays of pain in older children and adults.

While infants communicate pain when subjected to invasive procedures, they do not yet have the capacity for cognizing the significance of the experience. An infant's experience is dominated by sensory qualities and affective distress, which are perhaps all

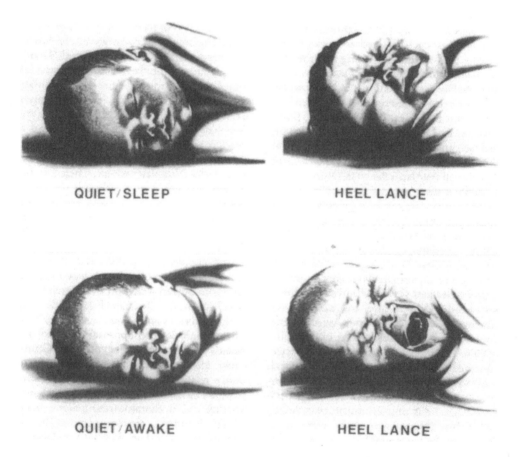

QUIET/SLEEP

HEEL LANCE

QUIET/AWAKE

HEEL LANCE

FIGURE 6.3. Infants' facial responses to the heel lance procedure vary with their behavioral state at the time of the lance. From Grunau and Craig (1987). Copyright 1987. Reprinted with permission from the International Association for the Study of Pain.

the more vivid because adult capacities for anticipating an end or exercising control are not available. The most compelling demonstration of the validity of infant facial coding as a pain index is a recent study showing that evoked cortical hemodynamic brain activity during blood collection in preterm infants was highly correlated with specific facial activity (r = .74, p = .0001; Slater et al., 2008).

There is prominent variation in facial activity correlated with gestational age at birth in preterm newborns. Facial reactions increase in vigor as infants approach term (Craig et al., 1993; Grunau et al., 2001; Johnston & Stevens, 1996; Johnston, Stevens, Yang, & Horton, 1995; Scott et al., 1999). However, the lesser reaction of preterm newborns to invasive procedures cannot be interpreted as signifying reduced pain. Fitzgerald and Macintosh (1989, p. 442) note that "the preterm infant is, if anything, supersensitive to painful stimuli when compared with the full term infant."

Other investigations have attributed infants' sensitivity of facial expression during painful events to individual differences and various interventions. Sensitivity of the NFCS measure to subtle individual differences is evident in, for example, the finding that maternal family history of hypertension attenuates the neonatal pain response (France, Taddio, Shah, Page, & Katz, 2009). In a number of studies, facial expression has provided an outcome index of pharmacological analgesia, including the impact of EMLA (a topical analgesic) during circumcision (Taddio, Katz, Ilershich, & Koren, 1997) and venipuncture (Larsson, Tannfeldt, Lagercrantz, & Olsson, 1998), fentanyl during mechanical ventilation of preterm infants (Guinsberg et al., 1998), and morphine during invasive procedures (Scott et al., 1999). Nonpharmacological interventions also have been evaluated. The food substance sucrose and rocking, as a simulation of the vestibular effects of carrying an infant, diminished the facial display of preterm neonates undergoing the routine heelstick procedure (Johnston, Stremler, Stevens, & Horton, 1997), as did sucrose alone with preterm neonates (Gasparado, Miyase, Chimello, Martinez, & Martins Linhares, 2008). Furthermore, both suckling and sucrose were demonstra-

bly analgesic with newborns (Blass & Watt, 1999).

Availability of a systematic measure of facial activity has allowed study of a variety of subtle influences on infant procedural pain. An enduring impact of early exposure to pain was demonstrated by Taddio, Katz, and colleagues (1997), who found that healthy 4- to 6-month-old boys who had been circumcised as neonates displayed a greater facial response, cried longer, and were judged as experiencing more pain in reaction to vaccination injections than did noncircumcised boys. As well, when premedication with the topical anesthetic EMLA was undertaken prior to the circumcision, there was a trend for EMLA-treated infants to have an intermediate pain response across all three measures of pain. Thus, there appeared to be a long-lasting effect of neonatal pain on subsequent infant pain behavior instigated by alterations in the infants' central neural processing of painful stimuli, with an analgesic capable of diminishing this sensitization to pain.

It is important to note that a small proportion of infants do not display facial reactions to invasive procedures (Grunau & Craig, 1987), particularly preterm infants born at extremely low gestational age (Craig et al., 1993). As well, cortical activation in the brain has been reported in preterm newborns during heelstick blood collection in the absence of change in facial behavior (Slater et al., 2008). Nevertheless, there are developmentally relevant motor behaviors seen in conjunction with procedural pain (Grunau, Holsti, Whitfield, & Ling, 2000; Holsti, Grunau, Oberlander, & Whitfield, 2004; Morison et al., 2003). Often, preterm newborns who show little or no facial change display specific hand movements of finger splay and/or fisting (Holsti & Grunau, 2007). This led to development of a scale—the Behavioral Indicators of Infant Pain (BIIP; Holsti, & Grunau 2007; Holsti, Grunau, Oberlander, & Osiovich, 2008)— that combines the five most salient pain facial actions from the NFCS (Grunau & Craig, 1987), with developmentally appropriate hand behaviors (finger splay and fisting) and ratings of sleep–wake state. Thus, preterm infants who communicate their pain with hand movements are not overlooked.

Because there are changes in facial anatomy during the transition from infancy to the toddler years (Oster & Rosenstein, 1993), development of the Child Facial Coding System (CFCS; Chambers, Cassidy, McGrath, Gilbert, & Craig, 1996) was based on FACS facial actions to focus on discrete facial actions that account for preschoolers' and older children's facial displays of pain. A constellation of actions similar to those observed in neonates and infants occurs consistently during invasive events (e.g., immunization injections, venipuncture, and finger lance; Chambers et al., 1996). Breau and colleagues (2001) reported a principal components analysis of CFCS coded reactions to immunization injections and concluded that a subset of actions (brow lowering, squinting, flared nostrils, nose wrinkling, lip corner pulling, and vertical mouth stretching) were sufficient to describe the children's display, with variability reflecting pain severity.

Facial activity has been incorporated as a primary or major component of most multidimensional behavioral checklists or rating scales for assessing pain in infants and children, whether or not they have acquired language skills. The Premature Infant Pain Profile (PIPP; Stevens, Johnston, Petryshen, & Taddio, 1996) provides a good illustration of a composite measure that effectively uses empirically derived characterization of the facial display of pain. Nurses and others assess pain by focusing on facial actions (brow bulge, eye squeezing, and nasolabial furrow) and physiological activity (heart rate and blood oxygen saturation), adjusted for gestational age of the infant and sleep–wake state. The PIPP has been used extensively to examine pharmacological, environmental, and behavioral control of infant pain (e.g., Axelin, Salantera, Kirjavainen, & Lehtonen, 2009). It is noteworthy that the Slater and colleagues (2008) study described earlier demonstrated that the pain signal in the cortex was more highly correlated with facial activity in preterm infants ($r = .74$, $p = .0001$) than physiological responses of heart rate/oxygen saturation ($r = .398$, $p = .04$), or total score on the PIPP ($r = .566$, $p = .001$).

Other coding systems requiring global judgments of an infant's face have been productive in understanding emotion and pain. Izard's (1979) Maximally Discriminative Facial Movement Coding System (MAX) requires coders to scan three regions of the face (brow, eyes, and mouth) for particular combinations of activity representing discrete emotional expressions of anger, fear, surprise, and joy, as well as pain. Several studies (e.g., Izard, Hembree, Dougherty, & Spizirri, 1983; Izard, Huebner, Risser, McGinness, & Dougherty, 1980) reported that during infancy, the early pattern of facial response to immunization injections predominantly suggests pain, but at around 6 to 8 months, the pattern becomes one of anticipatory fear prior to the injection, pain following the needle stick, and anger thereafter.

FACIAL EXPRESSION AS SOCIAL COMMUNICATION

So far we have emphasized encoding of the subjective experience of pain in facial expression. From a broader social communications perspective (Craig, 2009; Prkachin & Craig, 1995; Sullivan, 2008) it is important to understand how others attend to, interpret, and respond to specific cues or the configuration of pain. That which is salient and meaningful to an observer often does not correspond to objective features of the expression of pain. For example, health care professionals systematically have been found to estimate infant pain as lower than do family members (Pillai Riddell & Craig, 2007; Xavier Balda et al., 2000). Likewise, a complementary literature indicates that observers, including health care providers, underestimate the pain of adults (Kappesser, Williams, & Prkachin, 2006; Prkachin, Solomon, & Ross, 2007).

Cues Salient to Observers

The specific facial cues attended to by judges when assessing pain have been identified in several studies of adults and children. Brow lowering, eye blinking and narrowing, cheek raising, and upper-lip raising predicted 55% of the variance in ratings of adult pain (mean multiple $r = .74$) (Patrick et al., 1986). Prominent predictor variables for children tended to be taut tongue, open lips, latency to facial activity, vertically stretched mouth, and deepened nasolabial furrow (Craig, Grunau, & Aquan-Assee, 1988). These variables accounted for 43% of adult ratings of affective discomfort displayed by the children. Thus, there tends to be agreement on the pain cues that are salient to adult judges. This evidence suggests that naive judges make less than optimal use of the information available in facial expressions when drawing inferences about the pain of others. Objective coding of facial expression has been found to correspond more closely to self-report of pain than do observer judgments (Prkachin et al., 1994).

Voluntary Control of the Facial Expression of Pain

While displays are less subject to voluntary control than verbal report, children and adults can be relatively successful in faking, exaggerating, or suppressing facial displays of pain on demand when it seems in their interests (Craig, 2006; Hill & Craig, 2002; Prkachin, 2005). A judge's impressions tend to be consistent with the ways the individual presents himself or herself rather than in terms of the real experience (Hadjistavropoulos, Craig, Hadjistavropoulos, & Poole, 1996; Poole & Craig, 1992). Observers exceed chance in detecting faked or suppressed pain, but only marginally (Hadjistavropoulos et al., 1996; Hill & Craig, 2004; Prkachin, 1992). The pattern of display when people are fabricating pain tends to correspond to the spontaneous expression, but difficult-to-detect differences in structure and timing are evident on close study (Craig, Hyde, & Patrick, 1991; Prkachin, 1992). The faked or exaggerated pain display tends to be an overblown expression, with both facial actions typically associated with pain and those that do not appearing more frequently and with greater intensity; furthermore, the temporal pattern is disrupted, with facial actions displaying greater temporal contiguity during the spontaneous expression and the facial actions are more likely to be in sequence during the purposefully controlled display (Craig et al., 1991; Hill & Craig, 2002). Efforts to misrepresent oneself as not being in pain are associated with diminished reactivity, but not entirely so, because residual activity remains. The potential for misrepresentation is developed early in life (Larochette, Chambers, & Craig, 2006). Interestingly, children appear less successful in deceiving their parents than do adults in deceiving one and other, suggesting that skill in dissembling is acquired in the course of child development. The children were more adept at hiding pain than faking it, as indicated by both FACS coding and parental judgments.

Information Technology in the Assessment of Pain Expression

Facial expressions of pain are represented by distinct configurations of facial actions that vary in intensity, and unfold dynamically and rapidly over time. Until recently, this complexity has only been penetrable by human observers with skills in decoding pain and other expressions, yet the reliability of observations of components of pain expression is far from perfect. Humans are particularly limited in their ability to resolve changes in intensity of actions over the relatively brief time frames entailed in pain expression (movement dynamics). It has long been hoped that advances in information technology would supplement or supplant manual coding.

Since the 1990s, computer specialists have devoted attention to the problem of detecting facial features and facial expressions with increasing success (e.g., Bartlett, Ekman, Hager, & Sejnowski, 1999; Brahnam, Chuang, Sexton, & Shih, 2007; Brahnam, Chuang, Shih, & Slack, 2006; Cohn, Zlochower, Lien, & Kanade, 1999). Methodology in this field is evolving rapidly but typically involves several stages. First, researchers sample facial behavior using digital video capture. They extract facial features, such as eye, brow. and mouth activity, using such techniques as principal components analysis, or algorithms for identification of optical flow and edge detection. Image alignment is necessary due to common problems, such as motion of the head out of plane. The video data are then processed with a classification system based on machine learning procedures, such as neural nets trained to the task of recognizing facial actions or of classifying images previously identified as containing the signal of interest. The adequacy of the solution is tested by comparing performance with a test set of images that is independent of the training set. Using such techniques, investigators have demonstrated considerable success in identifying FACS Action Units in samples of video taken under optimal conditions, such as deliberately posed facial actions. Nevertheless, typical circumstances for assessing pain fall short of optimal for this type of detection, in part because the experience of pain itself produces movement of the trunk, body, and head.

To illustrate, Ashraf and colleagues (2009) used comparable procedures to develop a system for automatic detection of pain expression. Video recordings of patients with shoulder pain undergoing painful or not painful range-of-motion tests were processed using active appearance models (AAMs) and classified as demonstrating pain or no pain based on prediction scores derived from support vector machine classifiers. An optimized combination of AAMs resulted in a hit rate (correctly identifying sequences identified as painful) of 81% and an equal error rate (where false acceptances equal false rejections) of 19%. Figure 6.4 shows representative output, demonstrating how the score tracks variation in pain expression. This and related methodologies have potential to provide precise assessment of temporal and dynamic features of pain-related actions, and the ability to discriminate spontaneous and purposefully controlled facial displays (Bartlett et al., 1999).

Misleading Cues in Observational Behavioral Checklists and Rating Scales

Dramatically different and often inaccurate accounts of facial activity during pain appear in the clinical and research literatures. Charles Darwin long ago (1872/1965, pp. 69–70) described the pain expression as follows: "The mouth may be closely compressed, or more commonly, the lips are retracted, with the teeth clenched or ground together. . . . The eyes stare wildly as if in horrified astonishment." Recent systematic studies do not confirm this account. Rather, open lips and mouth, with the eyes narrowed or closed, are consistently observed.

Similar erroneous descriptions of the facial expression of pain can be found in observational checklists or rating scales to study pain in infants, young children, people with cognitive impairments, and older adults with dementias. These scales compound observer error when estimating pain in others by misrepresenting the empirically described display. Illustration of some difficulties is possible. The Faces, Legs, Activity, Cry, and Consolability Behavioral Pain Assessment Tool (FLACC; Merkel, Voepel-Lewis, Shayevitz, & Malviya, 1997) calls for observation of "frequent to constant quivering chin, clenched jaw" for the most severe pain

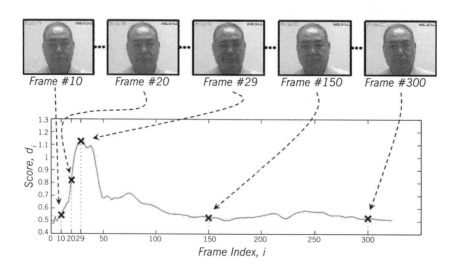

FIGURE 6.4. Automatic detection of pain expression; example of a video sequence prediction based on active appearance models. *Top*: Samples of a pain video sequence showing frame indices corresponding to highlighted points in *bottom*: support vector machine–derived scores for individual frames. From Ashraf et al. (2009). Copyright 2009. Reprinted with permission from Elsevier Science.

rating. However, these facial actions have rarely been reported as occurring during a child's pain. In another scale, "full cry expression" is said to be indicative of the most severe pain (Schade, Joyce, Gerkensmeyer, & Keck, 1996), yet crying is nonspecific and observed during many nonpainful events, including hunger, fear, anger, or general irritability. The Abbey Pain Scale (Abbey et al., 2004) asks the rater to look for "a tense, frowning, grimacing, and frightened facial expression" (p. 12), thereby compelling the observer to look for aversive feeling states that do not necessarily coincide with pain and that have facial characteristics inconsistent with pain. The most severe pain on the Doloplus–2 Scale (Lefebvre-Chapiro, 2001) is said to be represented by "a permanent and unusually blank look (voiceless, staring, looking blank)" (p. 192), again inconsistent with the facial display of pain. Interestingly, the Mahoney Pain Scale (Mahoney & Peters, 2008) includes *blank expression* in the following "pleasant, relaxed, or blank expression" (p. 258) as indicative of an absence of pain. Other scales choose to use vague and sometimes misleading terms such as "grimace," "tense face," "facial restlessness/tics," "looking sad/almost in tears," "frightened/fearful look," "trembling chin," "lips pucker up tight, pout or quiver," "wry mouth," "pout/lip purse," and so forth.

Low reliability in observer judgment is the likely consequence of vaguely defined actions or those that rarely occur, whereas higher reliability is associated with objectively defined actions that occur frequently during pain. Furthermore, actions that have not been associated with pain do not differentiate between painful and nonpainful conditions or they lead to false positives. For example, it is not unusual for children to be frightened or sad while in the hospital, but not in pain. Identifying a child as being in pain when this is not the case could lead to inappropriate treatment (e.g., use of analgesics) or failure to address nonpainful but important aversive states (fear, sadness). In general, we can expect observational scales that do not provide objective description of empirically derived facial actions of pain to be unreliable and insensitive and to underestimate or overestimate pain. Misleading and inaccurate cues likely lead to mistrust of scales and lack of use.

ESSENTIAL FEATURES IN CLINICAL CODING OF FACIAL EXPRESSIONS OF PAIN

Clinically useful, real-time assessment approaches are being developed, including simplified systems of facial coding and training that are compatible with clinicians' expectations. Based on the work indicating that adult pain expression consists largely of four consistent actions, Prkachin, Hughes, Schultz, Joy, and Hunt (2002) developed a protocol for training observers to perform real-time measurement of pain expression during physical examinations of patients with low back pain. Observers attended a 1-day workshop in which they learned to identify the core facial actions, to perform simple gradation of their intensity, and to integrate observations with key events in a standardized low back pain examination. The results indicated that observers could be trained to perform such assessments reliably and validly (Prkachin, Schultz, Berkowitz, Hughes, & Hunt, 2002). Evaluation of the properties of the measure indicated that patients' facial pain expressions were temporally reliable and more closely associated with different outcomes than other forms of pain behavior (Prkachin, Schultz, & Hughes, 2007).

In children, Rushforth, Griffiths, Thorpe, and Levene (1995) studied healthy infants undergoing heel lance. A single observer rated the occurrence of facial actions previously shown to be associated with pain in neonates (brow bulge, eye squeeze, deepened nasolabial furrow, and mouth open, as well as crying) in real time. Heel lancing and squeezing were associated with increases in facial actions in all 30 infants; however, data on validity and reliability were not reported. Grunau, Oberlander, Holsti, and Whitfield (1998) applied the NFCS to real-time assessment of 32- to 33-week postconceptional age infants undergoing heel lance procedures. Intercoder reliability was high (.83–.91, using the Ekman–Friesen formula), with four movements (brow-lower, eye squeeze, nasolabial furrow deepening, and open mouth) showing clear discrimination between painful and nonpainful phases of the procedure. Others have demonstrated high levels of intercoder reliability when observers trained in the use of the NFCS rated pain in children through direct observation (Guinsburg et al.,

1998, 2000). Given the minimal activity observed in preterm newborns' facial displays relative to those of term infants, special attention is required in assessment of pain in this population. Holsti and Grunau (2007) applied the BIIP (described earlier) in real time to video recordings of preterm infants at 25- to 32-weeks postconceptional age as they underwent heel lance procedures. This hybrid scale reliably differentiated painful from nonpainful phases of the heel lance procedure, scored by experienced and inexperienced raters.

Thus, contrary to arguments that complexity of the coding systems represents an excessive burden for routine clinical use of facial coding (Von Baeyer & Spragrud, 2007), brief description is possible, relatively brief training may suffice to eliminate the errors that follow from vague descriptions or lay understanding, and training improves measurement reliability and validity. The core features of the facial expression of pain can be captured with relatively few facial actions. With infants, the display is represented by NFCS items that focus on brow bulge, eye squeeze, nasolabial furrow, horizontal mouth stretch, and taut tongue (Peters et al., 2003). With children, CFCS items identifying brow lowering, squinting, flared nostril, nose wrinkle, lip corner pull, and vertical mouth stretch work well to identify pain (Breau et al., 2001; Gilbert, Lilley, Craig, McGrath, & Court, 2000). In adults, the subset of facial actions associated with pain appears best described by lowering of the brow, narrowing of the eyes by tightening the lids, and raising the cheeks in varying degrees, including fully closing the eyes, deepening the nasolabial fold, and wrinkling the nose, as well as opening the lips and mouth in varying degrees (Prkachin & Solomon, 2008; Simon et al., 2006).

We suggest that providing clinicians, researchers, family members, or others interested in pain assessment with guidance as to the specific actions associated with the facial display of pain would enhance the accuracy of judgments.

SUMMARY AND CONCLUSION

In the first edition of the *Handbook of Pain Assessment* (Turk & Melzack, 1992), the study of pain-related facial expression was in its infancy. Fine-grained approaches to characterizing facial actions during pain had only recently been developed, and there was little consensus among clinicians or researchers that specific information about pain was encoded in facial expression. Since then, pain expression has become a highly active area of pain research and practice. There is little doubt that considerable specific and important information is available about pain through observing facial expression, and that it may provide vital, if not exclusive, information about the experience of the person in pain. Advances in technology and validated psychometric instruments focusing on facial expression continue to improve both our ability to understand pain mechanisms and interpersonal processes related to pain, and clinical assessment and care.

ACKNOWLEDGMENTS

This work was supported, in part, through funding from the Social Sciences and Humanities Research Council of Canada (to Kenneth D. Craig and Ruth E. Grunau), the Canadian Institutes of Health Research (to Kenneth D. Craig, Kenneth M. Prkachin, and Ruth E. Grunau), the Michael Smith Foundation for Health Research (to Kenneth M. Prkachin), and the Kennedy Shriver National Institute of Child Health and Human Development (to Ruth E. Grunau).

REFERENCES

Abbey, J., Piller, N., Bellis, A., Esterman, A., Parker, D., Giles, L., et al. (2004). The Abbey Pain Scale: A 1-minute numerical indicator for people with end stage dementia. *International Journal of Palliative Nursing, 10,* 6–14.

Ashraf, A. B., Lucey, S., Cohn, J. F., Chen, T., Ambadar, Z., Prkachin, K., et al. (2009). The painful face: Pain expression recognition using active appearance models. *Image and Vision Computing, 27,* 1788–1796.

Axelin, A., Salantera, S., Kirjavainen, J., & Lehtonen, L. (2009). Oral glucose and parental holding preferable to opioid in pain management in preterm infants. *Clinical Journal of Pain, 25,* 138–145.

Bartlett, M. S., Ekman, P., Hager, J. C., & Sejnowski, T. J. (1999). Measuring facial expressions by computer image analysis. *Psychophysiology, 36,* 253–263.

Blass, E. M., & Watt, L. (1999). Suckling and sucrose-induced analgesia in human newborns. *Pain, 83,* 611–623.

Botvinick, M., Jha, A. P., Bylsma, L. M., Fabian, S. A., Solomon, P. E., & Prkachin, K. M. (2005). Viewing facial expressions of pain engages cortical areas involved in the direct experience of pain. *NeuroImage, 25,* 312–319.

Brahnam, S., Chuang, C. F., Sexton, R. S., & Shih, F. Y. (2007). Machine assessment of neonatal facial expressions of acute pain. *Decision Support Systems, 43,* 1242–1254.

Brahnam, S., Chuang, C. F., Shih, F. Y., & Slack, M. R. (2006). Machine recognition and representation of neonatal facial displays of acute pain. *Artificial Intelligence in Medicine, 36,* 211–222.

Breau, L. M., McGrath, P. J., Craig, K. D., Santor, D., Cassidy, K. L., & Reid, G. J. (2001). Facial expression of children receiving immunizations: A principal components analysis of the Child Facial Coding System. *Clinical Journal of Pain, 17,* 178–186.

Chambers, C. T., Cassidy, K. L., McGrath, P. J., Gilbert, C. A., & Craig, K. D. (1996). *Child Facial Coding System: A manual.* Halifax, Nova Scotia, Canada/Vancouver, British Columbia, Canada: Dalhousie University/University of British Columbia.

Chimello, J. T., Gaspardo, C. M., Cugler, T. S., Martinez, F. E., & Linhares, M. B. (2009). Pain reactivity and recovery in preterm neonates: Latency, magnitude, and duration of behavioral responses. *Early Human Development, 85,* 313–318.

Cohn, J. F., & Ekman, P. (2005). Measuring facial action. In J. A. Harrigan, R. Rosenthal, & K. R. Scherer (Eds.), *The new handbook of methods in nonverbal behavior research* (pp. 491–493). New York: Oxford University Press.

Cohn, J. F., Zlochower, A. J., Lien, J., & Kanade, T. (1999). Automated face analysis by feature point tracking has high concurrent validity with manual FACS coding. *Psychophysiology, 36,* 35–43.

Craig, K. D. (2006). Assessment of credibility. In R. F. Schmidt & W. D. Willis (Eds.), *The encyclopedia of pain* (pp. 491–493). New York: Springer.

Craig, K. D. (2009). The social communication model of pain. *Canadian Psychology, 50,* 22–32.

Craig, K. D., Grunau, R. V., & Aquan-Assee, J. (1988). Judgement of pain in newborns: Facial action and cry as determinants. *Canadian Journal of Behavioural Science, 20*(4), 442–451.

Craig, K. D., Hyde, S. A., & Patrick, C. J. (1991). Genuine, suppressed and faked facial behaviour during exacerbation of chronic low back pain. *Pain, 46,* 161–171.

Craig, K. D., & Patrick, C. J. (1985). Facial expressions during induced pain. *Journal of Personality and Social Psychology, 48,* 1080–1091.

Craig, K. D., Versloot, J., Goubert, L., Vervoort, T., & Crombez, G. (2010). Perceiving pain in others: Automatic and controlled mechanisms. *Journal of Pain, 11*(2), 101–108.

Craig, K. D., Whitfield, M. F., Grunau, R. V. E., Linton, J., & Hadjistavropoulos, H. (1993). Pain in the pre-term neonate: Behavioural and physiological indices. *Pain, 52,* 287–299.

Darwin, C. R. (1965). *The expression of emotions in man and animals.* Chicago: University of Chicago Press. (Original work published 1872)

Ekman, P., & Friesen, W. V. (1978). *Facial Action Coding System: A technique for the measurement of facial movement.* Palo Alto, CA: Consulting Psychologists Press.

Ekman, P., & Rosenberg, E. (Eds.). (2005). *What facial expression reveals about emotions, development, psychopathology and health* (2nd ed.). Oxford, UK: Oxford University Press.

Fitzgerald, M., & Macintosh, N. (1989). Pain and analgesia in the newborn. *Archives of Disease in Childhood, 64,* 441–443.

France, C. R., Taddio, A., Shah, V. S., Page, M. G., & Katz, J. (2009). Maternal family history of hypertension attenuates neonatal pain response. *Pain, 142,* 189–193.

Fridlund, A. J. (1994). *Human facial expression: An evolutionary view.* San Diego, CA: Academic Press.

Gaspardo, C. M., Miyase, C. I., Chimello, J. T., Martinez, F. E., & Martins Linhares, M. B. (2008). Is pain relief equally efficacious and free of side effects with repeated doses of oral sucrose in preterm neonates? *Pain, 137,* 16–25.

Gilbert, C. A., Lilley, C. M., Craig, K. D., McGrath, P. J., & Court, C. A. (2000). Postoperative pain expression in preschool children: Validation of the Child Facial Coding System. *Clinical Journal of Pain, 15,* 192–200.

Goubert, L., Craig, K. D., Vervoort, T., Morley, S., Sullivan, M. J. L., Williams, A. C. de C., et al. (2005). Facing others in pain: The effects of empathy. *Pain, 118,* 285–288.

Grunau, R. E., Holsti, L., Haley, D. W., Oberlander, T., Weinberg, J., Solimano, A., et al. (2005). Neonatal procedural pain exposure predicts lower cortisol and behavioral reactivity in preterm infants in the NICU. *Pain, 113,* 293–300.

Grunau, R. E., Holsti, L., Whitfield, M. F., & Ling, E. (2000). Are twitches, startles, and body movements pain indicators in extremely low birth weight infants? *Clinical Journal of Pain*, 16, 37–45.

Grunau, R. E., Oberlander, T. F., Whitfield, M. F., Fitzgerald, C., Morison, S. J., & Saul, J. P. (2001). Pain reactivity in former extremely low birth weight infants at corrected age 8 months compared with term born controls. *Infant Behavior and Development*, 24, 41–55.

Grunau, R. V., & Craig, K. D. (1987). Pain expression in neonates: Facial action and cry. *Pain*, 28, 395–410.

Grunau, R. V., Johnston, C. C., & Craig, K. D. (1990). Neonatal facial and cry responses to invasive and non-invasive procedures. *Pain*, 42, 295–305.

Grunau, R. V., Oberlander, T., Holsti, L., & Whitfield, M. F. (1998). Bedside application of the Neonatal Facial Coding System in pain assessment of premature neonates. *Pain*, 76, 277–286.

Guinsburg, R., de Araujo Peres, C., Branco de Almeida, M. F., de Cassia Xavier Balda, R., Cassia Berenguel, R., Tonelotto, J., et al. (2000). Differences in pain expression between male and female newborn infants. *Pain*, 85, 127–133.

Guinsburg, R., Kopelman, B. I., Anand, K. J., de Almeida, M. F., Peres, C. de A., & Miyoshi, M. H. (1998). Physiological, hormonal, and behavioral responses to a single fentanyl dose in intubated and ventilated preterm neonates. *Journal of Pediatrics*, 132, 954–959.

Hadjistavropoulos, H. D., & Craig, K. D. (1994). Acute and chronic low back pain: Cognitive, affective and behavioral dimensions. *Journal of Consulting and Clinical Psychology*, 62, 341–349.

Hadjistavropoulos, H. D., Craig, K. D., Grunau, R. E., & Whitfield, M. F. (1997). Judging pain in infants: Behavioral, contextual, and developmental determinants. *Pain*, 73, 319–324.

Hadjistavropoulos, H. D., Craig, K. D., Hadjistavropoulos, T., & Poole, G. D. (1996). Subjective judgments of deception in pain expression: Accuracy and errors. *Pain*, 65, 247–254.

Hadjistavropoulos, T., & Craig, K. D. (2002). A theoretical framework for understanding self-report and observational measures of pain: A communications model. *Behaviour Research and Therapy*, 40, 551–570.

Hadjistavropoulos, T., LaChapelle, D. L., Hadjistavropoulos, H. D., Green, S., & Asmundson, G. J. G. (2002). Using facial expressions to assess musculoskeletal pain in older persons. *European Journal of Pain*, 6, 179–187.

Hadjistavropoulos, T., LaChapelle, D. L., MacLeod, F. K., Snider, B., & Craig, K. D. (2000). Measuring movement-exacerbated pain in cognitively impaired frail elders. *Clinical Journal of Pain*, 16, 54–63.

Hale, C. J., & Hadjistavropoulos, T. (1997). Emotional components of pain. *Pain Research and Management*, 2, 217–225.

Hill, M. L., & Craig, K. D. (2002). Detecting deception in pain expressions: The structure of genuine and deceptive facial displays. *Pain*, 98, 135–144.

Hill, M. L., & Craig, K. D. (2004). Detecting deception in facial expressions of pain: Accuracy and training. *Clinical Journal of Pain*, 20, 415–422.

Holsti, L., & Grunau, R. E. (2007). Initial validation of the Behavioral Indicators of Infant Pain (BIIP). *Pain*, 132, 264–272.

Holsti, L., Grunau, R. E., Oberlander, T., & Osiovich, H. (2008). Is it painful or not?: Discriminant validity of the Behavioral Indicators of Infant Pain (BIIP) scale. *Clinical Journal of Pain*, 24, 83–88.

Holsti, L., Grunau, R. E., Oberlander, T. F., & Whitfield, M. F. (2004). Specific Newborn Individualized Developmental Care and Assessment Program movements are associated with acute pain in preterm infants in the neonatal intensive care unit. *Pediatrics*, 114, 65–72.

Iezzi, A., Adams, H. E., Bugg, F., & Stokes, G. S. (1991). Facial expressions of pain in muscle-contraction headache patients. *Journal of Psychopathology and Behavioral Assessment*, 13, 269–283.

Izard, C. E. (1979). *The Maximally Discriminative Facial Movement Coding System (MAX)*. Newark: University of Delaware Instructional Resources Center.

Izard, C. E., Hembree, E. A., Dougherty, L. M., & Spizirri, C. C. (1983). Changes in facial expressions of 2- to 19-month-old infants following acute pain. *Developmental Psychology*, 19, 418–426.

Izard, C. E., Huebner, R. R., Risser, D., McGinness, G. C., & Dougherty, L. M. (1980). The young infant's ability to produce discrete emotion expressions. *Developmental Psychology*, 16, 132–140.

Johnston, C. C., & Stevens, B. J. (1996). Experience in a neonatal intensive care unit affects pain response. *Pediatrics*, 98, 925–930.

Johnston, C. C., Stevens, B. J., Yang, F., & Horton, L. (1995). Differential response to pain by very premature neonates. *Pain*, 61, 471–479.

Johnston, C. C., & Strada, M. E. (1986). Acute pain response in infants: A multidimensional description. *Pain*, 24, 373–382.

Johnston, C. C., Stremler, R. L., Stevens, B. J., & Horton, L. J. (1997). Effectiveness of oral sucrose and simulated rocking on pain response in preterm neonates. *Pain*, 72, 193–199.

Kappesser, J., & Williams, A. C. de C. (2002). Pain and negative emotions in the face: Judgments by health care professionals. *Pain*, *99*, 197–206.

Kappesser, J., Williams, A. C. de C., & Prkachin, K. M. (2006). Testing two accounts of pain underestimation. *Pain*, *124*, 109–116.

Kleck, R. E., Vaughan, R. C., Cartwright-Smith, J., Vaughan, K. B., Colby, C. Z., & Lanzetta, J. T. (1976). Effects of being observed on expressive, subjective and physiological responses to painful stimuli. *Journal of Personality and Social Psychology*, *34*, 1211–1218.

Kunz, M., Chatelle, C., Lautenbacher, S., & Rainville, P. (2008). The relation between catastrophizing and facial responsiveness to pain. *Pain*, *140*, 127–134.

Kunz, M., Gruber, A., & Lautenbacher, S. (2006). Sex differences in facial encoding of pain. *Journal of Pain*, *7*, 915–928.

Kunz, M., Mylius, V., Schepelmann, K., & Lautenbacher, S. (2004). On the relationship between self-report and facial expression of pain. *Journal of Pain*, *5*, 368–376.

Kunz, M., Mylius, V., Schepelmann, K., & Lautenbacher, S. (2008). Impact of age on the facial expression of pain. *Journal of Psychosomatic Research*, *64*, 311–318.

Kunz, M., Prkachin, K., & Lautenbacher, S. (2009). The smile of pain. *Pain*, *145*, 273–275.

Kunz, M., Scharmann, S., Hemmeter, U., Schepelmann, K., & Lautenbacher, S. (2007). The facial expression of pain in patients with dementia. *Pain*, *133*, 221–228.

Labus, J. S., Keefe, F. J., & Jensen, M. P. (2003). Self-reports of pain intensity and direct observation of pain behavior: When are they correlated? *Pain*, *102*, 109–124.

Langford, D. J., Bailey, A. L., Chanda, M. L., Clarke, S. E., Drummond, T. E., Echols, S., et al. (2010). Coding of facial expressions of pain in the laboratory mouse. *Nature Methods*, *7*(6), 447–449.

Larochette, A. C., Chambers, C. T., & Craig, K. D. (2006). Genuine, suppressed and faked facial expressions of pain in children. *Pain*, *126*, 64–71.

Larsson, B. A., Tannfeldt, G., Lagercrantz, H., & Olsson, G. L. (1998). Venipuncture is more effective and less painful than heel lancing for blood tests in neonates. *Pediatrics*, *11*, 882–886.

Lefebvre-Chapiro, S. (2001). The Doloplus–2 Scale—evaluating pain in the elderly. *European Journal of Palliative Care*, *8*, 191–194.

Lehr, V. T., Zeskind, P. S., Ofenstein, J. P., Cepeda, E., Warrier, I., & Aranda, J. V. (2007). Neonatal facial coding system scores and spectral characteristics of infant crying during newborn circumcision. *Clinical Journal of Pain*, *23*, 417–424.

LeResche, L., & Dworkin, S. F. (1984). Facial expression accompanying pain. *Social Science and Medicine*, *19*, 1325–1330.

LeResche, L., & Dworkin, S. F. (1988). Facial expressions of pain and emotions in chronic TMD patients. *Pain*, *35*, 71–78.

Lilley, C. M., Craig, K. D., & Grunau, R. E. (1997). The expression of pain in infants and toddlers: Developmental changes in facial action. *Pain*, *72*, 161–170.

Lints-Martindale, A. C., Hadjistavropoulos, T., Barber, B., & Gibson, S. J. (2007). A psychophysical investigation of the Facial Action Coding System as an index of pain variability among older adults with and without Alzheimer's disease. *Pain Medicine*, *8*, 678–689.

Mahoney, A. E. J., & Peters, L. (2008). The Mahoney Pain Scale: Examining pain and agitation in advanced dementia. *American Journal of Alzheimer's Disease and Other Dementias*, *23*, 250–261.

Merkel, S. I., Voepel-Lewis, T., Shayevitz, J. R., & Malviya, S. (1997). The FLACC: A behavioral scale for scoring postoperative pain in young children. *Pediatric Nursing*, *23*, 293–297.

Messmer, R. L., Nader, R., & Craig, K. D. (2008). Judging pain intensity with autism undergoing venipuncture: The influence of facial activity. *Journal of Autism and Developmental Disorders*, *38*, 1391–1394.

Morison, S. J., Holsti, L., Grunau, R. E., Whitfield, M. F., Oberlander, T. F., Chan, H. W., et al. (2003). Are there developmentally distinct motor indicators of pain in preterm infants? *Early Human Development*, *72*, 131–146.

Nader, R., & Craig, K. D. (2008). *Infant pain expression throughout the first year of life*. Saarbrucken, Germany: VDM Verlag.

Nader, R., Oberlander, T. F., Chambers, C. T., & Craig, K. D. (2004). The expression of pain in children with autism. *Clinical Journal of Pain*, *20*, 88–97.

Oberlander, T. F., Grunau, R. E., Whitfield, M. F., Fitzgerald, C., Pitfield, S., & Saul, J. P. (2000). Biobehavioral pain responses in former extremely low birth weight infants at four months corrected age. *Pediatrics*, *105*, e6.

Oster, H., & Rosenstein, D. (1993). *Baby FACS: Analyzing facial movement in infants*. Unpublished manuscript, New York University.

Patrick, C. M., Craig, K. D., & Prkachin, K. M. (1986). Observer judgments of acute pain: Facial action determinants. *Journal of Personality and Social Psychology*, *50*, 1291–1298.

Peters, J. W. B., Koot, H. M., Grunau, R. E., de Boer, J., van Druenenen, M., Tibboel, D., et al.

(2003). Neonatal Facial Coding System for assessing postoperative pain in infants: Item reduction is valid and feasible. *Clinical Journal of Pain, 19,* 353–363.

Pillai Riddell, R. R., Badali, M. A., & Craig, K. D. (2004). Parental judgments of infant pain: Importance of perceived cognitive abilities, behavioural cues and contextual cues. *Pain Research and Management, 9,* 73–80.

Pillai Riddell, R. R., & Craig, K. D. (2007). Judgments of infant pain: The impact of caregiver identity and infant age. *Journal of Pediatric Psychology, 32,* 501–511.

Poole, G. D., & Craig, K. D. (1992). Judgments of genuine, suppressed and faked facial expressions of pain. *Journal of Personality and Social Psychology: Interpersonal Relations and Group Processes, 63,* 797–805.

Prkachin, K. M. (1992). The consistency of facial expressions of pain: A comparison across modalities. *Pain, 51,* 297–306.

Prkachin, K. M. (2005). Effects of deliberate control on verbal and facial expressions of pain. *Pain, 114,* 328–338.

Prkachin, K. M. (2009). Assessing pain by facial expression: Facial expression as nexus. *Pain Research and Management, 14,* 53–58.

Prkachin, K. M., Berzins, S., & Mercer, S. (1994). Encoding and decoding of pain expressions: A judgement study. *Pain, 58,* 253–259.

Prkachin, K. M., & Craig, K. D. (1995). Expressing pain: The communication and interpretation of facial pain signals. *Journal of Nonverbal Behavior, 19,* 191–205.

Prkachin, K., Hughes, E., Schultz, I., Joy, P., & Hunt, D. (2002). Real-time assessment of pain behavior during clinical assessment of low back patients. *Pain, 95,* 23–30.

Prkachin, K. M., & Mercer, S. R. (1989). Pain expression in patients with shoulder pathology: Validity, properties and relationship to sickness impact. *Pain, 39,* 257–265.

Prkachin, K. M., Schultz, I., Berkowitz, J., Hughes, E., & Hunt, D. (2002). Assessing pain behaviour in real time: Concurrent validity and examiner sensitivity. *Behaviour Research and Therapy, 40,* 595–607.

Prkachin, K. M., Schultz, I. Z., & Hughes, E. A. (2007). Pain behavior and the development of pain-related disability: The importance of guarding. *Clinical Journal of Pain, 23,* 270–277.

Prkachin, K. M., & Solomon, P. E. (2008). The structure, reliability and validity of pain expression: Evidence from patients with shoulder pain. *Pain, 139,* 267–274.

Prkachin, K. M., Solomon, P. E., & Ross, J. (2007). Underestimation of pain by healthcare providers: Towards a model of the process

of inferring pain in others. *Canadian Journal of Nursing Research, 39,* 88–106.

Rosenthal, R. (1993). *Judgment studies: Design, analysis, meta-analysis.* Cambridge, UK: Cambridge University Press.

Rushforth, J. A., Griffiths, G., Thorpe, H., & Levene, M. I. (1995). Can topical lignocaine reduce behavioural response to heel prick? *Archives of Disease in Childhood, 72*(1), F49–F51.

Saarela, M. V., Hlushchuk, Y., Williams, A. C. de C., Schurmann, M., Kalso, E., & Hari, R. (2007). The compassionate brain: Humans detect intensity of pain from another's face. *Cerebral Cortex, 17,* 230–237.

Schade, J. G., Joyce, B. A., Gerkensmeyer, J., & Keck, J. F. (1996). Comparison of three preverbal scales for postoperative pain assessment in a diverse pediatric sample. *Journal of Pain and Symptom Management, 12,* 348–359.

Schiavenato, M., Byers, J. F., Scovanner, P., McMahon, J. M., Xia, Y., Lu, N., et al. (2008). Neonatal pain expression: Evaluating the primal face of pain. *Pain, 138,* 460–471.

Scott, C. S., Riggs, K. W., Ling, E. W., Fitzgerald, C. F., Hill, M. L., Grunau, R. V. E., et al. (1999). Morphine pharmacokinetics and pain assessment in premature newborns. *Journal of Pediatrics, 135,* 423–429.

Sharek, P. J., Powers, R., Koehn, A., & Anand, K. J. (2006). Evaluation and development of potentially better practices to improve pain management of neonates. *Pediatrics, 18,* s78–s86.

Simon, D., Craig, K. D., Gosselin, F., Belin, P., & Rainville, P. (2008). Recognition and discrimination of prototypical dynamic expressions of pain and emotions. *Pain, 135,* 55–64.

Simon, D., Craig, K. D., Miltner, W. H. R., & Rainville, P. (2006). Brain responses to dynamic facial expressions of pain. *Pain, 126,* 309–318.

Slater, R., Cantarella, A., Franck, L., & Fitzgerald, M. (2008). How well do clinical pain assessment tools reflect pain in infants? *PLoS Medicine, 5,* 928–933.

Stevens, B., Johnston, C. C., Petryshen, P., & Taddio, A. (1996). Premature Infant Pain Profile: Development and initial validation. *Clinical Journal of Pain, 12,* 13–22.

Stevens, B., McGrath, P., Gibbins, S., Beyene, J., Breau, L., Camfield, C., et al. (2007). Determining behavioural and physiological responses to pain in infants at risk for neurological impairment. *Pain, 127,* 94–102.

Sullivan, M. J., Adams, H., & Sullivan, M. E. (2004). Communicative dimensions of pain catastrophizing: Social cueing effects on pain behaviour and coping. *Pain, 17,* 220–226.

Sullivan, M. J., Martel, M. O., Tripp, D., Savard, A., & Crombez, G. (2006). The relation between catastrophizing and the communication of pain experience. *Pain, 122,* 282–288.

Sullivan, M. J., Thorn, B., Haythornthwaite, J. A., Keefe, F., Martin, M., Bradley, L. A., et al. (2001). Theoretical perspectives on the relation between catastrophizing and pain. *Clinical Journal of Pain, 17,* 52–64.

Sullivan, M. J., Tripp, D., & Santor, D. (2000). Gender differences in pain and pain behavior: The role of catastrophizing. *Cognitive Therapy and Research, 24,* 121–134.

Sullivan, M. J. L. (2008). Toward a biopsychomotor conceptualization of pain. *Clinical Journal of Pain, 24,* 281–290.

Sweet, S. D., & McGrath, P. J. (1998). Relative importance of mothers' versus medical staff's behavior in the prediction of infant immunization pain behavior. *Journal of Pediatric Psychology, 23,* 249–256.

Taddio, A., Katz, J., Ilersich, A. L., & Koren, G. (1997). Effect of neonatal circumcision on pain response during subsequent routine vaccination. *Lancet, 349,* 599–603.

Taddio, A., Stevens, B., Craig, K. D., Rastogi, P., Ben David, S., Hennan, A., et al. (1997). Efficacy and safety of lidocaine–prilocaine cream for pain during circumcision. *New England Journal of Medicine, 336,* 1197–1201.

Turk, D. C., & Melzack, R. (Eds.). (1992). *Handbook of pain assessment.* New York: Guilford Press.

Vervoort, T., Goubert, L., & Crombez, G. (2009). The relationship between high catastrophizing children's facial display of pain and parental judgment of their child's pain. *Pain, 142,* 142–148.

Vervoort, T., Goubert, L., Eccleston, C., Verhoeven, K., De Clerq, A., Buysse, A., et al. (2008). The effects of parental presence upon the facial expression of pain: The moderating role of child pain catastrophizing. *Pain, 138,* 277–285.

Von Baeyer, C., & Spragrud, L. J. (2007). Systematic review of observational (behavioral) measures of pain for children and adolescents aged 3 to 18 years. *Pain, 127,* 140–150.

Williams, A. C. de C. (2002). Facial expression of pain: An evolutionary account. *Brain and Behavioral Science, 25,* 439–445.

Xavier Balda, R., Guinsburg, R., Almeida, M. F. B., Peres, C. A., Miyoshi, M. H., & Kopelman, B. I. (2000). The recognition of facial expression of pain in full-term newborns by parents and health professionals. *Archives of Pediatric and Adolescent Medicine, 154,* 1009–1016.

CHAPTER 7

Assessment of Pain Behaviors

Francis J. Keefe
Tamara J. Somers
David A. Williams
Suzanne J. Smith

Although pain is a personal and subjective experience, the fact that someone is experiencing pain is often apparent to others. People who have pain may vocalize their distress by talking about the pain or the pain-related distress they are experiencing. Alternatively, they may display paraverbal responses (e.g., moaning or groaning) or pain-related body postures or facial expressions. As a group, these verbal, paraverbal, and nonverbal behaviors have been called *pain behaviors*, because they serve to communicate the fact that pain is being experienced (Fordyce, 1976). The construct of pain behavior has emerged as a key component of behavioral formulations of chronic pain (Keefe & Gil, 1986). These formulations emphasize the role that social learning influences can play in the development and maintenance of pain behaviors (Fordyce, 1976; Keefe & Gil, 1986; Turk, Meichenbaum, & Genest, 1983). A patient with a low back injury, for example, may exhibit pain behavior long after the normal healing time if his or her spouse responds to pain behavior in an overly solicitous fashion.

The concept of pain behavior is particularly salient in the evaluation of patients with chronic pain who are seen in pain clinics and pain management programs (Keefe, 1989).

Many of these patients exhibit a maladaptive pattern of pain behavior that is characterized by an overly sedentary and restricted lifestyle, and excessive dependence on pain medications or family members. Behavioral interventions designed to modify this pain behavior pattern (e.g., activation programs, social reinforcement for engaging in adaptive well behaviors, and time-contingent delivery of pain medications) have been shown to reduce disability and improve psychological functioning of patients with chronic pain (Keefe & Gil, 1986; Turk et al., 1983).

Over the past 15 to 20 years, behavioral and cognitive-behavioral therapists have developed a number of strategies for assessing pain behavior. Assessing pain behavior is important for three main reasons (Labus, Keefe, & Jensen, 2003). First, clinicians often draw conclusions about patients' pain experience based on their observation of patients' pain behaviors. Second, direct observation of pain behavior is sometimes the only way to assess pain, such as when individuals cannot describe their pain (e.g., infants or small children, adults with severe cognitive deficits; see Rushkin, Amaria, Warnock, & McGrath, Chapter 11, and Hadjistavropoulos, Breau, & Craig, Chapter 13, this volume). Finally, understanding pain behaviors can inform pain theory. For example, the recently developed communication model of pain (Hadjistavropoulos & Craig, 2002) maintains that pain behaviors serve to encode internal pain experiences and provide potent signals for observers who need decode them to understand another's pain experience. Furthermore, the evolutionary theory of pain behaviors maintains that pain behaviors have emerged and played an active role in human survival because they are adaptive (i.e., they signal distress and elicit help from others; Williams, 2002).

A critical gap in the emerging literature on pain behavior observation, however, has been the lack of practical information on how one develops and carries out such behavioral assessments. Our purpose in this chapter is to provide clinicians and researchers with detailed information on pain behavior observation methods. The chapter guides the reader through the steps involved in developing an observation method and evaluating its reliability and validity. Although examples drawn from our own research on low back pain and arthritic pain are provided throughout, our intent is to provide guidelines for pain behavior assessment that are applicable to many chronic pain conditions.

The chapter is divided into four sections. In the first section we discuss basic elements of pain behavior observation, such as methods of sampling pain behavior, coding category definitions, and observer training. The second section describes an observation method we developed for osteoarthritis patients to illustrate practical aspects of each of the basic elements of observation. In the third section, we present some future directions for studying the behavior observations of pain. And in the final section, we consider important issues related to the application of pain behavior observation in clinical settings.

BASIC ELEMENTS OF PAIN BEHAVIOR OBSERVATION SYSTEMS

Although a variety of observational strategies can be used to record pain behavior, these strategies share certain basic elements. Five elements common to most observation methods are (1) a rationale for observation,

(2) a method for sampling pain behavior, (3) definitions of behavior codes, (4) a method for observer training, and (5) reliability and validity assessments.

Rationale for Observing Pain Behavior

Mr. Smith was having great difficulty tolerating the physical examination. Despite the fact that he had few physical findings, Mr. Smith complained bitterly of chronic back pain. He flinched visibly when the examiner palpated his back. His movements were slow, and he limped in an exaggerated fashion when asked to walk. He gave very detailed descriptions of his back pain and stated that he was not sure that he could cope with the pain much longer.

Most clinicians working in the pain management area have met patients like Mr. Smith. In a medical setting, the behavior of such a patient with chronic pain may influence decisions about the need for further assessment or treatment (Cailliet, 1968). Patients who show exaggerated or inconsistent pain behavior are often considered to be poor candidates for invasive diagnostic testing (e.g., electromyography), or medical or surgical interventions (Waddell, McCulloch, Kummel, & Venner, 1980). For a behavioral clinician, the behavior of a patient like Mr. Smith is interesting and important in and of itself.

One of the most common reasons to observe patients is to provide a detailed description of the patient's pain behavior. Descriptive data, for example, may be used to document the amount of time a patient spends up and out of the reclining position. *Actigraphy*, a validated measurement method of physical activity (Trost, McIver, & Pate, 2005), provides objective data on activity levels and is increasingly being used to record uptime in patients with pain (Kikuchi, Yoshiuchi, Ohashi, Yamamoto, & Akabayashi, 2007; Long, Palermo, & Manees, 2008; Murphy et al., 2008). Descriptive data may also provide a record of medication intake, or describe the verbal or nonverbal behaviors a patient displays during a physical examination. In behavioral assessment, such descriptive data are used for several purposes. First, descriptive data can pinpoint problem behaviors that may serve as targets for treatment efforts. Careful observations may reveal problem behaviors that patients are reluctant to report. A cancer patient, for example, may initially deny that pain is a problem, but when asked to swallow or cough, he or she may exhibit pain-related facial expressions suggesting that considerable pain is being experienced (Keefe, Brantley, Manuel, & Crisson, 1985; see also Craig, Prkachin, & Grunau, Chapter 6, this volume). Second, descriptive data can be used to establish an initial baseline measure against which the effects of treatment can be compared. By carrying out observations before treatment, after treatment, and at follow-up intervals, the clinician or investigator can evaluate the degree to which behavioral interventions can modify pain behavior. Finally, descriptive data on pain behavior may be used to predict a patient's response to treatment. Connolly and Sanders (1991), for example, found that overt pain behavior recorded prior to a lumbar sympathetic block predicted the amount of pain relief patients reported following initial and subsequent blocks.

The second reason to observe pain behavior is to analyze the variables controlling that behavior. This application of behavioral observation has been called *functional analysis* (Ferster, 1965) to contrast it with more descriptive, static analysis procedures. Functional analysis is designed to identify specific variables that seem to control pain behavior. Social and environmental variables often play an important role in eliciting pain behavior. A patient with an overly solicitous spouse, for example, may report a much higher level of pain in the presence of that spouse than when in the presence of a neutral observer, such as a ward clerk (Block, Kremer, & Gaylor, 1980; see also Romano, Cano, & Schmaling, Chapter 5, this volume). Pain behavior may also be affected by its consequences. White and Sanders (1986), for example, found that when an experimenter attended to chronic pain patients' discussions about pain, the patients' ratings of pain routinely increased.

The rationale for observing pain behavior is important in determining the specific methods to be used. If the goal is to provide descriptive data, the focus of observation is specific behaviors exhibited by the patient. Most of the current observation systems for

recording pain behavior provide data only on patient behavior. They are thus suitable for a static analysis of behavior. If the goal is to perform a functional analysis, however, the scope of observation must be expanded to include not only patient behavior but also social or environmental variables (e.g., spouse behavior) that may be controlling that behavior. Although observation systems for performing functional analysis have been used in behavior therapy research for the past 15 to 20 years, these methods were only recently extended to the chronic pain area in the 1990s (Romano et al., 1991, 1992, 1995).

Sampling and Recording Pain Behavior

One of the major decisions facing anyone who develops an observation system is how the behavior is to be sampled and recorded. There are five common options for sampling and coding behavior: (1) continuous observation, (2) duration recording, (3) frequency recording, and (4) interval recording.

In *continuous observation* the observer records any behaviors that occurred during the observation session. This approach provides rich detail on behavior and often yields important clues as to environmental variables controlling a particular behavior. For example, a continuous observation of a back pain patient in his home setting might suggest that downtime (i.e., reclining) and verbal pain behaviors (i.e., complaining of pain, requests for medications) were strongly influenced by the presence of the patient's spouse. Based on these findings, one could structure a behavioral treatment program that focuses on modifying not only the patient's behavior but also the spouse's response to that behavior. The major advantage of continuous observation is that it can capture complexity of behavior and requires minimal training. The major disadvantage is time and expense involved, and the difficulty of coding and reducing the enormous amount of information gathered. Because of these limitations, continuous observation is used sparingly, typically early in the course of assessment, when the evaluator is developing ideas about key target behaviors and controlling variables.

A second option for sampling and recording pain behavior is to take a *duration* measure, which involves simply recording the length of time the patient takes to perform a specific behavior. For example, when working with a patient who has become dependent on a back brace, one might record how much time the patient wears the brace each day. Alternatively, one could focus on measuring the duration of well behaviors (e.g., time spent walking or standing) that are incompatible with certain pain behaviors (e.g., time spent reclining) (Fordyce, 1976).

Duration measures provide a simple and practical means for directly observing pain behavior in naturalistic settings. Patients with chronic pain, for example, are often asked to complete diary records of their daily activities, so that the duration of time they spend sitting, standing, or walking (uptime) can be recorded. Staff members also may keep duration measures of the amount of time a patient takes to complete a physically demanding task, such as walking a series of laps around a track or climbing a set of stairs. The major disadvantage of duration measures is that someone must be physically present throughout the entire observation period to record behavior in a reliable and valid fashion. Although this is not a problem for behaviors that have a short duration (e.g., time taken to complete a set of 20 sit-ups), it is a serious disadvantage when recording behaviors that have a long duration (e.g., time spent reclining each day). Although the patient can be asked to observe and record his or her own behavior, the records provided may not be as reliable as those provided by independent observers.

Another option for observing pain behavior is to make *frequency counts*, in which one simply observes and records the number of instances of each target behavior. An observer might keep a frequency count of important pain behaviors, such as the number of times a patient requests medication or the number of times he or she complains of pain. The major limitation of frequency counts is that the observer may need to carry out observations over long time periods to gather reliable and valid data.

A fourth option for sampling and recording pain behavior is *interval recording*, in which the observation period (e.g., 10 minutes or several hours) is broken down into equal intervals (e.g., 30 seconds or 1 min-

ute long). The observer's task is to watch the patient throughout the interval and simply note at the end of the interval whether specific behaviors were or were not observed. Interval recording is often used in coding videotaped samples of behavior gathered during standardized or simulated tasks. For example, we have used interval recording methods to observe pain behaviors that occur in patients with chronic low back pain during videotaped sessions in which they are asked to sit, stand, walk, and recline (Keefe & Block, 1982). Using videotaped behavior samples for observation has many advantages. First, videotape provides a permanent record of the patient's behavior, enabling one to carry out repeated observations, check reliability, and refine or develop new coding systems. Second, one can structure a videotaped behavior sample to elicit pain behaviors. Patients can be observed as they engage in simple daily tasks that they tend to avoid doing, for example, walking, or transferring from a reclining to a standing position. Third, by applying interval recording methods to videotaped behavior samples, one can obtain data that are easily quantified.

There are several disadvantages of combining videotaped behavior sampling with interval recording methods. First, whenever a patient is being videotaped there is the potential for changes in behavior due to observation (Keefe, 1989). Some patients with chronic pain may inhibit their display of pain behavior during a videotaped observation session, whereas others may exaggerate their behavior. Changes in behavior due to observation can be minimized by (1) providing patients with minimal information on the categories of behavior being observed, and (2) avoiding interaction with the patient during observation of the effects of reactivity (Hartmann & Wood, 1982).

Definitions of Pain Behavior

A trainee who visited a pain management program during a midday break period was surprised that the patients failed to exhibit many observable signs that they were experiencing pain. Some patients were talkative; others were resting or reclining. They rarely displayed pain-related facial expressions or guarded movements indicative of pain.

One of the most important factors in observing pain behavior is how one defines pain behavior. The trainee, in the preceding example, implicitly defined pain behavior on the basis of facial expressions or guarded movements and failed to note the fact that, during the break period, patients had very low levels of activity and reclined most of the time. Thus, implicit assumptions about what constitutes pain behavior can determine whether an individual actually notices the presence of that pain behavior.

Implicit definitions of pain behavior can vary from one individual to another. Some base their judgments of pain behavior on a patient's medication intake, while others focus mainly on verbal complaints or motor behaviors indicative of pain. Fordyce (1976) originally defined *pain behaviors* as those behaviors that communicate to others the fact that pain is being experienced. This definition is a general one that encompasses behaviors ranging from verbal reports of pain to measures of the frequency of doctor visits. To develop a reliable and valid observation system, a more specific operational definition is required. An operational definition indicates precisely what the patient must do and what the observer must record. Thus, a good operational definition describes behavior in observable and measurable terms. It also specifies what aspect of the behavior is to be recorded, namely, frequency, duration, or intensity.

Several guidelines can be offered for developing operational definitions for pain behaviors. First, the behavior should occur with sufficient frequency that it can be observed. Behaviors that occur with very low frequency or that cannot be directly observed are generally not suitable for observation. Second, the definitions of the behavior should be written in simple, descriptive language that minimizes inference on the part of observers. This ensures that observers with different backgrounds can use the observation methodology. It also avoids the major problems that occur when observers are attempting to judge why a patient engaged in a particular behavior. Finally, the definition should be written down in a table or manual. Written definitions are particularly useful when multiple categories of behavior are being observed. In such a case, the written definitions provide the basis for initial training of observers.

Observer Training

There is growing recognition that observer training is important in the development of a psychometrically sound observation method (Hartmann & Wood, 1982). The amount of observer training generally varies with the complexity of the observation system. Observation methods that rely on duration measures or frequency counts rarely necessitate intensive observer training. Continuous and interval recording methods that require the coding of multiple categories of behavior, however, typically require a structured observer training program.

Hartmann and Wood (1982) have provided an extensive set of recommendations for training that include initially giving observers an opportunity to carry out observations on an informal basis, then following up with written materials detailing the procedures and coding categories the observers are expected to master. They also recommend having observers carry out practice coding sessions with an experienced observer. Hartmann and Wood suggest that observers reach a criterion level of reliability before starting data collection, and that periodic retraining sessions be conducted to check reliability. Finally, they suggest that observers be debriefed after they finish collecting observational data, to identify any problems that occur in coding behavior.

Assessing Reliability and Validity

If an observation method is to be truly useful in clinical or research settings, then it must be both reliable and valid. Data on the reliability and validity of direct observation methods have come primarily from studies that used trained observers to record pain behavior during videotaped behavior samples. In the early 1980s we carried out a series of studies evaluating the reliability and validity of an observation method for recording pain behavior in patients with low back pain (Keefe & Block, 1982). The observation method was designed to measure motor pain behaviors that occur during simple daily activities. Patients were asked to engage in a series of standardized tasks (walking, sitting, standing, and reclining) while being videotaped. The videotapes were subsequently scored by trained observers using an internal recording method. The categories of recorded pain behavior included guarding (stiff, interrupted, or rigid movement), bracing (pain-avoidant static posturing), rubbing of the painful area, facial grimacing, and sighing. A composite score, total pain behavior, was computed for each patient based on the sum of the number of occurrences of each pain behavior category. Trained observers were highly reliable in coding the pain behavior categories. This method also evidenced high interobserver reliability, sensitivity to detect changes in pain behavior following an intervention, good concurrent and construct validity, and adequate discriminant validity. Over the past 25 years, numerous studies have provided strong support for the reliability and validity of behavioral observation methods for assessing pain behavior. These include pain behavior observation studies carried out in patients with low back pain (Ohlund et al., 1994; Weiner, Peiper, McConnel, Martinez, & Keefe, 1996), rheumatoid arthritis (Anderson et al., 1987a, 1987b; Jawarski, Bradley, Heck, Roca, & Alarcon, 1995; McDaniel et al., 1986; Waters, Riordan, Keefe, & Lefebvre, 2008), osteoarthritis (Smith, Keefe, Caldwell, Romano, & Baucom, 2004), and in terminally ill cancer patients (Ahles et al., 1990).

DEVELOPMENT OF A PAIN BEHAVIOR OBSERVATION SYSTEM FOR RESEARCH

In this section we present general considerations, as well as practical details, to develop a standardized method for observing pain behavior. As an example, we describe a research system developed for observing pain behavior in patients with osteoarthritis (OA) of the knees.

Determining the Categories of Pain Behavior

Before categories of pain behavior can be selected, researchers must clarify their purpose in using such a system. For example, different behaviors might be selected if the intent is to differentiate the expression of pain from the expression of frustration or depression. Similarly, different behaviors might be selected if the intent is to study high-frequency versus low-frequency pain behaviors. Once the intent of the system is established, target

behaviors can be identified. Ideally, these are behaviors that (1) occur when pain is present but do not occur when pain is absent, (2) occur with sufficient frequency that the behaviors can be counted during the observation period, (3) may be easily elicited by routine daily tasks, and (4) may be reliably observed.

Since each patient population differs in how pain is expressed, focus groups can help identify potential behaviors for observation. Focus groups should consist of health care providers who are familiar with the patients with pain themselves, and the spouses of patients in pain. These focus groups work best when the mentioned parties meet separately, develop a list of potential behaviors indicative of pain, then meet as an aggregate to refine the list to those behaviors that all parties agree should be considered in the observation system. Although it may be tempting to retain all behaviors that might indicate pain, systems that use more than five to seven behaviors become cumbersome to raters, and reliability becomes difficult to maintain. It is usually best to retain only those behaviors that occur with high frequency and that clearly differentiate between pain and the expression of other affect. Once the focus groups develop a potential list of behaviors, pilot observations and videotapes should be made of patients displaying the targeted pain behaviors. The videotapes are used to verify empirically the opinions of the focus group members regarding the frequency, ability to observe, and the validity of certain behaviors as being indicative of pain expression.

Determining the Categories of Pain Behaviors for OA Pain

In the mid-1980s we developed an observation method to provide descriptive data on pain behavior in patients having osteoarthritis of the knees (Keefe et al., 1987). In this system, coding categories are separated into three major groups: (1) position codes, (2) movement codes, and (3) pain behavior. The *position codes* include three common but mutually exclusive body postures: sitting, standing, and reclining. The *movement codes* include pacing (walking) and shifting (moving from one position to another in the vertical plane). The position and movement codes are included in the observation system, so that the relationship among pain behavior, body posture, and dynamic movement can be studied.

The pain behavior coding categories used for patients with OA were identified by means of clinical observations and preliminary analysis of videotaped behavior samples. Five pain behaviors were exhibited by many patients and occurred with reasonable frequency: guarding, active rubbing of the knee, unloading the joint, rigidity, and joint flexing. Table 7.1 provides the operational definition for each of the pain behavior categories, as well as for the position and movement categories included in the scoring system.

Instructions

Some observation systems guide patients through a standardized set of tasks, so that each patient performs exactly the same set of tasks. When standardized tasks are used, it is essential that both patients and researchers adhere closely to a well-detailed protocol.

Instructions for the OA Behavioral Observation System

In order to elicit pain behavior, patients with OA are asked to perform a sequence of sitting, standing, walking, and reclining tasks. The tasks include 1- and 2-minute standing periods, 1- and 2-minute sitting periods, two 1-minute reclining periods, and two 1-minute walking periods. These tasks are appropriate for patients with OA for several reasons. First, the tasks are common daily activities. Second, a number of these tasks tend to increase arthritic pain mildly and provide a means of sampling pain behavior. Finally, the tasks are not so demanding that patients are unable to perform them. The order of the tasks is randomized for each patient with a set of cue cards that is shuffled after each observation session.

Before the observation session begins, the individual recording the session explains to the patient the tasks to be performed. The patient is then instructed to perform the task (i.e., sitting, standing, walking, or reclining) that appears on the first cue card for the specified length of time (1 or 2 minutes). Once

---

TABLE 7.1. Behavioral Categories of the Osteoarthritis Pain Behavior Observation System

Position codes	
Standing (std)	Patient is in an upright position with one or both feet on the floor for at least 3 sec.
Sitting (sit)	Patient is resting upon buttocks for at least 3 sec. If the patient is in the process of moving to or from a reclining position, do not score as a sit. Rather, this would be included in the shift (see below).
Reclining (rec)	Patient is resting in a horizontal position for at least 3 sec.
Movement codes	
Pacing (pce)	Moving two or more steps in any direction within the interval of 3 sec.
Shifting (sft)	Change in position upward or downward. (Example—changing from a sitting to a reclining position or a reclining to a standing position). A shift does not include the transition from standing to walking or walking to standing since no upward or downward shift is involved.
Pain behavior codes	
Guarding (gd)	Abnormally slow, stiff, interrupted, or rigid movement while shifting from one position to another or while walking.
Active rubbing (ar)	Hands moving over or grabbing the affected knee (knees) and the legs; hands must be palms down and rubbing must last 3 sec.
Unloading joint (unj)	Shifting of weight from one leg to the other during a stand.
Rigidity (rgd)	Excessive stiffness of the affected knee or knees during activities other than walking (during walking this would be scored as guarding).
Joint flexing (jf)	Flexing of the affected knee or knees while in a static position (i.e., during standing or sitting). This may take place in conjunction with unloading of a joint.

the time allotted to the task has expired, the patient is asked to perform the second task for the specified time period, then the third, and so on. In order to standardize the length of the observation session, patients are given only the allotted period of time to complete a given task. If they do not complete the task before the time period expires, they are instructed to move on to the next task.

Throughout the observation session, attempts are made to minimize conversation and contact with the patient. Conversation with the observer can be distracting to the patient and diminish the desire to express pain, if it is present. Similarly, conversation can impede sighing, grimacing, or verbal expressions of pain that are often categories in observation systems. Thus, the observer should simply verify that the patient is within the viewfinder of the camera and spend the remainder of the interval watching the stopwatch or ensuring that part of the subject's body is not cropped out of the picture when the task involves movement. Remote-controlled video equipment can eliminate the presence of the researcher altogether, and one can simply deliver instructions to the patient via speakers. Patients can be fitted with wireless microphones to record verbal and paraverbal pain behaviors. Web-based programs for recording and coding behaviors in real time are available and enable one to code observational data easily and obtain statistical summaries of that data.

Standardizing the Setting

One can gather observational data on pain behavior in almost any setting in which there is sufficient room. We have collected observational data in examination rooms, patients' hospital rooms, or the physical therapy area.

Standardized Setting Used with the OA System

The room in which observation sessions are conducted should have several features. First, it needs to have an examination table, a stool for stepping up onto the table, and a chair without arms. Patients are asked to recline on the examination table and to use the stool to help them get into the reclining position. This task is somewhat difficult for most patients with OA who have knee pain,

and it tends to elicit pain behavior. Transferring in and out of a chair that does not have arms can also be somewhat physically demanding for these patients, thus providing a good opportunity to observe pain behavior.

Second, the room should have adequate space so that patients can be asked to walk during the observation. A room that is at least 8- to 10-feet wide is required. Third, approximately 15 feet of space is needed so that the camera can be positioned in front of the patient. This camera placement enables one to keep most of the patient's body in the field of view of the camera. Finally, it is important that the room have adequate lighting and privacy.

Videotape Equipment

Digital videorecording or videotaping is necessary for research purposes. These approaches facilitate the assessment of interrater agreement and allow for the review of pain behavior in cases where raters disagree. Advances in digital technology have made the recording of pain behaviors much easier over the years. After the recording session is completed, the videorecording must be prepared for scoring by trained raters. The records are scored using an interval recording system. Each 10-minute sample is divided into 30-second intervals consisting of 20-second "observe" (i.e., instructing raters to watch the video for pain behavior), and 10-second "record" segments (i.e., instructing raters to record on the rating sheets any observed pain behavior).

Observer Training for the OA System

Observers can be research assistants or college undergraduates who go through a systematic training program that involves several steps. The first step involves learning the definitions of each coding category listed in Table 7.1. Observers study the definitions and are tested to ensure that they understand the definitions. Second, observers are instructed in the use of the scoring form, which provides space for each of 20 recording intervals and groups the individual coding categories into the three major groups (position, movement, and pain behaviors). During each scoring interval, observers simply circle the specific behavior coding categories observed. We use an interval recording method in which the observer simply notes the occurrence of a behavior. Thus, each behavior code is circled only once during any interval. Similar coding sheets can be created for online coding of digitally edited videotape.

The third phase of training involves practice scoring of videotapes. A previously trained observer (the master observer) conducts these practice sessions. The novice observers are shown several 30-second segments of a videotape and are asked to score the patient behaviors they observe. The novices then compare their scoring with that of the master observer. After each practice session, problem areas are addressed, and feedback is provided on the accuracy of coding. As the novices begin to develop their observation skills, the master observer gradually increases the number of intervals being scored. Typically, practice sessions begin with a single interval, and then progress to 5, 10, and 15 intervals. Eventually observers should be able to score an entire 20-interval session. Observers are required to score a practice series of 10-minute videotaped observation sessions and show acceptable reliability with the master observer (over 85% agreement) before they are considered fully trained.

The final step of training is to conduct periodic retraining sessions. These sessions are especially important in research applications in which the goal is to obtain reliable and accurate data. Retraining sessions help to prevent the phenomenon known as *observer drift*.

Reliability and Validity Data from the OA System

In our research with patients with OA, we carried out assessments of both the reliability and validity of the pain behavior observation method (Keefe et al., 1987). We calculated interobserver reliability by having observers independently and simultaneously score the same videotaped behavior sample. Interobserver reliability was very high (agreement = 93.7%). Second, in unpublished research we have evaluated the test–retest reliability of our observation method. Pain behavior observations were carried out on a group of 36 patients at baseline and 6 months later. Patients' total pain behavior at study entry cor-

related significantly with total pain behavior 6 months later ($r = .53$, $p < .005$). Third, we found that the observation method demonstrated good concurrent, discriminant, and construct validity in patients with OA (Keefe et al., 1987).

CLINICAL APPLICATIONS
OF BEHAVIORAL OBSERVATION:
ISSUES AND RECOMMENDATIONS

Although the research protocol just described offers rigor and control over tasks by giving participants specific instructions, this method can be criticized for being vulnerable to the effects of patient reactivity to the observation procedure. Reactivity is likely to be high given the presence of videotaping equipment, and the demand by the experimenter to adhere to a fixed activity protocol (Turk & Flor, 1987). When behavioral observation is conducted in the context of a clinical practice, naturalistic observation is generally preferred over the highly controlled standardized methods just described for research.

A number of important issues arise when one tries to incorporate behavioral observation methods into clinical practice settings. First is the issue of time. A commitment to gathering observational data usually means that a clinician needs to make adjustments in workload or shift priorities. Carrying out observations may mean that the practicing clinician has less available time to gather information with other assessment methods (e.g., interviews) or to carry out treatment procedures. One of the best ways to reduce the time demands of observation is to carry out preliminary observations before implementing data collection. These observations can help to pinpoint behaviors that can serve as the targets for behavioral observation. A patient, for example, may show one or two pain behaviors (e.g., excessive guarding or pain-avoidant posturing) that are particularly important targets for assessment and treatment efforts. Preliminary observations also can help to identify time periods during a clinical encounter when pain behaviors are most likely to occur. Observations in a physical therapy treatment session, for example, may reveal the specific times when patients are especially likely to exhibit pain behavior, perhaps when initiating new exercise regimens or initially teaching patients how to do transfers (e.g., transfer from a reclining to a standing position and vice versa). By restricting observation to key time periods, one can significantly reduce the costs of observation, while still obtaining an adequate sample of pain behavior.

A second issue in applying observation systems in clinical settings is the need for videotape equipment. Most of the sophisticated behavioral observation systems reviewed in this chapter have utilized video cameras and recording equipment. Although this equipment is useful in training observers and providing a permanent record of the observation session, it can be expensive and labor-intensive. The goals of behavioral observation can help clarify whether videotaping is needed. For example, if a permanent record is needed for research purposes or for training purposes, then videotape can be helpful. On the other hand, if the data are being used to make clinical decisions about a specific patient and will not be compared to others, then the utility of the videotape is negligible. In summary, we believe that videotape equipment is a helpful tool but not a necessity in performing observations. Research has shown that reliable and valid behavioral data can be collected without the assistance of videotape equipment (Hartmann & Wood, 1982). Live observations carried out in naturalistic settings can serve as a basis for defining pain behaviors, developing behavior sampling strategies, and training observers. Naturalistic observations are not only less expensive but they also may be less intrusive than videotaped observations. People new to the field of behavioral observation should be aware that most practicing behaviorally oriented clinicians rely on live, rather than videotaped, observation methods.

Live observation of pain behaviors have been carried out in patients with low back pain in the context of a physical examination. Keefe, Wilkins, Cook, Crisson, and Muhlbaier (1986) had trained observers code pain behaviors of patients with low back pain who were being evaluated for surgery. Observers were highly reliable in their coding, and the pain behaviors were meaningfully related to both medical variables and a psychological variable (depression). These findings suggest that physicians should consider depression, and psychologist need to be aware of the importance of evaluating pain and pain behavior in patients with low back pain. More recently, Prkachin, Schulz, and Hughes (2007) used a similar observation method to record pain behaviors exhibited by injured workers with low back pain. Of the pain behaviors displayed during a standardized physical exam, guarding was found to be highly predictive of return 3 months later. Patients who initially exhibited high levels of guarding also were found to miss more days of work and to report higher levels of disability. These results were apparent, even when they controlled for demographic, psychosocial, medical, and physical variables that might be important in explaining return to work and disability.

A third important issue for applying observation methods in clinical practice is the need for observer training. The complex and sophisticated behavioral observation methods used in research studies require extensive observer training. Individuals who gather data using these methods are recruited and trained specifically to serve as observers. In practice settings, one must usually rely on clinical staff to perform the functions of observers. Staff members usually do not have the time for intensive observer training, but they do have considerable clinical expertise, understand the concept of pain behavior, and are capable of providing high-quality observational data if adequately motivated. Brief periods of training can teach staff to use simple observation methods, such as duration measures or frequency counts. With periodic reliability checks and review of recording methods, reliable and valid data on pain behavior can be obtained for clinical use.

Clinical staff are sometimes resistant to carrying out behavioral observations. They may view observation as a burden that is imposed on their already busy work schedules. Although they may agree to collect data, the quality of the data may not be high. To avoid this problem, individual staff members who are to serve as observers need to be involved in the focus groups, the development, and the implementation of any pain behavior observation system. We think it is important to involve staff in writing definitions, setting schedules for observation, and checking reliability. Observation data should also be shared with the observers on a regular basis, so that they can be used in evaluating treatment outcome. If observation methods are to be integrated effectively into a pain unit or program, they must be viewed by all as contributing to the clinical management of the patient.

A Clinical Example

In 1990, Shutty, Cundiff, and DeGood developed a pain behavior observation system that could be used unobtrusively in an outpatient setting. While lacking some of the rigor necessary for a research protocol, this system offered the clinician a time-efficient method of obtaining a rating of pain behavior that could be used to help form his or her clinical impression of the patient. This system is described here in modified form so as to be applicable to patients with low back pain.

Coding for the Naturalistic Low Back Pain System

Unlike the OA system the naturalistic low back pain system (NLBPS) capitalizes on naturalistic observation in a standard clinic setting. The pain behavior coding categories used for clinical presentation of low back pain are again separated into three major groups: (1) position codes, (2) movement codes, and (3) pain behavior. The *position codes* include sitting, standing, and reclining. The *movement codes* include pacing (walking) and shifting (moving from one position to another in the vertical plane). Again, the position and movement codes are included in the observation system, so that the relationship of pain behavior to body posture and dynamic movement can be studied. The pain behaviors used with this system are similar to those used in the previously published low back pain behavior observation system (Keefe & Block, 1982) and include guarding, bracing, rubbing, grimacing, and sighing. A sixth behavior, "reliance on others," was added to this system. Table 7.2 provides the operational definition for each of the pain behavior categories for the NLBPS.

Instructions and Standardizing the Setting for the NLBPS

Whereas the OA system had observers giving instructions to patients to perform certain tasks to elicit pain behavior, the naturalistic system must rely on naturally occurring behaviors of the patient in the clinical setting. With a naturalistic approach, therefore, it is possible that patients will not perform tasks that elicit pain in the clinic. Clinicians, however, can capitalize on features of their own clinic that hold a higher than average likelihood of eliciting pain behavior in their patients. For example, staff can be instructed to watch for pain behavior when patients sit down in the waiting room. Given this approach, any norms that are established will, of course, apply only to other patients of the same clinic.

Most clinics offer an opportunity to observe pain behavior during the following common tasks: entering the waiting room (walking), checking in with the receptionist (standing), waiting for the doctor (transition from standing to sitting, and sitting), being called for the appointment (transition from sitting to standing), and leaving the waiting room with the doctor (walking). Nurses and or receptionists can be trained to observe pain behavior during these naturalistic events (see Figure 7.1).

Scoring the NLBPS

As with the OA system, the occurrence of a pain behavior is simply identified as present or absent during a specific episode. Thus, for example, there is no need to tally the number of guardings that occur in each episode; rather, one simply identifies guarding that occurred during the interval. A total pain behavior score can be summed across the four episodes. Clinicians may wish to establish norms for their individual offices and modify the observation episodes to fit their particular office environment.

FUTURE RESEARCH DIRECTIONS

There is a wide variety of important directions for future research on pain behavior observation. In this section we highlight five of these: applying pain behavior observation

TABLE 7.2. Behavioral Categories of the Naturalistic Low Back Pain Behavior Observation System

Position codes	
Standing (std)	Patient is in an upright position with one or both feet on the floor for at least 3 sec.
Sitting (sit)	Patient is resting upon buttocks for at least 3 sec. If the patient is in the process of moving to or from a reclining position, do not score as a sit. Rather, this would be included in the shift (see below).
Reclining (rec)	Patient is resting in a horizontal position for at least 3 sec.
Movement codes	
Pacing (pce)	Moving two or more steps in any direction within the interval of 3 sec.
Shifting (sft)	Change in position upward or downward. (Example—changing from a sitting to a reclining position or a reclining to a standing position.) A shift does not include the transition from standing to walking or walking to standing since no upward or downward shift is involved.
Pain behavior codes	
Guarding (gd)	Abnormally stiff, interrupted, or rigid movement while changing from one position to another (i.e., when recording sft) or during pacing. It includes patients who use canes or walkers, and cannot occur during a stationary position (i.e., sit, std, rec). The movement must be hesitant or interrupted, not merely slow.
Bracing (brc)	Position in which an almost fully extended limb supports and maintains an abnormal distribution of weight. It cannot occur during movement (i.e., pce, sft), and must be held for at least 3 sec. It most frequently is the gripping of the edge of a piece of furniture while sitting, but can also be grasping a table, cane, or walker while standing. What appears to be bracing during movement is termed *guarding*. It can occur with a leg if the patient leans against a wall using no other support but is not simply the shifting of weight while standing.
Rubbing (rb)	Touching, rubbing, or holding the affected area, which includes low back, hips, and legs for a minimum of 3 sec. It includes patients' hands in pockets or behind the back, but not the hands folded in a lap. It can occur during an interval of movement or nonmovement. Patients' palm(s) must be touching the affected area to be considered rubbing during a "sit." If a clear view is not available, a rub is recorded if touching can be reasonably inferred from the patient's position.
Grimacing (gr)	Obvious facial expression of pain, which may include furrowed brow, narrowed eyes, tightened lips, corners of mouth pulled back, and clenched teeth. It often resembles wincing. Observer must be alert to catch this behavior. It often occurs during a shift.
Sigh (si)	Obvious exaggerated exhalation of air, usually accompanied by shoulders first rising and then falling. Cheeks may be expanded.
Reliance on others (otr)	Obvious reliance on a companion or other person for performing tasks. If the patient is leaning on or using others for ambulating, then gd or brc should be used.

to new clinical populations, the use of novel palm-top computer approaches, emotional distress and pain behavior, and observational studies of patients and their spouses.

Applying Behavioral Observation to New Clinical Populations

Can behavioral observation methods be adapted to new clinical populations? Most of the observational methods discussed in this chapter have been used to record pain behavior in patients with persistent pain conditions, such as low back pain or arthritic pain. These methods, however, need not be restricted to these populations. Jay and Elliott (1984), for example, have demonstrated that observation methods can be used to record behavior in children who are experiencing acute pain due to medical procedures. We have demonstrated the utility of pain behavior observation in assessing back pain in community-dwelling older adults with OA (Weiner et al., 1996). Observation

Patient: _____ Observer: _____ Date: _____ Pain Location: _____

1. **Observation Episode 1**: Observe the behavior that occurs from the time the patient enters the waiting room to the time the patient checks in at the reception desk. (If the patient has a companion check in, score using the otr category.)

   std   sit   rec   pce   sft   gd   brc   rb   si   gr   otr

2. **Observation Episode 2**: Observe the behavior that occurs while the patient is standing at the reception desk to check in. (If the patient has a companion check in, score using the otr category.)

   std   sit   rec   pce   sft   gd   brc   rb   si   gr   otr

3. **Observation Episode 3**: Observe the behavior that occurs as the patient walks from the reception desk to a chair, sits down, and sits for 1 minute as he or she awaits to be called for the doctor visit.

   std   sit   rec   pce   sft   gd   brc   rb   si   gr   otr

4. **Observation Episode 4**: Observe the behavior that occurs after being called for the doctor visit. This includes rising from the chair, and walking out of the waiting room with the doctor or nurse.

   std   sit   rec   pce   sft   gd   brc   rb   si   gr   otr

FIGURE 7.1. Sample pain behavior scoring sheet for the Naturalistic Low Back Pain Behavior Observation System.

methods are potentially particularly helpful in patients with dementia who have difficulty describing their pain to others. Although several pain behavior assessment strategies have been proposed for this population, empirical work and reviews of the literature suggest that behavioral pain assessment strategies in older adult patients with dementia are still in development and refinement (Herr, Bjoro, & Decker, 2006; Horgas, Nichols, Schapson, & Vietes, 2008; Zwakhalen, Hamers, Abu-Saad, & Berger, 2006). Multidimensional pain assessments have been suggested as most desirable for older adult patients with compromised cognitive functioning. Finally, observational methods have also been used to record pain behavior in very ill patients, such as patients with terminal lung cancer (Ahles et al., 1990).

When adapting existent observational systems to new pain populations, there are two important considerations. First, tasks used to elicit pain behavior during a structured observation session must be relevant to the pain condition being studied. Walking or transferring from one position to another may elicit pain behavior in patients with low back pain, but may be of little value in eliciting pain behavior in a patient with facial pain. Preliminary observations may be needed to determine the best strategies for eliciting and sampling pain behavior.

Second, new coding categories may need to be developed. The topography of pain behaviors can vary from one clinical condition to another. Reviewing videotapes of patient behavior can be particularly useful in identifying coding categories for specific pain conditions.

Palm-Top Computer Technologies

Palm-top computers can help observers use pain behavior observation systems in the field when videotaping is not an option or paper-and-pencil recording sheets would be cumbersome. These handheld computers offer a high-tech method of recording pain behavior coding categories in digital form that can be tallied within the computer or quickly uploaded to a database. Such computers can be programmed to prompt the observer for "observe" and "record" intervals, thus eliminating the need for a stopwatch, and can facilitate the quantification of pain behavior data within the time frame of a patient visit. Thus, the clinician can have a measure of pain behavior immediately after the visit that is a part of his or her dictated report. The downside of this technology is obviously the cost and the need for a programmer to customize the software to capture the nuances of each behavioral observation system.

Emotional Distress and Pain Behavior

Patients who have difficulty dealing with pain-related emotions (i.e., who either inhibit their emotions or catastrophize) may be more prone to display behavior. Burns and colleagues (2008) examined the hypothesis that attempts to suppress angry thoughts during provocation increase subsequent pain intensity among patients with chronic low back pain. They found that patients who suppressed anger when provoked subsequently had greater anger, greater pain, and exhibited more pain behaviors. Keefe and colleagues (2000) found that women with OA were much more likely than men to exhibit pain behavior and that this finding was explained by women's propensity to engage in higher levels of pain catastrophizing. Interestingly, this result was obtained even after researchers controlled for the effects of depression.

Observational Studies of Patients and Spouses

Another emerging area of research incorporates spouses or significant others into the observation system. Pain behaviors provide a means of communicating the experience of pain to others, and are influenced by social and environmental consequences (Fordyce, 1976). Spouses play an especially significant role in this system due to their frequency of interaction with patients. The operant behavioral perspective of patient–spouse interaction asserts that if pain behaviors are followed by reinforcing consequences, the rate of pain behaviors will increase over time (Romano et al., 1992). For example, when a spouse responds to pain behaviors in a solicitous manner, such as expressing concern or providing assistance related to the patient's pain or disability, pain behavior is positively reinforced and increases. Conversely, when a spouse responds to the patient's pain behaviors in a more neutral and less reinforcing fashion, the behavior decreases. For example, if a spouse fails to pay much attention, the patient's pain behavior may be less likely to occur. Several studies have shown significant associations between spousal responses and patients' reports of pain and activity (Block et al., 1980; Flor, Kerns, & Turk, 1987; Kerns, Haythornthwaite, Southwick, & Giller, 1990; see also Romano et al., Chapter 5, this volume).

An analysis of spousal responses to pain behavior displays may have important clinical implications (see Romano et al., Chapter 5, this volume). First, by carefully assessing spousal response style, one may be able to distinguish between adaptive and maladaptive patient–spouse interactions. This information could be used by clinicians in advising patients and their spouses about interaction patterns that may have beneficial or deleterious effects on the pain experience. Second, early identification of maladaptive interventions may be useful in pinpointing couples who are likely to benefit from couple-based approaches to pain management (e.g., spouse-assisted pain coping skills training). By involving the spouse directly in pain management efforts, the spouse may not only learn more about the partner's pain but also learn how to prompt and reinforce adaptive behaviors, such as exercising and pacing activities.

Romano and colleagues (1991) were the first to develop a structured system for observing and recording the interactions of patients with chronic pain and their spouses. This system involves videotaping the couple in a series of household activities: sweeping a floor, changing bed sheets, bundling newspapers, and carrying logs across a room. These activities were chosen because they both elicit pain behaviors from patients and provide a context in which patient and spouse interact while working on a task together. The total time to complete these tasks was on average 20 minutes. Couples were instructed to perform the tasks together, with the patient taking the lead. The videotapes were then coded by trained observers using a modified version of the Living in Family Environments (LIFE; Hops et al., 1990) computer coding system. This system codes specified behaviors in a continuous, sequential stream in real time. Observers code verbal and nonverbal pain behaviors (e.g., comments referring to physical limitations, limping, stretching), as well as spousal response styles (e.g., facilitative, solicitous, aggressive).

Romano and her colleagues used this observation method to code the behaviors of patients with chronic low back pain and their spouses (Romano et al., 1991, 1992, 1995). Two interesting findings were obtained in this research. First, spousal solicitous behaviors have been shown both to precede and to follow patient nonverbal pain behaviors (Romano et al., 1992). Second, spousal solicitous responses have been found to be associated with greater frequency of reported pain and higher levels of disability (Romano et al., 1995). Both of these findings are consistent with operant behavioral theory and support the utility of this observational methodology as a research tool.

There is growing interest in the interpersonal context of pain behavior. One avenue of research has been to examine the links between pain behavior and the adjustment of significant others. In a study of older women with OA, Druley, Stephens, Matire, Ennis, and Wojno (2003) examined whether pain behavior was important in explaining the relationship between patients' depressive symptoms and their partners' levels of anger and depression. Pain behavior was found to be quite important. Specifically, in patients who engaged in high levels of pain behavior, there was a significant relationship between patients' depressive symptoms and their partners' depressive symptoms and anger. No such relationship was evident in patients who engaged in low levels of pain behavior. Although this study relied on self-reports of behavior, its findings suggest that pain behavior may set the stage for negative emotions in caregivers. An important future direction for this research is to replicate it using direct observation methods to record pain behavior.

Pain behavior can not only influence a significant other but it can also be influence by the behavior of a significant other. We conducted a study in which we observed patients with OA and their spouses interacting as they engaged in a standardized series of tasks (e.g., sweeping a floor, folding laundry, and carrying small artificial logs across a room) (Smith et al., 2004). We coded patient pain behaviors and spousal behaviors that might influence pain behavior. We were interested in solicitous behaviors (i.e., showing concern, encouraging the patient to do less, taking over for the patient) and facilitative behaviors (i.e., expressing support or approval). Data analyses examined the likelihood that spousal behaviors would precede or follow the patient pain behaviors. Interestingly, results showed that facilitative behavior (i.e., expressing approval, agreement, or support) preceded and followed patients'

pain behavior. This study also found that female spouses were much more likely to engage in facilitative behaviors both preceding and following male spouses' pain behavior than vice versa. This pattern of findings suggests that facilitative behavior, which is usually viewed as an adaptive spousal behavior, positively reinforces pain behavior. Educating spouses about the potential effects of facilitative behavior could be useful. Perhaps if facilitative behavior were shown less often in response to pain behavior and more often in response to adaptive, well behaviors, it would be less likely to serve as a prompt for pain behavior.

CLOSING COMMENT: THE ROLE OF PAIN BEHAVIOR OBSERVATION IN CLINICAL PRACTICE

Before completing our discussion of pain behavior observation, it is important to discuss the role that pain behavior plays in the overall assessment of the pain experience. Observations of pain behavior are meant to provide one measure of the pain experience. Pain behavior observations are designed to complement other forms of pain assessment. Empirical work suggests that pain behavior observation should not be used as a proxy for other pain assessments or vice versa (Hadjistavropolous & Craig, 2002; Labus et al., 2003). Chronic pain is a complex, multidimensional phenomenon (Melzack & Wall, 1965). Thus, pain behavior observation should be one component of a comprehensive assessment that includes the use of pain perception measures, standardized psychological tests, and a variety of medical evaluations. Thus, to analyze pain behavior, observational data need to be combined with information on the underlying tissue pathology, the perception of pain, and the degree of pain-related suffering (Fordyce, 1979). It is only by viewing pain behavior in its biopsychosocial context that we are likely to achieve significant advances in our ability to assess and treat chronic pain.

REFERENCES

Ahles, T. A., Coombs, D. W., Jensen, L., Stukel, T., Maurer, L. H., & Keefe, F. J. (1990). Development of a behavioral observation technique for the assessment of pain behaviors in cancer patients. *Behavior Therapy, 21*, 449–460.

Anderson, K. O., Bradley, L. A., McDaniel, L. K., Young, L. D., Turner, R. A., Agudelo, C. A., et al. (1987a). The assessment of pain in rheumatoid arthritis: Disease differentiation and temporal stability of a behavioral observation method. *Journal of Rheumatology, 14*, 700–704.

Anderson, K. O., Bradley, L. A., McDaniel, L. K., Young, L. D., Turner, R. A., Agudelo, C. A., et al. (1987b). The assessment of pain in rheumatoid arthritis: Validity of a behavioral observation method. *Arthritis and Rheumatism, 30*, 36–43.

Block, A. R., Kremer, E. F., & Gaylor, M. (1980). Behavioral treatment of chronic pain: Variables affecting treatment efficacy. *Pain, 8*, 367–371.

Burns, J. W., Quartana, P., Gilliam, W., Gray, E., Matsuura, J., Nappi, C., et al. (2008). Effects of anger suppression on pain severity and pain behaviors among chronic pain patients: Evaluation of an ironic process model. *Health Psychology, 27*, 645–652.

Cailliet, R. (1968). *Low back pain syndrome.* Philadelphia: Davis.

Connolly, G. H., & Sanders, S. H. (1991). Predicting low back pain patients' response to lumbar sympathetic nerve blocks and interdisciplinary rehabilitation: The role of pretreatment overt pain behavior and cognitive coping strategies. *Pain, 44*, 139–146.

Druley, J. A., Stephens, M. A. P., Matire, L .M., Ennis, N., & Wojno, W. C. (2003). Emotional congruence in older couples coping with wives' osteoarthritis: Exacerbating effects of pain behavior. *Psychology and Aging, 18*, 406–414.

Ferster, C. B. (1965). Classification of behavioral pathology. In L. Krasner & L. P. Ullman (Eds.), *Research in behavior modification* (pp. 6–26). New York: Holt, Rinehart & Winston.

Flor, H., Kerns, R. D., & Turk, D. C. (1987). The role of spouse reinforcement, perceived pain, and activity levels of chronic pain patients. *Journal of Psychosomatic Research, 31*, 251–259.

Fordyce, W. E. (1976). *Behavioral methods for chronic pain and illness.* St. Louis, MO: Mosby.

Fordyce, W. E. (1979). Environmental factors in the genesis of low back pain. In J. J. Bonica, J. E. Liebeskind, & D. G. Albe-Fessard (Eds.), *Advances in pain research and therapy* (Vol. 3, pp. 659 666). New York: Raven Press.

Hadjistavropoulos, T., & Craig, K. D. (2002). A theoretical framework for understanding self-report and observational measures of pain: A communications model. *Behaviour Research and Therapy, 40*, 551–570.

Hartmann, D. P., & Wood, D. D. (1982). Observational methods. In A. S. Bellack, M. Hersen, & A. E. Kazdin (Eds.), *International handbook of behavior modification and therapy* (pp. 109–138). New York: Plenum Press.

Herr, K., Bjoro, K., & Decker, S. (2006). Tools for assessment of pain in nonverbal older adults with dementia: A state-of-the-science review. *Journal of Pain and Symptom Management, 31*, 170–191.

Hops, H., Biglan, A., Tolman, A., Arthur, J., Sherman, L., Warner, P., et al. (1990). *Living in Family Environments (LIFE) coding system* (p. 66). Eugene: Oregon Research Institute.

Horgas, A. L., Nichols, A. L., Schapson, C. A., & Vietes, K. (2008) Assessing pain in person with dementia: relationships among the noncommunicative patient's pain assessment instrument, self-report, and behavioral observations. *Pain Management Nursing, 8*, 77–85.

Jawarski, T. M., Bradley, L. A., Heck, L. W., Roca, A., & Alarcon, G. S. (1995). Development of an observation method for assessing pain behaviors in children with juvenile rheumatoid arthritis. *Arthritis and Rheumatism, 38*, 1142–1151.

Jay, S. M., & Elliott, C. (1984). Behavioral observation scales for measuring children's distress: The effects of increased methodological rigor. *Journal of Consulting and Clinical Psychology, 52*, 1100–1107.

Keefe, F. J. (1989). Behavioral measurement of pain. In C. R. Chapman & J. D. Loeser (Eds.), *Issues in pain measurement* (pp. 405–424). New York: Raven Press.

Keefe, F. J., & Block, A. R. (1982). Development of an observation method for assessing pain behavior in chronic low back pain parents. *Behavior Therapy, 13*, 363–375.

Keefe, F. J., Brantley, A., Manuel, G., & Crisson, J. E. (1985). Behavioral assessment of head and neck cancer pain. *Pain, 23*, 327–336.

Keefe, F. J., Caldwell, D. S., Queen, R. T., Gil, K. M., Martinez, S., Crisson, S., et al. (1987). Osteoarthritic knee pain: A behavioral analysis. *Pain, 28*, 309–321.

Keefe, F. J., & Gil, K. M. (1986). Behavioral concepts in the analysis of chronic pain. *Journal of Consulting and Clinical Psychology, 54*, 776–783.

Keefe, F. J., Lefebvre, J. C., Egert, J. R., Affleck, G., Sullivan, M. J., & Caldwell, D. S. (2000). The relationship of gender to pain, pain behavior, and disability in osteoarthritis patients: The role of catastrophizing. *Pain, 87*, 325–334.

Keefe, F. J., Wilkins, R. H., Cook, W. A., Jr., Crisson, J. E., & Muhlbaier, L. H. (1986). Depression, pain, and pain behavior. *Journal of Consulting and Clinical Psychology, 54*, 665–669.

Kerns, R. D., Haythornthwaite, J., Southwick, S., & Giller, E. L. (1990). The role of marital interaction in chronic pain and depressive symptom severity. *Journal of Psychosomatic Research, 34*, 401–408.

Kikuchi, H., Yoshiuchi, K., Ohashi, K., Yamamoto, Y., & Akabayashi, A. (2007). Tension-type headache and physical activity: An actigraphic study. *Cephalalgia, 27*, 1236–1243.

Labus, J. S., Keefe, F. J., & Jensen, M. P. (2003). Self-reports of pain intensity and direct observation of pain behavior: When are they correlated? *Pain, 102*, 109–124.

Long, A. C., Palermo, T. M., & Manees, A. M. (2008). Brief report: Using actigraphy to compare physical activity levels in adolescents with chronic pain and healthy adolescents. *Journal of Pediatric Psychology, 33*, 660–665.

McDaniel, L. K., Anderson, K. O., Bradley, L. A., Young, L. D., Turner, R. A., Agudelo, C. A., et al. (1986). Development of an observation method for assessing pain behavior in rheumatoid arthritis patients. *Pain, 24*, 165–184.

Melzack, R., & Wall, P. D. (1965). Pain mechanisms: A new theory. *Science, 150*, 971–979.

Murphy, S. L., Strasburg, D. M., Lyden, A. K., Smith, D. M., Koliba, J. F., Dadabhoy, D. P., et al. (2008). Effects of activity strategy training on pain and physical activity in older adults with knee or hip osteoarthritis: A pilot study. *Arthritis Care and Research, 59*, 1480–1487.

Ohlund, C., Lindstrom, I., Areskoug, B., Eek, C., Peterson, L. E., & Nachemson, A. (1994). Pain behavior in industrial subacute low back pain: Part I. Reliability: concurrent and predictive validity of pain behavior assessments. *Pain, 58*, 201–209.

Prkachin, K. M., Schultz, I. Z., & Hughes, E. (2007). Pain behavior and the development of pain-related disability: The importance of guarding. *Clinical Journal of Pain, 23*, 270–277.

Romano, J. M., Turner, J. A., Friedman, L. S., Bulcroft, R. A., Jensen, M. P., & Hops, H. (1991). Observational assessment of chronic pain patient–spouse behavioral interactions. *Behavior Therapy, 22*, 549–567.

Romano, J. M., Turner, J. A., Friedman, L. S., Bulcroft, R. A., Jensen, M. P., Hops, H., et al. (1992). Sequential analysis of chronic pain behaviors and spouse responses. *Journal of Consulting and Clinical Psychology, 60*, 777–780.

Romano, J. M., Turner, J. A., Jensen, M. P., Friedman, L. S., Bulcroft, R. A., Hops, H., et al. (1985). Chronic pain patient–spouse behavioral interactions predict patient disability. *Pain, 63*, 353–360.

Shutty, M. S., Cundiff, G., & DeGood, D. E. (1990). *Development and validation of a brief pain behavior rating scale.* Unpublished manuscript.

Smith, S. J. A., Keefe, F. J., Caldwell, D. S., Romano, J., & Baucom, D. (2004). Gender differences in patient–spouse interactions: A sequential analysis of behavioral interactions in patients having osteoarthritic knee pain. *Pain, 112*, 183–187.

Trost, S. G., McIver, K. L., & Pate, R. R. (2005). Conducting accelerometer-based activity assessments in field-based research. *Medicine and Science in Sports and Exercise, 37*, S-31–S543.

Turk, D. C., & Flor, H. (1987). Pain behaviors: The utility and limitations of the pain behavior construct. *Pain, 31*, 277–295.

Turk, D. C., Meichenbaum, D., & Genest, M. (1983). *Pain and behavioral medicine: A cognitive-behavioral perspective.* New York: Guilford Press.

Waddell, G., McCulloch, J. A., Kummel, E., & Venner, R. M. (1980). Nonorganic physical signs in low-back pain. *Spine, 5*, 117–125.

Waters, S. J., Riordan, P. A., Keefe, F. J., & Lefebvre, J. C. (2008). Pain behavior in rheumatoid arthritis patients: Identification of pain behavior subgroups. *Journal of Pain and Symptom Management, 36*, 69–78.

Weiner, D., Peiper, C., McConnel, E., Martinez, S., & Keefe, F. J. (1996). Pain measurement in elders with chronic low back pain: Traditional and alternative approaches. *Pain, 67*, 461–467.

White, B., & Sanders, S. H. (1986). The influence of patients' pain intensity ratings of antecedent reinforcement of pain talk or well talk. *Journal of Behavior Therapy and Experimental Psychiatry, 17*, 155–159.

Williams, A. C. (2002). Facial expressions of pain: An evolutionary account. *Behavior and Brain Sciences, 25*, 429–488.

Zwakhalen, S. M. G., Hamers, J. P. H., Abu-Saad, H. H., & Berger, M. P. F. (2006). Pain in elderly people with severe dementia: A systematic review of behavioural pain assessment tools. *BMC Geriatrics, 6*, 3–18.

CHAPTER 8

Psychophysiological and Neuroimaging Measures in the Assessment of Patients with Chronic Pain

HERTA FLOR
PATRIC MEYER

In past decades, psychophysiological assessment methods have gained importance for both somatic and psychological disorders (Bingel & Tracey, 2008; Cacioppo, Tassinary, & Berntson, 2007; Tracey, 2008). They are primarily used as tools to determine the influence of psychological factors on bodily functioning, and specifically, to assess their contribution to the initiation and maintenance of symptoms. In many chronic pain syndromes, psychophysiological factors play a major role in the development and/or maintenance of the problem (e.g., Flor & Turk, 2006). Our purpose in this chapter are to provide an overview of the role of psychophysiological assessments in clinical pain syndromes and to suggest a framework for the integration of psychophysiological assessment data, including neuroimaging data within the comprehensive interdisciplinary assessment and treatment of pain. An overview of the use of psychophysiological measures in laboratory pain assessments is provided by several authors (e.g., Handwerker & Kobal, 1993; Niddam & Hsieh, 2009; Williams & Gracely, 2006). This chapter is divided into two sections: The first section discusses peripheral psychophysiological measures that are of primary importance in the assessment of chronic pain syndromes,

and the second section focuses on central psychophysiological measures that are increasingly gaining importance in clinical pain research.

First attempts to assess psychophysiological concomitants of pain were undertaken in the 1950s (e.g., Malmo, Shagass, & Davis, 1950) but became more accepted in the 1960s, when biofeedback methods came into wider use. Over the past 60 years, much evidence for the interaction of psychological and physiological variables in pain has accumulated (McMahon & Koltzenburg, 2005); thus, psychophysiological concepts of pain have gained importance (Apkarian, 2008; Flor & Turk, 2006). The quality of the measurements has been enhanced due to significant progress in electronics and computer technology. Despite these advances, much of the research related to the psychophysiology of pain still lacks adequate theoretical foundation and methodological rigor (cf. Apkarian, Bushnell, Treede, & Zubieta, 2005; Flor & Turk, 1989), thus presenting a challenge for future studies.

Psychophysiological data serve a number of useful functions in the assessment of chronic and acute pain states. They provide evidence on the role of psychological factors in maladaptive physiological functioning in specific patients. Moreover, results of psychophysiological recordings may be used for the differential indication of intervention methods. For example, Flor and Birbaumer (1993) employed psychophysiological responses to personal and general stress to classify patients into biofeedback responders versus responders to operant or cognitive-behavioral therapy. Psychophysiological assessments are, moreover, a necessary prerequisite for the use of biofeedback treatment. Psychophysiological measurements during treatment and posttreatment help to document the efficacy of the intervention, as well as generalization and transfer. They may also serve as predictors of treatment outcome (Flor & Birbaumer, 1993; Harris et al., 2008; Walitt et al., 2007).

Another important aspect of psychophysiological measurements is their motivational character. Patients may learn from the results that they are able to influence bodily processes by their own thoughts, emotions, and actions. Thus, feelings of helplessness may be reduced and the acceptance of psychological interventions may be increased not only in the patients but also in referring physicians to whom psychophysiological assessment data should be made available. In experimental pain research, psychophysiological data have been used to examine physiological concomitants of anxiety and general arousal associated with pain. They have also served as measures of central processes related to the pain experience (see the later section on central measures).

ELECTROMYOGRAPHIC RECORDINGS

Basic Issues

Elevated levels of muscle tension have been discussed as an etiological factor in a number of chronic pain syndromes (e.g., tension headache, temporomandibular pain and dysfunction, low back pain). Furthermore, it has been assumed that in any type of pain syndrome, reflex muscle spasm may develop that further increases pain. Thus, the surface electromyogram (EMG) is a frequently used psychophysiological parameter with chronic pain patients. In order to obtain EMG measures, muscle action potentials summed over a large area of the muscle are recorded as a voltage difference between adjacent sites. In

contrast to a neurological EMG that mainly serves the purpose of testing the function of motor neurons, psychophysiological EMG assessments are designed to record muscle tension related to psychological factors that may contribute to the pain experience. EMG evaluations are especially indicated for musculoskeletal pain syndromes such as chronic back pain (CBP), headache, or pain in the jaw and neck.

Several aspects of muscular function may be measured: elevated baseline levels, asymmetry of bilateral muscle tension, hyperreactivity to physical or psychological stress, time to return to baseline post stress, irregularities during movement, or aberrant frequency spectra (Flor & Turk, 1989; Graven-Nielsen & Arendt-Nielsen, 2008; Schwartz & Andrasik, 2005; van Dieën, Selen, & Cholewicki, 2003). These characteristics may be present singly, or they may appear in combination. A causal role of muscular dysfunctions has so far not been demonstrated for pain disorders. There is, however, conclusive evidence that pain may be maintained or exacerbated by increases in muscle tension (e.g., Glombiewski, Tersek, & Rief, 2008; Jensen, 1999; Strøm, Knardahl, Stanghelle, & Røe, 2009).

Whereas previously the frontalis muscle has most often been the target of measurements, based on the assumption that generalized hyperarousal is present in patients with chronic pain, today more emphasis is placed on localized increases in muscle tension levels. Therefore, measurements tend to be site-specific: the masseter and temporalis muscles are measured in patients with chronic temporomandibular pain and dysfunction, the erector spinae muscle in patients with lower back pain, the trapezius muscle in patients with upper back pain, and the splenius capitis, occipitalis, trapezius, or frontalis muscles for tension headache. There has also been a trend to assess several muscle groups at the same time, because this procedure yields information on the prime location of increased tension and permits an assessment of the generality or specificity of the response.

Methodological Considerations

Most physiological signals are quite weak and thus need sufficient amplification. The amplification factor of the EMG is usually around 100. Amplification that is too low leads to misinterpretations of the signal, because relevant EMG changes may not be detected (van Boxtel, 2001). Due to the high "noise" level that is present in unshielded clinical settings where most assessments are made, differential amplifiers with a high common mode rejection (80–100 decibels [dB]) are required. Thus, signals that act symmetrically on the electrodes and would lead to artifacts are suppressed. It is necessary that the impedance between the surface of the skin and the electrode not exceed 10 kilohms. The use of nonpolarizing silver/silver chloride (Ag/AgCl) electrodes is recommended. Amplifiers with very high input impedance allow for less strict skin preparation and permit the use of lower quality electrodes (see muscle scanning section below). The amplifiers need to have an adequate filtering range. Many biofeedback machines have a range of only 100–200 Hz, which is not sufficient for EMG dysfunction assessment (van Boxtel, 2001).

The raw EMG signal must be processed to receive adequate information about the state of muscle tension. Usually a root mean square integrated EMG is calculated from the raw data. It is important not to use too long integration intervals, because these will then disguise artifacts related to movements or other intrusions in the recording process. The raw EMG should always be displayed in order to detect artifacts. Another important aspect is the sampling rate of the signal. It must be at least two times higher than the highest frequency of the signal. If this requirement is not met, the signal will be distorted (*aliasing*). Cheaper biofeedback equipment usually does not have this high-speed sampling capability. Further details on recording sites, skin preparation, and further technical considerations may be found in Soderberg and Knutson (2001).

Resting Baseline Levels

In their critical review of 60 psychophysiological studies on chronic headache, back pain, and temporomandibular pain and dysfunction, Flor and Turk (1989) noted that although elevated resting baseline levels have sometimes been found, they are not a prime characteristic of patients with chronic pain. Overall, the evidence for permanently elevated baseline levels in patients with chronic musculoskeletal pain problems has been scarce. Although normative data for the EMG levels of various muscle groups have been established (e.g., Cram, 1990; Vaiman, Eviatar, & Segal, 2004), resting baseline levels must be interpreted with caution. Elevated levels may not always be considered abnormal, nor may low values be interpreted to be normal. In fact, in fibromyalgia syndrome, lower than normal EMG resting baseline levels were found (Thieme et al., 2006). Even though low baseline levels may be present, abnormal responses may be detected during movement or during psychological or physical stress. On the other hand, Wolf, Wolf, and Segal (1989) have shown that resting values may be inflated by slight changes in posture that are difficult to control. In three studies Lehman (2002) examined issues of EMG asymmetry and repeatability in populations with lower back pain and healthy controls. While the repeatability of the EMG signal during quiet stance was acceptable, bilateral asymmetry was not a definitive indicator of dysfunction. Tests that used the induction of acute pain and measured EMG resting levels found no significant relationship between increases in pain and resting muscle tension (e.g., Svensson, Graven-Nielsen, Matre, & Arendt-Nielsen, 1998). There are also doubts about the reliability of measurement in certain muscle groups, although the assessment of low back muscle tension in different postures has been demonstrated as reliable (Larivière et al., 2002).

Stress Reactivity

A possibly more important physiological parameter than the baseline value is the reactivity of the muscle during physical or psychological stress. EMG is assessed while the person is exposed to a somatic (e.g., a certain body position, writing on a computer keyboard) or a psychological stressor (e.g., stressful imagery, discussion of an emotionally involving event). The stressor should have personal relevance for the person. The superiority of personally relevant stressors has been demonstrated in various experiments (e.g., Ohrbach, Blascovich, Gale, McCall, & Dworkin, 1998; but see Glombiewski et al., 2008), and studies that used general stressors or only healthy controls often failed to find the proposed pain–tension relationship (e.g., Bansevicius, Westgaard, & Jensen, 1997). This point is underscored by a naturalistic examination of supermarket cashiers with frequent pain problems that revealed significantly elevated stress values at work, accompanied by elevated EMG levels in those with more musculoskeletal pain (Lundberg et al., 1999). In general, muscular work patterns seem to be predictive of future pain problems (e.g., Veiersted, Westgaard, & Andersen, 1993). However, it is quite possible that a certain vulnerability, as predicted by the diathesis–stress model of chronic pain, is a prerequisite for tension and pain levels to rise.

Several studies have shown that the EMG stress response is symptom-specific. In patients with CBP, the erector spinae muscles are most responsive to stress, whereas in patients with temporomandibular pain and dysfunction, the masseter muscle is most reactive but not vice versa (e.g., Flor, Birbaumer, Schugens, & Lutzenberger, 1992a; Glombiewski et al., 2008). In stress reactivity assessments, the question of norms and criteria for a stress response is still open. The best procedure is to employ both neutral and general, as well as stressful, stimuli and to assess person-specific differences in the response to all three types of stimuli. Stress reactivity seems to be especially high in patients with high levels of fear of movement or reinjury (Vlaeyen et al., 1999) as predicted by the diathesis–stress model of chronic pain (e.g., Flor & Turk, in press).

Overall, a number of empirical studies have demonstrated symptom-specific EMG hyperreactivity in CBP (e.g., Burns, 1997; DeGood, Stewart, Adams, & Dale, 1994; Flor, Turk, & Birbaumer, 1985; Flor et al., 1992). Similar results have been obtained for temporomandibular pain disorders (e.g., Flor, Birbaumer, Schulte & Roos, 1991; Gramling, Grayson, Sullivan, & Schwartz, 1997). There is also convincing evidence that symptom-specific responses are present in patients with chronic headache. In 29 of 37 studies reviewed by Flor and Turk (1989), at least one significant difference was found with respect to the muscular reactivity of patients with headache compared to healthy controls. Significant differences were especially present if the EMG was recorded from several muscles and personally relevant (e.g., socially involving situations) or physical stressors were used (e.g., Clark et al., 1997; Jensen, 1999). Reactivity is symptom-specific and not general, as has been shown by the assessment of additional physiological parameters, such as heart rate, blood pressure, and skin conductance.

Return to Baseline

An additional parameter, the time to return to baseline after the induction and termination of a stressor, has so far not been sufficiently assessed. Pritchard and Wood (1984) reported a slower return to baseline of the trapezius and frontalis EMG in patients with chronic tension headache; however, these results could not be replicated in other studies (cf. Feuerstein, Bush, & Corbisiero, 1982; Kröner, 1984). Flor and Turk (1989) presented a detailed analysis of the methodological problems, as well as suggestions for improved recording methods. Better controlled studies frequently resulted in extended returns to baseline (e.g., Flor et al., 1992).

Posture and Dynamic Movement

Wolf and Basmajian (1978) first reported that patients with CBP often show abnormal static posture. Similar results have been noted by Magnusson and colleagues (1996) and Cassisi, Robinson, O'Conner, and MacMillan (1999), but there have also been negative results (e.g., Miller, 1995). So far it is not known whether the changes in posture maintain or elicit pain problems, or whether they are a mere consequence of the pain and an adaptation in posture. It is also unclear whether too high or too low EMG levels during certain postures are the main problem. This problem is aggravated by the fact that normative data on static postures in healthy controls are only sparse (cf. Roy et al., 1997). In addition, evidence from experimental studies, as well as ambulatory monitoring, suggests that EMG alterations related to postural abnormalities may be a consequence rather than an antecedent of the experience of pain (e.g., Arendt-Nielsen, Graven-Nielsen, Svarrer, & Svensson, 1996; Jalovaara, Niikimaki, & Vanharanta,

1995). Differences in posture-related EMG also seem to be based on diagnostic subgroups. Arena, Sherman, Bruno, and Young (1989, 1991) showed that although patients with low back pain in general display higher EMG levels in a standing position, patients with intervertebral disc disorder are significantly different from other patients with back pain and healthy controls in that they exhibit higher EMG levels during supported sitting. On the one hand, this points to the necessity of a differential diagnostic assessment in these patients, and on the other, it supports the assumption that these postural EMG abnormalities may be reactive in nature.

Wolf, Nacht, and Kelly (1982, Wolf et al., 1989) have reported the presence of abnormal patterns of movement in patients with CBP. Follow-up studies confirmed that abnormal body motion patterns are present in patients with chronic pain (e.g., Cassisi et al., 1999; Rudy, Boston, Lieber, Kubinski, & Delitto, 1995), with most studies reporting deficient tension levels during movement. Based on these results, the authors suggested correcting these posture and movement abnormalities by a specific biofeedback training. It is, however, not clear to what extent abnormal movement patterns are an etiological factor or just a consequence of suffering from a chronic pain problem.

Muscle Scanning

EMG scanning is a quick and easy method to detect abnormal levels of muscle activity in patients with chronic pain (Cram & Steger, 1983). Using handheld electrodes, 22 muscle sites may be scanned in about 15 minutes. Bilateral recordings in a sitting and standing posture, with scan times of at least 2 seconds, are suggested. The values obtained are then compared to normative integrated EMG values from healthy controls. Due to the use of high-quality differential amplifiers the necessity of extensive skin abrasion is reduced. Test–retest reliability (Cram, Lloyd, & Cahn, 1994) and validity (Traue, Kessler, & Cram, 1992) of the measurements have been demonstrated. As noted earlier, the relationship of these elevated EMG levels to pain and psychological antecedents of pain has not been clarified; thus, the value of EMG scanning for the selection of psycho-

logical intervention methods still needs to be determined.

Analysis of EMG Frequency Patterns

Several authors have suggested that changes in the predominant EMG frequency might be more important for the development of back pain and other musculoskeletal disorders than alterations in integrated EMG levels (cf. Lundblad, Elert, & Gerdle, 1998; Mannion, Connolly, Wood, & Dolan, 1997; Oddson et al., 1997). Using spectral analysis of EMG patterns, Lundblad and colleagues (1998) showed that shifts in EMG frequency during certain movement tasks are correlated with complaints, with higher shifts being associated with fewer complaints.

Discrimination of Muscle Tension

Several authors have emphasized that the inadequate perception of bodily states, specifically, muscle tension levels, might contribute to the maintenance of chronic pain problems (e.g., Flor, Birbaumer, & Turk, 1990). We have examined the perception of physical symptoms and of muscle tension in patients with CBP, patients with temporomandibular disorders (TMD), and patients suffering from tension headache (Flor, Fürst, & Birbaumer, 1999; Flor, Schugens, & Birbaumer, 1992b). Patients with chronic pain were shown to be notoriously unable to correctly perceive muscle tension levels at not only the affected muscle but also at a muscle unrelated to the pain problem. On the other hand, they greatly overestimated physical symptoms related to the tension production tasks, rated the tasks as more aversive, and experienced more pain upon tensing their muscles. This inability to estimate the correct current muscle tension levels might contribute to the continued maintenance of high muscle tension levels after stressors have subsided. The high focus on bodily symptoms and their overestimation may contribute to the perception of pain even at low levels of stimulation. In psychophysiological assessments, a simple method can be used to estimate tension perception ability. Patients are presented with a bar of varying height on a video monitor and are asked to tense a muscle in accordance with the height of the bar (i.e., produce low tension with a low

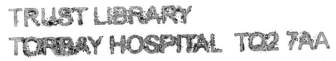

bar, and high tension with a high bar). Subsequently, the integrated EMG activity during the tension production procedure can be correlated with the height of the bar. Good tension discrimination yields a correlation greater than .80; bad tension discrimination ranges around .50 or lower.

Relationship of EMG and Pain Levels

Pain intensity and EMG levels are usually not systematically correlated at any given point in time (Geisser, Haig, Wallbom, & Wiggert, 2004; Mense & Hoheisel, 1999). Christensen (1986a, 1986b), among others, has shown that an elevation of muscle tension over an extended period of time leads to pain induction or an enhancement of already existing pain in the facial, back, or head muscles. In order to understand the relationship of pain and EMG levels better, extended EMG assessments with concurrent assessment of pain levels are necessary, preferably by using ambulatory monitoring devices. Attempts in this direction have been made by several groups (see Arena et al., 1994; Geisser, Robinson, & Richardson, 1995). Studies have provided evidence that pain may be induced by experimentally produced increases of muscle tension, and that there may be lag times of several days between the increase of muscle tension and the induction of pain (e.g., Feuerstein, Bortolussi, Houle, & Labbé, 1983). Finally, several authors have argued that there may be subgroups within certain diagnostic categories that may display specific patterns of psychophysiological abnormalities (e.g., Thieme & Turk, 2006).

AUTONOMIC MEASURES

Autonomic measures seem to be of little relevance in pain syndromes of a musculoskeletal nature. They may, however, play a major role in vascular pain problems (e.g., migraine headache or Raynaud's disease), as well as pain syndromes related to sympathetic dysfunction (e.g., complex regional pain syndromes). They have also been used in laboratory investigations with acute pain stimuli. Several methods are available to assess cardiovascular parameters: the electrocardiogram to measure heart rate; photoplethysmography, laser, or sonographic Doppler flowmetry to assess changes in blood flow; thermistor recordings or thermography to measure changes in skin temperature; and blood pressure recordings.

Measures of Blood Flow

Photoplethysmography involves the measurement of the volume of blood vessels using a light source directed at the vessel and a photosensitive plate that records the reflected light. When blood flow increases, the saturation with red blood cells increases and less light is reflected. *Tonic measurements* involve the changes in blood flow over time (blood volume recordings); *phasic measurements* are related to beat-to-beat variations in the force of flow (pulse volume recordings). Both blood and pulse volume are reduced with certain emotional responses (e.g., Coles, Donchin, & Porges, 1986a). Photopletysmographic measures have, however, the disadvantage that they can only display relative changes, not absolute values in volume.

Changes in blood volume are of special interest in migraine research based on etiological theories that assume an important role of vasomotor processes in the development of pain. Comparable to the results of EMG recordings in patients with tension headache, most controlled studies did not find baseline differences in vascular parameters in patients with migraine compared to healthy controls (for a summary, see Flor & Turk, 1989). Few specific differences with respect to EMG baseline values and vascular parameters have been reported for the different types of headaches (e.g., Arena, Blanchard, Andrasik, Appelbaum, & Myers, 1985). In patients with migraine, attacks could even be elicited by inducing spasms in the head muscles (Bakke, Tfelt-Hansen, Olesen, & Møller, 1982). The authors reported a high correlation between the onset of pain and peaks in EMG readings. This finding suggests that a muscular component in migraine pain may be relevant as well.

Studies on stress reactivity in patients with migraine point toward a functional abnormality of the major head arteries, particularly the temporal artery, especially when personally relevant stressors were used (e.g.,

Rojahn & Gerhards, 1986). The empirical results with respect to a slower return to baseline after stressors are controversial (see Flor & Turk, 1989, for a summary). Photoplethysmography of the temporal artery was used in several studies of patients with migraine as a biofeedback and assessment method. Patients were trained to reduce vascular contraction in order to block excessive dilation shortly before and during attacks. In a study on children with migraine, Hermann and Blanchard (1998) found no significant differences between patients and healthy controls with respect to several measures of autonomic reactivity, and suggested that assessments in children might provide a clearer picture of the psychophysiology of migraine because many chronicity-related factors are not yet present.

Peripheral sympathetic reflexes related to noxious stimulation as measured by photoplethysmography may be valid indicators of painful experiences. Significant abnormalities were observed in patients with complex regional pain syndrome (Birklein, Riedl, Neundörfer, & Handwerker, 1998).

Measurement of blood flow velocity with ultrasound Doppler sonography allows an indirect evaluation of cerebral circulation by measurement of cerebral blood flow velocity. Vasoreactivity or autoregulation mechanisms can be recorded and assessed with this noninvasive method (Nowak & Kacinski, 2009). Transcranial Doppler sonography uses high-frequency sound waves (above 20 kHz; for large vessels, 4–5 MHz) directed toward the vessel. The frequency of the reflection of the two slightly distant sound sources is proportional to the blood flow velocity (Anliker, Casry, Friedl, Kubli, & Keller, 1977). Laser Doppler flowmetry has been introduced as an alternative method (e.g., Eun, 1995). Migraine studies revealed abnormally increased flow velocity after presentation of stressful stimuli in people with migraine but not in controls (cf. Rieke et al., 1993). The interpretation of vascular parameters in clinical practice may be problematic, because the signals are very prone to artifact. Body temperature, the temperature of the environment, or the position of the body all may influence the recordings. Additional data on cerebral blood flow and pain are reported in the later section on neuroimaging.

Skin Temperature

Skin temperature is largely dependent on peripheral circulation. Vasoconstriction is associated with lower skin temperature, and vasodilation, with higher skin temperature. Usually, temperature-sensitive thermistors are used that measure temperature changes and convert them to changes in electrical resistance. However, recordings with thermistors are very prone to artifact, especially because they are easily disturbed by slight changes in temperature or air circulation in a room. Skin temperature does respond to stress. This is of special relevance in Raynaud's disease, which has been found to be associated with pain related to cold extremities (Block & Sequeira, 2001; Wigley, 2002). In a series of studies, Freedman and his coworkers (e.g., Freedman & Ianni, 1983; Jennings et al., 1999) showed that both emotional and physical stressors lead to more local vasoconstriction in patients with Raynaud's disease than in healthy controls. Consequently, temperature biofeedback has proven to be a very efficient treatment method (Karavidas, Tsai, Yucha, McGrady, & Lehrer, 2006).

In phantom limb pain, Sherman and his colleagues identified subgroups of patients with pain based on their psychophysiological responses (Sherman & Bruno, 1987; Sherman, Griffin, Evans, & Grana, 1992). Whereas burning, throbbing, and tingling phantom limb pain seems to covary with reduced temperature in the stump, cramping phantom limb pain was found to be related to and often preceded by decreases in muscle tension in the residual limb. These findings suggest differential treatments for these two patient subgroups.

Although temperature biofeedback has often been used in patients with migraine, the usefulness of temperature recordings has not yet been demonstrated for migraine headaches. The procedure is based on the observation that migraine attacks may improve with hand-warming biofeedback in attack-free periods. Studies that assessed the role of temperature and temperature reactivity in migraine headaches have not provided empirical evidence for a specific role in the therapeutic effect (for a summary, see Flor & Turk, 1989; Nestoriuc & Martin, 2007).

In thermography, infrared photography of the body surface measures vascular abnormalities related to pain (Ford & Ford, 1997; Friedman, 1994). Abnormally high, as well as low, temperatures may be associated with pain. Thermography has been widely used as both an assessment instrument and documentation of treatment-related changes (e.g., Sanchez et al., 2008; Uematsu, Hendeler, & Hungerford, 1981). Thermography is especially used in the assessment of pain caused by inflammatory processes, such as those in rheumatoid arthritis (MacDonald, Land, & Sturrock, 1994). Its usefulness as a psychophysiological research method has not yet been adequately assessed. Thermographic recordings have tended to suffer from inadequate analyses and may have little specificity (Leclaire, Esdaile, Hanley, Rossignol, & Bourdouxhe, 1996), although computerized thermographic recordings have yielded more reliable results (Bruehl, Lubenow, Nath, & Ivankovich, 1996; Sherman, Woerman, & Karstetter, 1996).

Thermographic recordings have also been used in the analysis of facial temperature in patients with migraine and patients with facial pain. Patients with TMD in high thermal asymmetry of the temporomandibular joint region was found compared to healthy controls (e.g., Graff-Radford, Ketelaer, Gratt, & Solberg, 1995). Nahm and colleagues (2007) found temperature differences between the opposite sides of the temporomandibular and masseter muscles in patients with TMD. Although the sensitivity of thermography in the diagnosis of TMD was low in their study, it had high specificity in the evaluation of TMD.

Heart Rate and Blood Pressure

The recording of heart rate is often used in psychophysiology, because it is a very easy to measure. Typically, the number of R-waves of the ECG is converted into beats per minute. Although frequently used in acute laboratory pain assessments, there is little research on the relationship of heart rate and chronic pain, and even less research on the relationship of blood pressure and chronic pain. Most of the research available is inconclusive. For example, Flor and colleagues (1985) reported no differences in heart rate during resting baseline or during various stressors (brief cold pressor, mental math, discussion of personally relevant stress and pain episodes) between patients with CBP and healthy controls. On the other hand, Arntz, Merckelbach, Peters, and Schmidt (1991) found lower heart rate reactivity to an extended cold pressor test, Flor, Birbaumer, and colleagues (1992) noted lower heart rate reactivity to personally relevant stress images in patients with CBP compared to healthy controls, and Kappel and colleagues (1989) reported less reactivity in patients with TMD compared to healthy controls. Both Arntz and colleagues and Flor, Birbaumer, and colleagues interpreted these findings as indicative of a lack of active coping in patients compared to controls. This hypothesis is based on Obrist's (1976) findings of a coupling of somatic and cardiovascular responses during active coping, and a decoupling during passive coping. This assumption is corroborated by the high negative correlation between heart rate reactivity and passive coping (catastrophizing) reported by Flor and colleagues. In fibromyalgia syndrome (FMS) altered autonomic reactivity has been reported (Thieme et al., 2006) with elevated baseline heart rate and higher skin conductance reactivity in the patients with FMS. Some authors have also suggested that lower heart rate variability might be associated with chronic pain; however, heart rate variability seems to be better correlated with impairment than with pain (cf. Gockel, Lindholm, Niemisto, & Hurri, 2008). Hassett and colleagues (2007) conducted biofeedback training in patients with FMS to manipulate suboptimal heart rate variability. They observed clinically significant decreases in depression and pain, and improvement in functioning from the first session to a 3-month follow-up. Heart rate variability and blood pressure variability increased during biofeedback tasks. These data suggest that heart rate variability biofeedback may be a useful treatment for FMS, perhaps mediated by autonomic changes. While heart rate variability effects were immediate, blood pressure, baroreflex, and therapeutic effects were delayed.

Heart rate has also frequently been used as a physiological correlate of acute pain intensity (Sternbach, 1968). However, increases in tonic heart rate have been related more to subjective pain ratings than to objective characteristics of the nociceptive stimulus (cf. Hampf, 1990; Moltner, Hölzl, & Strian, 1990). In studies of postoperative pain, cardiovascular measures have been used to document the effects of postoperative pain, as well as the favorable effects of psychological interventions. Both blood pressure and heart rate reductions have been reported more in patients who underwent psychological coping training than in patients not involved in these procedures (e.g., Wallace, 1984). However, in a prospective, observational study of a convenience sample of patients with acute pain presenting to an academic emergency department, Bossart, Fosnocht, and Swanson (2007) reported only a poor correlation between change in pain intensity and change in heart rate ($r = .08$).

In experimental pain studies, a negative correlation of blood pressure and pain experience has been established for participants with elevated tonic blood pressure, whereas this correlation is positive for normotensives (Larbig, Elbert, Rockstroh, Lutzenberger, & Birbaumer, 1985). The induction of elevated blood pressure levels by the use of baroreceptor stimulation leads to a reduction in pain sensitivity in borderline hypertensives and to an increase of pain sensitivity in normotensives (Dworkin et al., 1994). Similar blood pressure–related changes in pain sensitivity have also been reported for patients with chronic pain, but their practical relevance has not yet been established (Bruehl, McCubbin, & Harden, 1999). Light and colleagues (2009) examined cardiovascular responses in patients with FMS and healthy controls. Testing included baseline, postural, speech, and ischemic pain stressors. Patients with FMS showed lesser heart rate increases to posture challenge but greater blood pressure increases in reaction to postural and speech tasks than controls, as well as higher overall blood pressure and greater total vascular resistance than patients with TMD or controls. These findings support the hypothesis that both FMS and TMD may frequently involve dysregulation of beta-adrenergic activity that contributes to altered cardiovascular responses and to severity of clinical pain.

Pupil Size and Response Abnormalities

The literature suggests that there may also be pupil size and response abnormalities in patients with chronic pain. Harle, Wolff-sohn, and Evans (2005) used an infrared pupillometer to measure dynamic pupil responses to light in migraine sufferers (during nonheadache periods) and healthy controls. They found a significant increase in the absolute interocular difference of the latency of the pupil light response in the migraine group compared with the controls. Moreover, there was also a significant correlation between lateralization of headache and *anisocoria* (a condition characterized by an unequal size of the pupils). People with migraine with a habitual head pain side have more anisocoria, but this was not related to headache laterality. However, pupil changes were not correlated with the interval since the last migraine headache, the severity of migraine headache, or the number of migraine headaches per annum.

SKIN CONDUCTANCE MEASURES

Skin conductance may be viewed as a measure of general arousal. It changes with the activation of the sweat glands that are responsive to psychological stimuli (Fowles, 1986). Their activity is mediated by the sympathetic nervous system. Often-used parameters of the sympathetic activity of the skin are the tonic skin conductance level, or the phasic skin conductance response. Acute pain is associated with both increased heart rate and skin conductance levels (Tousignant-Laflamme, Goffaux, Bourgault, & Marchand, 2006). In certain pain syndromes, autonomic dysfunction seems to be of some importance (e.g., in complex regional pain syndromes or phantom limb pain). Here, measures of the activity of the sympathetic system, such as skin conductance level, seem indicated. However, results on the significance in skin conductance measures for chronic pain have been controversial. Peters and Schmidt (1991) reported increased skin conductance levels in response to stress in patients with low back pain, but these results were not confirmed by Flor and colleagues (1985; Flor, Birbaumer, et al., 1992). Jamner and Tursky (1987) reported that patients with pain show increased electrodermal activity in response to words that are relevant to their pain syndrome. The authors' suggestion to use this measure in the detection of deception in medicolegal cases has not been followed up.

Overall, responses to painful stimuli seem to be associated with characteristic peripheral physiological responses in the muscular, vascular, as well as the eccrine system. Further research is needed to determine the role of peripheral psychophysiological variables in chronic pain (see Petzke & Clauw, 2000, for a review).

RECOMMENDATIONS

Based on the methodological suggestions of Flor and Turk (1989), several guidelines for the assessment of psychophysiological variables in chronic pain syndromes have been established (see Table 8.1). First, the *type of pain problem* should be clearly described, and a differential diagnosis should be made. Only in conjunction with a *multiaxial evaluation* of the patient with chronic pain (cf. Gatchel, Peng, Peters, Fuchs, & Turk, 2007) can psychophysiological assessment data be interpreted in a valid manner. Moreover, the multiaxial assessment is necessary to identify physical or psychosocial stressors that are relevant for a given patient and can subsequently be used to test psychophysiological reactivity.

TABLE 8.1. Recommendations for Psychophysiological Assessment

- Use multiaxial classification of patients to know specific somatic and psychosocial characteristics of the patients.
- If possible, use normative data from controls.
- Control for pain status (i.e., test in a pain-free and painful state if possible).
- Control for medication (i.e., make sure patient has not taken analgesic or psychotropic medication for several days, if possible).
- Use sites proximal and distal to the painful site.
- Make sure that the measures you select are relevant for the specific type of pain you are studying (e.g., use temperature recordings for Raynaud`s syndrome rather than EMG levels).
- Use ecologically valid methods of stress induction (i.e., use self-selected stressors, test stressfulness by assessing subjective stress rating, heart rate, or skin conductance levels).
- Use sufficiently long adaptation phases and baselines.
- Use a syndrome-specific and a general autonomic measure.

Psychophysiological measurements should be tailored to the assumed *etiology of the pain* problem. Thus, EMG recordings seem to be of primary importance in chronic musculoskeletal pain problems, vascular measures in migraine headaches and Raynaud's disease, and vascular combined with skin conductance measures in neuropathic pain syndromes. Because we do not yet know enough about the role of symptom-specific and general arousal in patients with chronic pain, at least one specific and one general activation measure (skin conductance, heart rate) should be used. Following Dolce and Raczynski (1985), we recommend that EMG assessments should be accompanied by the recording of autonomic responses to identify patients who are generally overaroused and could profit from nonspecific stress management and relaxation. In patients with specific local dysfunctions, such as heightened stress reactivity of the back muscles or heightened vascular reactivity of the extremities, specific biofeedback is indicated (e.g., Flor & Birbaumer, 1991; Freedman, 1991). Feedback that includes stress exposure has a more favorable outcome than feedback aimed only at resting levels (e.g., Freedman, Ianni, & Wenig, 1983). Laboratory measures should be supplemented by field recordings with portable equipment in the natural environment.

One of the major problems in psychophysiological pain assessments is the frequent use of test stimuli that may not be relevant for the patient being tested. Whereas mental arithmetic may be a *personally relevant stressor* for a student, this type of stressor is most likely of no significance to a homemaker or a blue-collar worker. We have found it most useful to identify physical and psychological stressors from the pain assessment interview, then have the patient produce or report them during the assessment. It is also important to determine whether the stress induction was successful. This can be achieved by using subjective ratings of the stressfulness and personal relevance of the stressor. The validity of these ratings may be verified by the additional use of measures that represent autonomic activation such as heart rate or skin conductance levels.

Recordings from *several muscles* seem to be especially important, because several muscles may be involved in the disorder. In addition, recordings from a *distal site* should be made, because this allows conclusions about the site-specificity of the dysfunction and, again, has treatment implications. When choosing muscles from which to record, it is important to use a muscle site close to the site of pain, as well as a more distant muscle, to obtain comparison values about the generality or specificity of the response. Although EMG may often be the measure of choice in chronic pain syndromes, other variables may sometimes be more relevant for a specific pain syndrome. For example, in Raynaud's disease, peripheral temperature is a much more relevant variable to indicate deficient peripheral circulation. In patients with phantom limb pain, Sherman and Associates (1997) reported that changes in temperature of the stump may be related to throbbing, burning phantom limb pain, whereas increases in muscle tension may precede cramping, aching types of phantom pains, as discussed earlier.

Sufficient *adaptation* to the laboratory situation (about 15 minutes) and sufficiently long intertrial intervals (5–10 minutes) are required to allow for measures to return to baseline. Pretrial baselines should be recorded to take into account resting baseline changes due to different postures or lack of return to baseline on previous trials. Patients should refrain from taking analgesic and muscle-relaxing medication at least on the day of the assessment.

If possible, *normative data* from controls should be used to determine the extent to which a given level of psychophysiological reactivity is actually deviant. Published norms are available for a large number of patient samples and situations (Schwartz & Andrasik, 2005). A comparison of several tasks for a single patient may also be useful. It is also important to control for *pain status*. Ideally, patients with intermittent pain should be assessed in a pain-free and in a painful state. This allows determination of the role of pain in muscle tension levels and the significance of tonically elevated tension levels or heightened reactivity in pain-free states. Level of *medication* also needs to be controlled: as noted; both analgesic and psychotropic medication can influence muscle tension levels and lead to distorted recordings.

CASE STUDY

The following case is presented to demonstrate the integration of verbal–subjective, somatic–motor, and physiological–organic data into a comprehensive assessment profile that allows for specific treatment prescriptions.

Mr. F, a 55-year-old, married, blue-collar worker with a high school diploma, attended the pain outpatient clinic with facial pain. The pain began 5 years ago, when he was involved in an accident at his work site. Since then, his ability to work is greatly reduced (frequent days missed at work), and he has been informed that he might lose his job, although he is quite willing to work. After a comprehensive pain interview, the following assessment instruments were used: the Multidimensional Pain Inventory (Kerns, Turk, & Rudy, 1985), the Pain-Related Self-Statements Scale and the Pain-Related Convictions of Control Scale (Flor & Turk, 1988), the Brief Stress Questionnaire (Flor, 1991), and the Pain Behavior Scale (Feuerstein, Greenwald, Gamache, Papciak, & Cook, 1985).

Analysis of the questionnaires and interview data indicated that the patient's pain and interference levels were very high compared to other pain clinic patients. Both affective distress and depression scores were low. Life control, as well as active coping with the pain, were low; tendencies to catastrophize and to assume a helpless attitude toward the pain were high. Mr. F's spouse was supportive but showed little tendency to reinforce pain behaviors that, overall, were unremarkable. The patient experienced a high level of stress in his everyday life. He also noticed that anger or stress—especially at the work site—increased his pain. Additional factors that influenced the pain were heat and cold, changes in light, changes in mood, and high levels of concentration on a task. Overall, the patient attempted to ignore the pain or control it by rest and medication (narcotic and antidepressant). He reported sleep disturbances that he attributed to the pain. The patient seemed to be eager to work despite his incapacitating pain problem.

The psychophysiological assessment consisted of bilateral EMG measurements at the masseter, frontalis, and trapezius muscles, and recording of heart rate and skin conductance levels. Following a 10-minute adaptation and a 2-minute baseline, the patient imagined personally relevant pain and stress situations, and a neutral situation, participated in extended (10 minutes) mental arithmetic, and a 10-minute movement task. Each phase had 1-minute pre- and postbaseline recordings.

The resting values of the masseter, trapezius, and frontalis muscles were significantly elevated (EMG values > 15 microvolts), with a marked asymmetry especially at the frontalis muscle (related to damage during the accident). EMG levels at other sites, as well as heart rate and skin conductance levels, were not remarkable.

During stress testing, a marked response to the stressors was noted, with very high reactivity for the pain episode. Overall, the assessment revealed that the patient showed elevated facial muscle tension levels both in the resting state and during exposure to relevant stressors compared to healthy controls (see Figure 8.1). These increases in muscle tension were most likely a reaction to the pain problem, which was additionally exacerbated and maintained by them. This elevated tension also extended to the upper back, but not to the erector spinae muscle.

Based on these findings, the primary goal of the treatment was viewed as the reduction of tension in the relevant muscles and the alteration of the patient's response to aversive stimulation. The patient received EMG biofeedback training that focused on alternative ways of dealing with stressful situations. The patient imagined the aversive situations and simultaneously observed his EMG response in the masseter muscle and a "control" muscle of the lower back. Real-life exposure, such as aggressive verbalization of the therapist, was also combined with the task of bringing the EMG response of the masseter muscle back to the normal level of the "control" muscle as quickly as possible. Homework included the recording of stress episodes, the patient's response to them, and the generation of alternate responses.

CENTRAL MEASURES OF THE PAIN EXPERIENCE

Neuroimaging Methods

A variety of imaging techniques have been developed and used to study acute and chronic pain. The electroencephalogram (EEG) reflects fluctuations of voltage caused by changes of the summed ionic currents of

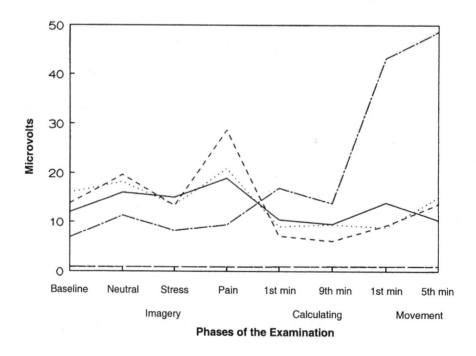

FIGURE 8.1. Psychophysiological profile of Mr. F.

billions of pyramidal cells of the cerebral cortex. Their dendrites in the apical layers (Layers I and II) of the cerebral cortex and their soma in the deeper brain structures (i.e., Layers III–V) generate an electrical dipole when there is input from thalamic or other brain structures. Thousands of pyramidal cells are simultaneously activated and create the potential changes on the cortical surface. The amplitude of the EEG is attenuated by the skull and the scalp, so that the normal EEG activity recorded from external electrodes ranges somewhere between one and several hundred microvolts. The EEG assesses changes in the electric potential of the cerebral cortex that may be related to subcortical activations whose activity is conducted as field potentials. The basis of neuroelectric source imaging of pain is the measurement of pain-related electric potentials. They must be extracted from the spontaneous EEG by averaging, and therefore require multiple stimulus presentations. After averaging the EEG to a stimulus, the resulting complex sequence of waves represents various physiological and psychophysiological events (Niedermeyer & Lopez da Silva, 2004).

Three types of evoked potentials have been identified as correlates of pain perception (they cannot be called measures of pain, because they are influenced by a number of factors, e.g., attention and general activation; Lorenz & Garcia-Larréa, 2003): brainstem potentials (10–15 msec after the application of the stimulus), potentials of short latency (15–20 msec after the application of the stimulus) that are probably based on thalamocortical sources, and long latency potentials (50–200 msec after the stimulus) that have a cortical basis (Chapman & Jacobson, 1984). Subjective pain perception correlates with the amplitude of the *evoked potential* in the 150–260 msec range that may provide information in addition to the subjective pain rating (Chapman et al., 1985). Dowman (1996) computed a difference potential between the evoked response at pain threshold versus that at noxious levels in the time range 75–240 msec poststimulus (sural nerve evoked potentials) and found evidence that this potential reflects exclusively Aδ nociceptive fiber activity.

EEG spectral analysis might also serve as a valuable tool to diagnose chronic pain. The EEG *power spectrum* provides a measure of the relative "power" of the EEG waves within a certain frequency band. Usually the band's delta (0.5 to 3.5 Hz—profound sleep and pathology), theta (3.5 to 7.5 Hz—deep sleep, but also focused attention if localized in the frontal area), alpha (8 to 12 Hz—relaxed wakefulness with eyes closed), and beta (13 to 30 Hz—eyes open, attentive) are discriminated.

The magnetoencephalogram (MEG) assesses magnetic fields in the brain that are based on electric potentials (Preissl, 2005). Highly sensitive detectors, so-called SQUIDS (superconducting quantum interference devices) positioned about 10–15 mm from the skull are able to detect the weak magnetic fields generated by electric dipoles of the brain. As in EEG measurements, activity peaks are usually determined by averaging over many stimulations. Since the MEG can be recorded without electrodes and are not distorted by skull and fluids, it is more accurate and more convenient for patient studies. However it has the disadvantage that only tangential components of the signal (i.e., those that are perpendicular to the surface of the cortex) can be measured. EEG and MEG have excellent time resolution and also quite good spatial resolution (1–4 mm for early components), but the location of the signal sources has to be reconstructed using mathematical models.

New methods of EEG and MEG analysis such as nonlinear *dimensional analysis* (Elbert et al., 1994), are other possible applications of central nervous system (CNS) recordings in the quantification of pain processing in the human brain. The use of nonlinear ("chaos") deterministic models allows the dimensional reduction of the EEG trace into a few basic factors (fractal dimensions) that determine the actual time series. Electro- and magnetoencephalography can also be helpful tools for the investigation of synchronous communication between cortical areas. In particular, time–frequency decomposition of signals recorded with these techniques seems to be a promising approach, because different pain-related oscillatory changes can be observed within different frequency bands, which are likely to be linked to specific sensory and motor functions (see Hauck, Lorenz, & Engel, 2008, for a review). Ploner, Gross, Timmermann, Pollok, and Schnitzler

(2006) used MEG to investigate the effects of pain on spontaneous brain rhythms. Their results showed that a focally applied, brief painful stimulus globally suppresses spontaneous oscillations in somatosensory, motor, and visual areas. This global suppression contrasted with the regionally specific suppressions of other modalities and suggests that pain induces a widespread change in cortical function and excitability. This global change in excitability may reflect the alerting function of pain, resulting in the processing of and reacting to relevant stimuli. In a more recent study, they observed that selective painful stimuli induce gamma oscillations between 60 and 95 Hz in primary somatosensory cortex (Gross, Schnitzler, Timmermann, & Ploner, 2007). Amplitudes of pain-induced gamma oscillations varied with objective stimulus intensity and subjective pain intensity. However, around pain threshold, perceived stimuli yielded stronger gamma oscillations than unperceived stimuli of identical stimulus intensity. These results demonstrate that pain induces gamma oscillations in primary somatosensory cortex that are particularly related to the subjective perception of pain. Consequently, the authors assumed that gamma oscillations are related to the internal representation of behaviorally relevant stimuli that should receive preferred processing.

Neuroelectric and neuromagnetic methods have the advantage that they assess neuronal activity rather than reflections of neuronal activity in metabolic changes. They have very high temporal resolution and are thus uniquely suited to measure quickly changing brain processes, but they have the disadvantage of a lower spatial resolution. The combination of multichannel EEG and MEG measurements with magnetic resonance imaging has led to the development of *neuroelectric and neuromagnetic source imaging* methods with a resolution of a few millimeters (2–5 mm, depending on the activity and measure used; cf. Hari & Forss, 1999; Kristeva-Feige et al., 1997). In addition, EEG, MEG, and functional magnetic resonance imaging (fMRI) methods have been combined in multimodal imaging studies, thus combining the advantages of high temporal and spatial resolution (e.g., Christmann, Koeppe, Braus, Ruf, & Flor, 2007; Mulert & Lemieux, 2009).

Several blood flow–based neuroimaging methods have been used in identifying the neuroanatomical correlates of pain. These measures include positron emission tomography (PET), single-photon emission computed tomography (SPECT), and fMRI. PET is based on the use of radio tracers, such as $H_2[^{15}O]$ or $[^{15}O]$butanol, that are usually introduced into the bloodstream and whose concentration is subsequently measured by a scanner that detects positrons emitted by the radioactive molecules. This determines which brain regions have taken up a radioactive substance and are thus active during a certain type of stimulation (Carson, Daube-Witherspoon, & Herscovitch, 1998; Valk, Dominique-Delbeke, & Bailey, 2006). Furthermore, ligand PET offers the opportunity to measure the regional distribution of different receptors (Sprenger et al., 2007). Ligand PET studies investigating chronic pain predominantly use ligands of the opioidergic system (Zubieta & Stohler, 2009). A drawback of the PET technique, however, is its relatively low temporal resolution, which is related to the fact that changes in metabolic activity occur very slowly (in the range of seconds), and that fairly long interstimulus intervals are needed to allow for return to baseline (several minutes). Moreover, the use of radioactive markers precludes in general repeat measurements in the same patient. PET is usually based on the analysis of group data. The relationship of blood flow changes and neuronal signals—that are the actual targets of the measurement—has not yet been sufficiently clarified. SPECT is similar to PET, in that it also uses radio tracers such as $[^{123}I]$iodoamphetamine, which emit signals that can be measured by photosensitive equipment. It has lower resolution and longer acquisition times than PET but has the advantage that no cyclotron is needed to produce the radioisotopes (English, 1996).

The fMRI method is rapidly gaining acceptance (cf. Belliveau et al., 1991; Huettel, Song, & McCarthy, 2009). fMRI is based on the application of a strong magnetic field through a person's head that leads to a spin of nuclei in hydrogen molecules with a particular orientation. Through application of high-frequency impulses, the relaxation times of the hydrogen protons can subsequently be measured. The relaxation times are dependent on the molecule density of the tissue. The most commonly used fMRI technique is based on the BOLD (blood oxygenation level dependent) contrast, in which a stimulus-associated reduction in the local concentration of deoxyhemoglobin is used as the measure of brain activation. The temporal resolution of fMRI is much better than that of PET, at around 2 seconds, and the spatial resolution is in the range of several millimeters (Villringer, 1997). Moreover, proton magnetic resonance spectroscopy enables quantitative measurement of defined metabolites in distinct brain regions. The most important signals obtained by proton nuclear magnetic resonance are from N-acetyl-aspartate (NAA), creatine and phosphocreatine (Cr), and choline-containing compounds (Cho). Also, resonances from glutamate (Glu), taurine (Tau), and inositol (Ino) are measurable in normal brain, while glutamine (Gln), gamma-aminobutyric acid (GABA), alanine (Ala), and lactate (Lac) can be identified in diverse pathological states. Recent advances have resulted in excellent proton nuclear magnetic resonance spectra being recorded from localized regions of the human brain, and marked abnormalities have been reported in the spectra of patients with cerebral disorders as varied as brain tumors, stroke, inborn genetic abnormalities, and neurodegenerative disorders (for a review, see Brandao & Doningues, 2003).

Changes in brain morphology can also be demonstrated using *diffusion tensor imaging* (DTI), which determines the mobility of water in the brain tissue as a function of the direction the water molecules can move. By this, it enables the measurement of the restricted diffusion of water in tissue to produce neural tract images. The resulting output is the *fractional anisotropy* (FA), an index of the extent of aligned structures ranging from 0 to 1. For isotropic water diffusion, the water displacements are equal in every direction and the FA value is 0, whereas diffusion in ordered structures has a higher FA (Mori, 2007).

Brain Areas Involved in the Perception and Evaluation of Pain

fMRI has been used intensively to investigate brain mechanisms underlying both acute and chronic pain. Despite various experimental paradigms and pain models, fMRI studies have consistently demonstrated an involvement of the thalamus, primary somatosensory cortex (S1), secondary somatosensory cortex (S2), insula, forebrain, and anterior cingulate cortex (ACC) during painful stimulation (for a review, see Apkarian et al., 2005; Tracey & Mantyh, 2007). These primary nociceptive areas are often termed the *pain matrix* (Melzack, 1999) (Figure 8.2). Accumulating evidence suggests that these areas process different aspects of pain (e.g., Hofbauer, Rainville, Duncan, & Bushnell, 2001). While the perception of sensory-discriminative features of pain is associated with the S1 and S2 cortices, the ACC and parts of the insula seem to be preferentially associated with the affective–motivational processing of pain (Price, 2000; Sewards & Sewards, 2002). Prefrontal cortical areas are supposed to be related to memory or stimu-

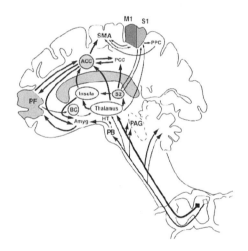

FIGURE 8.2. Cortical and subcortical regions involved in pain perception. The locations of the regions are superimposed onto a sample MRI. The areas primarily involved in pain perception are the primary somatosensory cortex (S1), the secondary somatosensory cortex (S2), the anterior cingulate cortex (ACC), the insula, the thalamus, the basal ganglia (BG), the prefrontal cortex (PF), and the primary motor cortex (M1). Other regions are the supplementary motor area (SMA), the posterior cingulate cortex (PCC), the amygdala (AMYG), the parabrachial nuclei (PB), and the periaqueductal gray (PAG). The schematic was originally published by Apkarian et al. (2005). Copyright 2005. Reprinted with permission from Elsevier Science and the authors.

lus evaluation processes, as well as pain anticipation (Apkarian et al., 2005; Porro, Cettolo, Francescato, & Baraldi, 2003).

Functional, Structural, and Biochemical Changes in the Brains of Patients with Chronic Pain

By use of neuroimaging methods, several cerebral mechanisms that have been found to be involved in chronic pain go beyond regular brain responses to acute pain (for a review, see Schweinhardt, Lee, & Tracey, 2006; Seifert & Maihöfner, 2009). At least six mechanisms seem to be essentially involved in the chronicity process: (1) *Activity increase in areas of the pain matrix* that are generally active during acute pain; (2) *recruitment of additional cortical areas beyond the classical pain matrix*; (3) *structural changes* in the brain, probably due to prolonged and sustained functional changes; (4) *disruption of the default network* of the brain; (5) *cortical reorganization and maladaptive neuroplasticity* as a consequence of the loss or the increase of peripheral input; and (6) *altered brain chemistry*. Key findings concerning those mechanisms and their implications for our understanding of chronic pain are summarized in the following paragraphs.

Using painful electric stimulation of the skin at the back or at the finger of patients with CBP during an MEG recording, Flor, Braun, Elbert, and Birbaumer (1997) showed significant brain activation differences between patients with CBP and healthy controls. Stimulation at the affected the back but not the finger led to a significantly higher magnetic field in the early time window (< 100 ms) for patients with CBP compared to controls. The signal strength in this time window and duration of pain were positively correlated, suggesting increased cortical responsivity with increasing chronicity. The source of this early activity originated from S1 and the localization of the fingers did not differ between patients and controls. However, the localization of the back was more inferior and medial in the patients. This indicates a shift and expansion toward the cortical representation of the leg (see Figure 8.3). This suggests that chronic pain leads to an expansion of the cortical representation zone related to nociceptive input, and that the amount of cortical reorganization increases with pain duration. This is much

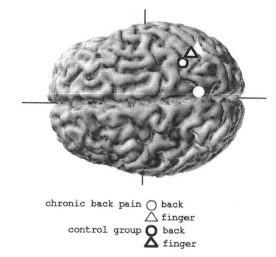

chronic back pain ○ back
△ finger
control group ● back
▲ finger

FIGURE 8.3. Localization of the digits and the back in patients with back pain and healthy controls in primary somatosensory cortex. Stimulation was on the left side of the body; the representations are on the hemisphere contralateral to the stimulation side. Note the shift of the back representation of the patients with back pain into a more medial position (i.e. toward the leg representation). The shift amounted to about 2–3 cm. Based on Flor et al. (1997).

like the expansions of cortical representations that have been documented to occur with other types of behaviorally relevant stimulation, and it differs from the changes that occur with deafferentation, in which the changes correlate with pain intensity rather than chronicity.

Flor, Diers, and Birbaumer (2004) used painful and nonpainful electric stimulation of the finger in patients with CBP, patients with headache, and controls. Only the patients with CBP displayed significantly lower pain thresholds and tolerance, as well as a reduced habituation (i.e., sensitization). Although the stimulation intensity for the three groups was different (i.e., lower in the CBP group), the patients with CBP showed equally high levels of evoked brain responses, as assessed by multichannel EEG recordings, suggesting also central sensitization. A later study by Diers and colleagues (2007) expanded these results to intramuscular recordings and observed both higher pain ratings (perceptual sensitization) over the course of the stimulation in the patients with

CBP and also enhanced CNS processing, as evidenced by an enhanced N80 component. Enhanced perceptual sensitization to tonic rather than phasic stimulation was found in patients with CBP (Kleinböhl et al., 1999). They used extended heat pain and a behavioral response as indicator of sensitization.

Giesecke and colleagues (2004) compared patients with CBP, patients with FMS, and healthy controls. During the fMRI measurements, they administered two kinds of painful stimulation to the thumbnails of participants: (1) stimuli of equal pressure and (2) equal subjective pain intensity. The pressure required to produce moderate pain was significantly higher for both patient groups than for the controls, indicating hyperalgesia. Equal amounts of pressure applied to the thumb revealed activation in five common brain regions for the two patients groups: contralateral S1, bilateral S2, the inferior parietal lobule, and the cerebellum. In healthy controls, this stimulation resulted only in activation of the contralateral S2. These results can be interpreted as increased central pain processing in CPB, even when the painful stimulus is at a site distant from the region involved in clinical pain. When subjects received a stimulus that resulted in the same amount of pain, all three groups showed activation in the central components of the pain matrix (S1, S2, insula, ACC, inferior parietal lobe), with the magnitude of activation being greater for the two patient groups.

Baliki and colleagues (2006) examined variations in habitual pain in patients with CBP. During the fMRI measurements, patients were asked to rate their habitual pain level continuously on a scale from 0 to 10. An increase of spontaneous pain in patients with CBP activated regions also seen in acute pain (i.e., the anterior and posterior insula, S2, the midcingulate cortex, S1, and the cerebellum). However, sustained high pain additionally engaged brain areas involved in emotion, cognition, and motivation, such as the medial prefrontal cortex, the rostral ACC, the posterior thalami, the ventral striatum, as well as the extended amygdala. Insular activity was also present and correlated with pain duration, leading the authors to conclude that it may reflect the chronicity of CBP. In contrast, activation of the medial prefrontal cortex correlated with the pain intensity ratings. In a later study Baliki, Geha, Apkarian, and Chialvo (2008) investigated two groups of patients with chronic pain: one with CBP and another with osteoarthritis (OA) of the knee. Both groups were placed in the fMRI scanner and rated the intensity of their pain with a finger-span logging device. The patients with CBP rated their current pain and its fluctuations, and the patients with OA rated their pain in response to pressure applied to their knee. During the pain-rating task patients with CBP reported fluctuations of their spontaneous pain intensity in the absence of any overt experimental stimulus. Activation related to these spontaneous fluctuations seemed to be mainly related to emotion/reward-mediating areas (i.e., the medial prefrontal cortex and the nucleus accumbens). Activations due to pressure pain in the OA group were found in S2, the insula, the supplementary motor area, the ACC, the medial frontal gyrus, the thalamus, the right putamen, and the left amygdala. This activation pattern was similar to that found in healthy subjects in response to acute pain (i.e., activation of the pain matrix). In a pre–post design these authors also investigated activation of brain regions before and after a 2-week treatment with a lidocaine patch applied to the painful body part.

On a behavioral level, patients with CBP experienced a robust decrease in pain intensity in response to the 2-week treatment. Before treatment, patients with CBP showed increased brain activity mainly in the frontal cortex (including the medial prefrontal cortex, rostral ACC, bilateral superior frontal gyrus, and the nucleus accumbens). Increased brain activity was also found in the inferior temporal gyrus and the left posterior parietal cortex. After treatment, the authors reported only one significant cluster of activation that showed increased activity for spontaneous pain, the left motor area (MT). The medial prefrontal cortex was the brain area the correlated best with the treatment effect. Baliki and colleagues (2008) concluded that the spontaneous pain appearing in patients with CBP was primarily of an emotional nature and assumed that lidocaine treatment decreased mainly emotional pain aspects.

Thunberg and colleagues (2005) also used PET in healthy volunteers and injected hypertonic saline into the right erector spinae muscle at the level of L3 in an attempt to mimic the pain of patients with CBP. The authors distinguished between two phases: an early acute phase (4 minutes after the start of the infusion) and a late tonic phase (21 minutes after the start of the infusion). They assumed that the latter should be a more realistic model of the chronic muscle pain found in patients. The cerebral response differed in the acute and tonic phases, and longer-lasting tonic muscle pain resulted in decreases in three clusters (left insula, right insula, and right cingulate cortex). Increases in regional cerebral blood flow (rCBF) were only found bilaterally in the occipital cortex. The authors interpret the decrease in subjective levels between the early phase and the late phase as a habituation effect and also attribute the changes in brain activity to this habituation. When the late phase was compared with baseline condition, regions implicated in the processing of all three components of pain (sensory–discriminative, motivational–affective, and cognitive–evaluative) were active. These included an increase of activation in the contralateral medial prefrontal cortex, as well as a decrease of activation in the insula, the ACC, and the dorsolateral prefrontal cortex of the ipsilateral hemisphere. The authors concluded that this dysfunction of the network may contribute to the development of chronic pain.

Recent studies have demonstrated that chronic pain also impairs cortical areas unrelated to pain itself (Acerra & Moseley, 2005; Apkarian et al., 2004). Chronic pain can alter the functional connectivity of cortical regions known to be active at rest (i.e., the components of the *default mode network* [DMN]) (Greicius, Krasnow, Reiss, & Menon, 2003; Raichle et al., 2001; Vincent et al., 2007). Using fMRI, Baliki and colleagues (2008) examined a group of patients with CBP and healthy controls while executing a simple visual attention task. They found that, despite performing the task equally well as controls, patients with CBP displayed reduced deactivation in several key DMN regions. A similar study by Cauda and colleagues (2009) compared the DMN of a sample of patients with diabetic neuropathic pain and that of controls by showing a reduced DMN and an increased resting

functional connectivity in some pain-related areas. These findings clearly demonstrate that chronic pain has a widespread impact on overall brain function. These disruptions are supposed to underlie the cognitive and behavioral impairments accompanying chronic pain.

SUMMARY

Our purpose in this chapter has been to demonstrate the usefulness of psychophysiological recording methods in the assessment of clinical pain syndromes. Whereas peripheral measures—especially the EMG and vascular parameters—have been widely used in the assessment of chronic pain, central measures, such as the spontaneous EEG, event-related potentials, PET, or fMRI, have so far mainly been limited to laboratory pain assessments. An integration of peripheral and central measures in clinical applications would be desirable. However, although neuroimaging methods are powerful tools for the analysis of central mechanisms contributing to the chronicity of pain, their diagnostic value in the assessment of a single patient must be regarded with caution. All reported data are the results of sophisticated averaging and statistical methods. There is obvious interindividual variability in brain response to identical noxious stimuli or brain correlates of similar levels of perceived pain. This concerns not only global changes in the intensity of the neuroimaging signals but also their localization and significance in specific brain regions. Thus, use of neuroimaging measures to diagnose a patient with chronic pain should not be the only method of choice and should always be combined with psychological and other psychophysiological assessments. Furthermore, the relationship of physiological measures and psychological processes should be further investigated. Many clinicians and researchers limit their endeavors to the assessment of abnormalities in physiological functioning of patients with pain, without relating them to psychological processes. A truly multidimensional assessment of pain must examine both physiological and psychological parameters of the pain experience and—most importantly—must elucidate their interrelationship.

ACKNOWLEDGMENT

The completion of this chapter was facilitated a grant from the State of Baden-Württemberg (Basic Research Award).

REFERENCES

Anliker, M., Casry, N., Friedl, P., Kubli, R., & Keller, H. (1977). Noninvasive measurement in blood flow. In N. H. Hwang & N. A. Norman (Eds.), *Cardiovascular flow dynamics and measurement* (pp. 177–198). Baltimore: University Park Press.

Apkarian, A. V. (2008). Pain perception in relation to emotional learning. *Current Opinion in Neurobiology, 18,* 464–468.

Apkarian, A. V., Bushnell, M. C., Treede, R. D., & Zubieta, J. K. (2005). Human brain mechanisms of pain perception and regulation in health and disease. *European Journal of Pain, 9,* 463–484.

Apkarian, A. V., Sosa, Y., Sonty, S., Levy, R. M., Harden, R. N., Parrish, T. B., et al. (2004). Chronic back pain is associated with decreased prefrontal and thalamic gray matter density. *Journal of Neuroscience, 24,* 10410–10415.

Arena, J. G., Blanchard, E. B., Andrasik, F., Appelbaum, K., & Myers, P. E. (1985). Psychophysiological comparisons of three kinds of headache subjects during and between headache states: Analysis of post-stress adaptation periods. *Journal of Psychosomatic Research, 29,* 427–441.

Arena, J. G., Bruno, G. M., Brucks, A. G., Searle, J. R., Sherman R. A., & Meador, K. J. (1994). Reliability of an ambulatory electromyographic activity device for musculoskeletal pain disorders. *International Journal of Psychophysiology, 17,* 153–157.

Arena, J. G., Sherman, R. A., Bruno, ..., & Young, T. R. (1989). E... graphic recordings of 5 types of ... pain subjects and non-pain contr... different positions. *Pain, 37,* 57–65.

Arena, J., Sherma... Bruno, M., & Young, T. R. (1991). ... graphic recording of low back pa... ...cts and non-pain controls in six different position: Effect of pain levels. *Pain, 45,* 23–28.

Arendt-Nielsen, L., Graven-Nielsen, T., Svarrer, H., & Svensson, P. (1996). The influence of low back pain on muscle activity and coordination during gait: A clinical and experimental study. *Pain, 64,* 231–240.

Arntz, A., Merckelbach, H., Peters, M. C., & Schmidt, A. J. M. (1991). Chronic low back pain, response specificity and habituation to painful stimuli. *Journal of Psychophysiology, 5,* 177–188.

Bakke, M., Tfelt-Hansen, P., Olesen, J., & Møller, E. (1982). Action of some pericranial muscles during provoked attacks of common migraine. *Pain, 14,* 121–135.

Baliki, M. N., Chialvo, D. R., Geha, P. Y., Levy, R. M., Harden, R. N., Parrish, T. B., et al. (2006). Chronic pain and the emotional brain: Specific brain activity associated with spontaneous fluctuations of intensity of chronic back pain. *Journal of Neuroscience, 26,* 12165–12173.

Baliki, M. N., Geha, P. Y., Apkarian, A. V., & Chialvo, D. R. (2008). Beyond feeling: Chronic pain hurts the brain, disrupting the default-mode network dynamics. *Journal of Neuroscience, 28,* 1398–1403.

Bansevicius, D., Westgaard, R. H., & Jensen, C. (1997). Mental stress of long duration: EMG activity, perceived tension, fatigue, and pain development in pain-free subjects. *Headache, 37,* 499–510.

Belliveau, J. W., Kennedy, D. N., Jr., McKinstry, R. C., Buchbinder, B. R., Weisskoff, R. M., Cohen, M. S., et al. (1991). Functional mapping of the human visual cortex by magnetic resonance imaging. *Science, 254,* 716–719.

Bingel, U., & Tracey, I. (2008). Imaging CNS modulation of pain in humans. *Physiology, 23,* 371–380.

Birklein, F., Riedl, B., Neundörfer, B., & Handwerker, H. O. (1998). Sympathetic vasoconstrictor reflex patterns in patients with complex regional pain syndrome. *Pain, 75,* 93–100.

Block, J. A., & Sequeira, W. (2001). Raynaud's phenomenon. *Lancet, 357,* 2042–2048.

...ssart, P., Fosnocht, D., & Swanson, E. (2007). Changes in heart rate do not correlate with changes in pain intensity in emergency department patients. *Journal of Emergency Medicine, 32,* 19–22.

Brandao, L. A., & Doningues, R. C. (2003). *MR spectroscopy of the brain.* Philadelphia: Lippincott Williams & Wilkins.

Bruehl, S., Lubenow, T. R., Nath, H., & Ivankovich, O. (1996). Validation of thermography in the diagnosis of reflex sympathetic dystrophy. *Clinical Journal of Pain, 12,* 316–325.

Bruehl, S., McCubbin, J. A., & Harden, R. N. (1999). Theoretical review: altered pain regulatory systems in chronic pain. *Neuroscience and Biobehavioral Reviews, 23,* 877–890.

Burns, J. (1997). Anger management style and hostility: Predicting symptom-specific physiological reactivity among chronic low back pain patients. *Journal of Behavioral Medicine, 20,* 505–522.

Cacioppo, J. T., Tassinary, L. G., & Berntson, G.

G. (Eds.). (2007). *Handbook of psychophysiology* (3rd ed.). Cambridge, UK: Cambridge University Press.

Carson, R. E., Daube-Witherspoon, M., & Herscovitch, P. (Eds.). (1998). *Quantitative functional brain imaging with positron emission tomography.* London: Academic Press.

Cassisi, J. E., Robinson, M. E., O'Conner, P., & MacMillan, M. (1999). Trunk strength and lumbar paraspinal muscle activity during isometric exercise in chronic low back pain patients and controls. *Spine, 18,* 245–251.

Cauda, F., Sacco, K., Duca, S., Cocito, D., D'Agata, F., Geminiani, G. C., et al. (2009). Altered resting state in diabetic neuropathic pain. *PLoS One, 4,* e4542.

Chapman, C. R., Casey, K. L., Dubner, R., Foley, K. M., Gracely, R. H., & Reading, A. E. (1985). Pain measurement: An overview. *Pain, 22,* 1–31.

Chapman, C. R., & Jacobson, R. C. (1984). Assessment of analgesic states: Can evoked potentials play a role? In B. Bromm (Ed.), *Pain measurement in man: Neurophysiological correlates of pain* (pp. 233–255). Amsterdam: Elsevier.

Christensen, L. V. (1986a). Physiology and pathophysiology of skeletal muscle contraction: Part 1. Dynamic activity. *Journal of Oral Rehabilitation, 13,* 451–461.

Christensen, L. V. (1986b). Physiology and pathophysiology of skeletal muscle contraction: Part 2. Static activity. *Journal of Oral Rehabilitation, 13,* 463–477.

Christmann, C., Koeppe, C., Braus, D. F., Ruf, M., & Flor, H. (2007). A simultaneous EEG-fMRI study of painful electric stimulation. *NeuroImage, 34,* 1428–1437.

Clark, G. T., Sakai, S., Merrill, R., Flack, V. F., McArthur, D., & McCreary, C. (1997). Waking and sleeping temporalis EMG levels in tension-type headache patients. *Journal of Orofacial Pain, 11,* 298–306.

Coles, M. G. H., Donchin, E., & Porges, S. W. (1986). *Psychophysiology: Systems, processes, and applications.* New York: Guilford Press.

Cram, J. R. (Ed.). (1990). *Clinical EMG surface recordings* (Vol. 2). Bothell, WA: Clinical Resources.

Cram, J. R., Lloyd, J., & Cahn, T. S. (1994). The reliability of EMG muscle scanning. *International Journal of Psychosomatics, 41,* 41–45.

Cram, J. R., & Steger, J. S. (1983). EMG scanning and the diagnosis of chronic pain. *Biofeedback and Self-Regulation, 8,* 229–242.

DeGood, D. E., Stewart, W. R., Adams, L. E., & Dale, J. A. (1994). Paraspinal EMG and autonomic reactivity of patients with back pain and controls to personally relevant stress. *Perceptual and Motor Skills, 79,* 1399–1409.

Diers, M., Koeppe, C., Diesch, E., Stolle, A. M., Hölzl, R., Schiltenwolf, M., et al. (2007). Central processing of acute muscle pain in chronic low back pain patients: An EEG mapping study. *Journal of Clinical Neurophysiology, 24,* 76–83.

Dolce, J. J., & Raczynski, J. M. (1985). Neuromuscular activity and electromyography in painful backs: Psychological and biomechanical models in assessment and treatment. *Psychological Bulletin, 97,* 502–520.

Dowman, R. (1996). Effects of operantly conditioning the amplitude of the P200 peak of the SEP on pain sensitivity and the spinal nociceptive withdrawal reflex in humans. *Psychophysiology, 33,* 252–261.

Dworkin, B. R., Elbert, T., Rau, H., Birbaumer, N., Pauli, P., Droste, C., et al. (1994). Central effects of baroreceptor activation in humans: Attenuation of skeletal reflexes and pain perception. *Proceedings of the National Academy of Sciences USA, 91,* 6329–6333.

Elbert T., Ray, W. J., Kowalik, Z. J., Skinner, J. E., Graf, K. E., & Birbaumer, N. (1994). Chaos and physiology: Deterministic chaos in excitable cell assemblies. *Physiological Reviews, 74,* 1–47.

English, R. J. (1996). *SPECT: Single-photon emission computed tomography: A primer.* Reston, VA: Society of Nuclear Medicine.

Eun, H. C. (1995). Evaluation of skin blood flow by laser Doppler flowmetry. *Clinical and Experimental Dermatology, 13,* 337–347.

Evers, S., Bauer, B., Grotemeyer, K. H., Kurlemann, G., & Husstedt, I. W. (1998). Event-related potentials (P300) in primary headache in childhood and adolescence. *Journal of Child Neurology, 13,* 322–326.

Feuerstein, M., Bortolussi, L., Houle, M., & Labbé, E. (1983). Stress, temporal artery activity, and pain in migraine headache: A prospective analysis. *Headache, 23,* 296–304.

Feuerstein, M., Bush, C., & Corbisiero, R. (1982). Stress and chronic headache: A psychophysiological analysis of mechanisms. *Journal of Psychosomatic Research, 26,* 167–182.

Feuerstein, M., Greenwald, M., Gamache, M. P., Papciak, A. S., & Cook, E. W. (1985). The Pain Behavior Scale: Modification and validation for outpatient use. *Journal of Psychopathology and Behavioral Assessment, 7,* 301–315.

Flor, H. (1991). *Psychobiologie des Schmerzes* [Psychobiology of pain]. Bern: Huber.

Flor, H., & Birbaumer, N. (1991). Comprehensive assessment and treatment of chronic back pain patients without physical disabilities. In M. Bond (Ed.), *Proceedings of the VIth World Congress on Pain* (pp. 229–234). Amsterdam: Elsevier.

Flor, H., & Birbaumer, N. (1993). Comparison of the efficacy of electromyographic biofeedback, cognitive-behavioral therapy, and conservative medical interventions in the treatment of chronic musculoskeletal pain. *Journal of Consulting and Clinical Psychology, 61,* 653–658.

Flor, H., Birbaumer, N., Schugens, M. M., & Lutzenberger, W. (1992). Symptom-specific psychophysiological responses in chronic pain patients. *Psychophysiology, 29,* 452–460.

Flor, H., Birbaumer, N., Schulte, W., & Roos, R. (1991). Stress-related EMG responses in chronic temporomandibular pain patients. *Pain, 46,* 125–142.

Flor, H., Birbaumer, N., & Turk, D. C. (1990). The psychobiology of chronic pain. *Advances in Behaviour Research and Therapy, 12,* 47–87.

Flor, H., Braun, C., Elbert, T., & Birbaumer, N. (1997). Extensive reorganization of primary somatosensory cortex in chronic back pain patients. *Neuroscience Letters, 224,* 5–8.

Flor, H., Diers, M., & Birbaumer, N. (2004). Peripheral and electrocortical responses to painful and non-painful stimulation in chronic pain patients, tension headache patients and healthy controls. *Neuroscience Letters, 361,* 147–150.

Flor, H., Fürst, M., & Birbaumer, N. (1999). Deficient discrimination of EMG levels and overestimation of perceived tension in chronic pain patients. *Applied Psychophysiology and Biofeedback, 24,* 55–66.

Flor, H., Schugens, M. M., & Birbaumer, N. (1992). Discrimination of muscle tension in chronic pain patients and healthy controls. *Biofeedback and Self-Regulation, 17,* 165–177.

Flor, H., & Turk, D. C. (1988). Chronic back pain and rheumatoid arthritis: Relationship of pain-related cognitions, pain severity, and pain behaviors. *Journal of Behavioral Medicine, 11,* 251–265.

Flor, H., & Turk, D. C. (1989). Psychophysiology of chronic pain: Do chronic pain patients exhibit symptom-specific psychophysiological responses? *Psychological Bulletin, 105,* 215–259.

Flor, H., & Turk, D. C. (2006). Cognitive and learning aspects. In S. McMahon & M. Koltzenburg (Eds.), *Wall and Melzack's textbook of pain* (5th ed., pp. 241–258). London: Elsevier.

Flor, H., & Turk, D. C. (in press). *A biobehavioral perspective of chronic pain and its management.* Seattle, WA: IASP Press.

Flor, H., Turk, D. C., & Birbaumer, N. (1985). Assessment of stress-related psychophysiological reactions in chronic back pain patients.

Journal of Consulting and Clinical Psychology, 53, 354–364.

Ford, R. G., & Ford, K. T. (1997). Thermography in the diagnosis of headache. *Seminars in Neurology, 17,* 343–349.

Fowles, D. (1986). The eccrine system and electrodermal activity. In M. G. H. Coles, E. Donchin, & S. W. Porges (Eds.), *Psychophysiology: Systems, processes, and applications* (pp. 51–96). New York: Guilford Press.

Freedman, R. R. (1991). Physiological mechanisms of temperature biofeedback. *Biofeedback and Self-Regulation, 16,* 95–115.

Freedman, R. R., & Ianni, P. (1983). Role of cold and emotional stress in Raynaud's disease and scleroderma. *British Medical Journal, 287,* 1499–1502.

Freedman, R. R., Ianni, P., & Wenig, P. (1983). Behavioral treatment of Raynaud's disease. *Journal of Consulting and Clinical Psychology, 51,* 539–549.

Friedman, M. S. (1994). The use of thermography in sympathetically maintained pain. *Iowa Orthopaedic Journal, 14,* 141–147.

Gatchel, R. J., Peng, Y. B., Peters, M. L., Fuchs, P. N., & Turk, D. C. (2007). The biopsychosocial approach to chronic pain: Scientific advances and future directions. *Psychological Bulletin, 133,* 581–624.

Geisser, M. E., Haig, A. J., Wallbom, A. S., & Wiggert, E. A. (2004). Pain-related fear, lumbar flexion, and dynamic EMG among persons with chronic musculoskeletal low back pain. *Clinical Journal of Pain, 20,* 61–69.

Geisser, M. E., Robinson, M. E., & Richardson, C. (1995). A time series analysis of the relationship between ambulatory EMG, pain, and stress in chronic low back pain. *Biofeedback and Self-Regulation, 20,* 339–355.

Giesecke, T., Gracely, R. H., Grant, M. A., Nachemson, A., Petzke, F., Williams, D. A., et al. (2004). Evidence of augmented central pain processing in idiopathic chronic low back pain. *Arthritis and Rheumatism, 50,* 613–623.

Glombiewski, J. A., Tersek, J., & Rief, W. (2008). Muscular reactivity and specificity in chronic back pain patients. *Psychosomatic Medicine, 70,* 125–131.

Gockel, M., Lindholm, H., Niemisto, L., & Hurri, H. (2008). Perceived disability but not pain is connected with autonomic nervous function among patients with chronic low back pain. *Journal of Rehabilitation Medicine, 40,* 355–358.

Graff-Radford, S. B., Ketelaer, M. C., Gratt, B. M., & Solberg, W. K. (1995). Thermographic assessment of neuropathic facial pain. *Journal of Orofacial Pain, 9,* 138–146.

Gramling, S. E., Grayson, R. L., Sullivan, T. N., & Schwartz, S. (1997). Schedule-induced masseter EMG in facial pain subjects versus no-pain controls. *Physiology and Behavior, 61*, 301–309.

Graven-Nielsen, T., & Arendt-Nielsen, L. (2008). Impact of clinical and experimental pain on muscle strength and activity. *Current Rheumatology Reports, 10*, 475–481.

Greicius, M. D., Krasnow, B., Reiss, A. L., & Menon, V. (2003). Functional connectivity in the resting brain: a network analysis of the default mode hypothesis. *Proceedings of the National Academy of Sciences USA, 100*, 253–258.

Gross, J., Schnitzler, A., Timmermann, L., & Ploner, M. (2007). Gamma oscillations in human primary somatosensory cortex reflect pain perception. *PLoS Biology, 5*, e133.

Hampf, G. (1990). Influence of cold pain in the hand on skin impedance, heart rate, and skin temperature. *Physiology and Behavior, 47*, 217–218.

Handwerker, H. O., & Kobal, G. (1993). Psychophysiology of experimentally induced pain. *Physiological Reviews, 73*, 639–671.

Hari, R., & Forss, N. (1999). Magnetoencephalography in the study of human somatosensory cortical processing. *Philosophical Transactions of the Royal Society London B: Biological Sciences, 354*, 1145–54.

Harle, D. E., Wolffsohn, J. S., & Evans B. J. (2005). The pupillary light reflex in migraine. *Ophthalmic and Physiological Optics, 25*, 240–245.

Harris, R. E., Sundgren, P. C., Pang, Y., Hsu, M., Petrou, M., Kim, S. H., et al. (2008). Dynamic levels of glutamate within the insula are associated with improvements in multiple pain domains in fibromyalgia. *Arthritis and Rheumatism, 58*, 903–907.

Hassett, A. L., Radvanski, D. C., Vaschillo, E. G., Vaschillo, B., Sigal, L. H., Karavidas, M. K., et al. (2007). A pilot study of the efficacy of heart rate variability (HRV) biofeedback in patients with fibromyalgia. *Applied Psychophysiology and Biofeedback, 32*, 1–10.

Hauck, M., Lorenz, J., & Engel, A. K. (2008). Role of synchronized oscillatory brain activity for human pain perception. *Reviews in the Neurosciences, 19*, 441–450.

Hermann, C., & Blanchard, E. B. (1998). Psychophysiological reactivity in pediatric migraine patients and healthy controls. *Journal of Psychosomatic Research, 44*, 229–240.

Hofbauer, R. K., Rainville, P., Duncan, G. H., & Bushnell, M. C. (2001). Cortical representation of the sensory dimension of pain. *Journal of Neurophysiology, 86*, 402–411.

Huettel, S. A., Song, A. W., & McCarthy, G. (Eds.). (2009). *Functional magnetic resonance imaging* (2nd ed.). New York: Palgrave Macmillan.

Jalovaara, P., Niikimaki, T., & Vanharanta, H. (1995). Pocket-size, portable EMG device in the differentiation of low back pain patients. *European Spine Journal, 4*, 210–212.

Jamner, L. D., & Tursky, B. (1987). Discrimination between intensity and affective pain descriptors: A psychophysiological evaluation. *Pain, 30*, 271–283.

Jennings, J. R., Maricq, H. R., Canner, J., Thompson, B., Freedman, R. R., Wise T., et al. (1999). A thermal vascular test for distinguishing between patients with Raynaud's phenomenon and healthy controls. Raynaud's Treatment Study Investigators. *Health Psychology, 18*, 421–426.

Jensen, R. (1999). Pathophysiological mechanisms of tension type headache: A review of epidemiological and experimental studies. *Cephalalgia, 19*, 602–621.

Karavidas, M. K., Tsai, P. S., Yucha, C., McGrady, A., & Lehrer, P. M. (2006). Thermal biofeedback for primary Raynaud's phenomenon: A review of the literature. *Applied Psychophysiology and Biofeedback, 31*, 203–216.

Kerns, R. D., Turk, D. C., & Rudy, T. E. (1985). The West Haven–Yale Multidimensional Pain Inventory (WHYMPI). *Pain, 23*, 345–356.

Kleinböhl, D., Hölzl, R., Moltner, A., Rommel, C., Weber, C., & Osswald, P. M. (1999). Psychophysical measures of sensitization to tonic heat discriminate chronic pain patients. *Pain, 81*, 35–43.

Kristeva-Feige, R., Grimm, C., Huppertz, H. J., Otte, M., Schreiber, A., Jager, D., et al. (1997). Reproducibility and validity of electric source localisation with high-resolution electroencephalography. *Electroencephalography and Clinical Neurophysiology, 103*, 652–660.

Kröner, B. (1984). Psychophysiologische Korrelate chronischer Kopfschmerzen. [Psychophysiological correlates of chronic headache]. *Zeitschrift für experimentelle und angewandte Psychologie, 31*, 610–639.

Larbig, W., Elbert, T., Rockstroh, B., Lutzenberger, W., & Birbaumer, N. (1985). Elevated blood pressure and reduction of pain sensitivity. In J. F. Orlebeke, G. Mulder, & L. J. P. van Doornen (Eds.), *Psychophysiology of cardiovascular control* (pp. 350–365). New York: Plenum Press.

Larivière, C., Arsenault, A. B., Gravel, D., Gagnon, D., Loisel, P., & Vadeboncoeur, R. (2002). Electromyographic assessment of back muscle weakness and muscle composition: Reliability and validity issues. *Archives of Physical Medicine and Rehabilitation, 83*, 1206–1214.

Leclaire, R., Esdaile, J. M., Hanley, J. A., Rossignol, M., & Bourdouxhe, M. (1996). Diagnostic accuracy of technologies used in low back pain assessment: Thermography, triaxial dynamometry, spinoscopy, and clinical examination. *Spine, 21*, 1325–1330.

Lehman, G. J. (2002). Clinical considerations in the use of surface electromyography: Three experimental studies. *Journal of Manipulative and Physiological Therapeutics, 25*, 293–299.

Light, K. C., Bragdon, E. E., Grewen, K. M., Brownley, K. A., Girdler, S. S., & Maixner, W. (2009). Adrenergic dysregulation and pain with and without beta-blockade in women with fibromyalgia and temporomandibular disorder. *Journal of Pain, 10*, 542–552.

Lorenz, J., & Garcia-Larréa, L. (2003). Contribution of attentional and cognitive factors to laser evoked brain potentials. *Journal of Clinical Neurophysiology, 33*, 293–301.

Lundberg, U., Dohns, I. E., Melin, B., Sandsjo, L., Palmerud, G., Kadefors, R., et al. (1999). Psychophysiological stress responses, muscle tension, and neck and shoulder pain among supermarket cashiers. *Journal of Occupational Health Psychology, 4*, 245–255.

Lundblad, I., Elert, J., & Gerdle, B. (1998). Worsening of neck and shoulder complaints in humans are correlated with frequency parameters of electromyogram recorded 1 year earlier. *European Journal of Applied Physiology, 79*, 7–16.

MacDonald, A. G., Land, D. V., & Sturrock, R. D. (1994). Microwave thermography as a noninvasive assessment of disease activity in inflammatory arthritis. *Clinical Rheumatology, 13*, 589–592.

Magnusson, M. L., Alkesiev, A., Wilder, D. G., Pope, M. H., Spratt, K., Lee, S. H., et al. (1996). Unexpected load and asymmetric posture as etiologic factors in low back pain. *European Spine Journal, 5*, 23–35.

Malmo, R. B., Shagass, C., & Davis, F. H. (1950). Symptom specificity and bodily reactions during psychiatric interview. *Psychosomatic Medicine, 12*, 362–372.

Mannion, A. F., Connolly, B., Wood, K., & Dolan, P. (1997). The use of surface EMG power spectral analysis in the evaluation of back muscle function. *Journal of Rehabilitation Research and Development, 34*, 427–439.

McMahon, S., & Koltzenburg, M. (Eds.). (2005). *Wall and Melzack's textbook of pain* (5th ed.). Edinburgh, UK: Churchill Livingstone.

Melzack, R. (1999). From the gate to the neuromatrix. *Pain Supplement, 6*, S121–S126.

Mense, S., & Hoheisel, U. (1999). New developments in the understanding of the pathophysiology of muscle pain. *Journal of Musculoskeletal Pain, 7*, 13–24.

Miller, D. J. (1995). Comparison of electromyographic activity in the lumbar paraspinal muscles of subjects with and without chronic low back pain. *Physical Therapy, 65*, 1347–1354.

Moltner, A., Hölzl, R., & Strian, F. (1990). Heart rate changes as an autonomic change measure of the pain response. *Pain, 43*, 81–89.

Mori, S. (2007). *Introduction to diffusion tensor imaging.* Oxford, UK: Elsevier Science.

Mulert, C., & Lemieux, L. (Eds.). (2009). *EEG–fMRI: Physiological basis, technique, and applications.* Berlin: Springer.

Nahm, F. S., Koo, M. S., Kim, Y. H., Suh J. H., Shin H. Y., Choi, Y. M., et al. (2007). Infrared thermography in the assessment of temporomandibular joint dysorder. *Korean Journal of Pain, 20*, 163–168.

Nestoriuc, Y., & Martin, A. (2007). Efficacy of biofeedback for migraine: A meta-analysis. *Pain, 128*, 111–127.

Niddam, D. M., & Hsieh, J. C. (2009). Neuroimaging of muscle pain in humans. *Journal of the Chinese Medical Association, 72*, 285–293.

Niedermeyer, E., & Lopes da Silva, F. (2004). *Electroencephalography: Basic principles, clinical applications, and related fields* (5th ed.). New York: Lippincott Williams & Wilkins.

Nowak, A., & Kacinski, M. (2009). Transcranial Doppler evaluation in migraineurs. *Polish Journal of Neurology and Neurosurgery, 43*, 162–172.

Obrist, P. A. (1976). The cardiovascular–behavioral interaction—as it appears today. *Psychophysiology, 13*, 95–107.

Oddson, L. I., Giphart, J. E., Buijs, R. J., Roy, S. H., Taylor, H. P., & De Luca, C. J. (1997). Development of new protocols and analysis procedures for the assessment of LBP by surface EMG techniques. *Journal of Rehabilitation Research and Development, 43*, 415–426.

Ohrbach, R., Blascovich, J., Gale, E. N., McCall, W. D., Jr., & Dworkin, S. F. (1998). Psychophysiological assessments of stress in chronic pain: Comparison of stressful stimuli and of response systems. *Journal of Dental Research, 77*, 1840–1850.

Peters, M., & Schmidt, A. J. (1991). Psychophysiological responses to repeated acute pain stimulation in chronic low back pain patients. *Journal of Psychosomatic Research, 35*, 59–74.

Petzke, F., & Clauw, D. J. (2000). Sympathetic nervous system function in fibromyalgia. *Current Rheumatology Reports, 2*, 116–123.

Ploner, M., Gross, J., Timmermann, L., Pollok, B., & Schnitzler, A. (2006). Pain suppresses spontaneous brain rhythms. *Cerebral Cortex, 16*, 537–540.

Porro, C. A., Cettolo, V., Francescato, M. P., & Baraldi, P. (2003). Functional activity mapping of the mesial hemispheric wall during anticipation of pain. *NeuroImage, 19*, 1738–1747.

Preissl, H. (Ed.). (2005). *Magnetoencephalography*. London: Academic Press.

Price, D. D. (2000). Psychological and neural mechanisms of the affective dimension of pain. *Science, 288,* 1769–1772.

Pritchard, D. W., & Wood, M. M. (1984). EMG levels in the occipito-frontalis muscles under an experimental stress condition. *Biofeedback and Self-Regulation, 8,* 165–175.

Raichle, M. E., MacLeod, A. M., Snyder, A. Z., Powers, W. J., Gusnard, D. A., & Shulman, G. L. (2001). A default mode of brain function. *Proceedings of the National Academy of Sciences USA, 98,* 676–682.

Rieke, K., Gallen, C. C., Baker, L., Dalessio, D. J., Schwartz, B. J., Torruella, A. K., et al. (1993). Transcranial Doppler ultrasound and magnetoencephalography in migraine. *Journal of Neuroimaging, 3,* 109–114.

Rojahn, J., & Gerhards, F. (1996). Subjective stress sensitivity and physiological responses to an aversive auditory stimulus in migraine and control subjects. *Journal of Behavioral Medicine, 9,* 203–212.

Roy, S. H., De Luca, C. J., Emley, M., Oddson, L. I., Buijs, R. J., Levins, J. A., et al. (1997). Classification of back muscle impairment based on the surface electromyographic signal. *Journal of Rehabilitation Research Development, 34,* 405–414.

Rudy, T. E., Boston, J. R., Lieber, S. J., Kubinski, J. A., & Delitto, A. (1995). Body motion patterns during a novel repetitive wheel-rotation task: A comparative study of healthy subjects and patients with low back pain. *Spine, 20,* 2547–2554.

Sanchez, B. M., Lesch, M., Brammer, D., Bove, S. E., Thiel, M., & Kilgore, K. S. (2008). Use of a portable thermal imaging unit as a rapid, quantitative method of evaluating inflammation and experimental arthritis. *Journal of Pharmacological and Toxicological Methods, 57,* 169–175.

Schwartz, M., & Andrasik, F. (2005). *Biofeedback: A practitioner's guide* (3rd ed.). New York: Guilford Press.

Schweinhardt, P., Lee, M., & Tracey, I. (2006). Imaging pain in patients: Is it meaningful? *Current Opinion in Neurology, 19,* 392–400.

Seifert, F., & Maihöfner, C. (2009). Central mechanisms of experimental and chronic neuropathic pain: Findings from functional imaging studies. *Cellular and Molecular Life Sciences, 66,* 375–390.

Sewards, T. V., & Sewards, M. A. (2002). The medial pain system: Neural representations of the motivational aspect of pain. *Brain Research Bulletin, 59,* 163–180.

Sherman, R., & Associates. (1997). *Phantom pain.* New York: Plenum Press.

Sherman, R. A., & Bruno, G. M. (1987). Concurrent variation of burning phantom limb and stump pain with near surface blood flow in the stump. *Orthopedics, 10,* 1395–1402.

Sherman, R. A., Griffin, V. D., Evans, C. B., & Grana, A. S. (1992). Temporal relationships between changes in phantom limb pain intensity and changes in surface electromyogram of the residual limb. *International Journal of Psychophysiology, 13,* 71–77.

Sherman, R. A., Woerman, A., & Karstetter, K. W. (1996). Comparative effectiveness of videothermography, contact thermography, and infrared beam thermography for scanning relative skin temperature. *Journal of Rehabilitation Research Development, 33,* 377–386.

Soderberg, G. L., & Knutson, L. M. (2000). A guide for use and interpretation of kinesiologic electromyographic data. *Physical Therapy, 80,* 485–498.

Sprenger, T., Henriksen, G., Valet, M., Platzer, S., Berthele, A., & Tolle, T. R. (2007). Positron emission tomography in pain research: From the structure to the activity of the opiate receptor system. *Schmerz, 21,* 503–513.

Sternbach, R. A. (1968). *Pain: A psychophysiological analysis.* New York: Academic Press.

Strøm, V., Knardahl, S., Stanghelle, J. K., & Røe, C. (2009). Pain induced by a single simulated office-work session: Time course and association with muscle blood flux and muscle activity. *European Journal of Pain, 13,* 843–852.

Svensson, P., Graven-Nielsen, T., Matre, D., & Arendt-Nielsen, L. (1998). Experimental muscle pain does not cause long-lasting increases in resting electromyographic activity. *Muscle and Nerve, 21,* 1382–1389.

Thieme, K., Rose, U., Pinkpank, T., Spies, C., Turk, D. C., & Flor, H. (2006). Psychophysiological responses in patients with fibromyalgia syndrome. *Journal of Psychosomatic Research, 61,* 671–679.

Thieme, K., & Turk, D. C. (2006). Heterogeneity of psychophysiological stress responses in fibromyalgia syndrome patients. *Arthritis Research and Therapy, 8*(1), R9.

Thunberg, J., Lyskov, E., Korotkov, A., Ljubisavljevic, M., Pakhomov, S., Katayeva, G., et al. (2005). Brain processing of tonic muscle pain induced by infusion of hypertonic saline. *European Journal of Pain, 9,* 185–194.

Tousignant-Laflamme, Y., Goffaux, P., Bourgault, P., & Marchand, S. (2006). Different autonomic responses to experimental pain in IBS patients and healthy controls. *Journal of Clinical Gastroenterology, 40,* 814–820.

Tracey, I. (2008). Imaging pain. *British Journal of Anaesthesia, 101,* 32–39.

Tracey, I., & Mantyh, P. W. (2007). The cerebral

signature for pain perception and its modulation. *Neuron, 55,* 377–391.

Traue, H. C., Kessler, M., & Cram, J. R. (1992). Surface EMG topography and pain distribution in pre-chronic back pain patients. *International Journal of Psychosomatics, 39,* 18–27.

Turk, D. C., & Flor, H. (1999) Chronic pain: A biobehavioral perspective. In R. J. Gatchel & D. C. Turk (Eds.), *Psychosocial factors in pain* (pp. 18–34*).* New York: Guilford Press.

Uematsu, S., Hendeler, N., & Hungerford, D. (1981). Thermography and electromyography in the differential diagnosis of chronic pain syndrome and reflex sympathetic dystrophy. *Electromyography and Clinical Neurophysiology, 21,* 165–182.

Vaiman, M., Eviatar, E., & Segal, S. (2004). Surface electromyographic studies of swallowing in normal subjects: A review of 440 adults: Report 2. Quantitative data: Amplitude measures. *Otolaryngology–Head and Neck Surgery, 131,* 773–780.

Valk, P. E., Dominique-Delbeke, D., & Bailey, D. L. (Eds.). (2006). *Positron emission tomography: Clinical practice.* Berlin: Springer.

van Boxtel, A. (2001). Optimal signal bandwidth for the recording of surface EMG activity of facial, jaw, oral, and neck muscles. *Psychophysiology, 38,* 22–34.

van Dieën, J. H., Selen, L. P., & Cholewicki, J. (2003). Trunk muscle activation in low-back pain patients, an analysis of the literature. *Journal of Electromyography and Kinesiology, 13,* 333–351.

Veiersted, K. B., Westgaard, R. H., & Andersen, P. (1993). Electromyographic evaluation of muscular work pattern as a predictor of trapezius myalgia. *Scandinavian Journal of Work and Environmental Health, 19,* 284–290.

Villringer, A. (1997). Understanding functional neuroimaging methods based on neurovascular coupling. *Advances in Experimental Medicine and Biology, 413,* 177–193.

Vincent, J. L., Patel, G. H., Fox, M. D., Snyder, A. Z., Baker, J. T., Van Essen, D. C., et al. (2007). Intrinsic functional architecture in the anaesthetized monkey brain. *Nature, 447,* 83–85.

Vlaeyen, J. W., Seelen, H. A., Peters, M., de Jong, P., Arntz, E., Beisiegel, E., et al. (1999). Fear of movement/(re)injury and muscular reactivity in chronic low back pain patients: An experimental investigation. *Pain, 82,* 297–304.

Walitt, B., Roebuck-Spencer, T., Esposito, G., Atkins, F., Bleiberg, J., Foster, G., et al. (2007). The effects of multidisciplinary therapy on positron emission tomography of the brain in fibromyalgia: A pilot study. *Rheumatology International, 27,* 1019–1024.

Wallace, L. M. (1984). Psychological preparation as a method of reducing the stress of surgery. *Journal of Human Stress, 10,* 62–77.

Wigley, F. M. (2002). Clinical practice: Raynaud's phenomenon. *New England Journal of Medicine, 347,* 1001–1008.

Williams, D. A., & Gracely, R. H. (2006). Biology and therapy of fibromyalgia: Functional magnetic resonance imaging findings in fibromyalgia. *Arthritis Research and Therapy, 8,* 224.

Wolf, S. L., & Basmajian, J. V. (1978). Assessment of paraspinal electromyographic activity in normal subjects and in chronic back pain patients using a muscle biofeedback device. In E. Asmussen & K. Jorgenson (Eds.), *Biomechanics: VI. Proceedings of the Sixth International Congress of Biomechanics* (pp. 315–324). Baltimore: University Park Press.

Wolf, S. L., Wolf, L. B., & Segal, R. L. (1989). The relationship of extraneous movements to lumbar paraspinal muscle activity: Implications for EMG biofeedback training applications to low back pain patients. *Biofeedback and Self-Regulation, 14,* 63–73.

Zubieta, J.-K., & Stohler, C. S. (2009). Neurobiological mechanisms of placebo responses. *Annals of the New York Academy of Sciences, 1156,* 198–210.

CHAPTER 9

Quantification of Function in Chronic Low Back Pain

PETER B. POLATIN
WHITNEY E. WORZER
EMILY BREDE
ROBERT J. GATCHEL

Chronic low back pain (CLBP) is the leading cause of disability among persons under the age of 45, and the third leading cause of disability in persons over the age of 45 (Gatchel, Polatin, et al., 1995), making it "the most expensive benign condition in America" (Mayer, Gatchel, et al., 1987, p. 1763; Woods, Kishino, et al., 2000). It is estimated that as many as 85% of people in industrialized countries will experience low back pain at some point in their lives (Andersson, 1999; Deyo, Cherkin, et al., 1991; Gatchel, 2004). The majority of such cases resolve within 3 months. However, for 2–7% of people, the condition will become chronic (Andersson, 1997). Patients with CLBP (those whose symptoms persist beyond 3 months) account for the largest expenditures in health care costs and have the poorest prognosis (Gatchel & Okifuji, 2006; Mayer & Gatchel, 1988). The National Center for Health Statistics (*www. cdc.gov/nchs/data/hus06_SpecialExcerpt. pdf*, 2006) reported low back related costs, including direct (co-pays, medications, etc.) and indirect costs (i.e., lost productivity and litigation) totaling between $50 billion and $100 billion each year. In fact, in the most recent survey of expenditures among adults

with back and neck problems, Martin and colleagues (2008) reported a 65% increase (adjusted for inflation) of expenditures from 1997 to 2005, which is a more rapid increase than overall health expenditures!

While surgery can be an option for some, little evidence supports patients with a low back episode actually benefiting from a surgical intervention (Glenn, 2002; Mayer, 2000; Mayer, Gatchel, et al., 1987). This places the treatment of CLBP primarily in the scope of conservative managed care, with programs aimed at helping patients experience less pain and disability, which in turn decrease losses in productivity, work absences, and health care–related costs. Programs that include interdisciplinary functional restoration are often recommended (Gatchel, Mayer, et al., 2006; Mayer & Gatchel, 1988). These programs provide initial assessments, such as a quantified functional evaluation (QFE), that measure physical capabilities of the lumbar spine and provide interdisciplinary treatment interventions, such as physical therapy, occupational therapy, psychosocial assessments and counseling, and assistance with work-related factors and education on health-related issues (Mayer & Polatin, 2000). Previous research has established the utility of measures that quantify lumbar function. Identifying deficits in function has proven to be predictive of, and associated with, disability and treatment outcomes. In studies that focus on reporting evidence-based outcomes, objective guidelines are not only especially important during assessment but they also aid in treatment and therapeutic goal setting (Flores, Gatchel, et al., 1997; Pransky, Shaw, et al., 2004; Proctor, Mayer, et al., 2005; Shaw, Means-Christensen, et al., 2007; Williams, 1998). Before further discussion of issues of disability, it is helpful to understand the meaning of disability for those suffering with pain. Stanos, McLean, and colleagues (2007) appropriately point out that the term *disability* can be better understood when considered in juxtaposition to similar concepts, such as impairment and handicap. The concept of disability is actually rooted in a pain patient's *impairment* (which refers to a deleterious change in either psychosocial or physical capacity associated with a pain condition). Thus, disability represents changes in the pain sufferer's ability to complete activities of daily living and tasks necessary to contribute to home, work, and recreation based on his or her impairment. *Handicap* is a broader concept used to describe the disruption of the pain sufferer's ability to fulfill his or her societal role due to disability-related obstacles in functional activity.

REASONS TO QUANTIFY FUNCTION

In documentation of pain and human suffering, the individual's subjective perception of pain has been used as a primary indicator. However, the inherently subjective nature of pain perception is influenced by many factors and although a strong correlation exists between measures of physical pain and treatment outcomes (Anagnostis, Mayer, et al., 2003; Beals, 1984; Becker, Sjogren, et al., 2000; Gatchel, Mayer, et al., 2006; McGeary, Mayer, et al., 2006; Sullivan, Feuerstein, et al., 2005), actual quantification of individual human perceptions has proven to be an elusive task. Individuals with similar physical injuries can have vastly different perceptions of pain, which reinforces the need for an objective way to quantify function. While standard self-report

measures of pain are clinically useful, they do not provide an objective assessment, and they limit the types of comparisons that can be made.

Disability often arises as a result of chronic pain and can be most easily defined in a behavioral context. When assessed in socio-economic terms, *decreased productivity* is used to measure disability and accounts for major societal losses (Gatchel, Mayer, et al., 1986; Levenstein & Kaplan, 1998). *Impairment in performance of functional tasks* defines the physical aspects of disability. Whereas psychosocial symptoms including depression, anxiety, somatization, and alcohol/drug abuse often accompany chronic pain, these symptoms by themselves also account for significant disability (Dersh, Mayer, et al., 2007; Fishbain, Cutler, et al., 1997; Kinney, Gatchel, et al., 1993; Polatin, Kinney, et al., 1993; Rush, Polatin, et al., 2000). Defining disability in legal terms involves *financial compensation* claims, which attempt to place blame for an injury that allegedly resulted in loss of the ability to work. Use of *physical function* to define disability is far less subjective than self-report and can be advantageous as long as certain criteria are met. Performance measures that address disability in a vocational context, as it relates to work, appeal to agencies involved in defining and treating disability.

CRITERIA FOR QUANTIFICATION TESTING

Certain requirements must be met when quantifying physical functioning (Gatchel, Polatin, et al., 1998; King, Tuckwell, et al., 1998; Mayer, Barnes, et al., 1988; Polatin, Gatchel, et al., 1989). Meaningful clinical interpretations can be made only when tests measuring physical functioning are relevant, valid, reproducible, reliable, capable of identifying suboptimal effort, and have a normative database. For a measure to have *physiological relevance*, a specific and defined capacity must be assessed, without reflecting additional unrelated information. For example, using a whole-body lifting task to assess a specific muscle group would not be a physiologically relevant task. Additionally, devices used to measure human performance must be accurate in their measurement to be *valid*. Precise measurement of clinical variables must be *reproducible* by the same tester (intratester reliability) and by different testers (intertester reliability). It is possible to have a valid test that lacks reproducibility, or to have a test that is reproducible but invalid.

It should also be kept in mind, as noted by Gatchel (2006), that a physical function measure is always more objective than a self-report or psychosocial measure:

No matter what the level of accuracy or sophistication of a mechanical device used in collecting physiologic measures, it's always the case that human interpretation ultimately must be used in the understanding of the resulting findings. In addition, it must be remembered that a patient's performance during a physical assessment protocol can be greatly influenced by fear of pain or injury, motivation, instructional set, etc. . . . (p. vi)

Validity of a test is paramount, because it is possible to address issues of reproducibility by adjusting the testing protocol. Once a functional measure of human performance meets these criteria, it is still necessary to have a way to identify suboptimal effort. Fear–avoidance, secondary gain, emotional distress, and other psychological factors can interfere with accurate assessment of function (Leeman, Polatin, et al., 2000; Rainville, Sobel, et al., 1997). Therefore, it is essential for each test of function to have a means to assess effort objectively. Finally, to make clinically meaningful interpretations, normative data are necessary. Access to a large, relevant *normative database* allows for extraction of meaningful information related to specific variables, such as age, gender, occupation, and type of injury (Keeley, 1997). Problems with obtaining large, normative databases have increased as technological advances have provided an abundance of new devices and variations in testing protocol. Therefore, clinicians must remain diligent in their efforts to provide relevant treatment while they collect normative data.

TESTS OF FUNCTIONAL CAPACITY IN THE LUMBAR SPINE

A comprehensive review of the various tests may be found in Gatchel (2006).

At the onset, it should be pointed out that assessing lumbar function clearly cannot be accomplished with any single test or measure of performance. However, combining individual physical evaluations provides valuable objective information regarding functional capacity (Flores, Gatchel, et al., 1997). See Table 9.1 for a summary of the functions to be measured, tests to be used, and appropriate references. Assessing *range of motion* provides information on the function of intervertebral discs and facet joints. *Surface electromyography* (SEMG) has become more widely used as an assessment of lumbar function, because it provides an objective means for quantification of muscle activity and fatigability (Arokoski, Airaksinen, et al., 2001). *Trunk strength* can be measured in a variety of ways, using devices that range in expense and sophistication. Multiple muscle groups are involved in trunk strength and function together to move the lumbar spine in various ways (abduction–adduction, flexion–extension, and rotation). Due to the involvement of the intrinsics (erector spinae, multifidus, quadratus lumborum, psoas, and deep interspinalis and intertransversales) and extrinsics (abdominals, gluteals, latissimus dorsi, and posterior thigh muscles), specific measures of trunk strength require the lumbopelvic unit to be isolated. Measurement of *lifting capacity* usually involves performance tasks and does not isolate the trunk. Lifting tests can provide information about maximum capacity, as well as endurance, based on the frequency with which lifting may be required. General physical condition is frequently assessed by measuring *aerobic capacity*. This provides an overall estimation of cardiovascular endurance and indicates the level of activity in which the body is able to participate. *Work capacity* tests do not specifically assess a particular lumbar function; rather, they address functional tasks related to job demands and include tasks such as bending, stooping, and crawling.

Range of Motion

A variety of techniques have been used in the past to assess lumbar range of motion (ROM), but many do not meet the criteria for quantification testing that we previously addressed. For example, the traditional "fin-

TABLE 9.1. Quantification of Lumbar Function

	Test	References
Range of motion (ROM)	• Dual inclinometry • AOMS (alteration of motion segment integrity)	• Nitschke, Nattrass, et al. (1999) • Mayer, Gatchel, et al. (1985) • Rondinelli, Genovese, et al. (2008)
Surface electromyography (SEMG)		• Ambroz, Scott, et al. (2000) • Donaldson, Donaldson, et al. (2003) • Watson, Booker, et al. (2007) • Geisser, Ranavauya, et al. (2005) • Pullman, Goodin, et al. (2000)
Trunk strength	• Isokinetic • Isoinertial • Isometric	• Newton & Waddell (1993) • Newton, Thow, et al. (1993) • Rissanen, Alaranta, et al. (1994)
Lifting capacity	• Isometric • Isokinetic • Progressive Isonertial Lifting Evaluation (PILE) • EPIC Lift Capacity Test	• National Institute for Occupational Sagety and Health (1983) • Hazard, Reeves, et al. (1992) • Kishino, Mayer, et al. (1985) • Mayer, Mooney, et al. (1991) • Mayer, Gatchel, et al. (1990) • Jay, Lamb, et al. (2000)
Aerobic capacity	• Submaximal treadmill, bicycle, or upper body ergometer	• Noonan & Dean (2000) • Hodselmans, Dijkstra, et al. (2008) • Cooper & Storer (2004)
Functional (work) capacity	• Functional capacity evaluations (FCEs)	• Vasudevan (1996) • Strong (2002) • Tuckwell, Straker, et al. (2002) • Rudy, Lieber, et al. (2003)

gertip to floor" technique does not account for the involvement of the hips, nor does it contain any assessment of effort. Currently, spinal ROM is most commonly measured with the *dual inclinometer technique*. The inclinometer measures angle, using either a fluid filled disc or a gravity sensor. Measurements are taken of the gross degree of flexion and the degree of hip/pelvic flexion, which is subtracted from the gross flexion to obtain the true lumbar flexion.

The first inclinometer is applied at the convex surface of the sacrum, parallel to the spine. The second inclinometer is applied over the T12–L1 spinous process, aligned in the sagittal plane. Both inclinometers are "zeroed," with the patient in a standing position. The patient is then asked to perform several movements: flexion (bend forward as far as you can); extension (bend backward as far as you can); lateral flexion (bend to the left or right side as far as you can); and rotation (turn to the left or right side as far as you can). Measurements are taken from

both inclinometers (Nitschke, Nattrass, et al., 1999). The first inclinometer gives the hip/pelvic flexion reading, and the second gives the gross flexion reading. Effort at the task can be assessed using a straight leg raising (SLR) test. With the patient supine, with both knees extended, the inclinometer is placed at the tibial spine. The patient is instructed to raise one leg in an extended position, stretching the hamstring. Once maximal stretch of the hamstring is achieved, the pelvis will flex until restrained by the hyperextension of the contralateral hip. SLR should closely correspond to hip flexion. Thus, if the tightest SLR exceeds total hip motion by more than 10 degrees, the patient has given suboptimal effort.

Although this technique has been shown to have adequate reliability and validity (Mayer, Gatchel, et al., 1985), the sixth edition of the American Medical Association's *Guides to the Evaluation of Permanent Impairment* (Rondinelli, Genovese, et al., 2008) no longer recommends this approach. Instead, an evaluation of alteration of motion segment integrity (AOMSI) under radiography is recommended, using a flexion–extension protocol. At levels L1–L5, a translation measurement of greater than 8 degrees anterior, or 9 degrees posterior, relative to the adjacent vertebrae on flexion or extension meets the criteria for AOMSI. At levels L5–S1, a translation measurement of greater than 6 degrees anterior, or 9 degrees posterior, on flexion or extension is required. AOMSI can also be diagnosed in the lumbosacral spine using angular motion. To meet the criteria for AMOSI, angular motion must exceed 15 degrees at L1–L2, L2–L3, or L4–L5, or 20 degrees at L4–L5, or 25 degrees at L5–S1, when compared with the angular motion at the adjacent level.

Surface Electromyography

The use of SEMG to evaluate CLBP has been met with considerable controversy. Unlike traditional EMG, in which needles are inserted into muscles to measure their electrical activity directly, SEMG involves the placement of electrodes on the skin that measure the sum of the action potentials generated by the group of muscles underlying the electrode (Ambroz, Scott, et al., 2000). Several abnormal findings have been hypothesized to be associated with CLBP. Researchers have examined resting muscle tension, asymmetry between left- and right-side muscle groups, delayed return of muscle activity to baseline, poor coordination between back and abdominal muscles, and the absence of the flexion–relaxation phenomenon (where paraspinal muscles relax at full forward flexion).

There are three main types of SEMG evaluations for CLPB (Donaldson, Donaldson, et al., 2003). The first is *static measurement*, in which activity of the paraspinal muscles is measured at rest, usually with the patient in either a sitting or standing posture. The second is *dynamic measurement*, in which muscle activity is measured during motion. This can involve isometric contraction of the muscles, either at maximal or submaximal intensity, or it can involve measurement of muscle activity during movements, such as stretches. The third approach combines static and dynamic measurement. An example of this is the measurement of the flexion–

relaxation phenomenon. Measurements are taken with the patient at rest in the standing position, during the motion of forward flexion, at rest during full flexion, and during the motion of reextension. These measurements are combined into ratios to determine the presence or absence of flexion–relaxation (Watson, Booker, et al., 1997).

Attempts to differentiate patients with low back pain from normal healthy subjects on the basis of SEMG have been inconsistent. A meta-analysis (Geisser, Ranavauya, et al., 2005) that included 44 studies on CLBP and SEMG concluded that measurements of static SEMG varied widely. Whereas some studies found increased muscle activity in CLBP patients, others found decreased muscle activity, or no difference from healthy subjects. Examination of SEMG during isometric contraction and muscle recovery were likewise inconsistent. The meta-analysis did find good support for the use of flexion–relaxation to differentiate CLBP patients from healthy subjects, with 76% accuracy.

The usefulness of SEMG data is highly dependent on the skill of the examiner. Electrodes must be placed correctly according to anatomical landmarks, and incoming raw data must be correctly filtered, smoothed, and interpreted. Although some clinicians find the addition of SEMG useful in the assessment of patients with low back pain, it has not been widely accepted, and the American Academy of Neurology does not recommend SEMG as a clinical tool in the evaluation of patients with low back pain (Pullman, Goodin, et al., 2000).

Trunk Strength

Isokinetic and isoinertial machines provide a rather sophisticated quantifiable measurement of trunk strength. However, to use these devices properly requires training, and they have limitations in terms of the quantity of normative data available for each individual new device (Newton & Waddell, 1993). *Trunk dynamometers* measure isometric and concentric strength, as well as muscular endurance of the extensors and flexors of the lumbar and thoracic spine. Lumbopelvic isolation is necessary to generate valid and reliable data (Newton, Thow, et al., 1993; Newton & Waddell, 1993). Accurate measures of torque can be gained with isokenetic devices, although they are not "true to life." The most well-established technique for measuring trunk strength is *isometric*, which measures the maximum force that a muscle, or group of muscles, can generate in contraction. However, it lacks dynamic measurement capability and also has an added risk for muscle strain when truly maximal effort is used. The derivations of average points curve (APC), maximum points curve, best work repetition curve, and power numbers can be generated by measuring trunk flexion, extension, and right and left torso rotation–peak torque (Rissanen, Alaranta, et al., 1994). When identical testing conditions are used on three separate tests, assessment of the effort given can be generated by a computer that analyzes discrepancies among the same points on three test curves and provides the *average-points variance* (AVP) (Newton, Thow, et al., 1993). For example, when using a Cybex Isokinetic TEF (torso extension–flexion) and torso rotation device, an AVP greater than 20 degrees indicates suboptimal effort. As previously discussed, EMG has also recently become an important quantifiable measure of strength of individual trunk muscles.

Lifting Capacity

Lifting capacity is considered to be a "whole-body activity," and devices that assess this function provide additional information related to strength but do not isolate individual trunk muscles. However, to provide precise and reproducible measures, restrictions on variables such as acceleration or position exist in isometric and isokinetic lifting tests. The National Institute for Occupational Safety and Health (NIOSH) standardizes the isometric devices they use in lift procedures by requiring patients to pull a bar from a predetermined height from a number of positions (i.e., straight back, bent knee, straight knee, bent back). More dynamic lifting is measured with isokinetic devices, because a greater variety of body positions and lifting styles is possible when a lifting handle is on a cable attached to a dynamometer. When the force exerted (along the cable and in line with the dynamometer) is recorded after speed and acceleration are controlled, then peak force, shape curve, work performed, and power consumed are derived; AVP can

also be calculated as an effort assessment (Hazard, Reeves, et al., 1992). As previously explained, it remains necessary to have normative databases when using these devices. For example, the Cybex Liftask utilizes a three-speed (18 in/sec, 30 in/sec, and 36 in/sec) testing protocol (Kishino, Mayer, et al., 1985), and a normative database continues to expand to include different job categories and comparative norms (Mayer, Mooney, et al., 1991).

Additional tests that more directly address task performance and neuromuscular coordination do not place restrictions on activity. The Progressive Isoinertial Lifting Evaluation (PILE) and the EPIC Lift Capacity Test (Employment Potential Improvement Corp., Santa Ana, CA) are examples of such functional dynamic evaluation tools (Jay, Lamb, et al., 2000; Mayer, Gatchel, et al., 1990). These tests use standardized protocols that involve lifting increases in load increments from various heights. The protocol for the PILE involves lifting a receptacle filled with varying amounts of weights from floor to waist and from waist to shoulder height. Weight increases incrementally at specific rates, and the patient remains "blind" to the actual amount of weight being lifted. The test has three ways in which it can end, and termination of the tests occurs when any of the three are first achieved. The endpoints are (1) psychophysical (fatigue or pain), (2) aerobic (reaching 85% of age determined maximum heart rate), or (3) safety (predetermined safe limits of 45–55% of body weight).

Results reveal maximum weight lifted, as well as endurance, and since distance and repetition are known, work and power consumption can be calculated and may be normalized to body weight. Normative databases exist for this test, and an assessment of effort is made by comparing target heart rate with final heart rate, measured at the completion of the test. This is a useful measure that can be directly related to job requirements, because it provides an objective measure of frequent lifting capacity.

Aerobic Capacity

Aerobic capacity is measured during the assessment of low back pain to determine the degree of total body deconditioning as a result of disability. Patients with chronic pain are prone to inactivity due to pain symptoms and fear–avoidance (Hodselmans, Dijkstra, et al., 2008). This leads to decreased physical fitness and cardiovascular endurance over time (Protas, Mayer, et al., 2004). Most rehabilitation programs include some type of aerobic conditioning, and initial fitness levels must be assessed to prescribe an appropriate treatment regimen.

Although a direct measurement of aerobic capacity obtained though maximal exercise testing is most accurate, this type of testing poses cardiovascular risk to the deconditioned patient, and it requires close supervision by medical professionals (Cooper & Storer, 2004). Maximal exercise testing is also highly dependent on patient effort to obtain accurate results, and is often poorly tolerated by deconditioned patients. Thus, submaximal testing is more often used in the rehabilitation setting. Most submaximal test results can be converted into an estimate of maximal aerobic capacity using either formulas or nomograms (Noonan & Dean, 2000). Reliable and valid protocols have been developed for treadmills, bicycle ergometers, and upper body ergometers. Most patients with back pain find the bicycle ergometer the most tolerable.

Testing with either the bicycle or upper body ergometer begins with a warm-up phase. Then, the workload and speed are increased at predetermined intervals depending on the physical condition of the patient. If the patient is extremely deconditioned, workload increases may be adjusted for lean body mass (Hodselmans, Dijkstra, et al., 2008). The test concludes when the target heart rate (85% of age-related maximum) is reached. Maximum oxygen consumption can be estimated using final heart rate and workload (Noonan & Dean, 2000). Time to complete the test is also noted; a total test time of 8–12 minutes has been shown to be ideal (Cooper & Storer, 2004).

Functional Capacity

Work capacity is less directly related to low back pain. However, the measurement of functional tasks is frequently used when assessing work-related back pain (Feuerstein & Zastowny, 1996). Functional capacity evaluations (FCEs) attempt to measure the ability to perform the physical demands required on the job in a systematic and comprehensive manner (Strong, 2002; Tuckwell, Straker, et al., 2002; Vasudevan, 1996). FCEs typically focus on the performance of job demands listed in the *Dictionary of Occupational Titles* (DOT), including activities such as sitting, standing, walking, carrying, pushing, pulling, kneeling, and stooping. FCEs have become widely used by many agencies, including workers' compensation authorities, insurance companies, welfare systems, government entities (e.g., the Occupational Safety and Health Administration and the Social Security Administration), as well as other regulator agencies interesting in determining precise levels of disability (Harten, 1998; Innes & Straker, 2002). The most common application of FCEs is to determine an injured worker's ability to return to work, and although evaluations are based primarily on assessing impairment of physical abilities, psychosocial factors have been proven to greatly influence performance (Rudy, Lieber, et al., 2003). Many different types of FCEs exist and have been beneficial in assessing limitation in function as it relates to work demands. FCEs typically contain components and questionnaires to assess psychosocial factors, such as fear of pain, but still have limitations, and the specific battery of tests and testing protocols can vary between different FCEs. Ideally, a single, standardized battery of tests would be used to assess all functional capacity. However, due to various dynamics, this has not been achieved.

INTERNATIONAL CLASSIFICATION OF FUNCTIONING

There has been a desire to obtain a single, standardized model for assessing function that would allow for consistency in measuring and reporting health components involved in functioning and disability. Due to the variability in evaluations, there has not been a way to compare disability information in a global manner. In response to this, the World Health Organization (WHO) created a new paradigm at the World Health Assembly on May 22, 2001, when it approved the International Classification of Functioning, Disability and Health (ICF; WHO, 2001). The ICF does not specifically measure disability; rather, it classifies functional abilities in various domains. The ICF contains components of body functions and structures, activities, and participation. Functioning and disability are assessed in the context of environmental and personal factors, taking into account the social aspects of disability. Individual abilities and limitations are viewed as interactive and dynamic rather than linear or static, and emphasis is placed on function rather than on condition or disease (Wind, Gouttebarge, et al., 2005). The framework of this classification system measures health and disability at individual levels, as well as population levels, and recognizes that disability can impact anyone. All health conditions are viewed in the same context, which allows use of a common metric when comparing health and disability. ICF *activities* are defined as the actions people accomplish without assistance or barriers, and they range from basic to complex. Activities include basic actions, such as dressing, eating, and bathing, or more complex actions, including work, school, and civic activities. *Participation* refers to functioning and accounts for the impact of barriers in the environment (WHO, 2001).

The ICF-specific classification for activities and participation includes learning and applying knowledge, general tasks and demands, communication, movement, self-care, domestic life areas, interpersonal interactions, major life areas, and community and social/civic life. Empirical evidence supports a distinction between activity and participation dimensions within the ICF, measuring factors of mobility activities, daily activities, and social life/participation (Jette, Haley, et al., 2003).

The ICF was developed to aid in providing a scientific basis for assessing the impact of health conditions. It also establishes the capability to communicate and compare data between countries and health care disciplines. However, it should be noted that a recent Delphi Survey Study by Soer, van der Schans, Groothoff, Geertzen, and Reneman (2008) revealed that experts around the world agree on using the IFC as a conceptual framework for FCE, as well as the terms defined in the IFC. However, "no consensus was reached on the term FCE itself. Even though consensus was reached on the different terms that comprise FCS, no con-

sensus was reached for one single definition of FCE" (p. 394). They go on to indicate the two definitions with the highest points scored (p. 395):

- An FCE is an evaluation designed to document and describe a person's current safe work ability from a physical ability and motivational perspective, with consideration given to any existing medical impairment and/or syndromes. (38% agreement)
- An FCE is an evaluation of capacity of activities used to make recommendations for participation in work, while considering the person's body functions and structures, environmental factors, personal factors, and health status. (63% agreement)

As can be seen, in both definitions, multiple biopsychosocial variables (personal, body functioning, environmental, etc.) need to be taken into account. This is no easy task, as we discuss in the next section. Nevertheless, for the time being, Soer, van der Schans, and colleagues (2008) appropriately recommended that "authors define definitions they use in future research in order to permit comparison of data and serve as the use of a common language" (p. 395).

SUMMARY AND CONCLUSIONS

The biopsychosocial model is now viewed as the most heuristic approach in the assessment and treatment of chronic pain disorders such as CLBP (Gatchel, 2005; Gatchel & Bruga, 2005; Turk & Monarch, 2002). As such, three broad categories of measures—physical, psychological, and socioeconomic—all have been used to assess patients with CLBP. However, these three major measurement categories (or biopsychosocial referents) may not always display high concordance with one another when measuring a construct such as CLBP or disability (e.g., Gatchel, 2006). Indeed as Flores, Gatchel, and colleagues (1997) noted:

Such less-than-perfect concordance among these behavioral referents of a construct . . . is not unique to the area of spinal disorders or rehabilitation medicine in general. It has long been noted in the psychological literature, for example, that self-report, overt behavior and physiological indices of behavior sometimes show how correlations among one another. Therefore, if one uses a self-report measure as a primary index of a construct and compares it to the overt behavioral or physiological index for the same construct, direct overlap cannot automatically be expected. In addition, two different self-report indices or physiological indices of the same constructs may not be as highly correlated as one would desire. What has plagued the evaluation arena in general has been the lack of agreement in the wide variation of measures used to document a construct such as pain and disability, as well as changes in that construct. Therefore, the literature is replete with many different measurement techniques and tests of a construct such as function. (pp. v–vi)

Now, 30 years later, this quotation still rings true, even though the literature is beginning to demonstrate that some measures are more reliable and valid than others (Gatchel, 2006). In terms of quantification of function in patients with chronic pain, one must be aware that there is no totally valid "gold standard" measure of it. Clinicians/researchers must be mindful of clearly defining operationally how they are measuring function, as well as using the most reliable measurement devices. Because a device is mechanical does not automatically rule out psychosocial factors (fear–avoidance, patient motivation, etc.) that may affect final performance. Again, a more comprehensive biopsychosocial approach needs to be employed, in which physical function is just one component of the overall evaluation process (Gatchel, 2006).

REFERENCES

Ambroz, C., Scott, A., et al. (2000). Chronic low back pain assessment using surface electromyography. *Journal of Occupational and Environmental Medicine, 42*(6), 660–669.

Anagnostis, C., Mayer, T. G., et al. (2003). The Million Visual Analog Scale: Its utility for predicting tertiary rehabilitation outcomes. *Spine, 28,* 1–10.

Andersson, G. B. J. (1997). The epidemiology of spinal disorders. In J. W. Frymoyer (Ed.), *The adult spine: Principles and practice* (pp. 93–133). New York: Raven Press.

Andersson, G. B. J. (1999). Epidemiological features of chronic low back pain. *Lancet, 354,* 581–585.

Arokoski, J. P., Airaksinen, V. T., et al. (2001). Back and abdominal muscle function during stabilization exercises. *Archives of Physical Medicine and Rehabilitation, 82,* 1089–1098.

Beals, R. (1984). Compensation and recovery from injury. *Western Journal of Medicine, 140,* 233–237.

Becker, N., Sjogren, P., et al. (2000). Treatment outcome of chronic non-malignant pain patients managed in a Danish multidisciplinary pain centre compared to general practice: A randomised controlled trial. *Pain, 84*(2–3), 203–211.

Cooper, C. B., & Storer, T.W. (2004). *Exercise testing and interpretation: A practical approach.* Cambridge, UK: Cambridge University Press.

Dersh, J., Mayer, T., et al. (2007). Do psychiatric disorders affect functional restoration outcomes in chronic disabling occupational spinal disorders? *Spine, 32,* 1045–1051.

Deyo, R. A., Cherkin, D., et al. (1991). Cost, controversy, crisis: Low back pain and the health of the public. *Annual Review of Public Health, 12,* 141–156.

Donaldson, S., Donaldson, M. S., et al. (2003). SEMG evaluations: An overview. *Applied Psychophysiology and Biofeedback, 28*(2), 121–127.

Feuerstein, M., & Zastowny, T. R. (1996). Occupational rehabilitation: Multidisciplinary management of work related musculoskeletal pain and disability. In R. J. Gatchel & D. C. Turk (Eds.), *Psychological approaches to pain management: A practitioner's handbook* (pp. 458–485). New York: Guilford Press.

Fishbain, D. A., Cutler, R., et al. (1997). Chronic pain-associated depression: Antecedent or consequence of chronic pain?: A review. *Clinical Journal of Pain, 13,* 116–137.

Flores, L., Gatchel, R. J., et al. (1997). Objectification of functional improvement after nonoperative care. *Spine, 22*(14), 1622–1633.

Gatchel, R. J. (2004). Musculoskeletal disorders: Primary and secondary interventions. *Journal of Electromyography and Kinesiology, 14,* 161–170.

Gatchel, R. J. (2005). *Clinical essentials of pain management.* Washington, DC: American Psychological Association.

Gatchel, R. J. (Ed.). (2006). *Compendium of outcome instruments.* LeGrange, IL: North American Spine Society.

Gatchel, R. J., & Bruga, D. (2005, September/October). Multidisciplinary intervention for injured workers with chronic low back pain. *SpineLine*, pp. 8–13.

Gatchel, R. J., Mayer, T., et al. (2006). The Pain Disability Questionnaire: Relationship to one-year functional and psychosocial rehabilitation outcomes. *Journal of Occupational Rehabilitation*, 16, 75–94.

Gatchel, R. J., Mayer, T. G., et al. (1986). Quantification of lumbar function: Part VI. The use of psychological measure in guiding physical functional restoration. *Spine*, 11, 36–42.

Gatchel, R. J., & Okifuji, A. (2006). Evidence-based scientific data documenting the treatment- and cost-effectiveness of comprehensive pain programs for chronic nonmalignant pain. *Journal of Pain*, 7(11), 779–793.

Gatchel, R. J., Polatin, P., et al. (1995). The dominant role of psychosocial risk factors in the development of chronic low back pain disability. *Spine*, 20(24), 2702–2709.

Gatchel, R. J., Polatin, P. B., et al. (1998). Use of the SF-36 Health Status Survey with a chronically disabled back pain population: Strengths and limitations. *Journal of Occupational Rehabilitation*, 8, 237–246.

Geisser, M. E., Ranavauya, M., et al. (2005). A meta-analytic review of surface electromyography among persons with low back pain and normal, healthy controls. *Journal of Pain*, 6(11), 711–726.

Glenn, B. A. (2002). Process and outcome of multidisciplinary pain treatment: An evaluation of a stage of change model. *Dissertation Abstracts International: B: Sciences and Engineering*, 62(11-B), 5373.

Harten, J. A. (1998). Functional capacity evaluation. *Occupational Medicine*, 13, 209–212.

Hazard, R. G., Reeves, V., et al. (1992). Lifting capacity: Indices of subject effort. *Spine*, 17, 1065–1070.

Hodselmans, A. P., Dijkstra, P. U., et al. (2008). Exercise capacity in non-specific chronic low back pain patients: A lean body mass-based Åstrand bicycle test; Reliability, validity, and feasibility. *Journal of Occupational Rehabilitation*, 18, 282–289.

Innes, E., & Straker, L. (2002). Workplace assessments and functional capacity evaluations: Current practices for therapists in Australia. *Work*, 18(1), 51–66.

Jay, M. A., Lamb, J. M., et al. (2000). Sensitivity and specificity of the indicators of sincere effort of the EPIC lift capacity test on a previously injured population. *Spine*, 25(11), 1405–1412.

Jette, A. M., Haley, S., et al. (2003). Are the ICF Activity and Participation dimensions distinct? *Journal of Rehabilitation Medicine*, 35(3), 145–149.

Keeley, J. (1997). Quantification of function. In T. G. Mayer, V. Mooney, & R. J. Gatchel (Eds.), *Contemporary conservative care for painful spinal disorders* (pp. 290–307). Philadelphia: Lea & Febiger.

King, P. M., Tuckwell, N., et al. (1998). A critical review of functional restoration. *Physical Therapy*, 78(8), 852–866.

Kinney, R. K., Gatchel, R. J., et al. (1993). Prevalence of psychopathology in acute and chronic low back pain patients. *Journal of Occupational Rehabilitation*, 3(2), 95–103.

Kishino, N. D., Mayer, T. G., et al. (1985). Quantification of lumbar function: Part 4. Isometric and isokinetic lifting simulation in normal subject and low-back dysfunction patients. *Spine*, 10, 921–927.

Leeman, G., Polatin, P., et al. (2000). Managing secondary gain in patients with pain-associated disability: A clinical perspective. *Journal of Workers Compensation*, 9, 25–44.

Levenstein, S. K., & Kaplan, G. A. (1998). Socio-economic status and ulcer. A prospective study of contributory risk factors. *Journal of Clinical Gastroenterology*, 26(1), 14–17.

Martin, B. I., Deyo, R. A., et al. (2008). Expenditures and health status among adults with back and neck problems. *Journal of the American Medical Association*, 299(6), 656–664.

Mayer, T. G. (2000). Quantitative physical and functional capacity assessment. In T. G. Mayer, R. J. Gatchel, & P. B. Polatin (Eds.), *Occupational musculoskeletal disorders: function, outcomes and evidence* (pp. 266–284). Philadelphia: Lippincott Williams & Wilkins.

Mayer, T. G., Barnes, D., et al. (1988). Progressive isoinertial lifting evaluation: Part I. A standardized protocol and normative database. *Spine*, 13, 993–997.

Mayer, T. G., Gatchel, R. J., et al. (1985). Objective assessment of spine function following industrial injury: A prospective study with comparison group and one-year follow-up. *Spine*, 10, 482–493.

Mayer, T. G., Gatchel, R. J., et al. (1987). A prospective two year study of functional restoration in industrial low back injury utilizing objective assessment. *Journal of the American Medical Association*, 258, 1763–1767.

Mayer, T. G., & Gatchel, R. J. (1988). *Functional restoration for spinal disorders: The sports medicine approach*. Philadelphia: Lea & Febiger.

Mayer, T. G., Gatchel, R., et al. (1990). Safety of the dynamic Progressive Isoinertial Lifting Evaluation (PILE) test [Letter]. *Spine*, 15(9), 985–986.

Mayer, T. G., Mooney, V., et al. (Eds.). (1991). *Contemporary conservative care for pain-*

ful spinal disorders. Philadelphia: Lea & Febiger.

Mayer, T. G., & Polatin, P. B. (2000). Tertiary nonoperative interdisciplinary programs: The functional restoration variant of the outpatient chronic pain management program. In T. G. Mayer, R. J. Gatchel, & P. B. Polatin (Eds.), *Occupational musculoskeletal disorders: Function, outcomes and evidence* (pp. 639–649). Philadelphia: Lippincott Williams & Wilkins.

McGeary, D. D., Mayer, T. G., et al. (2006). High pain ratings predict treatment failure in chronic occupational musculoskeletal disorders. *Journal of Bone and Joint Surgery, 88*(2), 317–325.

Newton, M., Thow, M., et al. (1993). Trunk strength testing with iso-machines: Part 2. Experimental evaluation of the Cybex II back testing system in normal subjects and patients with chronic low back pain. *Spine, 18,* 812–824.

Newton, M., & Waddell, G. (1993). Trunk strength testing with iso-machines: Part 1. Review of a decade of scientific evidence. *Spine, 18,* 801–811.

Nitschke, J. E., Nattrass, C. L., et al. (1999). Reliability of the American Medical Association Guides' model for measuring spinal range of motion. *Spine, 24,* 262–268.

Noonan, V., & Dean, E. (2000). Submaximal exercise testing: Clinical application and interpretation. *Physical Therapy, 80*(8), 782–807.

Polatin, P. B., Gatchel, R. J., et al. (1989). A psychosociomedical prediction model of response to treatment by chronically disabled workers with low back pain. *Spine, 14,* 956–961.

Polatin, P. B., Kinney, R., et al. (1993). Psychiatric illness and chronic low back pain: The mind and the spine—Which goes first? *Spine, 18,* 66–71.

Pransky, G., Shaw, W. S., et al. (2004). Disability prevention and communication among workers, physicians, employers, and insurers: Current models and opportunities for improvement. *Disability and Rehabilitation, 26*(11), 625–634.

Proctor, T. J., Mayer, T. G., et al. (2005). Failure to complete a functional restoration program for chronic musculoskeletal disorders: A prospective one-year outcome study. *Archives of Physical and Rehabilitation Medicine, 86,* 1509–1515.

Protas, E. J., Mayer, T. G., et al. (2004). Relevance of aerobic capacity measurements in the treatment of chronic work-related spinal disorders. *Spine, 19,* 2158–2160.

Pullman, S. L., Goodin, D. S., et al. (2000). Clinical utility of surface EMG: Report of the Therapeutics and Technology Assessment Subcommittee of the American Academy of Neurology. *Neurology, 55,* 171–177.

Rainville, J., Sobel, J., et al. (1997). The effect of compensation involvement of the reporting of pain and disability by patients referred for rehabilitation of chronic low back pain. *Spine, 22*(17), 2016–2024.

Rissanen, A., Alaranta, H., et al. (1994). Isokinetic and non-dynamometric tests in low back pain patients related to pain and disability index. *Spine, 19,* 1963–1967.

Rondinelli, R. D., Genovese, E., et al. (Eds.). (2008). *Guides to the evaluation of permanent impairment.* Chicago: American Medical Association.

Rudy, T. E., Lieber, S. J., et al. (2003). Psychosocial predictors of physical performance in disabled individuals with chronic pain. *Clinical Journal of Pain, 19,* 18–30.

Rush, A., Polatin, P., et al. (2000). Depression and chronic low back pain: Establishing priorities in treatment. *Spine, 25,* 2566–2571.

Shaw, W. S., Means-Christensen, A., et al. (2007). Shared and independent associations of psychosocial factors on work status among men with subacute low back pain. *Clinical Journal of Pain, 23*(5), 409–416.

Soer, R., van der Schans, C. P., et al. (2008). Towards consensus in operational definitions in functional capacity evaluation: A Delphi Survey. *Journal of Occupational Rehabilitation, 4,* 389–400.

Stanos, S. P., McLean, J., et al. (2007). Physical medicine rehabilitation approach to pain medical clinics of North America. *Pain Management, 91*(1), 57–95.

Strong, S. (2002). Functional capacity evaluation: The good, the bad, and the ugly. *Occupational Therapy Now, 6,* 5–9.

Sullivan, M. J. L., Feuerstein, M., et al. (2005). Integrating psychosocial and behavioral interventions to achieve optimal rehabilitation outcomes. *Journal of Occupational Rehabilitation, 15*(4), 475–489.

Tuckwell, N. L., Straker, L., et al. (2002). Test-retest reliability on nine tasks of the physical work performance evaluation. *Work, 19,* 243–253.

Turk, D. C., & Monarch, E. S. (2002). Biopsychosocial perspective on chronic pain. In D. C. Turk & R. J. Gatchel (Eds.), *Psychological approaches to pain management: A practitioner's handbook* (pp. 346–364). New York: Guilford Press.

Vasudevan, S. V. (1996). Role of functional capacity assessment in disability evaluation. *Journal of Back and Musculoskeletal Rehabilitation, 6,* 237–248.

Watson, P. J., Booker, C. K., et al. (1997). Surface electromyography in the identification of chronic low back pain patients: The development of the flexion–relaxation ration. *Clinical Biomechanics, 12*(3), 165–171.

Williams, C. (1998). Evidence-based health care: Applying fine words to one's fingertips. *Pain Forum, 7*(1), 55–57.

Wind, H., Gouttebarge, V., et al. (2005). Assessment of functional capacity of the musculoskeletal system in the context of work, daily living, and sport: A systematic review. *Journal of Occupational Rehabilitation, 15*(2), 253–272.

Woods, C. S., Kishino, N. D., et al. (2000). Effects of subacute versus chronic status of low back pain patients' response to a functional restoration program. *Journal of Occupational Rehabilitation, 10*(3), 229–233.

World Health Organization. (2001). *International classification of functioning, disability and health.* Geneva, Switzerland: Author.

CHAPTER 10

Assessment of Patients with Chronic Pain
A Comprehensive Approach

DENNIS C. TURK
JAMES P. ROBINSON

Chronic pain affects approximately 20–30% of the adult population in Western countries (Verhaak, Kerssens, Dekker, Sorbi, & Bensing, 1998). In the United States, the National Center for Health Statistics (2006) estimates that about 25% of the adult American population has chronic or recurrent pain, 10% reported having pain that lasted a year or more, and 40% stated that the pain has a moderate or severe degrading impact on their lives. In a World Health Organization (WHO) survey of primary care patients in 15 countries, 22% of patients reported pain present for 6 months or longer that required medical attention or medication or interfered significantly with daily activities (Gureje, 1998). According to the National Headache Foundation (2005) more than 45 million American experience chronic headaches. Chronic pain is also prevalent children. Chronic or recurrent pain is a common occurrence among children and adolescents, affecting as much as 25% of the pediatric population (Perquin et al., 2000). Approximately 3.5 million people in the United States have cancer, with moderate to severe pain reported by 35–45% at the intermediate stage of the disease and 60–85% in advanced stages of cancer (Raj, 1990), and with over 40% not experiencing sufficient relief from their pain treatments

(Olivier, Kravitz, & Kaplan, 2001). These astronomical figures do not accurately communicate the impact of pain and related suffering on the individual patients aggregated in the impersonal statistics.

For individuals experiencing chronic back pain, there is a continuing quest for relief that remains elusive as they trek from doctor to doctor and diagnostic test to diagnostic test in a continuing search to have their pain diagnosed and successfully treated. They may also develop treatment-related complications along the way. Moreover, the experience of *medical limbo* (i.e., the presence of a painful condition that eludes diagnosis and that carries the implication of either psychiatric causation or malingering on the one hand, or an undiagnosed potentially disabling condition on the other) is itself the source of significant stress and can initiate psychological dysfunction.

For many, the pain becomes the central focus of their lives as they confront not only the stress of pain but also a cascade of ongoing problems (e.g., financial, familial). As people with pain withdraw from society, they lose their jobs, alienate family and friends, and become isolated. They may become enmeshed in a legal system that prolongs and compounds their distress. Pain affects their ability to sleep, to function, and compromises the quality of all aspects of their lives. In this ongoing and often elusive quest for relief, it is hardly surprising that they experience feelings of frustration, helplessness, hopelessness, demoralization, and outright depression. In short, living with persistent pain conditions requires considerable emotional resilience and tends to deplete people's emotional reserves, and taxes not only the individual but also the capacity of family, friends, coworkers, and employers to provide support.

Furthermore, the average age of patients treated at multidisciplinary pain rehabilitation facilities is 44 years old (Flor, Fydrich, & Turk, 1992), and the average duration of their symptoms prior to treatment was 7 years. Thus, prior to the pain onset, these people had histories spanning 37 years; therefore, their prior experiences are important in understanding how they respond to their symptoms and plight. Moreover, most people live a social context. Significant people in patients' lives likely influence their adaptation and, conversely, are impacted by living with a person with chronic pain. Thus, it is important to include history and context in understanding people with chronic pain and treatment planning.

Based on the scenario outlined here, it is apparent that although biomedical factors, in the majority of cases, appear to instigate the initial report of pain; over time, psychosocial and behavioral factors may serve to maintain and exacerbate the level of pain, influence adjustment, and contribute to excessive disability. Given this broad perspective, pain that persists should not be viewed as solely physical or solely psychological; the experience of pain is maintained by an interdependent set of biomedical, psychosocial, and behavioral factors.

In this volume, a number of chapters address diagnostic populations with specific chronic pain, for example, back pain, headache, fibromyalgia syndrome, cancer-related pain. Each of these chapters provides information about specific medical diagnostic assessment procedures. The nature of the diagnostic procedures vary depending on the medical conditions being evaluated; that is, the medical evaluation of a patient who presents with pain—whether acute or chronic—is generally specific, and is directed toward discovering biomedical derangements that can reasonably explain the pain. In contrast, the evaluation of functional, psychosocial, and behavioral factors involved in chronic pain involves common themes that transcend the specific problem.

Our intent in this chapter is to focus on a conceptual framework that can be used in the comprehensive assessment of patients with chronic pain. We outline the components of the assessment that should be integrated with medical diagnostic information in decision making, developing an appropriate treatment plan, and as means to monitor patients during and at the termination of treatment. At times we mention various assessment procedures and instruments as illustrations, but more extended descriptions and discussions of the psychometric properties of these measures are contained in other chapters. We discuss several areas that might be particularly relevant for assessment of patients with chronic pain, namely, substance abuse, fear, malingering, and cognitive factors (e.g., attention, memory, concentration).

GENERAL ISSUES

There are three very general questions regarding the assessment of chronic pain:

1. What variables or factors should be assessed?
2. What methods should be used to assess the variables?
3. What type of training should the assessor have?

Table 10.1 lists the categories of factors that we believe should be considered in a comprehensive evaluation of a patient with chronic pain. These are covered in more depth below. However, in discussing them, it is useful to begin with the concept of pain behaviors. These are the behaviors of an individual when he or she is in pain. Pain behaviors include verbal behaviors (i.e., statements about pain), as well as nonverbal behaviors that may indicate a person is experiencing pain, such as limping or wincing. These pain behaviors signal to others that an individual is experiencing pain.

The challenge for an examiner is to interpret the pain behaviors of a patient. Although

TABLE 10.1. Areas Addressed in Extended Psychological Interviews

Experience of pain and related symptoms

- Location and description of pain (e.g., "sharp," "burning")
- Onset and progression
- Perception of cause (e.g., trauma, virus, stress)
- What has the patient been told about the symptoms and condition? Does the patient believe that this information is accurate?
- Exacerbating and relieving factors (e.g., exercise, relaxation, stress, massage)
- Pattern of symptoms (e.g., worse certain times of day or following activity or stress)
- Sleep habits (e.g., difficulty falling to sleep or maintaining sleep, sleep hygiene)
- Thoughts, feelings, and behaviors that precede, accompany, and follow fluctuations in symptoms

Treatments received and currently receiving

- Medication (prescribed and over-the-counter). How helpful have these been?
- Pattern of medication use (as-needed basis, time-contingent), changes in quantity or schedule
- Physical modalities (e.g., physical therapy). How helpful have these been?
- Exercise (e.g., Do they participate in a regular exercise routine? Is there evidence of deactivation and avoidance of activity due to fear of pain or exacerbation of injury?). Has the pattern changed (increased, decreased)?
- Complementary and alternative (e.g., chiropractic manipulation, relaxation training). How helpful have these been?
- Which treatments have they found the most helpful?
- Compliance (adherence) with recommendations of health care providers
- Attitudes toward previous health care providers

Compensation and litigation

- Current disability status (e.g., receiving or seeking disability, amount, percent of former job income, expected duration of support)
- Current or planned litigation

Responses by patient and significant others

- Typical daily routine
- Changes in activities and responsibilities (both positive and obligatory) due to symptoms
- Changes in significant other's activities and responsibilities due to patient's symptoms
- Patient's behavior when pain increases or flares up
- Significant others' responses to behavioral expressions of pain
- What does the patient do when pain is not bothering him or her (uptime activities)?
- Significant other's response when patient is active
- Impact of symptoms on interpersonal, family, marital, and sexual relations (e.g., changes in desire, frequency, or enjoyment)
- Activities that patient avoids because of symptoms
- Activities continued despite symptoms
- Pattern of activity and pacing of activity (can use activity diaries that ask patients to record their pattern of daily activities [e.g., sitting, standing, walking] for several days or weeks)

Coping

- How does the patient try to cope with his or her symptoms? Does patient view him- or herself as having any role in symptom management? If so, what role?
- Current life stresses
- Pleasant activities

Educational and vocational history

- Level of education completed, including any special training
- Work history
- How long at most recent job?
- How satisfied with most recent job and supervisor?
- What does the patient like least about most recent job?
- Would the patient like to return to most recent job? If not, what type of work would the patient like?
- Current work status, including homemaking activities
- Vocational and avocational plans

(cont.)

TABLE 10.1. *(cont.)*

Social history

- Relationships with family or origin
- History of pain or disability in family members
- History of substance abuse in family members
- History of, or current, physical, emotional, and sexual abuse. Was the patient a witness to abuse of someone else?
- Marital history and current status?
- Quality of current marital and family relations

Alcohol and substance use

- Current and history of alcohol use (quantity, frequency)
- History and current use of illicit psychoactive drugs
- History and current use of prescribed psychoactive medications
- Consider the CAGE questions as a quick screen for alcohol dependence (Mayfield, McLeod, & Hall, 1974). Depending on response consider, other instruments for alcohol and substance abuse (Allen & Litten, 1998).

Psychological dysfunction

- Current psychological symptoms/diagnosis (depression including suicidal ideation, anxiety disorders, somatization, posttraumatic stress disorder). Depending on responses, consider conducting structured interview such as the Structured Clinical Interview for DSM-IV-TR (SCID; American Psychiatric Association, 1997).
- Is the patient currently receiving treatment for psychological symptoms? If yes, what treatments (e.g., psychotherapy or psychiatric medications). How helpful are the treatments?
- History of psychiatric disorders and treatment including family counseling
- Family history of psychiatric disorders

Concerns and expectations

- Patient concerns/fears
- Explanatory models of pain held by the patient
- Expectations regarding the future and treatment (will get better, worse, never change)
- Attitude toward rehabilitation versus "cure"

Treatment goals

---

pain behaviors are sometimes determined entirely by an abnormal biological process in a patient's body, they are typically also influenced by various psychological factors and by the social environment of the patient. Thus, an examiner has to consider the role of multiple factors that may be influencing the pain behaviors of a patient he or she is evaluating. A useful way to conceptualize this challenge is to think of a regression (prediction) equation with multiple unknowns:

$$PB = f(Xa1, Xa2 \ldots, Xan1;$$
$$Xb1, Xb2 \ldots, Xbn2;$$
$$Xc1, Xc2 \ldots, Xcn3;$$
$$Xd1, Xd2 \ldots, Xdn4)$$

where PB is the pain behavior that a patient demonstrates, and predictor variables are organized into four categories, such that $Xa1$, $Xa2 \ldots, Xan1$ refer to biomedical factors at the end organ where the patient reports pain; $Xb1, Xb2 \ldots, Xbn2$ refer to alterations in nervous system function that perpetuate pain after nociceptive impulses from the end organ have diminished or ceased; $Xc1, Xc2 \ldots, Xcn3$ refer to psychological variables; and $Xd1, Xd2 \ldots, Xdn4$ refer to systems or contextual variables that influence pain reports (Turk & Robinson, 2008).

The equation emphasizes the multiplicity of factors that influence patients' expressions of pain, and highlights the dilemma facing an evaluating physician. The dilemma is that it is extremely difficult to determine the weights that should be assigned to various factors for an individual patient. To make matters even worse, there is no real consensus about what the possible variables within various categories are (e.g., to specify the types of psychological factors that may affect a patient's pain behavior).

MEDICAL FACTORS

A careful medical evaluation is crucial to the assessment of a patient with chronic pain. The primary purpose of such an evaluation is to identify a pathophysiological process that accounts for the patient's pain. For the most part, medical evaluations focus on the identification of peripheral generators of nociceptive signals, and embody the assumption that patients experience pain because of dysfunction in the organs or body parts where they report experiencing their pain (Robinson & Apkarian, 2009). Sometimes, a medical evaluation leads to a diagnosis that implies a patient's pain reflects altered nervous system functioning, as opposed to nociception from the body part that is painful. For example, a physician might diagnose a peripheral neuropathy or multiple sclerosis. In general, though, medical evaluations are not particularly effective in identifying altered nervous system functioning as a cause of chronic pain (see below).

Medical evaluations are almost always specific, in the sense that different evaluations are done for different chronic pain problems. For example, the evaluation procedures for patients with chronic low back pain, chronic interstitial cystitis, and chronic headaches are completely different.

In an ideal world, a medical evaluation would lead to a precise diagnosis to explain a patient's chronic pain, and the diagnosis would pave the way to effective treatment of the pain. In reality, medical evaluations of patients with chronic pain often yield ambiguous results, and do not lead to dramatically effective treatment. In fact, the frequent failure of traditional medical evaluations to yield useful information about patients with chronic pain has played a major role in stimulating broader approaches to the evaluation of these patients.

Altered Nervous System Functioning

As noted earlier, the traditional medical approach to patients with chronic pain is to search for dysfunction in the region where a patient reports pain. This approach embod-

ies the assumption that patients' perceptions of pain reflect nociceptive input from an abnormal organ or body part, with straightforward nervous system processing of the nociceptive signals (Robinson & Apkarian, 2009; Robinson, Turk, & Loeser, 2005). However, this assumption has been challenged by several lines of research. In particular, research dating back to the 1980s has demonstrated that tissue damage and associated nociception can produce sensitization of the peripheral nervous system and the central nervous system, and that this sensitization can subserve a dissociation between tissue injury and pain (Curatolo, Arendt-Nielsen, & Petersen-Felix, 2004, 2006; Ji, Kohno, Moore, & Woolf, 2003). More recently, research using functional magnetic resonance imaging (fMRI) procedures has demonstrated distinctive patterns of brain activity in patients with chronic pain (Baliki et al., 2006; Geha et al., 2008; Metz, Yau, Centeno, Apkarian, & Martina, 2009).

It is beyond the scope of this chapter to discuss the vast literature on altered nervous system functioning (ASNF) in chronic pain in any detail. However, three observations are particularly relevant to the chapter. First, ASNF has recently been proposed as an explanation of several chronic pain syndromes whose pathophysiology has been difficult to elucidate via conventional medical approaches. Examples include complex regional pain syndrome (Harden, 2005), chronic headache (Welch, 2003), fibromyalgia syndrome (Staud, Price, Robinson, Mauderli, & Vierck, 2004; Staud & Rodriguez, 2006), and chronic spinal pain (Brisby, 2006). Second, ANSF provides an alternative to the two types of explanations that have dominated analyses of chronic pain—explanations based on traditional medical evaluations (focused on end-organ dysfunction), and ones emphasizing psychological dysfunction. Finally, it is important to emphasize that the procedures (e.g., fMRI) used to identify altered nervous system functioning in research settings are not available to clinicians. Thus, although we believe that clinicians should be aware of the possibility of ASNF as an explanation for chronic pain, we cannot outline procedures for making this determination in clinical settings, for the simple reason that clinically applicable procedures have not been developed.

PSYCHOLOGICAL FACTORS

General Considerations

Generally, a referral for evaluation may be indicated when disability greatly exceeds what would be expected, based on physical findings alone; when the patient makes excessive demands on the health care system; when the patient persists in seeking medical tests and treatments that are not indicated; when the patient displays significant emotional distress (e.g., depression or anxiety); or when the patient displays evidence of addictive behaviors, there are concerns about substance abuse, or there is continual non-adherence to the prescribed regimen. Table 10.1 contains a detailed outline of areas that should be addressed in a more extensive psychological interview for patients with pain (see also DeGood & Cook, Chapter 4, this volume).

Depending on the results of such a brief screening (e.g., ACT-UP; see Table 10.2 and below), the provider may undertake additional psychological evaluation or refer the patient for a more comprehensive evaluation for which the provider may not have the time or expertise. If a patient is referred for a comprehensive psychosocial evaluation, then a number of potentially relevant issues enumerated in Table 10.1 will be covered. Reports based on extensive psychological evaluation should inform the provider as to what factors will play a role in the patient's response to treatment, and they should be addressed by either the primary care provider or a referral agent.

TABLE 10.2. Brief Psychosocial Screening: ACT-UP

1. *Activities*: How is your pain affecting your life (i.e., sleep, appetite, physical activities, relationships)?
2. *Coping*: How do you deal/cope with your pain (What makes it better–worse)?
3. *Think*: Do you think your pain will ever get better?
4. *Upset*: Have you been feeling worried (anxious)/depressed (down, blue)?
5. *People*: How do people respond when you have pain?

Note. From Turk and Robinson (2010). Copyright by Lippincott Williams & Wilkins. Reprinted by permission.

Patients' beliefs about the cause of symptoms, their trajectory, and beneficial treatments will have important influences on emotional adjustment and adherence to therapeutic interventions. Maladaptive thoughts may contribute to a sense of hopelessness, dysphoria, and unwillingness to engage in activity. These reactions, in turn, deactivate the patient and severely limit his or her physical and emotional adaptation. The provider should also determine both the patient's and the significant others' expectancies and goals for treatment. An expectation that all symptoms will be eliminated completely may be unrealistic and will have to be addressed to prevent discouragement when this outcome does not occur. Setting appropriate and realistic goals is an important process in pain rehabilitation that requires the patient to attain better understanding of chronic pain.

Once a comprehensive medical and psychosocial assessment has been completed and the diagnosis confirmed, the clinician can begin to formulate a treatment plan. The plan should take into consideration the patient's current circumstances and capabilities.

Purposes of Psychological Assessment

Based on the integrated, comprehensive perspective espoused in this chapter, clinicians need to examine not only the physical source of the pain through examination and diagnostic tests but also the patient's mood, fears, expectancies, coping efforts, resources, responses of significant others, and the impact of pain on the patient's life.

In short, the examiner must evaluate the "whole patient," not just a primary symptom or the site of pain. Regardless of whether an organic basis for the pain can be documented, or whether psychosocial problems preceded or resulted from the pain, the evaluation process can be helpful in identifying how biomedical, psychosocial, and behavioral factors interact to influence the nature, severity, and persistence of symptoms and disability.

Interviews

A psychological interview with patients is typically semi-structured (see chapter 4 by DeGood & Cook, this volume). A structured psychiatric interview (e.g., Structured Clinical Interview for DSM-IV Disorders [SCID]; American Psychiatric Association, 1997) can be incorporated as a tool to examine psychopathology. However, in patients with pain, a psychological interview needs to go beyond an assessment of psychopathology, since its main purpose is to assess a wide range of psychosocial factors (not just psychopathology) related to patients' symptoms and disability.

When conducting an interview with patients who have chronic pain, the examiner should focus on not only on gathering information provided by the patient but also observing patients' pain behaviors and the manner in which they convey information. Patients' beliefs about the cause of symptoms, their trajectory, and beneficial treatments have important influences on emotional adjustment and adherence to therapeutic interventions. A habitual pattern of maladaptive thoughts may contribute to a sense of hopelessness, dysphoria, and unwillingness to engage in activity. These reactions, in turn, deactivate the patient and severely limit his or her coping efforts and resources. The interviewer should also determine both the patient's and the significant other's expectancies and goals for treatment. An expectation that pain will be eliminated completely may be unrealistic and will have to be addressed to prevent discouragement when this outcome does not occur. Setting appropriate and realistic goals is an important process in pain rehabilitation that requires the patient to attain better understanding of chronic pain and goes beyond the dualistic, traditional medical model.

In order to help the patient with musculoskeletal pain understand the psychosocial aspects of pain, attention should focus on the patient's reports of specific thoughts, behaviors, emotions, and physiological responses that precede, accompany, and follow pain episodes or exacerbation, as well as the environmental conditions and consequences associated with cognitive, emotional, and behavioral responses in these situations. To establish salient features of the target situations, including the controlling variables, during the interview the clinician should attend to the temporal association of these cognitive, affective, and behavioral events, their specificity versus generality across situations, and the frequency of their occurrence. The interviewer seeks information that assists in the development of potential alternative responses, appropriate goals for the patient, and possible reinforcers for these alternatives.

Standardized Assessment Instruments

In addition to interviews, a number of assessment instruments that have been developed and published to evaluate patients' attitudes, beliefs, and expectancies about themselves, their symptoms, and the health care system are described throughout this volume. One survey (Piotrowski, 2007) of clinicians who treat pain indicated that the most frequently used published instruments in the assessment of pain, in order of frequency, are as follows: McGill Pain Questionnaire (Melzack, 1975); Beck Depression Inventory (BDI; Beck, Ward, Mendelson, Mock, & Erbaugh, 1961; Beck, Steer, Ball, & Ranieri, 1996), Multidimensional Pain Inventory (MPI; Kerns, Turk, & Rudy, 1985); and the Coping Strategies Questionnaire (Rosenstiel & Keefe, 1983; for critiques of these and other standardized measures, see DeGood & Cook, Chapter 4, this volume).

Standardized instruments have advantages over semistructured and unstructured interviews. They are easy to administer and require less time, they assess a wide range of behaviors, obtain information about behaviors that may be private (sexual relations) or unobservable (thoughts, emotional arousal) and, most importantly, they can be submitted to analyses that permit determination of their reliability and validity. These instruments should not be viewed as alternatives to interviews; rather, they may suggest issues to be addressed in more depth during an interview or investigated with other measures.

A word of caution should be offered in interpreting the results of self-report inventories. Studies of the psychometric properties of self-report inventories typically involve data collection from a large number of patients. Because reliability estimates are influenced by sample size, it follows that the measurement error of questionnaire data from one person should be expected to be much greater than that found in reports based on group data. One way to address concerns about reliability with some measures is to collect data at multiple points over time rather than simply comparing pretreatment and posttreatment data.

INAPPROPRIATE MEDICATION USE, MISUSE, AND SUBSTANCE ABUSE

Patients with widespread pain often consume a variety of medications not only for their pain but also for the myriad comorbid symptoms associated with their chronic pain syndromes. It is important to discuss a patient's medications during the interview, because many pain medications (particularly opioids) are associated with side effects that may mimic emotional dysfunction. A clinician, for example, should be familiar with medication-induced side effects such as fatigue, sleep difficulties, and mood changes to avoid misdiagnosis of depression. A general understanding of commonly used medications for chronic pain (opioids; nonsteroidal antiinflamatory medications, anticonvulsants, antidepressants) is important, because some patients also may use opioid analgesics to manage mood. During the interview, potential psychological dependence on pain-relieving medications and engagement in aberrant drug-seeking behaviors should be evaluated. When patients make frequent requests for increased or stronger medications, rely solely on medications for relief, or when there are indications that the patient may be overmedicated (e.g., the patient can no longer do his job because he or she is too sedated), a thorough evaluation for chemical dependence may be warranted.

Assessment of Chemical Dependence

Patients with chronic pain, like a significant minority of people in general, might use a variety of licit and illicit substances in inappropriate ways. However, the primary concern in relation to patients with chronic pain involves opioid use for the simple reason that pain physicians often prescribe opioids for chronic pain.

There is ample evidence that consumption of prescription opioids has increased markedly since the early 1990s (Gilson et al., 2004; Reid et al., 2002). Along with this increase in availability, large-scale data have emerged that indicate misusing prescrip-

tion opioids has occurred more frequently over time and represents a significant public health problem (Gilson, Maurer, & Joranson, 2005; Soderstrom et al., 2001). Also, there has been a rise in opioid-related deaths (Franklin et al., 2005). On a smaller scale, several researchers have reported data on small cohorts of patients with pain, indicating that inappropriate or aberrant use of prescription opioids is far more common than physicians supposed during the 1980s and 1990s (Chabal, Erjavec, Jacobson, Mariano, & Chaney, 1997; Passik & Kirsh, 2004; Webster & Webster, 2005).

A key problem in the clinical assessment of patients who might be using opioids inappropriately is that there are no agreed-upon criteria for diagnosing opioid abuse or dependence in patients with chronic pain (Saxon, Robinson, & Sullivan, in press). In practice, pain physicians typically rely on indirect indicators when they make inferences about opioid dependence in patients with chronic pain (Ballantyne & LaForge, 2007; Webster & Webster, 2005). For example, they are likely to suspect such dependence when patients engage in aberrant behaviors, demonstrate poor judgment in relation to opioids (e.g., drive while heavily sedated), or insist on increasing doses of opioids despite behaviors that suggest drug toxicity.

In the absence of agreed-upon criteria for diagnosing opioid abuse or opioid dependence in chronic pain patients, it is not possible to specify appropriate assessment methods with certainty. For example, several attempts have been made to develop procedures to identify patients with chronic pain who are high risk for substance abuse. Both structured interviews and self-report questionnaires have been used for this purpose. Although some methods show promising results, each of the measures used has limitations (Turk, Swanson, & Gatchel, 2008). At this point, no measure that has been published meets appropriate psychometric standards for predicting misuse or abuse among opioid-naive patients with chronic pain, and if used, these measures should be used with caution, followed by additional assessment.

Despite these caveats, it is possible to identify principles of assessment of patients with pain that should be followed in the evaluation for opioid abuse and dependence. First, the examiner should ask straightforward questions regarding patients' present and past use of both licit and illicit substances. Second, interview data should be supplemented by questionnaires supported by at least some validity data. Examples include the CAGE (Cut down, Annoyed, Guilty, Eye-opener; Mayfield, McLeod, & Hall, 1974) questions, the Opioid Risk Tool (ORT; Webster & Webster, 2005), and the Screener and Opioid Assessment for Patients with Pain (SOAPP; Butler, Budman, Fernandez, & Jamison, 2004). Third, the medical evaluation of a patient with chronic pain should examine markers of inappropriate drug use, including evidence of intoxication in a mental status examination, evidence of acute drug withdrawal (e.g., mydriasis and hyperreflexia), presence of needle tracks, and laboratory data (e.g., liver function tests). Finally, a thorough evaluation for possible opioid abuse or dependence in a patient receiving opioids for chronic pain should include consideration of collateral information (e.g., records from the treating physician and from the pharmacy where prescriptions are filled). Finally, the examiner should strongly consider ordering or recommending urine toxicology screening.

ASSESSMENT OF EMOTIONAL DISTRESS

The results of numerous studies suggest that chronic pain is often associated with emotional distress, particularly depression, anxiety, anger, and irritability. The presence of emotional distress in people with chronic pain presents a challenge when assessing symptoms such as fatigue, reduced activity level, decreased libido, appetite change, sleep disturbance, weight gain or loss, and memory and concentration deficits. These symptoms are often associated with pain and have also been considered "vegetative" symptoms of depressive disorders. Improvements or deterioration in such symptoms, therefore, can be a result of changes in either pain or emotional distress.

The BDI and BDI-2 (Beck et al., 1961, 1996) and the Profile of Mood States (POMS; McNair, Lorr, & Droppleman, 1971) have well-established reliability and validity in the assessment of symptoms of depression and emotional distress, and they have been used in numerous psychiatric clinical tri-

als and an increasing number of studies of patients with chronic pain (Kerns, 2003). These two measures have been recommended for the assessment of emotional distress in clinical trials (Dworkin et al., 2005). In psychiatric and chronic research, the BDI provides a well-accepted criterion of the level of psychological distress in a sample and its response to treatment. The POMS (McNair et al., 1971) assesses six mood states— tension–anxiety, depression–dejection, anger–hostility, vigor–activity, fatigue– inertia, and confusion–bewilderment—and also provides a summary measure of total mood disturbance. Although the discriminant validity of the POMS scales in patients with chronic pain has not been adequately documented, it has scales for the three most important dimensions of emotional functioning in patients with chronic pain (Depression, Anxiety, Anger) and also assesses three other dimensions that are very relevant to chronic pain and its treatment, including a Positive Mood scale of vigor–activity. Moreover, the POMS has demonstrated beneficial effects of treatment in some (but not all) recent chronic pain trials (e.g., Dworkin et al., 2003; Rowbotham et al., 1998). For these reasons, the BDI and the POMS are reasonable choices as brief measures of emotional distress.

As noted earlier, various symptoms of depression (e.g., decreased libido, appetite or weight changes, fatigue, memory and concentration deficits) are also commonly believed to be consequences of chronic pain and the medications used for its treatment (Gallagher & Verma, 2004). It is unclear whether the presence of such symptoms in patients with chronic pain (and other medical disorders) should nevertheless be considered evidence of depressed mood, or whether the assessment of mood in these patients should emphasize symptoms that are less likely to be secondary to physical disorders (Wilson, Mikail, D'Eon, & Minns, 2001).

ASSESSMENT OF FEAR

Many patients who have sustained musculoskeletal injuries are fearful of engaging in activities that they believe may either contribute to injury or exacerbate their symptoms. Avoidance of activities may, in the short term, lead to symptom reduction. Over time, restriction of activities is likely to lead to decreased functional capacities as a result of deconditioning. Also, avoidance of activity has the unfortunate consequence of preventing corrective feedback. Health care providers may inadvertently contribute to avoidance of activity by providing patients with cervical collars that restrict neck movements and advising them to avoid activities that hurt (hurt = harm). They may contribute to patients' anxiety that something is seriously wrong with their bodies by continuing to order sophisticated diagnostic tests in search of occult physical pathology. Assessment of fear seems particularly relevant for people who have sustained a trauma; thus, we examine methods of assessment in some depth.

The fear–avoidance model (Vlaeyen, Kole-Snijders, Boeren, & van Eek, 1995) emphasizes the importance of fear that physical activity will cause pain and (re)injury. The central features of this model are that certain cognitive responses (e.g., catastrophizing) following painful experiences lead to fear of movement. This fear of movement induces the person to avoid activities that he or she *believes* will aggravate the injury and cause pain.

Several different measures have been used to assess fear of pain and injury in research on the fear–avoidance model. The most commonly used measure, the Tampa Scale of Kinesiophobia (TSK; Kori, Miller, & Todd, 1990), comprises 17 items and employs a 4-point Likert-type scale. Summing all items creates a Total Score, with higher scores indicating greater fear of movement. Although the TSK was initially developed in 1990, it was not published in a readily accessible form. In 1995, the measure was translated into Dutch by Vlaeyen and colleagues (Vlaeyen, Kole-Snijders, Boeren, et al., 1995; Vlaeyen, Kole-Snijders, Rooteveel, Ruesink, & Heuts, 1995), who explored the psychometric properties of the TSK.

Test–retest reliability and internal consistency of the TSK are reasonably good (Peters, Vlaeyen, & van Drunen, 2000; Swinkels-Meewisse, Swinkels, Verbeek, Vlaeyen, & Oostendorp, 2003; Vlaeyen, Kole-Snijders, Boeren, et al., 1995). Concurrent validity has been demonstrated through correlations between the TSK Total Score and other measures of fear–avoidance beliefs, fear of bodily injury–illness–death (Vlaeyen, Kole-Snijders, Boeren, et al., 1995), and social phobia and agoraphobia (Vlaeyen, Kole-Snijders, Boeren, et al., 1995), although coefficients were weak to moderate in magnitude (.33–.39).

The Pictorial Fear of Activity Scale—Cervical (PFActS-C; Turk, Robinson, Sherman, Burwinkle, & Swanson, 2008) was designed to assess fear of movement by having patients respond to concrete, pictorial stimuli rather than to abstract verbal statements. This approach can be contrasted with the TSK, which includes more general questions, some of which are not specially related to fear of movement as implied by the title of the TSK (Burwinkle, Robinson, & Turk, 2005). Discussions with physicians and physical therapists who treat patients with cervical pain led to the identification of 72 specific movements that are likely to elicit fear of movement in patients with cervical pain. Photographs that depicted a plainly clothed female model performing each of the 72 potentially stressful "active" movements were taken. The 72 pictures represented systematic variation of four factors in a 6 × 2 × 2 × 3 design. The factors varied were Direction of Movement (flexion, extension, right and left rotation, and right and left lateral bending), Extremity of Movement (moderate vs. extreme), Loading (lifting an object vs. not lifting anything) and Arm Position (at sides, at shoulder height, overhead). Additionally, 11 other photographs were taken. Unlike the rest of the photographs that showed distinct neck movements, five "control" photographs showed the model with arms at her sides performing leg movements that were expected not to stress the neck. Six "neutral" photographs showed a model performing the same activities (e.g., arms raised, loaded), but with no neck movements. We expected that both control and neutral photographs would elicit low fear ratings among people with whiplash-associated disorders (WADs).

Examples of PFActS-C photographs in each of these domains are displayed in Figure 10.1. The psychometric properties of the PFActS-C are excellent, with good internal consistency and test–retest reliability. The construct validity has also been shown to be quite good (Turk, Robinson, et al., 2008).

Arms at side Unloaded Lt
Rotation Extreme

Arms extended shoulder
Unloaded Rt Rotation Minimal

Arms overhead Loaded Flexion
Extreme

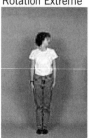 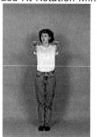 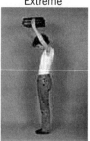

FIGURE 10.1. Example of items from the Pictorial Fear of Activities Scale—Cervical (PFActS-C). From Turk, Robinson, Sherman, Burwinkle, and Swanson (2008). Reprinted with permission from the International Association for the Study of Pain. The figure may not be reproduced for any other purpose without permission.

ASSESSMENT OF PAIN BEHAVIORS

As noted previously, patients display a broad range of responses communicating to others that they are experiencing pain, distress, and suffering. Some of these pain behaviors may be controllable by the person, whereas others are not. Although there is no one-to-one relationship between these pain behaviors and self-report of pain, they are at least modestly correlated. Informally, a health care provider can observe patients' behaviors during their interviews and examinations. Because patients know that they are being observed in these contexts, we have found it is also useful to observe patients' behaviors in the waiting room, when they walk to the examination or interview room, and when they exit. It is also useful to observe patients in the presence of their significant others, both to observe patient behaviors and to observe how the significant others respond to those behaviors.

A number of different observational procedures have been developed to identify and quantify pain behaviors (see Keefe, Somers, Williams, & Smith, Chapter 7, this volume). Structured methods that require patients to engage in a set of behaviors while their behavior is observed and rated have been proposed by Keefe and Block (1982; Keefe, Williams, & Smith, 2001). Such structured approaches may be useful in research studies but can be cumbersome in clinical settings. Several investigators have developed observational pain behavior checklists (e.g., Rich-

ards, Nepomunceno, Riles, & Suer, 1992; Turk, Wack, & Kerns, 1985) that can be used in any setting. Although they have the advantage of efficiency, these methods may be less appropriate for comparisons among patients who are viewed in different contexts (e.g., during a physical examination or interview).

The context may influence the behaviors observed. For example, the nature of pain behaviors observed might be quite different during a stressful physical examination than during an interview. The number and nature of pain behaviors might be influenced by the presence of a significant other during the observation period. At a minimum, it is important to note the context in which the behaviors were observed. Studies using pain behavior checklist have found a significant association between these self-reports and behavioral observations. A variant of this observational procedure was developed by Kerns and colleagues (1991), who developed a self-report version in which patients endorsed specific behaviors in which they engaged when experiencing pain.

Uses of the health care system and analgesic medication are other ways to assess pain behaviors. Patients can record the times when they take medication over a specified interval, such as a week. Diaries not only provide information about the frequency and quantity of medication but may also permit identification of the antecedent and consequent events of medication use. Antecedent events might include stress, boredom, or activity. Examination of antecedents is useful in identifying patterns of medication use that may be associated with factors other than pain per se. Similarly, patterns of response to the use of analgesic may be identified. Does the patient receive attention and sympathy whenever he or she is observed by significant others taking medication? That is, do significant others provide positive reinforcement for the taking of analgesic medication and thereby unwittingly increase medication use?

ASSESSMENT OF COPING AND PSYCHOSOCIAL ADAPTATION TO PAIN

Historically, psychological measures designed to evaluate psychopathology have been used to identify specific individual differences associated with reports of pain, even though these measures were usually neither developed for nor standardized on samples of medical patients. However, it is possible that responses by medical patients may be distorted as a function of the disease or the medications that they take. For example, common measures of depression ask patients about their appetites, sleep patterns, and fatigue. Because disease status and medication can affect responses to such items, medical patients' scores may be elevated, thereby distorting the meaning of their responses. As a result, a number of measures have been developed for use specifically with patients with pain. Instruments have been developed to assess psychological distress; the impact of pain on patients' lives; a feeling of control; coping behaviors; and attitudes about disease, pain, and health care providers and the patient's plight (see DeGood & Cook, Chapter 4, this volume, for an extensive review and discussion).

ASSESSMENT OF COGNITIVE FUNCTIONING

Adaptability to stress includes completing tasks under stress. For vocational evaluations, it is helpful to know how the patient responds to cognitive demands associated with work. Many patients with chronic pain report having difficulties related to cognitive functioning. Review of relevant research reveals that some patients with chronic pain,

who have not suffered from traumatic brain injuries or neurological disorders, display deficits in attentional capacity, processing speed, and psychomotor speed (Hart, Martelli, & Zasler, 2000). Several measures that appear to be reasonable for assessing neuropsychological impairments in patients with chronic pain include the Wechsler Memory Scales–III—General and Delayed Memory (Grace, Berg, & Nielson, 1995), the Paced Auditory Serial Addition Test (Grace, Nielson, Hopkins, & Berg, 1999; Taylor, Cox, & Mailis, 1996), and the Wechsler Adult Intelligence Scale—Digit Symbol (Grace et al., 1999; Schmand et al., 1998).

A gross assessment of mental status can be obtained with very brief measures such as the Mini-Mental State Examination (Folstein, Folstein, & McHugh, 1975). When patients with pain perform below expected levels on cognitive tests, however, results need to be interpreted in light of their pain medication use, potentially disrupted sleep, emotional factors, and other symptoms.

Busy clinicians may feel that they do not have time to cover all of the areas just described. A brief screening may be all they feel they have time for, and based on such a screening they may refer patients with chronic pain for a more comprehensive evaluation. A useful procedure to help the clinician decide what areas should be covered in more depth is captured in the acronym, ACT-UP (Turk & Robinson, 2010). Table 10.2 outlines the questions that facilitate decisions about subsequent assessment.

SOCIAL FACTORS

Social factors are construed as factors in the social environment that influence people, independent of their individual psychological characteristics. A good example is the receipt of workers' compensation benefits. There is good evidence that injured workers respond less well to a variety of treatments than do individuals with similar medical conditions who do not have workers' compensation claims (Harris, Mulford, Solomon, van Gelder, & Young, 2005). Although participation in the workers' compensation system exerts its negative influence through effects on the perceptions, goals, and attitudes of injured workers, the influence appears to be robust and not dependent on any particular psychological characteristics of affected individuals.

Another social factor that has received a great deal of attention is participation in litigation (e.g., Mendelson & Mendelson, 1991). Much of the research in this area deals with WAD injuries from motor vehicle collisions (MVCs). This emphasis reflects the facts that whiplash injuries occur fairly frequent in MVCs, and that a significant proportion of such individuals file personal injury claims. Research on the relation between litigation and clinical course in WAD injuries has been contradictory. For example, whereas several recent studies have reported a negative effect of attorney involvement and litigation on recovery from WAD injuries (Dufton et al., 2006; Gun et al., 2005), Scholten-Peeters and colleagues (2003) concluded in a comprehensive review that "often mentioned factors like age, gender, and compensation do not seem to be of prognostic value" (p. 320) in relation to the clinical course of whiplash injuries. It is beyond the scope of this chapter to review the often contentious literature on the effect of litigation/attorney involvement on outcomes of WAD injuries (e.g., Cassidy et al., 2000; Merskey & Teasell, 2000). Our interpretation is that this literature on balance supports the hypothesis that attorney involvement and participation in litigation is a negative prognostic factor for individuals with WAD injuries.

Social factors include influences from an individual's immediate social environment. For example, there is good evidence that patients with pain generally demonstrate more dramatic pain behaviors when they are in the presence of solicitous spouses (e.g., Thieme, Spies, Sinha, Turk, & Flor, 2005). Social factors also include demographic variables that influence the presentation and clinical course of people with painful conditions. In particular, research indicates that an individual's clinical presentation is associated with his or her age, gender, ethnicity (Hernandez & Sachs-Ericsson, 2006; Watson, Latif, & Rowbotham, 2005), and education level (Berglund, Bodin, Jensen, Wiklund, & Alfredsson, 2006; Holm, Carroll, Cassidy, & Ahlbom, 2006).

BURDEN OF ILLNESS: PAIN SEVERITY AND DISABILITY BECAUSE OF PAIN

A major focus of the preceding discussion has been the identification of factors underlying patient symptoms. It is important to note, though, that identification of factors that qualitatively play a role in patient symptoms is not the same as explanation of the severity of these symptoms, or the extent to which the patient is disabled by such symptoms. Thus, we recommend that an evaluation of any patient with chronic pain should assess the extent to which the patient is affected by his or her symptoms. The issue of severity of symptoms and disability is particularly important, because it is often left out in traditional medical evaluations. There is a tendency throughout medicine to place great emphasis on diagnosis, and to deemphasize evaluation of the extent to which an individual is incapacitated by his or her medical condition. Among patients with chronic pain, however, severity/disability assessment is often at least as revealing as diagnostic assessment. One reason for this is that it is often difficult to make a precise diagnosis that accounts even qualitatively for the symptoms of a patient with chronic pain. A second and more typical reason is that even if a diagnosis can be made, the diagnosed condition is usually compatible with a wide range of functional capabilities. For example, whereas some individuals return to professional sports after decompressive lumbar spine surgery, others remain virtually bedridden. The patients who come to the attention of pain physicians are those who demonstrate high levels of disability relative to the diagnosed medical condition. It is important to evaluate two aspects of the burden of illness borne by a chronic pain patient—the severity of his or her pain, and the effect of the pain on his or her ability to function.

ASSESSMENT OF PAIN

Assessment of patients with chronic pain often begins with attempts to clarify the severity and qualities of pain. Although a ubiquitous phenomenon, pain is inherently subjective. The only way to know about others' pain is by what they say or show by their behavior. Because there is no "objective" method for assessing pain, self-report serves as the "gold standard" in assessments of pain and its characteristics. Pain assessment therefore requires that patients and participants in clinical trials describe their own experiences. Although individuals interpret measures of pain in different and somewhat idiosyncratic ways, these interpretations can be expected to remain relatively constant within people over time. As a result, they can also provide valid measures of change in pain due to treatment or time.

Pain Intensity

Self-report measures of pain often ask patients to quantify their pain by providing a single, general rating of pain: "Is your usual level of pain 'mild,' 'moderate,' or 'severe?'" or "Rate your typical pain on a scale from 0 to 10, where 0 equals 'no pain' and 10 is the 'worst pain you can imagine.'" A number of simple methods can be used to evaluate current pain intensity—numerical scales (NRSs), verbal ratings scales (VRSs), and visual analogue scales (VASs).

Each commonly used method of rating pain intensity (NRS, VRS, or VAS) appears sufficiently reliable and valid, and no single method consistently demonstrates greater responsiveness in detecting improvements associated with pain treatment (Jensen & Karoly, 2001; see Chapter 2 by Jensen & Karoly, this volume). However, there are important differences among NRS, VRS, and VAS measures of pain intensity with respect to missing data, stemming from failure to complete the measure, patient preference, ease of data recording, and ability to administer the measure by telephone or with electronic diaries. NRS and VRS measures tend to be preferred over VAS measures by patients, and VAS measures usually demonstrate more missing data than do NRS measures. Greater difficulty completing VAS measures is associated with increased age and greater opioid intake, and cognitive impairment has been shown to be associated with inability to complete NRS ratings of pain intensity (Jensen & Karoly, 2001). Patients who are unable to complete NRSs may be able to complete the VRS (e.g., "none,"

"mild," "moderate," "severe"). Other measures are available to assess pain in children and in those who are unable to communicate verbally (e.g., stroke patients, mentally impaired) (Hadjistavropoulos, von Baeyer, & Craig, 2001).

There has been some concern that retrospective reports may not be valid, because they may reflect current pain severity that serves as an anchor for recall of pain severity over some interval (Gendreau, Hufford, & Stone, 2003; Stone & Shiffman, 2002). More valid information may be obtained by asking about the current level of pain, pain over the past week, worst pain of the last week, and lowest level of severity over the last week. This has also led to the use of daily diaries, which are believed to be more accurate because they are based on real time rather than recall. For example, patients are asked to maintain regular diaries of pain intensity, recording ratings several times each day (e.g., at meals and bedtime) for several days or weeks. One problem noted with the use of paper-and-pencil diaries is that patients may not follow the instruction to provide ratings at specified intervals. Rather, patients may complete diaries in advance ("fill forward') or shortly before seeing a clinician ("fill backward") (Stone, Shiffman, Schwartz, Broderick, & Hufford, 2003). These two reporting approaches undermine the putative validity of diaries. As an alternative to paper-and-pencil diaries, a number of commentators have advocated for the use of electronic devices that can prompt patients for ratings and "time-stamp" the actual ratings, thus facilitating real-time data capture. Although there are numerous advantages to the use of advanced technology to improve the validity of patient ratings, they are not without potential problems, including hardware, software, and user problems (Turk, Burwinkle, & Showlund, 2007). These methods are also costly and, although they may be appropriate for research studies, their usefulness in clinical settings may be limited.

Pain Quality

Pain is known to have different sensory and affective qualities, in addition to its intensity, and measures of these components of pain may more fully describe an individual's pain experience (Melzack & Torgerson, 1971; Price, Harkins, & Baker, 1987). It is possible that the efficacy of pain treatments varies for different pain qualities. Therefore, measures of pain quality may identify treatments that are efficacious for certain types of pain but not for overall pain intensity. Assessment of specific pain qualities at baseline also makes it possible to determine whether certain patterns of pain quality moderate the effects of treatment. The Short-Form McGill Pain Questionnaire (SF-MPQ; Melzack, 1987) assesses 15 sensory and affective pain descriptors, and its Sensory and Affective subscales have demonstrated responsivity to treatment in a number of clinical trials (e.g., Dworkin et al., 2003; Rowbotham et al., 1998; see Katz & Melzack, Chapter 3, this volume).

Recently, the SF-MPQ was developed to incorporate a set of descriptors of neuropathic pain that were thought to be lacking (Dworkin et al., 2009). The SF-MPQ-2 not only expands the descriptors but modifies the response scale from a 0- to 3-point scale to a 0- to 10-point scale. This modification permits detection of smaller yet meaningful differences that may occur over in the natural course of a disease or in response to treatment (see Katz & Melzack, Chapter 3, this volume).

Pain Modifiers

For the majority of people with chronic, widespread pain, pain severity varies. Thus, it is useful to ask the patient what makes his or her pain worse. For example, do specific activities result in an increase in symptoms? Do certain circumstances contribute to exacerbation of pain, such as stress in the form of interpersonal conflicts? Does pain vary with time of day? For example, does the patient notice that his or her pain is worse in the morning or later in the day? In the same way that it is important to identify factors that magnify or initiate pain episodes, it is important to ask about factors that result in reductions of pain. For example, do medication, rest, heat or cold, distraction, or exercise result in reductions of pain severity or even elimination of symptoms for some period?

ASSESSMENT OF THE ABILITY TO FUNCTION

Typically, assessments of the ability of a patient to function are described as assessments of disability, thus emphasizing limitations in the patient's functional capacities. It is helpful to distinguish two different "types" of disability, and to assess both. One type of disability involves limitations in the ability to perform activities of daily living (ADLs). The other relates to inability to perform adult roles, and in particular, the ability to work.

Assessment of Limitations in ADLs

In assessing disability in the sense of ADL limitations, an examiner should ask whether a patient has to lie down during a typical day, whether he or she is independent in basic self-care (e.g., dressing), and whether he or she needs assistance with household chores. In addition to informal questions about activity limitations, evaluators should strongly consider using formal instruments designed for this purpose. Self-report measures have been developed to assess peoples' reports of their abilities to engage in a range of functional activities, such as the ability to walk up stairs, to sit for specific periods of time, to lift specific weights, and to perform ADLs. These measures are also designed to evaluate the severity of the pain experienced upon the performance of these activities. There are a number of well-established, psychometrically supported generic (e.g., Short-Form 36 Health Survey [SF-36]; Ware & Sherbourne, 1992) and pain-specific (e.g., Brief Pain Inventory Interference scale [Cleeland & Ryan, 1994]; Pain Disability Index [Pollard, 1984]; MPI Interference scale [Kerns et al., 1985]), and neck-pain-specific (Neck Disability Index [Vernon, 1996]; Fibromyalgia Impact Questionnaire [Burckhardt, Clark, & Bennett, 1991]) measures of functional status.

In general, disease-specific measures are designed to evaluate the specific effects of a disorder that may not be assessed by a generic measure (Dworkin et al., 2005). In addition, responses on disease-specific measures generally do not reflect the effects of comorbid conditions on physical functioning, which may confound the interpretation of change occurring over the course of a trial when generic measures are used. Disease-specific measures may be more sensitive to the effects of treatment on function, but generic measures provide information about physical functioning and treatment benefits that can be compared across different conditions and studies (Dworkin, Nagasako, Hetzel, & Farrar, 2001; Guyatt, Feeney, & Patrick, 1993). Each of these approaches has strengths. Decisions regarding whether to use a disease-specific or a generic measure, or some combination of the two, depend on the purpose of the assessment. For individual patients in a clinical practice it would be most appropriate to use measures developed on samples with comparable characteristics. If the clinician wishes to compare across a group of patients, then one of the broader based pain-specific measures should be considered. If the assessment is being performed as part of a research study, some combination might be appropriate to compare chronic pain samples with a larger sample with diverse medical diseases (e.g., SF-36).

Assessment of Work Disability

We are not aware of validation of an instrument assessing work disability in relation to chronic widespread pain. In the absence of a standard instrument, we recommend that clinicians who assess these patients address the following issues:

1. Is the patient currently working?
2. If the patient is not working, is this related to his or her health, and more specifically, to any specific injury?
3. How long has the patient been out of the workforce?
4. Is he or she receiving any kind of work disability benefits? Which ones?

PATIENT CREDIBILITY

A fundamental feature of pain is that it is a private experience. Since an examiner cannot directly experience or measure the pain a patient reports, he or she must rely in large part on the patient's statements about the pain. This raises an obvious question: Are the patient's reports credible? Sometimes

the credibility of a patient's reports is questionable, because the patient has cognitive difficulties that impair the ability to communicate his or her experiences accurately. Examples include patients who are intoxicated or demented. But most discussions of patient credibility address the issue of conscious or unconscious elaboration of symptoms by patients who have no known cognitive limitations. In this setting, questions about malingering or secondary gain arise.

The term *malingering* refers to deliberate, planned deception by a patient to achieve some kind of reward—typically, a monetary one. The definition of *secondary gain* is less clear (Robinson & Loeser, in press). In a general way, it refers to behaviors on the part of a patient that appear to be influenced by potential monetary award but are not consciously planned, or at least are not as deliberate as the behaviors that are markers of malingering. Robinson and Loeser (in press) differentiate the two as follows:

> Some observers emphasize that secondary gain describes the behavior of claimants who are influenced unconsciously by potential rewards in their environment. . . . The idea that secondary gain involves unconscious behavior makes it morally less objectionable than malingering, which refers to conscious fabrication in order to achieve some reward. However, this seemingly clear distinction between secondary gain and malingering has been challenged by other writers. . . . The disagreements among different observers in the conceptualization of secondary gain highlight the elusiveness of the concept. It is best to think of the terms "malingering" and "secondary gain" as alternative ways to describe the effect of environmental rewards on the behavior of claimants, with the difference being one of the moral opprobrium assigned to a claimant's behavior. While neither term is flattering, a clinician or adjudicator who accuses a claimant of malingering is rendering a much harsher judgment than one who says the claimant's behavior is motivated by secondary gain.

Controversy abounds regarding the prevalence of malingering and secondary gain, and the appropriate methods for identifying their presence. Many third-party payers believe that patients who report pain in the absence of sufficient objective physical pathology are frequently motivated by secondary gains, especially financial compensation. In contrast, some observers have found that the base rate for malingering in chronic pain is quite low (e.g., Mendelson, 1986). Dramatic cases, however, are very salient and induce high levels of suspicion. Uncertainties about the base rate for malingering, along with the difficulties of interpreting evidence for and against it in relation to an individual patient, make the task of identifying malingerers extremely difficult.

When asked to address the question of malingering, the clinician needs to rely on multiple convergent sources of information, including archival data (previous history), collateral sources of information, knowledge of incentives, litigation status, responsiveness to previous treatments, evidence of physical pathology, performance of tasks of physical functioning, observable behavior in the interview and other unobtrusive situations (e.g., observation of patient in waiting room, as exiting the office), facial expressions, self-reports during an interview (i.e., content, quality, and clarity of information provided), and responses on self-report questionnaires that can be compared to appropriate comparison groups or that include "validity scales." Each of these sources of information and the consistency among them contribute to the clinician's determination of the credibility of the patient's report.

Given the psychometric limitations of tests of malingering and the inherent difficulty with finding appropriate criterion groups for research in this area, it is best to rely on behavioral decision rules. Williams (1998) suggested that psychologists should use three major areas in which discrepancies occur to construct a malingering index for traumatic brain injury. Some of these concepts are also relevant for patients with chronic pain. The first is the relationship of injury severity to cognitive functioning. The severity of the injury is directly related to the severity of the expected impairment. The second area involves noting the interrelationship of the tests and subtests. Williams opined, "Inconsistencies are expressed as scores that are sufficiently disparate that they violate the known relationships between the tests" (p. 122). The third area involved the relationship between preinjury status and current test results, and, by extension, current functioning. In a forensic report the psychol-

ogist may point out inconsistencies but leave the determination of veracity to the "trier of fact."

Conscious dissimulation on any self-report measure is possible. This dissimulation is often referred to as *response bias*. This is particularly a concern when there is an incentive, such as disability compensation, based on performance deficits. Highly contentious situations often surround assessment of pain-related impairment and disability such as workers' compensation, Social Security disability, veterans' disability compensation, civil litigation related to accidental injuries (e.g., MVCs, product liability), and access to controlled substances. This is the reason the validity scales have been developed for instruments such as the Minnesota Multiphasic Personality Inventory (MMPI) and the Eysenck Personality Questionnaire (Eysenck & Eysenck, 1975) and the Variable Response scale for the MPI (Bruehl, Lofland, Sherman, & Carlsom, 1998). In a preliminary study, Lofland, Semenchuk, and Cassisi (1995) concluded the MPI "appears to be a good screening measure to detect patients who are exhibiting symptom exaggeration."

There have been a number of attempts to identify specific psychological profiles of litigation- and compensation-prone patients. There is, however, no conclusive evidence that specific characteristics differentiate those who are litigating or receiving disability compensation from those who are not (Kolbison, Epstein, & Burgess, 1996).

Turk, Robinson, and Aulet (2002) conducted a preliminary study comparing three groups of people with chronic pain to determine whether a group evaluated by physicians performing an independent medical examination (IME) that completed a self-report measure assessing pain, emotional distress, and functional limitations (Impairment Impact Inventory; Turk, Robinson, Loeser, Cocchiarella, & Hunt, 2001) responded differently than groups of patients with chronic pain being treated in rehabilitation facilities (a group of patients with fibromyalgia and a heterogeneous group of patients with chronic pain attending an interdisciplinary pain clinic). The authors found no difference in responses to any of the three sections of the instrument—Pain Severity, Emotional Distress, and Functional Activities. The authors concluded that clinicians should not assume that patients who potentially have something to gain by poor performance (disability seeking) will inevitably exaggerate the burden of their pain and the resultant disability.

Others investigators have examined facial expressions of people in pain and the ability of observers to distinguish exaggerated pain expressions from healthy subjects and pain sufferers' *real* expressions of pain (Craig, Hyde, & Patrick, 1991; Poole & Craig, 1992).

Physical tests to evaluate suboptimal performance have also been used to detect malingering (Robinson, O'Connor, Riley, Kvaal, & Shirley, 1994). Some researchers ask patients to repeat standard physical tasks and use discrepancy of performance (index of congruence) as an indication of motivated performance. Reviewing efforts to detect deception led Craig, Hill, and McMurtry (1999) to the following conclusion: "Definitive, empirically validated procedures for distinguishing genuine and deceptive report are not available and current approaches to the detection of deception remain to some degree intuitive" (p. 41).

Waddell, McCulloch, Kummel, and Venner (1980) developed a system of "nonorganic" signs that could be assessed during the physical examination of patients with low back pain. These were physical findings judged not to be characteristic of known organic pathology in the lumbar spine. Subsequent research demonstrated that patients with high scores on the "Waddell signs" typically suffered from emotional distress. Main and Waddell (1998) deplored the tendency for participants in adversarial proceedings to interpret the presence of nonorganic signs as an indicator of malingering.

A growing body of information concerns the ability of neuropsychological tests to detect malingering. The Letter Memory Test and the Digit Memory Test appear to have the best "hit" rates for the detection of malingering (Inman & Berry, 2002). Additional research is needed before strong conclusions should follow from performance even on these measures. At best, performance on these tests should be combined with other confirmatory information.

Finally, it should be noted that most of the research on secondary gain and malingering has been funded by insurance carriers (Robinson & Loeser, in press). This research has shone an unflattering light on injured workers and litigants. However, workers' compensation claims and litigation involve adversarial relationships in which all parties may maneuver to gain advantage. Virtually no systematic research has examined the frequency with which insurance adjusters, employers, or defense attorneys distort information to minimize their financial liability in contested claims. Research on the behavior of all participants in contested claims is needed before we can get an accurate grasp of the frequency with which these actors engage in deceptive behavior.

WHO SHOULD PERFORM CHRONIC PAIN ASSESSMENTS?

As discussed earlier, the assessment of a patient with chronic pain involves multiple domains. It is difficult, if not impossible, for a single professional to have expertise in all these domains. Thus, the best way to perform comprehensive evaluations of patients with chronic pain is via a multidisciplinary team. Such teams exist in multidisciplinary pain rehabilitation centers (Robinson, Leo, Wallach, McGough, & Schatman, in press). These centers differ somewhat in the composition of their multidisciplinary evaluating teams, but most teams include a physician, a psychologist, and a vocational rehabilitation counselor. Typically, members of a team evaluate a patient individually, then confer to develop a composite picture of the patient.

CONCLUDING COMMENTS

Abundant scientific evidence supports the view that chronic pain is a complex phenomenon that incorporates physical, psychosocial, and behavioral factors. Failure to incorporate each of these factors leads to an incomplete understanding and thereby an inadequate treatment.

Our goal in this chapter has been to outline a comprehensive approach to the evaluation of patients with chronic pain. Specifically, we have focused on the components of a psychosocial and behavioral assessment. The information derived from this assessment should be integrated with information from patients' histories, physical evaluation, and medical evaluation described in other chapters in this volume. Depending on the diagnosis, some specific measures have been developed to assess psychosocial factors. These are described in other chapters in this volume. Treatment plan development should be based on each of the factors described to improve clinical outcomes and reduce disability.

REFERENCES

Allen, J. P., & Litten, R. Z. (1998). Screening instruments and biochemical screening. In A. W. Graham, T. K. Schultz, & B. B. Wilford (Eds.), *Principles of addiction medicine* (pp. 263–272). Annapolis Junction, MD: American Society of Addiction Medicine.

American Psychiatric Association. (1997). *User's guide for the Structured Clinical Interview for DSM-IV Axis I Disorders SCID-1: Clinician version.* Washington, DC: American Psychiatric Press.

Baliki, M. N., Chialvo, D. R., Geha, P. Y., Levy, R. M., Harden, R. N., Parrish, T. B., et al. (2006). Chronic pain and the emotional brain: Specific brain activity associated with spontaneous fluctuations of intensity of chronic back pain. *Journal of Neuroscience, 26,* 12165–12173.

Ballantyne, J. C., & LaForge, K. S. (2007). Opioid dependence and addiction during opioid treatment of chronic pain. *Pain, 129,* 235–255.

Beck, A. T., Steer, R. A., Ball, R., & Ranieri, W. F. (1996). Comparison of Beck Depression Inventories -IA and -II in psychiatric outpatients. *Journal of Personality, 67,* 588–597.

Beck, A. T., Ward, C. H., Mendelson, M., Mock, J., & Erbaugh, J. (1961). An inventory for measuring depression. *Archives of General Psychiatry, 4,* 561–571.

Berglund, A., Bodin, L., Jensen, I., Wiklund, A., & Alfredsson, L. (2006). The influence of prognostic factors on neck pain intensity, disability, anxiety and depression over a 2-year period in subjects with acute whiplash injury. *Pain, 125,* 244–256.

Brisby, H. (2006). Pathology and possible mechanisms of nervous system response to disc degeneration. *Journal of Bone and Joint Surgery, 88,* 68–71.

Bruehl, S., Lofland, K. R., Sherman, J. J., & Carlson, C. R. (1998). The Variable Responding scale for detection of random responding

on the Multidimensional Pain Inventory. *Psychological Assessment, 10,* 3–9.

Burckhardt, C. S., Clark, S. R., & Bennett, R. M. (1991). The Fibromyalgia Impact Questionnaire: Development and validation. *Journal of Rheumatology, 18,* 728–733.

Burwinkle, T., Robinson, J. P., & Turk, D. C. (2005). Fear of movement: Factor structure of the Tampa Scale of Kinesiophobia in patients with fibromyalgia syndrome. *Journal of Pain, 6,* 384–391.

Butler, S. F., Budman, S. H., Fernandez, K., & Jamison, R. N. (2004). Validation of a screener and opioid assessment measure for patients with chronic pain. *Pain, 112,* 65–75.

Cassidy, J. D., Carroll, L. J., Cote, P., Lemstra, M., Berglund, A., & Nygren, A. (2000). Effect of eliminating compensation for pain and suffering an outcome of insurance claims for whiplash injury. *New England Journal of Medicine, 342,* 1179–1186.

Chabal, C., Erjavec, M. K., Jacobson, L., Mariano, A., & Chaney, E. (1997). Prescription opiate abuse in chronic pain patients: clinical criteria, incidence, and predictors. *Clinical Journal of Pain, 13,* 150–155.

Cleeland, C. S., & Ryan, K. M. (1994). Pain assessment: Global use of the Brief Pain Inventory. *Annals of Academic Medicine, 23,* 129–138.

Craig, K. D., Hill, M. L., & McMurtry, B. W. (1999). Detecting deception and malingering. In A. R. Block, E. F. Kremer, & E. Fernandez (Eds.), *Handbook of pain syndromes* (pp. 41–58). Mahwah, NJ: Erlbaum.

Craig, K. D., Hyde, S., & Patrick, C. J. (1991). Genuine, suppressed, and faked facial behavior during exacerbation of chronic low back pain. *Pain, 46,* 161–172.

Curatolo, M., Arendt-Nielsen, L., & Petersen-Felix, S. (2004). Evidence, mechanisms, and clinical implications of central hypersensitivity in chronic pain after whiplash injury. *Clinical Journal of Pain, 20,* 469–476.

Curatolo, M., Arendt-Nielsen, L., & Petersen-Felix, S. (2006). Central hypersensitivity in chronic pain: Mechanisms and clinical implications. *Physical Medicine and Rehabilitation Clinics of North America, 17,* 287–302.

Dufton, J. A., Kopec, J. A., Wong, H., Cassidy, J. D., Quon, J., McIntosh, G., et al. (2006). Prognostic functions associated with minimal improvement following acute whiplash-associated disorders. *Spine, 31,* E754–E765; discussion E766.

Dworkin, R. H., Corbin, A. E., Young, J. P., Sharma, U., LaMoreaux, L., Bockbrader, H., et al. (2003). Pregabalin for the treatment of postherpetic neuralgia: A randomized, placebo-controlled trial. *Neurology, 60,* 1274–1283.

Dworkin, R. H., Nagasako, E. M., Hetzel, R. D., & Farrar, J. T. (2001). Assessment of pain and pain-related quality of life in clinical trials. In D. C. Turk & R. Melzack (Eds.), *Handbook of pain assessment* (2nd ed., pp. 659–692). New York: Guilford Press.

Dworkin, R. H., Turk, D., Farrar, J., Haythornthwaite, J., Jensen, M., Katz, N., et al. (2005). Core outcome measures for chronic pain clinical trials: IMMPACT recommendations. *Pain, 113*, 9–19.

Dworkin, R. H., Turk, D. C., Revicki, D. A., Harding, G., Coyne, K. S., Peirce-Sandner, S., et al. (2009). Development and initial validation of an expanded and revised version of the Short-Form McGill Pain Questionnaire (SF-MPQ-2). *Pain, 144*, 35–42.

Eysenck, H. J., & Eysenck, S. B. G. (1975). *The manual of the Eysenck Personality Questionnaire.* London: Hodder & Stoughton.

Flor, H., Fydrich, T., & Turk, D. C. (1992). Efficacy of multidisciplinary pain treatment centers: A meta-analytic review. *Pain, 49*, 221–230.

Folstein, M. F., Folstein, S. E., & McHugh, P. R. (1975). "Mini-Mental State": A practical method for grading the cognitive of patients for the clinician. *Journal of Psychiatric Research, 12*, 189–198.

Franklin, G. M., Mai, J., Wickizer, T., Turner, J. A., Fulton-Kehoe, D., & Grant, L. (2005). Opioid dosing trends and mortality in Washington State Workers' Compensation, 1996–2002. *American Journal of Industrial Medicine, 48*, 91–99.

Gallagher, R. M., & Verma, S. (2004). Mood and anxiety disorders in chronic pain. In R. H. Dworkin & W. S. Breitbart (Eds.), *Psychosocial aspects of pain: A handbook for health care providers* (pp. 589–606). Seattle, WA: IASP Press.

Geha, P. Y., Baliki, M. N., Harden, R. N., Bauer, W. R., Parrish, T. B., & Apkarian, A. V. (2008). The brain in chronic CRPS pain: Abnormal gray-white matter interactions in emotional and autonomic regions. *Neuron, 60*, 570–581.

Gendreau, M., Hufford, M. R., & Stone, A. A. (2003). Measuring clinical pain in chronic widespread pain: Selected methodological issues. *Best Practices in Research and Clinical Rheumatology, 17*, 575–592.

Gilson, A. M., Maurer, M. A., & Joranson, D. E. (2005). State policy affecting pain management: Recent improvements and the positive impact of regulatory health policies. *Health Policy, 74*, 192–204.

Gilson, A. M., Ryan, K. M., Joranson, D. E., & Dahl, J. L. (2004). A reassessment of trends in the medical use and abuse of opioid analgesics and implications for diversion control: 1997–2002. *Journal of Pain Symptom Management, 28*, 176–188.

Grace, G. M., Berg, M. A., & Nielson, W. (1995). Assessment of attention, concentration, and memory in patients with fibromyalgia. *Journal of the International Neuropsychological Society, 1*, 137.

Grace, G. M., Nielson, W. R., Hopkins, M., & Berg, M. A. (1999). Concentration and memory deficits in patients with fibromyalgia syndrome. *Journal of Clinical and Experimental Neuropsychology, 21*, 477–487.

Gun, R. T., Ost, O. L., O'Riordan, A., Mpelasoka, F., Eckerwall, C. G., & Smyth, J. F. (2005). Risk factors for prolonged disability after whiplash injury: A prospective study. *Spine, 30*, 386–391.

Gureje, O. (1998). Persistent pain and well-being: A World Health Organization study in primary care. *Journal of the American Medical Association, 280*, 147–151.

Guyatt, G. H., Feeney, D. H., & Patrick, D. L. (1993). Measuring health-related quality of life. *Annals of Internal Medicine, 118*, 622–629.

Hadjistavropoulos, T., von Baeyer, C., & Craig, K. D. (2001). Pain assessment in persons with limited ability to communicate. In D. C. Turk & R. Melzack (Eds.), *Handbook of pain assessment* (2nd ed., pp. 134–152). New York: Guilford Press.

Harden, R. N. (2005). Pharmacotherapy of complex regional pain syndrome. *American Journal of Physical Medicine and Rehabilitation, 84*(Suppl. 3), S17–S28.

Harris, I., Mulford, J., Solomon, M., van Gelder, J. M., & Young, J. (2005). Association between compensation status and outcome after surgery: A meta-analysis. *Journal of the American Medical Association, 293*, 1644–1652.

Hart, R. P., Martelli, M. F., & Zasler, N. D. (2000). Chronic pain and neuropsychological functioning. *Neuropsychology Review, 10*, 1231–1249.

Hernandez, A., & Sachs-Ericsson, N. (2006). Ethnic differences in pain reports and the moderating role of depression in a community sample of Hispanic and Caucasian participants with serious health problems. *Psychosomatoc Medicine, 68*, 121–128.

Holm, L. W., Carroll, L. J., Cassidy, J. D., & Ahlbom, A. (2006). Factors influencing neck pain intensity in whiplash-associated disorders. *Spine, 31*, E98–E104.

Inman, T. H., & Berry, D. T. R. (2002). Cross-validation of indicators of malingering: A comparison of nine neuropsychological tests, four test of malingering, and behavioral observations. *Archives of Clinical Neuropsychology, 17*, 1–23.

Jensen, M. P., & Karoly, P. (2001). Self-report scales and procedures for assessing pain in adults. In D. C. Turk & R. Melzack (Eds.), *Handbook of pain assessment* (2nd ed., pp. 15–34). New York: Guilford Press.

Ji, R. R., Kohno, T., Moore, K. A., & Woolf, C. J. (2003). Central sensitization and LTP: Do pain and memory share similar mechanisms? *Trends in Neurosciences, 26,* 696–705.

Keefe, F. J., & Block, A. R. (1982). Development of an observation method for assessing pain behavior in chronic low back pain. *Behavior Therapy, 12,* 363–375.

Keefe, F. J., Williams, D. A., & Smith, S. J. (2001). Assessment of pain behaviors. In D. C. Turk & R. Melzack (Eds.), *Handbook of pain assessment* (2nd ed., pp. 170–188). New York: Guilford Press.

Kerns, R. D. (2003, April). *Assessment of emotional functioning in pain treatment outcome research.* Paper presented at the second meeting of the Initiative on Methods, Measurement, and Pain Assessment in Clinical Trials (IMMPACT-II). Available online at *www.immpact.org/meetings.html.*

Kerns, R. D., Haythornthwaite, J., Rosenberg, R., Southwick, S., Giller, E. L., & Jacob, M. C. (1991). The Pain Behavior Checklist (PBCL)— Function, structure and psychometric properties. *Journal of Behavioral Medicine, 14,* 155–169.

Kerns, R. D., Turk, D. C., & Rudy, T. E. (1985). The West Haven–Yale Multidimensional Pain Inventory (WHYMPI). *Pain, 23,* 345–356.

Kolbison, D. A., Epstein, J. B., & Burgess, J. A. (1996). Tempormandibular disorders, headaches, and neck pain following motor vehicle accidents and the effects of litigation: Review of the literature. *Journal of Orofacial Pain, 10,* 101–125.

Kori, S., Miller, R., & Todd, D. (1990, January/February). Kinisophobia: A new view of chronic pain behavior. *Pain Management,* pp. 35–43.

Lofland, K. R., Semenchuk, E. M., & Cassisi, J. E. (1995, November). *The Multidimensional Pain Inventory and symptom exaggeration in chronic low back pain patients.* Paper presented at the 14th Scientific Meeting of the American Pain Society, Los Angeles.

Main, C. J., & Waddell, G. (1998). Behavioral responses to examination. A reappraisal of the interpretation of "nonorganic signs." *Spine, 23,* 2367–2371.

Mayfield, D., McLeod, G., & Hall, P. (1974). The CAGE questionnaire. *American Journal of Psychiatry, 131,* 1121–1123.

McNair, D. M., Lorr, M., & Droppleman, L. F. (1971). *Profile of Mood States.* San Diego, CA: Educational and Industrial Testing Service.

Melzack, R. (1975). The McGill Pain Questionnaire: Major properties and scoring methods. *Pain, 1,* 277–299.

Melzack, R. (1987). The Short-Form McGill Pain Questionnaire. *Pain, 30,* 191–197.

Melzack, R., & Torgerson, W. S. (1971). On the language of pain. *Anesthesiology, 34,* 50–59.

Mendelson, G. (1986). Chronic pain and compensation: A review. *Journal of Pain and Symptom Management, 1,* 135–144.

Mendelson, G., & Mendelson, D. (1991). Legal aspects of the management of chronic pain. *Medical Journal of Australia, 155,* 640–642.

Merskey, H., & Teasell, R. W. (2000). Effects of eliminating compensation for pain and suffering an outcome of insurance claims. *New England Journal of Medicine, 343,* 1119.

Metz, A. E., Yau, H. J., Centeno, M. V., Apkarian, A. V., & Martina, M. (2009). Morphological and functional reorganization of rat medial prefrontal cortex in neuropathic pain. *Proceedings of the National Academy of Science USA, 106,* 2423–2428.

National Center for Health Statistics. (2006). Health, United States, 2006 with chartbook on trends in the health of Americans. Hyattsville: Author.

National Headache Foundation. (2005). Fact Sheet: January 1, 2003. Available online at *www.headaches.org/consumer/presskit/factsheet.pdf.*

Olivier, J. W., Kravitz, R. L., & Kaplan, S. H. (2001). Individualized patient education and coaching to improve pain control among cancer outpatients. *Journal of Clinical Oncology, 19,* 2206–2212.

Passik, S. D., & Kirsh, K. L. (2004). Opioid therapy in patients with a history of substance abuse. *CNS Drugs, 18,* 13–25.

Perquin, C. W., Hazebroek-Kampscheur, A. A., Hunfeld, J. A., Bohnen, A. M., van Suijlekom-Smit, L. W., Passchier, J., et al. (2000). Pain in children and adolescents: A common experience. *Pain, 87,* 51–58.

Peters, M. L., Vlaeyen, J. W. S., & van Drunen, C. (2000). Do fibromyalgia patients display hypervigilance for innocuous somatosensory stimuli?: Application of a body scanning reaction time paradigm. *Pain, 86,* 283–292.

Piotrowski, C. (2007). Review of the psychological literature on assessment instruments used with pain patients. *North American Journal of Psychology, 9,* 303–306.

Pollard, C. A. (1984). Preliminary validity study of the Pain Disability Index. *Perceptual and Motor Skills, 59,* 974.

Poole, G. D., & Craig, K. D. (1992). Judgments of genuine, suppressed, and faked expressions of pain. *Journal of Personality and Social Psychology, 63,* 797–805.

Price, D. D., Harkins, S. W., & Baker, C. (1987). Sensory–affective relationships among different types of clinical and experimental pain. *Pain, 28,* 297–307.

Raj, P. P. (1990). Pain relief: Fact or fancy? *Regional Anesthesia, 15,* 157–169.

Reid, M. C., Engles-Horton, L. L., Weber, M. B., Kerns, R. D., Rogers, E. L., & O'Connor, P. G. (2002). Use of opioid medications for chronic noncancer pain syndromes in primary care. *Journal of General Internal Medicine, 17,* 173–179.

Richards, J. S., Nepomunceno, C., Riles, M., & Suer, Z. (1992). Assessing pain behavior: The UAB Pain Behavior Scale. *Pain, 14,* 313–338.

Robinson, J. P., & Apkarian, A. V. (2009). Low back pain. In E. A. Mayer & M. C. Bushnell (Eds.), *Functional pain syndromes: Presentation and pathophysiology* (pp. 23–53). Seattle, WA: IASP Press.

Robinson, J. P., Leo, R., Wallach, J., McGough, E., & Schatman, M. (in press). Rehabilitative treatment for chronic pain. In C. Stannard, E., Kalso, & J. Ballantyne (Eds.), *Evidence-based chronic pain management.* Philadelphia: Lippincott Williams & Wilkins.

Robinson, J. P., & Loeser, J. D. (in press). Effects of workers' compensation systems on recovery from disabling injuries. In M. Hasenbring, A. Rusu, & D. C. Turk (Eds.), *From acute to chronic back pain: Risk factors, mechanisms and clinical implications.* Oxford, UK: Oxford University Press.

Robinson, J. P., Turk, D. C., & Loeser, J. D. (2005). Pain, impairment, and disability in the AMA Guides. *Journal of Law, Medicine, and Ethics, 32,* 315–326.

Robinson, M. E., O'Connor, P. D., Riley, J. L., Kvaal, S. A., & Shirley, F. R. (1994). Variability of isometric and isotonic leg exercise: Utility for detection of submaximal efforts. *Journal of Occupational Rehabilitation, 4,* 163–169.

Roland, M., & Morris, R. (1983). A study of the natural history of back pain: Part I. Development of a reliable and sensitive measure of disability in low back pain. *Spine, 8,* 141–144.

Rosenstiel, A. K., & Keefe, F. J. (1983). The use of coping strategies in chronic low back pain patients. *Pain, 17,* 33–44.

Rowbotham, M. C., Harden, N., Stacey, B., Bernstein, P., Magnus-Miller, L., & the Gabapentin Postherpetic Neuralgia Study Group. (1998). Gabapentin for the treatment postherpetic neuralgia: A randomized controlled trial. *Journal of the American Medical Association, 280,* 1837–1842.

Saxon, A. J., Robinson, J. P., & Sullivan, M. D. (2010). Assessment and treatment of chemical dependency. In J. C. Ballantyne, J. P. Rathmell,

& S. M. Fishman (Eds.), *Bonica's management of pain* (4th ed., pp. 1330–1345). Philadelphia: Lippincott Williams & Wilkins.

Schmand, B., Lindeboom, J., Schagen, S., Heijt, R., Koene, T., & Hamburger, H. L. (1998). Cognitive complaints of patients after whiplash: The impact of malingering. *Journal of Neurology, Neurosurgery, and Psychiatry, 64,* 339–343.

Scholten-Peeters, G. G. W., Verhagen, A. P., Berkkeving, G. E., Vandrwindt, D. A. W. M., Barnsley, L., Oostendorp, R. A. B., et al. (2003). Prognostic factors of whiplash-associated disorders: A systematic review of prospective cohort studies. *Pain, 164,* 303–322.

Soderstrom, C. A., Dischinger, P. C., Kerns, T. J., Kufera, J. A., Mitchell, K. A., & Scalea, T. M. (2001). Epidemic increases in cocaine and opiate use by trauma center patients: Documentation with a large clinical toxicology database. *Journal of Trauma, 51,* 557–564.

Staud, R., Price, D. D., Robinson, M. E., Mauderli, A. P., & Vierck, C. J. (2004). Maintenance of windup of second pain requires less frequent stimulation in fibromyalgia patients compared to normal controls. *Pain, 110,* 689–696.

Staud, R., & Rodriguez, M. E. (2006). Mechanisms of disease: Pain in fibromyalgia syndrome. *Nature Clinics in the Practice of Rheumatology, 2,* 90–98.

Stone, A. A., & Shiffman, S. (2002). Capturing momentary, self-report data: A proposal for reporting guidelines. *Annals of Behavioral Medicine, 24,* 236–243.

Stone, A. A., Shiffman, S., Schwartz, J. E., Broderick, J. E., & Hufford, M. R. (2003). Patient compliance with paper and electronic diaries. *Control Clin Trials, 24,* 182–199.

Swinkels-Meewisse, E. J., Swinkels, R. A., Verbeek, A. L., Vlaeyen, J. W., & Oostendorp, R. A. (2003). Psychometric properties of the Tampa Scale for Kinesiophobia and the Fear–Avoidance Beliefs Questionnaire in acute low back pain. *Manual Therapy, 8,* 29–36.

Taylor, A. E., Cox, C. A., & Mailis, A. (1996). Persistent neuropsychological deficits following whiplash: Evidence for chronic mild traumatic brain injury? *Archives of Physical Medicine and Rehabilitation, 77,* 529–535.

Thieme, K., Spies, C., Sinha, P., Turk, D. C., & Flor, H. (2005). Predictors of pain behaviors in fibromyalgia syndrome patients. *Arthritis Care and Research, 53,* 343–350.

Turk, D. C., Burwinkle, T., & Showlund, M. (2007). Assessing the impact of chronic pain in real-time. In A. Stone, S. Shiffman, A. Atienza, & L. Nebeling (Eds.), *The science of real-time data capture: Self-reports in health research* (pp. 204–228). New York: Oxford University Press.

Turk, D. C., & Robinson, J. P. (2008). Assessment of patients with whiplash-associated disorders consequent to motor vehicle collisions: A comprehensive approach. In M. P. Duckworth, A. Iezzi, & W. O'Donohue (Eds.), *Motor vehicle collisions: Medical, psychosocial, and legal consequences* (pp. 187–227). New York: Elsevier.

Turk, D. C., & Robinson, J. P. (2010). Multidisciplinary assessment of patients with chronic pain. In J. Ballantyne, J. Rathmell, & S. Fishman (Eds.), *Bonica's management of pain* (4th ed., pp. 288–301). Philadelphia: Lippincott Williams & Wilkins.

Turk, D. C., Robinson, J. R., & Aulet, M. R. (2002). Impairment Impact Inventory (I³): Comparison of responses by treatment-seekers and claimants undergoing independent medical examinations. *Journal of Pain, 3*(Suppl. 1), 1.

Turk, D. C., Robinson, J. R., Loeser, J. D., Cocchiarella, L., & Hunt, S. (2001). Pain. In L. Cocchiarella & S. Lord (Eds.), AMA Guides: Vol. 5. *A medical and legal transition to the Guides to the Evaluation of Permanent Impairment* (pp. 277–325). Chicago: AMA Press.

Turk, D. C., Robinson, J. P., Sherman, J. J., Burwinkle, T. M., & Swanson, K. S. (2008). Assessing fear in patients with cervical pain: Development and validation of the Pictorial Fear of Activity Scale—Cervical (PFActS-C). *Pain, 139,* 55–62.

Turk, D. C., Swanson, K. S., & Gatchel, R. J. (2008). Predicting opioid misuse by chronic pain patients: A systematic review and literature synthesis. *Clinical Journal of Pain, 24,* 497–508.

Turk, D. C., Wack, J. T., & Kerns, R. D. (1985). An empirical examination of the "pain behavior" construct. *Journal of Behavioral Medicine, 9,* 119–130.

Verhaak, P. F., Kerssens, J. J., Dekker, J., Sorbi, M., & Bensing, M. (1998). Prevalence of chronic benign pain disorder among adults: A review of the literature. *Pain, 77,* 231–239.

Vernon, H. (1996). The Neck Disability Index: Patient assessment and outcome monitoring whiplash. *Journal of Musculoskeletal Pain, 4,* 95–104.

Vlaeyen, J. W. S., Kole-Snijders, A., Rooteveel, A., Ruesink, R., & Heuts, P. (1995). The role of fear of movement/(re)injury in pain disability. *Journal of Occupational Rehabilitation, 5,* 235–252.

Vlaeyen, J. W. S., Kole-Snijders, A. M., Boeren, R. G. B., & van Eek, H. (1995). Fear of movement/(re)injury in chronic low back pain and its relation to behavioral performance. *Pain, 62,* 363–372.

Waddell, G., McCulloch, J. A., Kummel, E., & Venner, R. M. (1980). Nonorganic physical signs in low-back pain. *Spine, 5,* 117–125.

Ware, J. E., & Sherbourne, C. D. (1992). The MOS 36-Item Short-Form Health Survey (SF-36). *Medical Care, 30,* 473–483.

Watson, P. J., Latif, R. K., & Rowbotham, D. J. (2005). Ethnic differences in thermal pain responses: A comparison of South Asian and White British healthy males. *Pain, 118,* 194–200.

Webster, L. R., & Webster, R. M. (2005). Predicting aberrant behaviors in opioid-treated patients: Preliminary validation of the Opioid Risk Tool. *Pain Medicine, 6,* 432–442.

Welch, K. M. (2003). Contemporary concepts of migraine pathogenesis. *Neurology, 28,* 61(Suppl. 4), S2–S8.

Williams, J. (1998). The malingering of memory disorder. In C. Reynolds (Ed.), *Detection of malingering during head injury litigation* (pp. 73–89). New York: Plenum Press.

Wilson, K. G., Mikail, S. F., D'Eon, J. L., & Minns, J. E. (2001). Alternative diagnostic criteria for major depressive disorder in patients with chronic pain. *Pain, 91,* 227–234.

PART III

ASSESSMENT OF SPECIAL POPULATIONS

CHAPTER 11

Assessment of Pain in Infants, Children, and Adolescents

DANIELLE A. RUSKIN
KHUSH A. AMARIA
FAY F. WARNOCK
PATRICIA A. MCGRATH

The field of pediatric pain assessment is enormous—spanning the developmental continuum from preterm infants to adolescents, ranging widely from simple hand signals that can be used clinically in developing countries to sophisticated physiological imaging techniques primarily used in research, and targeting the diverse array of acute and chronic pains that children can experience. Pain assessment is a dynamic component of pediatric clinical care—beginning with an initial diagnostic examination, extending throughout children's treatment, and culminating with evidence that pain has improved sufficiently. The assessment tools we use differ depending on our clinical objectives: to capture pertinent diagnostic information, to document pain features and symptoms related to different disease conditions, to monitor pain intensity routinely during treatment, to quantify functional impairment, or to assess the psychosocial factors that can exacerbate pain and distress. To achieve these varied objectives, more than 100 pain measures have been developed for infants, children, and adolescents.

Several authors carefully reviewed different pediatric measures (e.g., Champion, Goodenough, von Baeyer, & Thomas, 1998; Cohen et al., 2008; Duhn & Medves, 2004; Hummel & van Dijk, 2006; P. J. McGrath, 1998; Royal College of Nursing Institute, 1999; Stinson, Kavanagh, Yamada, Gill, & Stevens, 2006; Sweet & McGrath, 1998; von Baeyer & Spagrud, 2007) and we provided annotated details of the then roughly 60 measures in the previous edition of this text (McGrath & Gillespie, 2001). In this chapter, we build on information provided from research and clinical practice to describe a practical, evidence-based approach for assessing children's pain. We first describe the situational and developmental factors unique for children so as to provide a framework for choosing among the myriad pain measures based on a child-centered clinical model. We then review the validated pain scales for infants and children, used to assess acute pain and chronic pain, and conclude with suggestions for a versatile set of assessment tools for clinical practice and for conducting research studies to evaluate different therapies.

CHILDREN—"NOT SIMPLY LITTLE ADULTS"

Unprecedented attention has focused on children's pain during the last two decades, so that our knowledge of how children perceive pain and how we can alleviate their suffering has dramatically improved (McGrath, 2005; Schechter, Berde, & Yaster, 2003). As in adults, a child's pain depends on complex neural interactions, where impulses generated by tissue damage are modified by both ascending systems activated by innocuous stimuli and by descending pain-suppressing systems activated by various situational and psychological factors. However, children are not "little adults" with respect to how they perceive pain. The developing nociceptive system responds differently to injury (i.e., increased excitability and sensitization) when compared to the mature adult system. Moreover, children's pain intensity and their pain-related disability is very plastic or modifiable in comparison to that of adults.

Developmental Considerations

Although it is possible to assess distress and pain from infancy throughout adolescence, developmental differences guide our selection of pain measures. Infants exhibit an array of distress behaviors and physiological changes in response to tissue damage. Basic nociceptive connections are formed before birth, so that even the youngest of infants experience pain, but these systems undergo rapid structural and functional maturation, particularly during the neonatal period (Fitzgerald, 1993). Neurophysiological studies in animal models reveal that both high threshold Aδ and low threshold Aβ mechanoreceptors respond at birth with lower firing frequencies than those in the adult animal. Aβ afferents extend dorsally into laminae II and I along with C fibers, rather than into only laminae III and IV, as in the adult animal. Activation of these Aβ afferents evokes excitatory responses more typical of those evoked by Aβ and C fibers in the adult animal. In addition, the receptive fields of dorsal horn cells and somatosensory cortical cells are larger in the newborn. With these larger receptive fields and the dominant A-fiber input, there is an increased likelihood that central cells will be excited by peripheral sensory stimulation, thereby increasing the sensitivity of infant sensory reflexes to stimulation (for review, see Fitzgerald & Walker, 2009). Moreover, descending inhibitory mechanisms are not functional at birth (Boucher, Jennings, & Fitzgerald, 1998), so that an important en-

dogenous analgesic system is lacking, and noxious input may affect neonates more than adults. The immaturity of synaptic connections and integrated circuitry in the newborn means that the infant pain experience is more diffuse and less spatially focused than that in adults, and since it is also under less endogenous control, the system is therefore potentially more powerful. As a result, newborns may be more sensitive to the effects of noxious stimulation and may thus exhibit a stronger behavioral response to pain that is diffuse, inconsistent, and unpredictable compared to that of older children and adults (Fitzgerald & Walker, 2009). As infants mature, the nature and magnitude of their distress responses also change throughout the neonate to infant period.

We must rely on physiological changes and behavioral signals to indicate pain in infants and children who are unable to communicate verbally. However, such signals may be variable in infants and toddlers depending on their pain history and the maturity of their central nervous systems (for a review, see Walker, 2008). For example, repeated exposure to heel lances can cause sensitization to subsequent tissue injury during infancy (Fitzgerald, 1993). This alteration may help explain why some preterm infants exposed to multiple care procedures fail to exhibit a pain response (Johnston et al., 1999; Johnston & Stevens, 1996) and why some full-term infants with a history of repeated pain exposure react more to subsequent heel lance than do infants without that pain exposure (Taddio & Katz, 2005; Taddio, Shah, Gilbert-MacLeod, & Katz, 2002). Full-term newborns with repeated exposure to short-term pain may also learn to anticipate pain before invasive procedures. These newborns exhibit a behavioral response indicative of pain to even the non-noxious cleansing phase of subsequent heel lances (Taddio et al., 2002). Prematurity, low birthweight, age of gestation, and illness severity are additional co-occurring factors that may further hamper the infant's ability to self-regulate in response to routine pain procedures, resulting in heightened vulnerability to pain and individual differences in pain expression (Anand, 1998). Distinguishing pain or evaluating the effects of pain treatment in critically ill infants and toddlers is challenging. These children often display contradictory pain behaviors—agitation, diminishment in pain behavior, or variability in physiological responses due to their illness severity or sedation level (for review, see Ramelet, Abu-Saad, Rees, & McDonald, 2004). Health and developmental factors have implications for infant pain measurement. It is essential to recognize that developmental neurobiological mechanisms and prior pain experience may alter pain experience and pain expression.

Most healthy infants communicate their distress very clearly to their parents, although they do not communicate the nature of their distress. Parents infer that infants have pain based on their cries, behaviors, and the environmental context. When children begin to speak, they communicate more directly the source of their distress—that they are hurt rather than hungry or fearful. Gradually children's understanding of pain and communication develops as they mature and experience various types of pain. Children learn to describe different amounts of pain as they experience new pains that vary in cause, location, strength, quality, and duration. The specific words children use to communicate about pain—where it hurts, how much it hurts and what it feels like—increase as in all language acquisition through children's direct experience and vicarious learning within a particular family and culture. Children's level of cognitive development determines how they are able to understand their sensory experiences and how to communicate with health care providers about their pains. It is essential to use children's own terminology in communicating with them about pain. Because children's concepts of pain follow a consistent developmental pattern (Gaffney, 1988; Harbeck & Peterson, 1992), we should select pain measures that are age-appropriate. For example, most toddlers (approximately 2 years of age) can communicate the presence of pain, using words learned from their parents to describe the sensations they feel when they hurt themselves. They use concrete analogies to describe their perceptions. Gradually children learn to differentiate and describe three levels of pain intensity—basically "a little," "some" or "medium," and "a lot." By the age of 5, most children can differentiate a wider range of pain intensities and use simple quantitative scales to rate their pain

intensity. Thus, administration of a pain measure for children requires a basic appreciation of children's different developmental stages and their cognitive levels.

Factors That Modify Children's Pain and Disability

In comparison to that of adults, a child's pain appears to have a greater degree of plasticity—more influenced by cognitive, behavioral, and emotional factors. "How much it hurts" depends on not only the severity of tissue damage but also psychological factors, such as the meaning or the relevance of the pain, expectations for obtaining eventual recovery and pain relief, and children's coping abilities (McGrath & Dade, 2004). The model shown in Figure 11.1 lists the key situational factors that can modify pain, distress, and pain-related disability. Child characteristics (shown in the lower box), such as age, cognitive level, sex and gender, underlying physical and mental health, prior pain experience, temperament, family, and cultural background generally shape how children experience the various nociceptive or neuropathic sensations evoked by tissue damage (Helgadottir & Wilson, 2004; LeResche, Mancl, Drangsholt, Saunders, & Korff, 2005; Logan & Scharff, 2005). In contrast, the cognitive, behavioral, and emotional factors (listed in the shaded boxes) interact with the child experiencing pain, and the unique and dynamic context in which the pain is experienced (McGrath & Hillier, 2001; Ross & Ross, 1988). What children understand, what they do, and how they feel profoundly impacts their pain experience. For example, children who are well prepared for an invasive procedure and have some control (e.g., choosing which arm to use and engaging in an effective distraction technique during the injection) typically experience significantly less pain than do children who lack information and control.

Cognitive factors encompass parents' and children's beliefs about the cause of pain and its likely time course, expectations for pain control and recovery, knowledge of effective pain control strategies (especially practical strategies children can use independently), and expectations and relevance of pain to children's lives. The aversive relevance may vary from a mild interruption from play for an acute pain caused by an injury to an

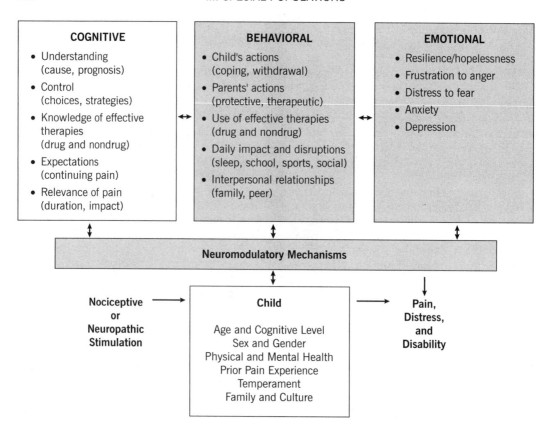

FIGURE 11.1. Situational factors that modify a child's pain.

overwhelming concern that children's lives will be altered forever by disease or chronic pain. Behavioral factors are what children and parents do to prevent and relieve pain, or to protect children from further harm. Specific behaviors vary widely, from a mother providing comfort and reassurance to a toddler who falls while learning to walk, to a family actively seeking extensive medical investigations for a child with unexplained pain. Protective behaviors appropriate for children with acute pain may prolong pain-related disability for children with chronic pain, such as when parents withdraw children from certain activities rather than helping them to participate as much as possible (McGrath & Dade, 2004). Implementation of pain treatments and possible disruptions to family relationships and daily activities are also behavioral factors. Emotional factors include parents' and children's feelings about their pain, underlying health condition (if present), and their feelings about the

adverse impact for the entire family. In addition, some children may have pain caused, significantly exacerbated, or maintained by psychological factors such as anxiety or depression. Children's emotions affect their ability to understand what is happening, their ability to cope positively, their behaviors, and ultimately their pain. Children's immediate emotional reactions to a painful procedure may vary from a relatively neutral acceptance to annoyance, anxiety, fear, frustration, anger, or sadness.

In summary, many children's and parents' beliefs guide children's behaviors and shape their emotional responses to a pain problem. These situational factors affect not only the immediate perception of pain through neuromodulatory mechanisms but also influence a child's pain-related disability and subsequent distress. Thus, assessment should include an appraisal of whether the factors depicted in Figure 11.1 contribute to children's pain, distress, and the quality of their lives.

Acute and Chronic Pain

Most pain measures can be used for many different types of pain, even though very different situational factors are relevant for acute pain from injuries, acute pain from medical treatments, and chronic pain (McGrath & Dade, 2004). The vast majority of pains that infants, children, and adults experience are acute pains caused by injuries. Acute pains usually have a rapid onset and a protective significance, warning children to avoid further physical harm. These pains are symptoms that diminish progressively as injuries heal. A wide array of over-the-counter analgesics provides effective pain relief. Children usually do not experience any prolonged emotional distress, because acute pains are understandable and can be controlled easily. Thus, through experience, children gain an accurate understanding of the pain source and positive expectations for pain relief.

In contrast, children generally approach invasive procedures, such as injections, sutures, and endoscopic procedures, with some trepidation. They often do not know what to expect (with respect to the quality or intensity of the sensations they will feel), they do not know whether the pain will be well controlled; they may believe that they have little control during the procedure, or be worried about how they will cope during the procedure; they may anxiously watch staff to assess how well the procedure is proceeding; and they may be very fearful about an underlying health problem. Thus, the situational factors associated with acute procedural pains are often negative—uncertainty, little perceived control, apprehension, fear, anxiety, and distress.

Unlike acute pain, chronic pain is not always a symptom of active disease or injury. Chronic pain may have multiple sources that comprise nociceptive and neuropathic components rather than a single nociceptive source. The pain often lacks a protective biological significance. Even when triggered by injury, the pain may not lessen progressively as the injury heals. Treatments that relieve acute pain may be wholly ineffective, so that individuals do not know whether they will ever be pain-free again. The continuing pain adversely affects all interpersonal relationships and all aspects of life—family, social, sports, school, and, for adolescents, role functioning at work and in romantic relationships. Children with chronic pain may experience prolonged psychological distress, impaired physical functioning, decreased independence, and often an uncertain prognosis.

Although most pediatric pain measures were developed to assess acute pain, many may also be used to monitor pain intensity and behavioral distress in children with chronic pain. However, increasing attention has focused on the need to develop broader assessment techniques for chronic pain that also capture information about relevant psychosocial, disability, and situational factors.

Properties of Pediatric Pain Scales

Some pain measures are indirect, in that we monitor children's distress behaviors (e.g., facial expression) or physiological indices (e.g., their heart or respiration rates), then infer the presence or strength of pain. In contrast, self-report measures can provide direct information about many subjective dimensions of pain, such as its strength and quality, as well as information about psychosocial factors and the impact of pain for children and families.

Validated pain measures unequivocally quantify a specific dimension of a child's pain, so that changes in a child's pain ratings reflect meaningful differences in a child's pain experience. They provide consistent and trustworthy pain ratings regardless of the time of testing, the clinical setting, or who is administering the measure. Versatile clinical measures are practical for assessing different types of pain and for use in diverse clinical settings.

While several methods have been used to validate pain scales for infants and children, construct or content validity is the most common method. Pain scores are compared before and after children experience a painful stimulus (e.g., heel lance, immunization injection, surgery) and after children receive analgesics to show that pain scores change accordingly. Concurrent validity is demonstrated by showing that pain scores derived on the "newly developed scale" are comparable to ratings on an already validated scale, such as the visual analogue scale. Discriminant validity is established when the pain measure can differentiate among known patient groups that differ in pain experience. The reliability of pain scales is usually determined by comparing the pain scores obtained by different raters for the same child (interrater reliability) and by correlating the scores among individual items or subscales (internal consistency). The psychometric properties of pain scales, as well as the methods used to determine validity and reliability, are provided in the original citations for pediatric pain measures included in Tables 11.1–11.5. Health care providers should use consistent criteria for monitoring children, scoring behavioral and physiological changes, and tabulating data to derive a child's pain score. Pain scores obtained from different pain scales are not necessarily equivalent, so that a "4" may be strong pain on one scale but represent moderate pain on another. Some scales use numbers to represent different pain intensity levels (e.g., "no pain" = 0, "mild pain" = 1, "moderate pain" = 2, and "strong pain" = 3). The numbers are often interpreted as if they represent absolute and accurate amounts of pain. Unless an investigator studies the relationship between a child's pain level and the numbers he or she uses to rate it, we only know that larger numbers mean stronger pain; however, we do not know *how much* stronger. As a result, when evaluating treatment effects, we cannot assume that a child who reports that a treatment lessened a pain from a score of 2 to 1 ("moderate" to "mild") is equivalent to a reduction from 3 to 2 ("strong" to "moderate") for another child. Similarly, when a child rates a pain as a 3, the pain level may not really be three times the strength of the pain he or she rates as a 1. Nevertheless, most pain scores are interpreted as if they represent numbers on equal interval or ratio scales.

PAIN SCALES FOR INFANTS AND TODDLERS

Behavioral and Composite Pain Scales

An extensive array of pain scales has been developed and validated for use with infants and toddlers (for review, see Crellin, Sullivan, Babl, O'Sullivan, & Hutchinson, 2007; Duhn & Medves, 2004; Hummel & van Dijk, 2006; Stevens, Pillai Riddell, Oberlander, & Gibbons, 2007). In this section, we summarize key information on available

measures that may be used clinically for infants and toddlers. Infant pain measures include both behavioral scales that comprise behavioral distress indices, such as crying, facial action, motor movement, and sleep state, as listed in Table 11.1, and various composite scales that also include physiological indices, such as changes in heart rate (HR), oxygen saturation, and blood pressure from baseline, as shown in Table 11.2. Pain scales are listed according to developmental age from preterm to toddler, with the formal name of the scale, acronym, citation; the age of the child, the type of pain measured, and condition of the infant; and the number of distress behaviors or physiological indicators monitored. Of special note, in the last two columns of Tables 11.1 and 11.2, we provide practical information about scales, including (1) whether items are operationally defined and thus provide clear criteria for rating behaviors, (2) whether scales are easy to use and require minimal training, and (3) whether additional scoring equipment is required (e.g., audio- or videotape).

The number of distress indicators varies widely across scales, from 3 to 13. For example, the *Postoperative Pain Score* (POPS; Barrier, Attia, Mayer, Amiel-Tison, & Shnider, 1989), measures 10 behavioral distress indicators, including sleep during the proceeding hour, facial expression, quality of cry, consolability, sociability, sucking, spontaneous excitability, spontaneous motor activity, flexion of fingers and toes, and tone. Other, shorter scales typically measure a few basic indices (e.g., cry, facial expression, and movement), such as the *Modified Behavioral Pain Scale* (MBPS; Taddio & Katz, 2005). Of note, some scales include items that are age-specific. For example, sleep–wake state is typically included in scales developed for preterm infants but is not regularly included in scales for full-term infants. State regulation occurs by approximately 27–30 weeks' gestational age (Curzi-Dascalova et al., 1993), thus stabilizing neurological, physiological, and stress subsystems (Als, 1982). However, regulation may be immature in the preterm infant and easily disrupted. The inclusion of this item enables clinicians to measure the effect of pain stimuli on a variable important to the development of the preterm and can help guide pain-reducing treatments that include reducing environ-

TABLE 11.1. Behavioral Pain Measures for Infants and Toddlers (Listed According to Age)

Measure	Age group Infant	Age group GA (wk)	Age group Months	Age group Years	Type of pain/ condition	Number of indicators	Operational definition	Clinical ease/ equipment
Douleur Aigue du Nouveau-né (DAN; Carbajal et al., 1999)	PT	23–41			P, PO/M	3	OD	
Behavioral Indicators of Infant Pain (BIIP; Holsti & Grunau, 2007)	PT	24–31			P	13	OD	V
Neonatal Pain and Discomfort Scale (EDIN; Debillon et al., 2001)	PT	25–36			P/I	5	OD	
Neonatal Infant Pain Scale (NIPS; Lawrence et al., 1993)	PT/FT	28–34	0–2		P/M, I	6	OD	E
Behavior Pain Score (BPScore; Pokela, 1994)	PT/FT	31	0–1		P/M, I	4		
Modified Postoperative Comfort Score (PCS; Guinsberg et al., 1998)	PT	≤32			PO/M, I	7		V
ABC Pain Scale (Bellieni et al., 2005)	PT/FT	34±2	0–1		P	3		A
Neonatal Facial Coding System (NFCS; Grunau & Craig, 1987)	PT/FT		0–18		P, PO	10	OD	E/V
Modified Behavioral Pain Scale (MBPS; Taddio et al., 1995)	FT		1–6		P	3	OD	
Liverpool Infant Distress Scale (LIDS; Horgan & Choonara, 1996)	FT				PO	9		
Children's and Infants' Postoperative Pain Scale (CHIPPS; Büttner & Finke, 2000)	FT			0–5	PO	5	OD	E
Postoperative Pain Score (POPS; Barrier et al., 1989)	FT			T[a]	PO	10	OD	E
Riley Infant Pain Scale (RIPS; Schade et al., 1996)	FT			T[a]	PO	6	OD	E
Nursing Assessment of Pain Intensity (NAPI; Stevens, 1990)	FT			T[a]	PO	4	OD	E
Behavioral Pain Scale (BPScale; Robieux et al., 1991)	FT			T	P/CI	3		E
Pain Observation Scale for Young Children (POCIS; Boelen-van der Loo et al., 1999)	FT			1–4	PO	7	OD	E/V
Toddler/Preschool Postoperative Pain Tool (TPPPS; Tarbell et al., 1991)	FT			1–5	P, PO	7	OD	E
Face, Legs, Activity, Cry, Consolability (FLACC; Merkel et al., 1997)	FT			1–5[b]	PO	5	OD	E

Note. PT, preterm; FT, full-term; GA, gestational age (provided in weeks); T, toddlers; P, procedural pain; PO, postoperative pain; M, mechanically intubated; I, ill or critically ill; CI, chronically ill; OD, operational definitions are provided; E, clinical ease (requires short training and/or easy to use) is reported in at least one study; V, special video recording equipment required; A, special audio recording equipment required.

[a]Can be used with nonverbal children of any age with cerebral palsy.

[b]Can be used with nonverbal children with mild or severe cognitive impairment.

219

TABLE 11.2. Composite Pain Measures for Infants and Toddlers (Listed According to Age)

Measure	Age group Infant	GA (wk)	Months	Years	Type of pain/ condition	Number of indicators	Operational definition	Clinical ease/ equipment
Neonatal Pain, Agitation, and Sedation Scale (N-PASS; Hummel & Puchalski, 2002)	PT/FT	23–40			PO/I, CI	5 (4/1)	OD	
Scale for Use in Newborns (SUN; Blauer & Gerstmann, 1998)	PT/FT	24–40			P/I, CI	6 (4/2)		E
Nepean Neonatal Intensive Care Unit Pain Assessment Tool (NNICUPAT; Marceau, 2003)	PT/FT	26–35			P/M, I	7 (4/3)	OD	
Pain Assessment in Neonates (PAIN; Hudson-Barr et al., 2002)	PT	26–47			—/I	7 (5/2)		
Pain Assessment Tool (PAT; Hodgkinson et al., 1994; Spence et al., 2005)	PT/FT	27–40			PO/M, I	10 (7/3)	OD	E
Premature Infant Pain Profile (PIPP; Stevens et al., 1996)	PT	28–42			P, PO	7 (4/3)	OD	E
Crying, Requires Oxygen, Increased Vital Signs, Expression, Sleepless (CRIES; Krechel & Bildner, 1995)	PT/FT	32–60	0–3		PO/I	5 (2/3)	OD	E
Multidimensional Assessment Pain Scale (MAPS; Ramelet et al., 2007)	FT		0–31		P, PO/I	5 (4/1)	OD	
COMFORT Scale (Ambuel et al., 1992)	FT		0–36		P, PO/M	9 (7/2)	OD	E
Modified Infant Pain Scale (MIPS; Buchholz et al., 1998)	FT		1–8		PO	13 (10/2)		E
Preverbal, Early-Verbal Pediatric Pain Scale (PEPPS; Schultz et al., 1999)	FT			T	PO	7 (6/1)		E/V
Objective Pain Scale/or Pain Discomfort Scale (OPS); Broadman et al., 1988)	FT			1–13	PO	5 (4/1)		E

Note. PT, preterm; FT, full-term; GA, gestational age (provided in weeks); T, toddlers; P, procedural pain; PO, postoperative pain; M, mechanically intubated; I, ill or critically ill; CI, chronically ill; —, no additional information provided; OD, operational definitions are provided; E, clinical ease (requires short training and/or easy to use) is reported in at least one study; V, special video recording equipment required mental stimuli, such as sound, and instituting comfort measures, such as containment. For postoperative scales that include sleep–wake state, it is recommended that baseline assessment of this indicator be taken 1 hour before surgery, because sleep patterns in the first hour following surgery are influenced by prior general anesthesia (van Dijk, Peters, Boumeester, & Tibboel, 2002).

All infant pain scales were validated for either procedural (P) or postoperative pain (PO), as designated in Tables 11.1 and 11.2. Postoperative scales are useful to assess acute pain and prolonged pain, while procedural scales are useful for brief, acute pains caused by tissue injury from diagnostic heel lances, venipunctures, and distress-provoking care events, such as suctioning. As shown in Tables 11.1 and 11.2, the majority of scales for preterm infants were designed to assess procedural pain. Of the scales validated for preterm infants, seven are for mechanically intubated preterm infants, 11 are for critically ill preterms, and three are for chronically ill preterms. The majority of scales that assess postoperative pain were developed for full-term infants and toddlers.

Some scales provide operational definitions of complex behaviors, such as grimacing and breathing patterns on the *Neonatal Infant Pain Scale* (NIPS; Lawrence et al., 1993). These definitions enhance objective and unbiased measurement. Operational definitions are not a simple listing of pain indicators. Rather, they are formal explanations written so that the meaning of the indicator can be commonly understood and measured. For example, while the behavioral item "grimacing" is simply listed in some scales, the operational definition "tight facial muscles furrowed brow chin jaw (negative facial expression—nose mouth brow)" in the NIPS allows raters to know exactly what to look for when scoring an infant's pain. Clear, unambiguous definitions of a scale's various distress behaviors are critical, because they enable health care providers to use uniform criteria rather than only their interpretation of children's distress when they rate pain levels. In the second to last column of Tables 11.1 and 11.2, we denote scales that provide operational definitions with the letters "OD."

Health care providers must be adequately trained to follow each scale's guidelines on how long to monitor infants and how often to repeat scoring. Frequent time sampling usually enhances accuracy in measurement, because more assessments are made during the period of observation, enabling one to capture changes in pain more accurately. Scales differ in terms of the training and equipment required for their use. For example, one single assessment of the *Children's and Infants' Postoperative Pain Scale* (CHIPPS; Büttner & Finke, 2000) takes only 15 seconds to identify the presence and intensity of an operationally defined behavior. Scales that require minimal training and no special equipment are likely most advantageous for nursing staff with multiple care responsibilities.

Other scales, such as the *Neonatal Facial Coding System* (NFCS; Grunau & Craig, 1987), the *Behavioral Indicators of Infant Pain* (BIIP; Holsti & Grunau, 2007), and the ABC Pain Scale (Bellieni et al., 2005), require the use of sophisticated recording equipment since they consist of behaviors such as changes in facial action or crying that occur too rapidly or are too detailed to code accurately via direct observation or listening. Their application requires extensive training of raters to ensure that coding of prerecorded behaviors between raters is systematically derived, unbiased, and reliable. These scales also necessitate blinding so that pain raters do not know the particular context (e.g., before or after analgesic administration). At present, such scales are best suited for research, although the NFCS has also been tested for bedside application with premature infants (Grunau, Oberlander, Holsti, & Whitfield, 1998) and BIIP workshops and video training have been developed for its clinical use. Scales that have been reported in at least one study as demonstrating clinical ease are denoted in the final column of Tables 11.1 and 11.2 with the letter "E." Those that require use of special equipment are denoted with the letter "V" for videotape or "A" for audiotape. We recommend that clinicians consider the time intensity and the availability for training when deciding to use such scales.

As shown in Table 11.2, composite scales also vary in terms of the types of behaviors and physiological parameters depending on age, illness severity, and types of pain monitored. Typical physiological indices include blood pressure, HR, and oxygen saturation level. For example, the (Crying, Requires Oxygen, Increased Vital Signs, Expression, Sleepless) *CRIES* scale (Krechel & Bildner, 1995) requires assessment of oxygen saturation, HR, blood pressure, sleeplessness, and crying. In contrast to behavioral scales, the majority of composite scales pertain to critically ill infants born prematurely and/ or infants with low birthweight and those requiring mechanical ventilation, including toddlers. Critically ill infants and children who require mechanical ventilation and/or sedation often exhibit responses that range from agitation to immobility, which makes it difficult to distinguish acute or prolonged pain from general distress. Almost all pain scales may be used with critically ill children but two. The *Neonatal Pain, Agitation, and Sedation Scale* (N-PASS; Hummel & Puchalski, 2002) and the *COMFORT* Scale (Ambuel, Hamlett, Marx, & Blumer, 1992) were specifically developed or validated to assess prolonged pain and distress in critically ill, mechanically ventilated, and/or sedated infants. These composite scales differ from scales used with healthy infants, in that they require scoring sedation levels, in addition to behavioral and physiological pain items. Concurrent scoring of pain and sedation is essential, because these infants are at increased risk for the adverse consequences of pain, and mechanical ventilation and sedation can mask their overt pain responses. These scores also help in determining the demand and effects of pharmacological pain treatment. For example, the Total Pain score derived from the N-PASS is used not only to assess the infant's response to stimuli but also to determine the optimal level of sedation (Hummel & Puchalski, 2002).

The combinations of behavioral and physiological measures may also yield a more sensitive pain score for newborns and young children following major surgery. For example, van Dijk and colleagues (2001) found low to moderate correlations between COMFORT behavior scores and mean arterial pressure variability in children ages 0–3 years following major surgery, independent of gender, physical condition, surgical stress, or morphine condition/dose. As the level of pain increased, the behavior–physiology correlations increased. Hence, although behavioral pain scales are generally recommended

for children ages 0–3 following minor surgery (without arterial line), the combination of physiological and behavioral measures is preferred following major surgery, especially when the child's behavioral pain response appears strong (van Dijk et al., 2001). Additionally, physiological indicators are primarily used for assessing pain in preterm infants following surgery because of high variability in their behavioral expression of pain over time, and because physiological measures help guide pharmacological pain treatment.

Some scales, such as the *Premature Infant Pain Profile* (PIPP; Stevens, Johnston, Petryshen, & Taddio, 1996), incorporate baseline information on gestation age and HR so that infants' Total Pain score can be adjusted. For example, the pain responses of infants of very low gestational age (e.g., < 27 weeks gestation) are less intense and sustained, making it difficult to detect pain-related changes in their HR. Thus, adjusting for gestation age avoids interpreting that infants are "pain-free."

As shown, behavioral and composite scales vary widely in terms of their characteristics and features. Hence, utility depends on whether a scale provides necessary operational definitions, clear instructions on sampling, and time required for training, and the required type of equipment requirements.

Selecting a Pain Scale for Infants and Toddlers: Special Considerations

At present, no single scale is appropriate for all infants and toddlers. Instead, scales should be selected on the basis of infant age, health condition, the type of pain to be assessed, and the clinical or research perspective. Of the 30 scales listed in Tables 11.1 and 11.2, 19 pertain to infants, nine to toddlers, and three to a wider age range that includes infants, toddlers, and children. Although all the scales may be used throughout a prolonged observation period to assess acute and chronic pain, almost all of these measures were initially validated as tools to assess the strength of acute pain caused by invasive procedures or postoperatively in healthy infants and toddlers. However, 19 scales have been developed or tested for use with preterm infants, and infants and toddlers with complex conditions, and/or were developed to assess prolonged or chronic pain and distress. Health care providers could use these scales in a time sampling manner and monitor infants throughout a prolonged period.

Health care providers should recognize the impact of an infant's health state when selecting a pain measure. Although moderate associations have been demonstrated between behavioral and physiological parameters for acute pain in premature infants (Johnston, Stevens, Yang, & Horton, 1995), associations are weaker for some critically ill infants because of central nervous system (CNS) immaturity, age, severity of illness, exposure to repeated pain procedures, and concomitant stress (Barr, 1998). The use of composite rather than behavioral pain scales is recommended for these children. However, because some preterm infants exhibit a weak or a subtle HR change in response to painful procedures, it is important to know the potential limitations of composite measures. In these infants, change in facial action may be more robust; hence, this indicator may receive more weight than HR when the total composite score is calculated. As a result, the interpretation of the total composite score may be more based on change in facial action and an underestimation of pain related changes in HR. This has implications for pain care decision making and for determining the effects of pain treatment. For these reasons, we recommend that separate measures of HR be taken when using a composite pain scale with critically ill preterm infants. We also recommend supplemental measures when assessing pain intensity in critically ill children who are mechanically ventilated. In these children, physiological adaptation occurs rapidly, and sedation may blunt pain response (Brinker, 2004). Although sedation and mechanical ventilation affect physiological pain indices, we recommend that composite scales be used for critically ill children, because both behavioral and physiological indices provide valuable information about pain and stress dysregulation that may not be captured by behavioral scales alone (Ramelet et al., 2004). Sedation level should also be measured.

We have the tools to regularly assess pain for infants and toddlers. However, challenges remain for health care providers in judging pain as it relates to infant age. Older infants are generally judged to have more pain than younger infants despite controlling for vigor in behavior pain response (Craig, Korol, & Pillai, 2002). The underestimate of pain in younger children by clinicians may be due to observer bias, which may occur for several reasons. Some clinicians may still believe that younger children experience less pain than older children. Others may lack knowledge about the unpredictable and variable nature of pain expression in younger children and the many factors that may influence it. Clinicians' frequency of exposure to the pain in others is also thought to have a conditioning effect that may result in less sensitivity in pain rating (Craig et al., 2002). It is essential to recognize the potential impact of observer bias and the clinical environment in interpreting an infant's pain score. Health care providers should base treatment decisions on not only the pain score but also their clinical judgment about key health factors that may influence scores. Existing infant pain scales do not yet incorporate weighting factors to account for the effects of the clinical environment on pain response. Preliminary data suggest that ambient sound (Warnock & Sandrin, 2004) and increased handling (Holsti, Grunau, Oberlander, & Whitfield, 2005) can prolong pain reactivity and regulation in infants. Such contextual factors will probably be included in future scale revisions as we continue to gain new knowledge about their importance in mediating pain responses.

PAIN SCALES FOR CHILDREN

The vast majority of pain scales for children were validated initially as measures of pain intensity for acute pain caused by invasive medical treatments. The noxious stimulus is evident, the evoked pain is brief, and children should be able to distinguish pain-free periods before and after the painful medical treatment enabling investigators to determine the validity of the measure. Then, the scale could be used to assess the intensity of other types of pain at discrete intervals. Pain scales for children include a diverse array of behavioral scales, self-report scales measuring pain intensity, and psychosocial pain questionnaires and interviews that assess multiple dimensions of children's pain experiences.

Behavioral Pain Scales

Several behavioral pain scales were developed to quantify children's pain at discrete time intervals during invasive procedures and to monitor children's pain intensity after surgery. Comparable to infant pain scales, most of these scales require health care providers and, in some cases, parents to document specified distress behaviors (e.g., crying, muscle tension, flailing). Behavioral scales are particularly useful for assessing pain in children who cannot reliably communicate pain via self-report, such as children who are preverbal, cognitively impaired, or restricted by bandages, ventilators, or immobilizing medications. For children who can communicate, behavioral measures are a valuable adjunct to self-report scales when subjective pain ratings are regarded as exaggerated or minimized because of cognitive, emotional, or behavioral factors (von Baeyer & Spagrud, 2007).

In general, behavioral scales for children differ with respect to the number of behaviors recorded (varying from 3 to 20), whether raters also rank the intensity of each behavior, such as rating "cry" from 0 = *no cry* to 3 = *full-lunged cry* on the *Children's Hospital of Eastern Ontario Pain Scale* (CHEOPS; P. J. McGrath et al., 1985), and whether assessors assign predetermined weights to behaviors to reflect different pain intensities, so that "scream" receives a higher weight than "quiet crying sounds" on the *Observational Scale of Behavioral Distress* (OSBD; Jay, Ozolins, Elliott, & Caldwell, 1983). All behavioral scales yield a numerical pain score—either the sum of all observed behavioral indicators or a composite pain score derived from the weighted scores for each observed behavior.

In Table 11.3 we list 23 behavioral pain scales for children, noting whether the scale is scored simply during routine care with minimal training, or whether the scale requires intensive training, along with specialized monitoring and scoring equipment. For each scale, we provide the formal scale name and acronym, the number of distress indicators monitored, whether or not distress indicators are operationally defined, the type of pain measured, and the age range for which the scale was developed. As seen in the second column of Table 11.3, some pain scales,

such as the *Douleur de L'Enfant Goustave-Roussy* (DEGR; Gauvain-Piquard, Rodary, Rezvani, & Lemerle, 1987), also include distress indicators that reflect children's anxiety and mood.

The number of distress indicators varies widely across scales, from three to 20. For example, the *Procedure Behavior Checklist* (PBCL; LeBaron & Zeltzer, 1984) measures eight behaviors, including muscle tension, screaming, crying, restraint used, pain verbalized, anxiety verbalized, verbal stalling, and physical resistance. The *Child–Adult Medical Procedure Interaction Scale—Revised* (CAMPIS-R; Blount et al., 1997) contains many of these same distress indicators (e.g., scream, cry, and verbal resistance, to name a few) and also includes intricate coding to assess children's coping and neutral behaviors, as well as adult coping promoting, distress promoting, and neutral behaviors. In general, most scales measure basic distress indices, such as cry, facial expression, and movement. Behavioral ratings are typically made by health care providers, but several scales can be rated by staff or parents, including the *Paediatric Pain Profile* (PPP; Hunt et al., 2004), *Paediatric Observational Quality of Life Questionnaire* (PQL; Myatt & Myatt, 1998), *Individualized Numeric Rating Scale* (INRS; Solodiuk & Curley, 2003), *Revised Faces, Legs, Activity, Cry and Consolability Behavioral Pain Assessment Tool* (FLACC; Malviya, Voepel-Lewis, Burke, Merkel, & Tait, 2006), and *Non-Communicating Children's Pain Checklist* (NCCPC; Breau, McGrath, Camfield, Rosmus, & Finley, 2000). The *Parents' Postoperative Pain Measure* (PPPM; Chambers, Finley, McGrath, & Walsh, 2003) is only parent-rated.

Behavioral scales for children differ in terms of how well behavioral distress indicators are operationally defined. All scales listed in Table 11.3 provide some definition of the behaviors to be rated. However, definitions vary such that some leave minimal room for interpretation, whereas others require coders to draw on their own experience or frame of reference to make ratings. For example, the OSBD (Jay et al., 1983) provides clear criteria on which to rate a child's verbal pain:

> any words, phrases, or statements which refer to pain, damage or being hurt, or discomfort.

TABLE 11.3. Behavioral Pain Measures for Children (Listed by Date)

Measure	Number of pain/distress indicators	Quality of operational definition	Type of pain	Age (yr)
Scales that require minimal training				
Procedural Behavioral Rating Scale—Revised (PBRS-R; Katz, Kellerman, & Siegel, 1980)	13	I	P	6–10
Children's Hospital of Eastern Ontario Pain Scale (CHEOPS; P. J. McGrath et al., 1985)	6	I	PO	1–7
Behavioral Approach–Avoidance and Distress Scale (BAADS; Hubert et al., 1988)	3; approach–avoidance items	II	P	3–7
Groningen Distress Scale (GDS; Humphrey et al., 1992)	3	II	P	2.5–18
Princess Margaret Hospital Pain Assessment Tool (PMH-PAT; Robertson, 1993)	5	II	PO	7–14
FLACC (Facial expression, Leg movement, Activity, Cry, Consolability; Merkel et al., 1997)	5	II	P	2–7
Paediatric Observational Quality of Life Questionnaire (PQL; Myatt & Myatt, 1998)	8	I	PO	2–13
Pain Observation Scale for Young Children (POCIS; Boelen-van der Loo et al., 1999)	7	I	PO/R	1–4
Non-Communicating Children's Pain Checklist (NCCPC; Breau et al., 2000)	7	I	R	3–44[a]
Parents' Postoperative Pain Measure (PPPM; Chambers et al., 2003)	15	I	PO	2–12
Derbyshire Children's Hospital Pain Tool (DPC; Peden et al., 2003)	3	II	PO	1–5
Alder Hey Triage Pain Score (AHTPS; Stewart et al., 2004)	5	II	ER	0–16
Paediatric Pain Profile (PPP; Hunt et al., 2004)	20	II	R	1–18[a]
Behavioural Observational Pain Scale (BOPS; Hesselgard et al., 2007)	3	II	PO	1–7
Individualized Numeric Rating Scale (INRS; Solodiuk & Curley, 2003)	Pain behavior specific to child stratified from 0–10	—	R	> 3[a]
Scales that require additional equipment/training				
Observational Scale of Behavioral Distress (OSBD; Jay et al., 1983)	11	I	P	6–10
Procedure Behavior Checklist (PBCL; LeBaron & Zeltzer, 1984)	8	I	P	6–18
Douleur de l'enfant Goustave-Roussy (DEGR; Gauvain-Piquard et al., 1987)	7; mood and anxiety items	I	R	2–6
Child–Adult Medical Procedure Interaction Scale—Revised (CAMPIS-R; Blount et al., 1997)	6; child coping items	I	P	2–13
Child Facial Coding System (CFCS; Gilbert et al., 1999)	13	I	PO	1–6
Child–Adult Medical Procedure Interaction Scale—Short Form (CAMPIS-SF; Blount et al., 2001)	4; child coping items	I	P	3–7
Brief Behavioral Distress Scale (BBDS; Tucker et al., 2001)	4	I	P	2–1
Revised FLACC (Malviya et al., 2006)	5	II	PO	4–19[a]

Note. I, very good (well defined); II, good (defined; some room for interpretation); P, procedural; PO, postoperative; R, recurrent; ER, emergency room.
[a]Scales validated for children with cognitive impairment.

Must be intelligible. May be in *any tense.* Can be anticipatory as well as actual. Has to be a statement, *not a question.* This category is distinguishable from "cry" by coding discrete intelligible *words* as pain ("owh," "ouch") and non-word crying sounds as "cry." Only exception is groans without crying are coded as verbal pain ("ahhh"). (Jay & Elliott, 1986, p. 2, original emphasis)

In contrast, an item on the *Princess Margaret Hospital Pain Assessment Tool* (PMH-PAT; Robertson, 1993) requires a nurse to assess a child's level of pain with instructions as follows: *Using your previous experience, decide how much pain you think the child has. Input from the parent may also be used at this time.* A child's pain is then rated in intervals of 0.5 from 0 = "no pain" to 2 = "severe pain." The reliability and validity of this scale may be compromised, because ratings vary depending on a rater's prior experience and on contextual factors, such as whether a parent is in the room, or whether the rater is familiar with the child. For situations where multiple staff members evaluate a child's pain, it is necessary to use scales with well-defined criteria to promote consistency across raters.

A major feature that distinguishes among the varied behavioral pain scales is whether health care providers can use the scale quickly and easily in clinical practice. Some scales involve time-consuming procedures, such as intensive training of raters, videotaping events, and subsequent transcribing and coding of tapes. To help readers select scales suitable for their individual goals and settings, the pain scales in Table 11.3 are stratified according to whether the scale can be simply scored and requires minimal equipment or training. For example, CAMPIS-R (Blount et al., 1997) yields rich information about children's distress and coping during acute procedures but is not yet suitable for most clinical situations given extensive time demands associated with videotaping, transcribing, and coding behaviors. To address this limitation, a short form of the CAMPIS-R was developed that reduces coding requirements but still requires videotape (Blount, Bunke, Cohen, & Forbes, 2001). In contrast, the Procedural Behavior Rating Scale—Revised (PBRS-R; Katz, Kellerman,

& Siegel, 1980) is easily scored in real-time situations (e.g., patient's room), does not need any special equipment, and requires minimal training.

Many of the behavioral items across scales listed in Table 11.3 are very similar to one another, because they have been revised with use to better reflect our increased understanding of how children express pain through their behaviors and our practical experience using these scales in different clinical settings. For example, the PBRS (Katz et al., 1980), one of the first scales to measure procedural distress, was revised to increase its sensitivity and validity by including continuous recording of behavior (vs. recording only specific events) and weighting behaviors (vs. simply coding the presence or absence of behavior). This revised version, which retains many PBRS items, was named the *Observational Scale of Behavioral Distress* (OSBD; Jay et al., 1983). As more studies were published using the OSBD, it became evident that researchers varied considerably in defining the phase (i.e., anticipatory, procedural, recovery) and duration of the medical procedure during which child behaviors were coded (Blount, Sturges, & Powers, 1990). The OSBD was thus modified so that coding of behaviors occurred during discrete procedural events (e.g., "cleaning injection site" or "needle insertion"), resulting in a more consistent coding framework that could be used across settings, independent of a procedure's sequence or duration. The revised scale was termed the *Brief Behavioral Distress Scale* (BBDS; Tucker, Slifer, & Dahlquist, 2001).

Only recently have efforts turned to validating behavioral scales for assessing pain in children with cognitive impairment. Children with cognitive delays are at greater risk for receiving inadequate pain treatment in comparison to normally developing peers, who more easily express their pain (Malviya et al., 2001; Stallard, Williams, Lenton, & Velleman, 2001). Assessing pain-related distress in children with cognitive impairment is complicated by the fact that "typical" pain behaviors, such as moaning and facial changes, are frequently exhibited by these children in the absence of pain (Breau et al., 2000). Observational scales have thus been modified or developed, often with input from parents, to include pain behaviors specific to children with cognitive delays. Three such scales are identified in the Table 11.3 footnote. The NCCPC (Breau et al., 2000) has been revised to assess postoperative pain (Breau, McGrath, Camfield, & Finley, 2002) and a short-form version has received preliminary validation (Breau, Camfield, McGrath, Rosmus, & Finley, 2001). Because scales for children with cognitive impairment generally depend on parents' knowledge of their child to make a judgment, reliability of scores may be reduced when behaviors are rated by nonparents.

The majority of scales listed in Table 11.3 measure either procedural or postoperative pain, with some exceptions. The *Alder Hey Triage Pain Score* (AHTPS; Stewart, Lancaster, Lawson, Williams, & Daly, 2004) evaluates pain in children admitted to the emergency room. Pain assessment scales for children with cognitive impairment are designed to assess children's recurrent pains and pain during hospital admissions (as on the NRS; Solodiuk & Curley, 2003). In general, procedural pain scales assess behaviors that occur during procedural phases, for example, before, during, and after a needle stick on the CAMPIS-R (Blount et al., 1997), and either use short time intervals (e.g., 2–3 minutes) or continuous recording to assess behaviors during each phase. Postoperative pain scales use longer time intervals, for example, morning, afternoon, and evening on the PPPM (Chambers et al., 2003), since they are not anchored by discrete procedural events.

A final point concerns whether behavioral scales may be used to assess chronic pain. Scales listed in Table 11.3 generally measure the robust, reflexive responses displayed by otherwise healthy children during acute pain (e.g., withdrawal, vocalizing, grimacing). As noted by von Baeyer and Spagrud (2007), these behaviors can rapidly attenuate in children with chronic pain and be replaced by more covert responses, such as rigidity, silence, and guarding the painful area. Thus, children with chronic pain may not score as high as children with acute pain despite comparable pain levels. Behavioral scales that assess the affective impact of pain, such as Depression and Anxiety on the DEGR (Gauvain-Piquard et al., 1987) or behavioral scales that measure coping, such as the CAMPIS-R (Blount et al., 1997), may be most appropriate for assessing behaviors related to the impact of chronic pain.

Despite the many benefits of using behavioral scales, scores should be interpreted with some caution. All children do not consistently display the same type of distress behavior in direct proportion to the intensity of their pain experience. Behavioral pain scores do not always correlate with children's own pain ratings (Walco, Conte, Labay, Engel, & Zeltzer, 2005). Some children may behave stoically but still experience pain, whereas others may exhibit many distress behaviors in clinics even before a scheduled painful treatment. Children's cultural backgrounds may underlie these differences given recent research indicating that culture can affect a child's pain expression, especially the intensity of pain behaviors (Finley, Kristjansdottir, & Forgeron, 2009). Ultimately, the relationship between children's pain and their behaviors is influenced by the situational factors shown in Figure 11.1. Thus, it is important to interpret children's pain scores within the context in which they experience pain, their cultural background, and within the limitations of behaviors they display.

Self-Report Measures

As the "gold standard" in pain assessment, self-report measures enable children to communicate directly about their pain experience and its impact on their lives. Many analog scales, facial scales, word checklists, pain diaries, clinical interviews, and pain questionnaires are used clinically to assess children's pain. Most health care providers ask children directly about their pain features—onset, location, intensity, quality, and pattern (as depicted in Figure 11.2). Pain clinics typically document pain history and treatment efficacy using a standardized format that might include several complementary pain measures for children and parents.

Since Eland's pivotal studies of childhood pain and her development of the *Eland Color Tool* (Eland & Anderson, 1977), a body outline on which children colored their pain using different colors to indicate different intensities, much research has investigated developing pain intensity measures

Pain History	• Onset • Investigations conducted • Radiological and laboratory results • Consult results • Analgesic and adjuvant medications (type, dose, frequency, route)		
Location(s)	☐ single or ☐ multiple sites		
	☐ head	☐ arm or hand	☐ pelvis
	☐ oral/facial	☐ back	☐ genital, perineal, anal
	☐ neck or shoulder	☐ abdomen	☐ leg or foot
Intensity	Current _____ ; Usual _____ ; Range: Min _____ to Max _____ Note: At rest/On activity		
Temporal Pattern	☐ Constant		
	☐ Daily episodes	☐ 1 time/week	☐ 2–3 times/week
	☐ 1–2 times/month	☐ other _____	
	Episode length:		
	☐ few minutes	☐ ½ hour	☐ couple hours (2–3)
	☐ several hours (4–6)	☐ all day (12)	☐ other _____
Quality	☐ aching	☐ hot	☐ stabbing
	☐ burning	☐ pounding	☐ stinging
	☐ cold	☐ sharp	☐ throbbing
	☐ cutting	☐ shooting	☐ tingling
	☐ dull	☐ squeezing	☐ other _____

FIGURE 11.2. Components of pain assessment.

for children. We know that children can use many different scales to rate the intensity of their pain. In response to "How much does it hurt?", children can choose a position along a continuum or a level on a scale that best describes the strength of their own pain. Often children are asked to choose a number from 0, representing "no pain," to 10, representing "strongest pain possible," choose a face that depicts distress, or choose a term, from "a little, or mild" to "a lot, or intense." All pain intensity scales yield a numerical score and are generally easy to administer, requiring only a few seconds to complete once children understand how to use the scale. They are versatile and can assess acute and chronic pain in diverse clinical and home settings. Given the plethora of pain intensity scales currently available, in Table 11.4 we provide a sampling of commonly used and clinically valid pain intensity scales that represent the variations in analogue and categorical scales in use. Although all provide useful informa-

tion about a child's pain intensity for acute and chronic pain, they have different limitations depending on one's clinical or research objectives.

Analogue scales provide a continuum of possible pain intensities using a ratio scale, such as on the 14.5-cm wedge on the *Coloured Analogue Scale* (CAS; McGrath et al., 1996). Ratio or analogue scales indicate that there is a set position or order between numbers, that the magnitude of the difference between numbers is the same (i.e., a difference in pain score between 8 and 9 is equivalent to the difference between 3 and 4), and that the numbers reflect actual ratios of magnitudes and allow for comparisons across children. Precise conclusions about how much different pains vary in strength or how much a child's pain has lessened after treatment are valid when ratio scales are used. In contrast, rating scales that include a discrete number of levels (e.g., "none," "mild," "moderate," "strong," "intense")

TABLE 11.4. Self-Report Pain Intensity Scales for Children

Measure	Pain score	Ages (yr)
Analogue scales		
Pain Ladder (Hester et al., 1990)	0–10	5–13
Coloured Analogue Scale (CAS; McGrath et al., 1996)	0–10	5–18
Visual Analogue Scale (VAS; P. A. McGrath et al., 1985)	0–100	5 +
Oucher NRS[a] (Beyer & Aradine, 1986)	0–100	6 +
Numerical Rating Scale (NRS; Amaria et al., 2010)	0–10	8 +
Object scales	Stimulus	
Glasses Rating Scale (Whaley & Wong, 1987)	7 pictures of glasses	3–18
Multiple Size Poker Chip Tool (MSPCT; St. Laurent-Gagnon et al., 1999)	4 varying-sized poker chips	4–6
Tactile Scale (TaS; Westerling, 1999)	9 balls	4–6
Poker Chip Tool[b] (Hester, 1979)	5 poker chips	4–7
Children's Global Rating Scale (CGRS; Carpenter, 1990)	4 wavy lines	4–8
Facial scales		
Oucher[c] (Beyer, 1984)	6 photographed child faces ("neutral" to "pain")	3–12
Faces Pain Scale[d] (Bieri et al., 1990)	7 hand-drawn adult faces ("neutral" to "pain")	3–15
Wong–Baker FACES Pain Rating Scale (Wong & Baker, 1988)	6 cartoon faces ("smiling" to "crying")	3–18
Children's Anxiety and Pain Scale (CAPS; Kuttner & LePage, 1989)	5 hand-drawn child faces ("neutral" to "distress")	4–10
Facial Affective Scale (FAS; P. A. McGrath et al., 1985)	9 cartoon faces ("smiling" to "crying")	5 +
Word scales		
Word–Descriptor Scale (Whaley & Wong, 1987)	6 descriptors ("no pain" to "worse pain")	3–7
4-point Verbal Descriptor Scale (Goodenough et al., 1997)	4 descriptors ("not at all" to "most hurt possible")	4–6
Word–Graphic Rating Scale (WGRS; Tesler et al., 1991)	5 descriptors ("no pain" to "worse pain")	5 +
Simple Descriptor Scale (SDS; Wong & Baker, 1988)	5 descriptors ("no pain" to "excruciating")	Not provided

[a]Should be used by older children and not in conjunction with the Oucher facial scale (Beyer, 1984).
[b]Also known as Pieces of Hurt Tool (Hester et al., 1990).
[c]European American version; African American (Beyer, Denyes, & Villarruel, 1992) and Hispanic (Villarruel & Denyes, 1991) alternative versions are available.
[d]The Face Pain Scale—Revised (Hicks et al., 2001) uses six faces.

are described as category scales. The numbers assigned to each word or level on a categorical scale is arbitrarily assigned by the investigator and usually reflect increasing intensity (i.e., order) but may not represent true differences beyond intensity order. A pain level scored at 3 may not represent three times the strength of a pain scored as 1 on a categorical scale.

In Table 11.4, the number of possible pain levels for each scale is listed under Pain Score. In general, the larger the possible response continuum, the more sensitive the pain measure, because children have more options to match the particular strength of their pain on the scale. Both types of scales provide valid information, but the potential increased sensitivity afforded by analogue scales make them preferable in certain situations, such as an outcome measure in randomized controlled trials to evaluate analgesic efficacy. A major consideration in selecting among self-report measures is how the pain ratings will be used—for example, to determine whether an individual child is improving, or to compare pain ratings among children receiving different types of treatment. In the latter situation, scales that provide pain ratings on a ratio scale are preferable.

We list five examples of analogue scales in Table 11.4 that yield pain scores with ratio properties (Beyer & Aradine, 1986; Hester, Foster, & Kristensen, 1990; McGrath, deVeber, & Hearn, 1985; McGrath et al., 1996). The 0- to 10-point numerical rating scale (NRS) is an analogue scale and probably the most commonly used pain measure in clinical practice, as most readers will appreciate from their own experiences in the health care system. NRSs are sensitive pain measures for adults and are less subject to error when used by adult patients in comparison to traditional visual analogue scales (Jensen, 2003). In their study of children's pain experience, Ross and Ross (1982) showed children a 0- to 10-point scale and asked them if they knew what a Richter scale was. The study was conducted in California, and almost all children knew the meaning of points on the Richter. After this was established, the children were asked to rate a few common pain experiences (e.g., scraped knee, finger stick) using the NRS. Ross and Ross found that children easily used the NRS. Current research shows that children's

chronic pain ratings on a 0- to 10-point NRS are positively correlated with their ratings on an analogue scale (Amaria et al., 2010). Yet very few studies have published NRS instructions, validity, or reliability information relevant to children, and we lack a consensus on standardized age-appropriate guidelines for its use with children (von Baeyer et al., 2009).

As listed in Table 11.4, categorical scales have been developed with a multitude of creative stimuli (objects, faces, words). In contrast to analogue scales, these scales typically provide a more limited set of discrete pain levels (from 4 to 9), so that children are more restricted in matching their pain to a level on the scale. These scales provide health care providers with a valid pain score for an individual child. However, the difference in "pain" depicted between two categories, for example, a difference of 1 point between the pain scores of face 4 and face 5 on a facial scale, may not be equivalent to a difference of 1 point between the pain scores depicted by face 1 and face 2 on the same scale. While caution must be used when statistically interpreting levels (or numerical anchors) on category scales across groups of children, these scales are particularly useful for children who are young, who have limited pain experience, or who have cognitive difficulties.

Children generally prefer to use facial scales. Various examples of clinically useful facial scales are listed in Table 11.4 (Fogel-Keck, Gerkensmeyer, Joyce, & Schade, 1996; Goodenough et al., 2005; West et al., 1994; Wong & Baker, 1988). Facial scales comprise cartoon faces (e.g., *Wong–Baker FACES Pain Rating Scale*; Wong & Baker, 1988), hand-drawn realistic depictions (e.g., *Faces Pain Scale*; Bieri, Reeve, Champion, Addicoat, & Ziegler, 1990), and photographs of actual children in distress (e.g., *Oucher*; Beyer, 1984). The Oucher scale has been modified and validated for different ethnic groups using photographs of African American children (Beyer, Denyes, & Villarruel, 1992) and Hispanic children (Villarruel & Denyes, 1991) to improve its cultural sensitivity. Facial scales differ with respect to the severity of emotional distress depicted (e.g., *Children's Anxiety and Pain Scale* [CAPS]; Kuttner & LePage, 1989) and the inclusion of positive faces (e.g., Wong–

Baker FACES Pain Rating Scale; Wong & Baker, 1988). Facial scales can have different mathematical properties depending on the number of faces used, anchoring levels, and use of neutral faces (Chambers, Giesbrecht, Craig, Bennett, & Huntsman, 1999).

Several adjective, verbal descriptor, or word scales are included in interviews and questionnaires to assess varied pain characteristics, such as frequency (e.g., "all the time," "one to two times per day"), quality (e.g., "stinging," "pounding"), affect (e.g., "sad," "worried"), as well as pain intensity. In our clinical and research experience, children's spontaneous descriptions of their pain are extremely valuable in helping us to understand their sensory experiences. While analogue pain scales constitute our main intensity measure, we also use the word scale "a little bit," "medium," "a lot," "a real lot" for young children and "slight," "mild," "moderate," "strong," "intense" for older children (McGrath & Koster, 2001). Words may be added as "markers" on visual analogue scales to provide children with reference points for their pain ratings, such as on the Word–Graphic Rating Scale (WGRS; Tesler et al., 1991), where intensity adjectives are placed at approximately equal intervals along a 100-mm line. Children may find graphic scales easier with such reference points, but the psychometric properties of the scale are no longer than those of an analogue scale. Children's pain ratings may reflect values for a category scale where there are not equal intervals between words, even though they are spaced equally along the scale.

Pain intensity scales are an essential component of pain diaries, enabling children to record the type, intensity, and frequency of their pain (McGrath, 1990). Pen-and-paper diaries may be copied from blank appointment calendars or downloaded from the Internet and personalized for children's treatment monitoring. Clinicians ask children to record whatever is most relevant for their clinical management: pain episodes, pain intensity, medication use, at-home physiotherapy sessions, or school attendance. Electronic diaries provide an advanced technique for capturing real-time data. Most children enjoy and are extremely competent in using computers, personal digital assistants (PDAs), cell phones, and iPods, and

might be more compliant in recording pain and health data with "more fun" devices. Recent research shows that compliance for daily pain diaries improves with the use of electronic diaries (Palermo, Valenzuela, & Stork, 2004) and that e-diaries are well liked by adolescents (e.g., Stinson et al., 2008). A difficulty in our clinical experience is cost to provide systems to all children and troubleshooting data collection that requires technical support. Yet, e-recording is a creative and valuable tool for assessing many aspects of children's pain.

Several studies have compared pain intensity scales to determine the correlations among different measures and to explore whether one measure may represent a more valid index of pain than another. The results of most studies show positive correlations among pain scales, with no unequivocal demonstration that one scale is best (e.g., Goodenough et al., 2005, von Baeyer & Spagrud, 2007). Recent evidenced-based reviews of pain intensity scales for clinical practice (i.e., Cohen et al., 2008) and clinical trials (i.e., Stinson et al., 2006) concur with our previous conclusion "that no one scale is appropriate for all children and for all situations in which they experience pain" (McGrath & Gillespie, 2001, p. 111). Clinicians and researchers should choose an intensity scale based on the age and cognitive development of the child, the sensitivity needed to achieve clinical or scientific objectives (i.e., tracking an individual child's pain throughout treatment or comparing pain scores among children), and practical logistic considerations based on available resources and clinic environment.

Multidimensional Pain Scales and Interviews

Clinical interviews are an essential component of pain assessment, enabling children to describe directly what they feel in their own words. Health care providers should ask children directly about the onset, location, quality, intensity, and duration or frequency of pain using a semistructured format—that is, a few basic questions asked in a consistent manner, with different follow-up questions depending on the child's responses. Such information, along with children's physical signs and symptoms, is critical for accurately determining the etiology of a child's pain (e.g., nociceptive vs. neuropathic) and prescribing appropriate treatment.

For children with chronic pain, semistructured conversations about their pain history and its impact on their daily activities enable health care providers to evaluate the extent to which cognitive, behavioral, and emotional factors may exacerbate pain, emotional distress, or disability. Three early clinical interviews were developed to capture information about chronic pain from a biopsychosocial perspective: the *Varni–Thompson Pediatric Pain Questionnaire* (PPQ; Varni, Thompson, & Hanson, 1987), the *Children's Comprehensive Pain Questionnaire* (CCPQ; McGrath, 1990), and the *Adolescent Pediatric Pain Tool* (APPT; Savedra, Holzemer, Tesler, & Wilkie, 1993). All interviews originated from clinical experience treating children with chronic pain problems and provide rating scales to quantify varied pain characteristics. However, they differ in the extent to which they assess situational factors that may modify children's pain. The PPQ evaluates socioenvironmental factors (e.g., life stressors and family responses) that influence a child's pain, and assesses pain characteristics and pain-related disability. The CCPQ, an in-depth interview for children and parents, enables a trained interviewer to evaluate the cognitive, behavioral, and emotional factors outlined in Figure 11.1. This interview has been revised and condensed for use with chronic pain but still requires a trained interviewer (McGrath & Hillier, 2001). In contrast, the APPT is a self-completed questionnaire for which adolescents select words from a sensory list (e.g., "aching"), an evaluative list (e.g., "annoying"), and an affective list (e.g., "awful"). More recently, formal multidimensional pain questionnaires have been validated for use as a discrete chronic pain measure or as a complement to clinical interviews, as listed in Table 11.5. They provide a standardized format for collecting data on pain characteristics, child characteristics, psychosocial factors, and the impact of pain on children and families.

Chronic pain questionnaires vary with respect to the targeted age range, the respondent (child or parent), language, and the primary focus: pain, disability, and/or psychosocial factors. Some questionnaires are self-administered, require no training,

and yield easily interpretable outcomes, as listed in the first section of Table 11.5; others require administration, as listed in the next section, and still others are semistructured interviews that require a trained interviewer, as listed in the last section. Data from these questionnaires permit us to gain information on possible risk and prognostic factors for chronic pain, both for individuals and for specific subgroups. For example, increasing research focuses on identifying various correlates of childhood chronic pain to understand better the factors that may place certain subgroups at risk for developing particular pain conditions (e.g., females and preteens for complex regional pain syndrome Type 1).

Almost all chronic pain questionnaires include a measure of disability, but scales vary widely with respect to the nature of "disability" assessed—physical activity, sleep disturbance, social withdrawal, or school absences. Wide variation is also seen in the time frames used to assess disability—from "today" to over the past 3 months, as noted by the superscripts in Table 11.5. Disability is a key outcome to evaluate regularly throughout a child's treatment program. In our experience, we select the time frame that is most appropriate based on a child's particular treatment plan and the frequency of a child's follow-up appointments. For example, disability may be assessed daily for a child in a randomized clinical trial but be assessed after a 6-week period for a child enrolled in multiple treatments (e.g., physiotherapeutic, psychological, and pharmacological) through a multidisciplinary program. Since interventions may reduce disability in one area but not others (e.g., sleep may improve but not school absences), some aspect of physical limitations, sleep disturbance, school attendance, and social disability should be evaluated.

For the most accurate ratings of disability, it is critical to provide clear criteria to guide ratings. Most scales in Table 11.5 assess disability on continuous or Likert-type scales, such as on the *Pain Experience Questionnaire* (PEQ; Hermann, Hohmeister, Zohsel, Tuttas, & Flor, 2008), where children's level of disability is rated on a 7-point scale, anchored by "*not at all*" to "*very much*." Raters use their subjective judgment to determine a child's *level* of impairment. In our

TABLE 11.5. Multidimensional Pain Scales and Interviews

Measure	Age (yr)	Respondent	Pain features	Disability	Psychosocial factors
Self-report format					
Childhood Health Assessment Questionnaire (CHAQ; Singh et al., 1994)	1–19	Child; parent if child < 9	Intensity[b]	Physical activity[b]	Not assessed
Pain Experience Questionnaire (PEQ; Hermann et al., 2008)	7–18	Child; parent (German)	Intensity[b]	School, social, physical activity[b]	Child's mood, anxiety; parental support during pain; parents' general mood, coping, and anxiety about pain
Bath Adolescent Pain Questionnaire (BAPQ; Eccleston et al., 2005)	11–17	Child; parent	Not assessed	Social, physical activity[c]	Pain-related and general anxiety; impact of pain on family functioning and child's development
Children's Headache Assessment Scale (CHAS; Budd et al., 1994)	6–16	Parent	Not assessed	School, social, physical activity[e]	Pain triggers; parent response to pain medication use
Child Activity Limitations Interview—Self Report (Palermo et al., 2008)	8–18	Child; parent	Not assessed	Sleep, school, social, physical activity[d]	Not assessed
Requires administrator					
Adolescent Pediatric Pain Tool (APPT; Savedra et al., 1989)	8–17	Child	Location, intensity,[a] quality	Not assessed	Pain-related affect
Pediatric Quality of Life Inventory (PedsQL; Varni et al., 1999)	8–18	Child; parent	Location, intensity[a,b]	Sleep, school, social, physical activity[d]	Anxiety related to treatment, pain, underlying health; cognitive problems; perceived physical appearance; physician–nurse communication
MultiDimensional Measure for Recurrent Abdominal Pain (MM-RAP; Malaty et al., 2005)	4–18	Child; parent	Intensity[a,f]	School, physical activity[a,b,f]	Not assessed
Functional Disability Inventory (FDI; Walker & Greene, 1991)	8–16	Child	Not assessed	Sleep, school, social, physical activity[c]	Not assessed
Interview requiring training/administration					
Varni–Thompson Pediatric Pain Questionnaire (PPQ; Varni et al., 1987)	4–19	Child; parent	Location, intensity,[b] quality	Sleep, school, social, physical activity[g]	Situational stressors and pain triggers; child and family responses to pain; pain-related affect
Children's Comprehensive Pain Questionnaire (CCPQ; McGrath, 1990)	5–19	Child; parent	Location, intensity, quality[i]	School, social, physical activity[i]	Pain triggers; child and parent beliefs about/responses to pain; pain-related affect

Note. Time period of assessment: *a*, current; *b*, past week; *c*, past 2 weeks; *d*, past month; *e*, past 2 months; *f*, past 3 months; *g*, past 3 months reported on parent form; *h*, no time frame provided; *i*, time frame selected by assessor.

233

clinic, we use a clinical measure, the *Sick Kids Life Disruption Scale* (see Figure 11.3 for a sample question), which includes clear, objective criteria for evaluating children's level of disability at each level of a 5-point scale.

Almost all chronic pain questionnaires provide some quantitative outcomes (i.e., numerical totals or subscale scores). In general, higher scores indicate more pain and more disability. Some scales, such as the APPT (Savedra, Tesler, Holzemer, Wilkie, & Ward, 1989), the PPQ (Varni et al., 1987), and the CCPQ (McGrath, 1990), yield nonnumerical information, such as pain location or word descriptors, that can be used to assess important temporal or treatment-related changes in children's pain experience. These types of data, along with numerical outcomes, can be easily compared at different time periods for individual children to monitor treatment efficacy, and across children to evaluate differences among pain groups. For example, significant, clinically meaningful differences in children's disability scores on the *Children's Health Assessment Questionnaire* (CHAQ; Singh, Athreya, Fries, & Goldsmith, 1994) were noted for pre- and post–corticosteroid therapy treatment (Feldman et al., 1995). Similarly, the responsiveness of the *Pediatric Quality of Life Inventory* (PedsQL; Varni, Seid, & Rode, 1999) was demonstrated through patient change over time following clinical intervention (Varni et al., 2002). Future research is expected to demonstrate the responsiveness and predictive validity of more recently developed scales listed in Table 11.5, such as the *Bath Adolescent Pain Questionnaire* (BAPQ; Eccleston et al., 2005) and the PEQ (Hermann et al., 2008).

Qualitative pain and psychosocial data accrued as part of interviews such as the PPQ (Varni et al., 1987) and CCPQ (McGrath, 1990) provide rich and detailed information about children's pain and its impact on their lives, but require specialized interviewers to code and quantify children's information. In our clinic, psychologists interview children with a recently revised version of the CCPQ, then complete a report documenting the extent to which factors, such as those listed in Figure 11.1, may contribute to children's pain and disability.

In selecting a pain questionnaire for a child with chronic pain, it is essential to consider which scale best satisfies treatment or research objectives. To obtain a quantitative pain score, it may be best to select a simple pain intensity rating scale and a disability scale. However, to obtain broader-based estimates of a child's emotional state, functional disability, and impact of pain, assessment may include administration of an interview such as the CCPQ (McGrath, 1990). When assessing changes in chronic pain, it is essential to specify a particular time frame for monitoring children, and health care providers should use the same time period for which the scale was developed.

SUMMARY

The vast array of behavioral and self-report measures validated for use with infants, children, and adolescents provides a versatile repertoire of pain measures for almost any clinical situation or research study. The choice of a particular measure is guided by the child's age and cognitive level. Behavioral measures must be used for infants and

Rate most typical, recent week . . .
School Attendance (e.g., absences due to pain)
0   No disruption (regular attendance)
1   Mild disruption (misses < 1 day/week)
2   Moderate disruption (misses 1–2 days/week)
3   Major disruption (misses > 3 days/week)
4   Severe disruption (complete withdrawal for at least 1 week)

FIGURE 11.3. Sample question from the Sick Kids Life Disruption Scale.

for children who are unable to communicate about their pain. Yet health care providers should also consider the potential impact of developmental age, health status, and immediate clinical context (e.g., multiple invasive procedures in a critical care unit) on the resulting behavioral pain score. The optimal evaluation of pain for infants may require the use of concurrent physiological and behavioral indices to provide a composite score with reference to gestation age and health status.

Since children ages 1 to 4 may not be able to use quantitative rating scales, behavioral scales can provide numerical estimates for their pain-related distress. However, whenever children are able to understand differences in intensity, they should be asked directly about their pain and rate how strong it feels using a validated pain intensity scale. For clinical situations in which several different health care providers obtain children's pain ratings at different times, health care providers should select a scale that is practical, that can be administered consistently over time, and that yields a pain score with minimal coding and scoring requirements. For research studies, especially randomized clinical trials, investigators should use analogue pain intensity scales that provide the highest sensitivity and psychometric properties. However, pain assessment for children with chronic pain should be broader than the assessment of pain intensity. Administration of clinical interviews and pain questionnaires allows health care providers to document the sensory features of a child's pain, evaluate the impact of pain on the child and family, and assess the extent to which key situational factors may be affecting pain and pain-related disability.

While no single pain measure is perfectly appropriate for all children and for all situations in which they experience pain, unprecedented research in the field of pediatric pain measurement has yielded a rich array of validated pain scales, interviews, and questionnaires that cover the age span from neonates to adolescents, are appropriate for acute and chronic pain, and satisfy our clinical and scientific objectives. Thus, health care providers can assemble a versatile battery consisting of a behavioral measure, a few pain rating scales (to cover the sensory components), a standardized clinical interview, and a few broader questionnaires to assess the factors that influence chronic pain and its impact on children's lives.

AUTHOR NOTE

Danielle A. Ruskin, Khush A. Amaria, and Patricia A. McGrath contributed to sections on pain assessment in children and adolescents. Fay F. Warnock contributed to the section on pain assessment in infants.

REFERENCES

Als, H. (1982). Toward a synactive theory of development: Promise for the assessment and support of infant individuality. *Infant Mental Health Journal, 3,* 229–243.

Amaria, K., Kewley, E., Brown, S., Campbell, F., Jeavons, M., Stinson, J., et al. (2010, April). *Validation of the 0–10 Numerical Rating Scale for Children with Chronic Pain.* Poster session presented at the annual conference of the Canadian Pain Society, Calgary, Alberta.

Ambuel, B., Hamlett, K. W., Marx, C. M., & Blumer, J. L. (1992). Assessing distress in pediatric intensive care environments: The COMFORT scale. *Journal of Pediatric Psychology, 17*(1), 95–109.

Anand, K. J. (1998). Clinical importance of pain and stress in preterm neonates. *Biology of the Neonate, 73*(1), 1–9.

Barr, R. G. (1998). Reflections on measuring pain in infants: Dissociation in responsive systems and "honest signalling." *Archives of Disease in Childhood Fetal Neonatal Edition, 79*(2), F152–F156.

Barrier, G., Attia, J., Mayer, M. N., Amiel-Tison, C., & Shnider, S. M. (1989). Measurement of post-operative pain and narcotic administration in infants using a new clinical scoring system. *Intensive Care Medicine, 15*(Suppl. 1), S37–S39.

Bellieni, C. V., Bagnoli, F., Sisto, R., Neri, L., Cordelli, D., & Buonocore, G. (2005). Development and validation of the ABC Pain Scale for healthy full-term babies. *Acta Paediatrica, 94*(10), 1432–1436.

Beyer, J. E. (1984). *The Oucher: A user's manual and technical report.* Evanston, IL: Judson.

Beyer, J. E., & Aradine, C. R. (1986). Content validity of an instrument to measure young children's perceptions of the intensity of their pain. *Journal of Pediatric Nursing, 1*(6), 386–395.

Beyer, J. E., Denyes, M. J., & Villarruel, A. M. (1992). The creation, validation, and continuing development of the Oucher: A measure of pain intensity in children. *Journal of Pediatric Nursing, 7*(5), 335–346.

Beyer, J. E., & Wells, N. (1989). The assessment of pain in children. *Pediatric Clinics of North America, 36*(4), 837–854.

Bieri, D., Reeve, R. A., Champion, G. D., Addicoat, L., & Ziegler, J. B. (1990). The Faces Pain Scale for the self-assessment of the severity of pain experienced by children: Development, initial validation, and preliminary investigation for ratio scale properties. *Pain, 41*(2), 139–150.

Blauer, T., & Gerstmann, D. (1998). A simultaneous comparison of three neonatal pain scales during common NICU procedures. *Clinical Journal of Pain, 14*(1), 39–47.

Blount, R. L., Bunke, V., Cohen, L. L., & Forbes, C. J. (2001). The Child–Adult Medical Procedure Interaction Scale—Short Form (CAMPIS-SF): Validation of a rating scale for children's and adults' behaviors during painful medical procedures. *Journal of Pain and Symptom Management, 22*(1), 591–599.

Blount, R. L., Cohen, L. L., Frank, N. C., Bachanas, P. J., Smith, A. J., Manimala, M. R., et al. (1997). The Child–Adult Medical Procedure Interaction Scale—Revised: An assessment of validity. *Journal of Pediatric Psychology, 22*(1), 73–88.

Blount, R. L., Sturges, J. W., & Powers, S. W. (1990). Analysis of child and adult behavioral variations by phase of medical procedure. *Behavior Therapy, 21*, 33–48.

Boelen-van der Loo, W. J., Scheffer, E., de Haan, R. J., & de Groot, C. J. (1999). Clinimetric evaluation of the pain observation scale for young children in children aged between 1 and 4 years after ear, nose, and throat surgery. *Journal of Developmental and Behavioral Pediatrics, 20*(4), 222–227.

Boucher, T., Jennings, E., & Fitzgerald, M. (1998). The onset of diffuse noxious inhibitory controls in postnatal rat pups: A C-Fos study. *Neuroscience Letters, 257*(1), 9–12.

Breau, L. M., McGrath, P. J., Camfield, C., Rosmus, C., & Finley, G. A. (2000). Preliminary validation of an observational pain checklist for persons with cognitive impairments and inability to communicate verbally. *Developmental Medicine and Child Neurology, 42*(9), 609–616.

Breau, L. M., McGrath, P. J., Camfield, C. S., & Finley, G. A. (2002). Psychometric properties of the Non-Communicating Children's Pain Checklist—Revised. *Pain, 99*(1–2), 349–357.

Brinker, D. (2004). Sedation and comfort issues in the ventilated infant and child. *Critical Care Nursing Clinics of North America, 16*(3), 365–377, viii–ix.

Broadman, L. M., Rice, L. J., & Hannallah, R. S. (1988). Testing the validity of an objective pain scale for infants and children. *Anesthesiology, 69*(3A), A770.

Buchholz, M., Karl, H. W., Pomietto, M., & Lynn, A. (1998). Pain scores in infants: A modified infant pain scale versus visual analogue. *Journal of Pain and Symptom Management, 15*(2), 117–124.

Budd, K. S., Workman, D. E., Lemsky, C. M., & Quick, D. M. (1994). The Childrens Headache Assessment Scale (CHAS)—factor structure and psychometric properties. *Journal of Behavioral Medicine, 17*(2), 159–179.

Büttner, W., & Finke, W. (2000). Analysis of behavioural and physiological parameters for the assessment of postoperative analgesic demand in newborns, infants and young children: A comprehensive report on seven consecutive studies. *Paediatric Anaesthesia, 10*(3), 303–318.

Carbajal, R., Chauvet, X., Couderc, S., & Olivier-Martin, M. (1999). Randomised trial of analgesic effects of sucrose, glucose, and pacifiers in term neonates. *British Medical Journal, 319*, 1393–1397.

Carpenter, P. J. (1990). New method for measuring young children's self-report of fear and pain. *Journal of Pain and Symptom Management, 5*(4), 233–240.

Chambers, C. T., Finley, G. A., McGrath, P. J., & Walsh, T. M. (2003). The Parents' Postoperative Pain Measure: Replication and extension to 2-6-year-old children. *Pain, 105*(3), 437–443.

Chambers, C. T., Giesbrecht, K., Craig, K. D., Bennett, S. M., & Huntsman, E. (1999). A comparison of faces scales for the measurement of pediatric pain: Children's and parents' ratings. *Pain, 83*(1), 25–35.

Champion, G. D., Goodenough, B., von Baeyer, C. L., & Thomas, W. (1998). Measurement of pain by self-report. In G. A. Finley (Ed.), *Measurement of pain in infants and children* (pp. 123–160). Seattle, WA: IASP Press.

Cohen, L. L., Lemanek, K., Blount, R. L., Dahlquist, L. M., Lim, C. S., Palermo, T. M., et al. (2008). Evidence-based assessment of pediatric pain. *Journal of Pediatric Psychology, 33*(9), 939–956.

Craig, K. D., Korol, C. T., & Pillai, R. R. (2002). Challenges of judging pain in vulnerable infants. *Clinics in Perinatology, 29*(3), 445–457.

Crellin, D., Sullivan, T. P., Babl, F. E., O'Sullivan, R., & Hutchinson, A. (2007). Analysis of the validation of existing behavioral pain and distress scales for use in the procedural setting. *Paediatric Anaesthesia, 17*(8), 720–733.

Curzi-Dascalova, L., Figueroa, J. M., Eiselt, M.,

Christova, E., Virassamy, A., d'Allest, A. M., et al. (1993). Sleep state organization in premature infants of less than 35 weeks' gestational age. *Pediatric Research*, *34*(5), 624–628.

Debillon, T., Zupan, V., Ravault, N., Magny, J. F., & Dehan, M. (2001). Development and initial validation of the EDIN scale, a new tool for assessing prolonged pain in preterm infants. *Archives of Disease in Childhood Fetal Neonatal Edition*, *85*(1), F36–F41.

Duhn, L. J., & Medves, J. M. (2004). A systematic integrative review of infant pain assessment tools. *Advances in Neonatal Care*, *4*(3), 126–140.

Eccleston, C., Jordan, A., McCracken, L. M., Sleed, M., Connell, H., & Clinch, J. (2005). The Bath Adolescent Pain Questionnaire (BAPQ): Development and preliminary psychometric evaluation of an instrument to assess the impact of chronic pain on adolescents. *Pain*, *118*(1–2), 263–270.

Eland, J. M., & Anderson, J. E. (1977). The experience of pain in children. In *Pain: A source book for nurses and other health professionals* (pp. 453–471). Boston: Little, Brown.

Feldman, B. M., Ayling-Campos, A., Luy, L., Stevens, D., Silverman, E. D., & Laxer, R. M. (1995). Measuring disability in juvenile dermatomyositis: Validity of the Childhood Health Assessment Questionnaire. *Journal of Rheumatology*, *22*(2), 326–331.

Finley, G. A., Kristjansdottir, O., & Forgeron, P. A. (2009). Cultural influences on the assessment of children's pain. *Pain Research and Management*, *14*(1), 33–37.

Fitzgerald, M. (1993). Development of pain pathways and mechanisms. *Pain Research and Clinical Management*, *5*(4), 19–37.

Fitzgerald, M., & Walker, S. M. (2009). Infant pain management: A developmental neurobiological approach. *Nature Clinical Practice Neurology*, *5*(1), 35–50.

Fogel-Keck, J., Gerkensmeyer, J. E., Joyce, B. A., & Schade, J. G. (1996). Reliability and validity of the Faces and Word Descriptor scales to measure procedural pain. *Journal of Pediatric Nursing*, *11*(6), 368–374.

Gaffney, A. (1988). How children describe pain: A study of words and analogies used by 5–14 year olds. In R. Dubner, G. Gebhart, & M. Bond (Eds.), *Pain research and clinical management* (Vol. 3, pp. 341–347). Amsterdam: Elsevier.

Gauvain-Piquard, A., Rodary, C., Rezvani, A., & Lemerle, J. (1987). Pain in children aged 2–6 years: A new observational rating scale elaborated in a pediatric oncology unit—preliminary report. *Pain*, *31*(2), 177–188.

Gilbert, C. A., Lilley, C. M., Craig, K. D., McGrath, P. J., Court, C. A., Bennett, S. M., et al. (1999). Postoperative pain expression in preschool children: Validation of the Child Facial Coding System. *Clinical Journal of Pain*, *15*(3), 192–200.

Goodenough, B., Addicoat, L., Champion, G. D., McInerney, M., Young, B., Juniper, K., et al. (1997). Pain in 4- to 6-year-old children receiving intramuscular injections: A comparison of the Faces Pain Scale with other self-report and behavioral measures. *Clinical Journal of Pain*, *13*(1), 60–73.

Goodenough, B., Piira, T., von Baeyer, C. L., Chua, K., Wu, E., Trieu, J. D. H., et al. (2005). Comparing six self-report measures of pain intensity in children [Electronic version]. *The Suffering Child*, *8*, 1–30.

Grunau, R. E., Oberlander, T., Holsti, L., & Whitfield, M. F. (1998). Bedside application of the Neonatal Facial Coding System in pain assessment of premature neonates. *Pain*, *76*(3), 277–286.

Grunau, R. V., & Craig, K. D. (1987). Pain expression in neonates: Facial action and cry. *Pain*, *28*(3), 395–410.

Guinsburg, R., Kipelman, B. I., Anand, K. J., de Almeida, M. F., Peres, C., & Miyoshi, M. H. (1998). Physiological, hormonal, and behavioral responses to a single fentanyl dose in intubated and ventilated preterm neonates. *Journal of Pediatrics*, *132*(6), 954–959.

Harbeck, C., & Peterson, L. (1992). Elephants dancing in my head: A developmental approach to children's concepts of specific pains. *Child Development*, *63*(1), 138–149.

Helgadottir, H. L., & Wilson, M. E. (2004). Temperament and pain in 3 to 7-year-old children undergoing tonsillectomy. *Journal of Pediatric Nursing*, *19*(3), 204–213.

Hermann, C., Hohmeister, J., Zohsel, K., Tuttas, M. L., & Flor, H. (2008). The impact of chronic pain in children and adolescents: Development and initial validation of a child and parent version of the Pain Experience Questionnaire. *Pain*, *135*(3), 251–261.

Hesselgard, K., Larsson, S., Romner, B., Stromblad, L. G., & Reinstrup, P. (2007). Validity and reliability of the Behavioural Observational Pain Scale for postoperative pain measurement in children 1–7 years of age. *Pediatric Critical Care Medicine*, *8*(2), 102–108.

Hester, N., Foster, R., & Kristensen, K. (1990). Measurement of pain in children: Generalizability and validity of the Pain Ladder and Pieces of Hurt Tool. *Advances in Pain Research and Therapy*, *15*, 79–84.

Hester, N. K. (1979). The preoperational child's reaction to immunization. *Nursing Research*, *28*, 250–255.

Hicks, C. L., von Baeyer, C. L., Spafford, P. A., van Kovlaar, I., & Goodenough B. (2001). The

Faces Pain Scale—Revised: Toward a common metric in pediatric pain measurement. *Pain, 93*(2), 173–183.

Hodgkinson, K., Bear, M., Thorn, J., & Van Blaricum, S. (1994). Measuring pain in neonates: Evaluating an instrument and developing a common language. *Australian Journal of Advanced Nursing, 12*(1), 17–22.

Holsti, L., & Grunau, R. E. (2007). Initial validation of the Behavioral Indicators of Infant Pain (BIIP). *Pain, 132*(3), 264–272.

Holsti, L., Grunau, R. E., Oberlander, T. F., & Whitfield, M. F. (2005). Prior pain induces heightened motor responses during clustered care in preterm infants in the NICU. *Early Human Development, 81*(3), 293–302.

Horgan, M., & Choonara, I. (1996). Measuring pain in neonates: An objective score. *Paediatric Nursing, 8*(10), 24–27.

Hubert, N. C., Jay, S. M., Saltoun, M., & Hayes, M. (1988). Approach–avoidance and distress in children undergoing preparation for painful medical procedures. *Journal of Clinical Child Psychology, 17*, 194–202.

Hudson-Barr, D., Capper-Michel, B., Lambert, S., Palermo, T. M., Morbeto, K., & Lombardo, S. (2002). Validation of the Pain Assessment in Neonates (PAIN) scale with the Neonatal Infant Pain Scale (NIPS). *Neonatal Network, 21*(6), 15–21.

Hummel, P., & Puchalski, M. (2002). Establishing initial reliability and validity of the N-PASS: Neonatal Pain, Agitation, and Sedation Scale—a pilot study. *Newborn and Infant Nursing Reviews, 1*(2), 114–121.

Hummel, P., & van Dijk, M. (2006). Pain assessment: Current status and challenges. *Seminars in Fetal and Neonatal Medicine, 11*(4), 237–245.

Humphrey, G. B., Boon, C. M., van Linden van den Heuvell, G. F., & van de Wiel, H. B. (1992). The occurrence of high levels of acute behavioral distress in children and adolescents undergoing routine venipunctures. *Pediatrics, 90*(Pt. 1), 87–91.

Hunt, A., Goldman, A., Seers, K., Crichton, N., Mastroyannopoulou, K., Moffat, V., et al. (2004). Clinical validation of the Paediatric Pain Profile. *Developmental Medicine and Child Neurology, 46*(1), 9–18.

Jay, S. M., & Elliott, C. (1986). *Observational Scale of Behavioral Distress—Revised manual*. Los Angeles: Children's Hospital of Los Angeles.

Jay, S. M., Ozolins, M., Elliott, C. H., & Caldwell, S. (1983). Assessment of children's distress during painful medical procedures. *Health Psychology, 2*(2), 133–147.

Jensen, M. P. (2003). The validity and reliability of pain measures in adults with cancer. *Journal of Pain, 4*(1), 2–21.

Johnston, C. C., & Stevens, B. J. (1996). Experience in a neonatal intensive care unit affects pain response. *Pediatrics, 98*(5), 925–930.

Johnston, C. C., Stevens, B. J., Franck, L. S., Jack, A., Stremler, R., & Platt, R. (1999). Factors explaining lack of response to heel stick in preterm newborns. *Journal of Obstetric, Gynecologic, and Neonatal Nursing, 28*(6), 587–594.

Johnston, C. C., Stevens, B. J., Yang, F., & Horton, L. (1995). Differential response to pain by very premature neonates. *Pain, 61*(3), 471–479.

Katz, E. R., Kellerman, J., & Siegel, S. E. (1980). Behavioral distress in children with cancer undergoing medical procedures: Developmental considerations. *Journal of Consulting and Clinical Psychology, 48*(3), 356–365.

Krechel, S. W., & Bildner, J. (1995). CRIES: A new neonatal postoperative pain measurement score: Initial testing of validity and reliability. *Paediatric Anaesthesia, 5*(1), 53–61.

Kuttner, L., & LePage, T. (1989). Face scales for the assessment of pediatric pain: A critical review. *Canadian Journal of Behavioral Sciences, 21*, 198–209.

Lawrence, J., Alcock, D., McGrath, P., Kay, J., MacMurray, S. B., & Dulberg, C. (1993). The development of a tool to assess neonatal pain. *Neonatal Network, 12*(6), 59–66.

LeBaron, S., & Zeltzer, L. (1984). Assessment of acute pain and anxiety in children and adolescents by self-reports, observer reports, and a behavior checklist. *Journal of Consulting and Clinical Psychology, 52*(5), 729–738.

LeResche, L., Mancl, L. A., Drangsholt, M. T., Saunders, K., & Korff, M. V. (2005). Relationship of pain and symptoms to pubertal development in adolescents. *Pain, 118*(1–2), 201–209.

Logan, D. E., & Scharff, L. (2005). Relationships between family and parent characteristics and functional abilities in children with recurrent pain syndromes: An investigation of moderating effects on the pathway from pain to disability. *Journal of Pediatric Psychology, 30*(8), 698–707.

Malaty, H. M., Abudayyeh, S., O'Malley, K. J., Wilsey, M. J., Fraley, K., Gilger, M. A., et al. (2005). Development of a multidimensional measure for recurrent abdominal pain in children: Population-based studies in three settings. *Pediatrics, 115*(2), 210–215.

Malviya, S., Voepel-Lewis, T., Burke, C., Merkel, S., & Tait, A. R. (2006). The revised FLACC observational pain tool: Improved reliability and validity for pain assessment in children with cognitive impairment. *Paediatric Anaesthesia, 16*(3), 258–265.

Malviya, S., Voepel-Lewis, T., Tait, A. R., Merkel, S., Lauer, A., Munro, H., et al. (2001). Pain management in children with and without cognitive impairment following spine fusion surgery. *Paediatric Anaesthesia, 11*(4), 453–458.

Marceau, J. (2003). Pilot study of a pain assessment tool in the neonatal intensive care unit. *Journal of Paediatrics and Child Health, 39*(8), 598–601.

McGrath, P. A. (1987). The multidimensional assessment and management of recurrent pain syndromes in children. *Behaviour Research and Therapy, 25*(4), 251–262.

McGrath, P. A. (2005). Pain assessment: Children. In R. F. Schmidt & W. D. Willis (Eds.), *Encyclopedic Reference of Pain* (pp. 1644–1648). New York: Springer-Verlag.

McGrath, P. A. (1990). *Pain in children: Nature, assessment and treatment.* New York: Guilford Press.

McGrath, P. A., & Dade, L. A. (2004). Strategies to decrease pain and minimize disability. In D. Price & M. C. Bushnell (Eds.), *Psychological methods of pain control: Basic science and clinical perspectives* (Vol. 29, pp. 73–96). Seattle, WA: IASP Press.

McGrath, P. A., de Veber, L. L., & Hearn, T. H. (1985). Multidimensional pain assessment in children. In H. R. Fields, R. Dubner, & F. Cervero (Eds.), *Advances in pain research and therapy* (Vol. 9, pp. 387–393). New York: Raven Press.

McGrath, P. A., & Gillespie, J. M. (2001). Pain assessment in children and adolescents. In D. C. Turk & R. Melzack (Eds.), *Handbook of pain assessment* (2nd ed., pp. 97–118). New York: Guilford Press.

McGrath, P. A., & Hillier, L. M. (Eds.). (2001). *The child with headache: Diagnosis and treatment* (Vol. 19). Seattle, WA: IASP Press.

McGrath, P. A., & Koster, A. L. (2001). Headache measures for children: A practical approach. In P. A. McGrath & L. M. Hillier (Eds.), *The child with headache: Diagnosis and treatment* (pp. 29–56). Seattle, WA: IASP Press.

McGrath, P. A., Seifert, C. E., Speechley, K. N., Booth, J. C., Stitt, L., & Gibson, M. C. (1996). A new analogue scale for assessing children's pain: An initial validation study. *Pain, 64*(3), 435–443.

McGrath, P. J. (1998). Behavioral measures of pain. In G. A. Finley (Ed.), *Measurement of pain in infants and children* (pp. 83–102). Seattle, WA: IASP Press.

McGrath, P. J., Johnson, G., Goodman, J. T., Shillinger, J., Dunn, J., & Chapman, J. A. (1985).

CHEOPS: A behavioral scale for rating postoperative pain in children. In H. Fields (Ed.), *Advances in pain research and therapy* (Vol. 9, pp. 395–401). New York: Raven Press.

Merkel, S. I., Voepel-Lewis, T., Shayevitz, J. R., & Malviya, S. (1997). The FLACC: A behavioral scale for scoring postoperative pain in young children. *Pediatric Nursing, 23*(3), 293–297.

Myatt, H. M., & Myatt, R. A. (1998). The development of a paediatric quality of life questionnaire to measure post-operative pain following tonsillectomy. *International Journal of Pediatric Otorhinolaryngology, 44*(2), 115–123.

Palermo, T. M., Lewandowski, A. S., Long, A. C., & Burant, C. J. (2008). Validation of a self-report questionnaire version of the Child Activity Limitations Interview (CALI): The CALI-21. *Pain, 139*(3), 644–652.

Palermo, T. M., Valenzuela, D., & Stork, P. P. (2004). A randomized trial of electronic versus paper pain diaries in children: Impact on compliance, accuracy, and acceptability. *Pain, 107*(3), 213–219.

Peden, V., Vater, M., & Choonara, I. (2003). Validating the Derbyshire Children's Hospital Pain Tool: A pilot study. *Paediatric Anaesthesia, 13*(2), 109–113.

Pokela, M. L. (1994). Pain relief can reduce hypoxemia in distressed neonates during routine treatment procedures. *Pediatrics, 93*(3), 379–383.

Ramelet, A. S., Abu-Saad, H. H., Rees, N., & McDonald, S. (2004). The challenges of pain measurement in critically ill young children: A comprehensive review. *Australian Critical Care, 17*(1), 33–45.

Ramelet, A. S., Rees, N., Mcdonald, S., Bulsara, M., & Abu-Saad, H. H. (2007). Development and preliminary psychometric testing of the Multidimensional Assessment of Pain Scale: MAPS. *Paediatric Anaesthesia, 17*(4), 333–340.

Robertson, J. (1993). Pediatric pain assessment: Validation of a multidimensional tool. *Pediatric Nursing, 19*(3), 209–213.

Robieux, I., Kumar, R., Radhakrishnan, S., & Koren, G. (1991). Assessing pain and analgesia with a lidocaine–prilocaine emulsion in infants and toddlers during venipuncture. *Journal of Pediatrics, 118*(6), 971–973

Ross, D. M., & Ross, S. A. (1982). A study of the pain experience in children (Final Report, Ref. No. 1 R01 HD 13672-01). Bethesda, MD: National Institute of Child Health and Human Development.

Ross, D. M., & Ross, S. A. (1988). *Childhood pain: current issues, research, and management.* Baltimore: Urban & Schwarzenberg.

Royal College of Nursing Institute. (1999). *Clinical guideline for the recognition and assessment of acute pain in children: Recommendations*. London: Author.

Savedra, M. C., Holzemer, W. L., Tesler, M. D., & Wilkie, D. J. (1993). Assessment of postoperation pain in children and adolescents using the Adolescent Pediatric Pain Tool. *Nursing Research, 42*(1), 5–9.

Savedra, M. C., Tesler, M. D., Holzemer, W. L., Wilkie, D. J., & Ward, J. A. (1989). Pain location: Validity and reliability of body outline markings by hospitalized children and adolescents. *Research in Nursing and Health, 12*(5), 307–314.

Schade, J. G., Joyce, B. A., Gerkensmeyer, J., & Keck, J. F. (1996). Comparison of three preverbal scales for postoperative pain assessment in a diverse pediatric sample. *Journal of Pain and Symptom Management, 12*(6), 348–359.

Schechter, N. L., Berde, C. B., & Yaster, M. (Eds.). (2003). *Pain in infants, children, and adolescents* (2nd ed.). Philadelphia: Lippincott Williams & Wilkins.

Schultz, A. A., Murphy, E., Morton, J., Stempel, A., Messenger-Rioux, C., & Bennett, K. (1999). Preverbal, early verbal pediatric pain scale (PEPPS): Development and early psychometric testing. *Journal of Pediatric Nursing, 14*(1), 19–27.

Singh, G., Athreya, B. H., Fries, J. F., & Goldsmith, D. P. (1994). Measurement of health status in children with juvenile rheumatoid arthritis. *Arthritis and Rheumatism, 37*(12), 1761–1769.

Solodiuk, J., & Curley, M. A. (2003). Pain assessment in nonverbal children with severe cognitive impairments: The Individualized Numeric Rating Scale (INRS). *Journal of Pediatric Nursing, 18*(4), 295–299.

Spence, K., Gillies, D., Harrison, D., Johnston, L., & Nagy, S. (2005). A reliable pain assessment tool for clinical assessment in the neonatal intensive care unit. *Journal of Obstetric, Gynecologic, and Neonatal Nursing, 34*(1), 80–86.

Stallard, P., Williams, L., Lenton, S., & Velleman, R. (2001). Pain in cognitively impaired, non-communicating children. *Archives of Disease in Childhood, 85*(6), 460–462.

Stevens, B. (1990). Development and testing of a pediatric pain management sheet. *Pediatric Nursing, 16*(6), 543–548.

Stevens, B., Johnston, C., Petryshen, P., & Taddio, A. (1996). Premature Infant Pain Profile: Development and initial validation. *Clinical Journal of Pain, 12*(1), 13–22.

Stevens, B., Pillai Riddell, R., Oberlander, T., & Gibbons, S. (2007). Assessment of pain in neonates and infants. In K.J. Anand (Ed.), *Pain in neonates and infants* (3rd ed., pp. 67–90). Philadelphia: Elsevier.

Stewart, B., Lancaster, G., Lawson, J., Williams, K., & Daly, J. (2004). Validation of the Alder Hey Triage Pain Score. *Archives of Disease in Childhood, 89*(7), 625–630.

Stinson, J. N. (2009). Improving the assessment of pediatric chronic pain: Harnessing the potential of electronic diaries. *Pain Research and Management, 14*(1), 59–64.

Stinson, J. N., Kavanagh, T., Yamada, J., Gill, N., & Stevens, B. (2006). Systematic review of the psychometric properties, interpretability and feasibility of self-report pain intensity measures for use in clinical trials in children and adolescents. *Pain, 125*(1–2), 143–157.

Stinson, J. N., Stevens, B. J., Feldman, B. M., Streiner, D., McGrath, P. J., Dupuis, A., et al. (2008). Construct validity of a multidimensional electronic pain diary for adolescents with arthritis. *Pain, 136*(3), 281–292.

St. Laurent-Gagnon, T., Bernard-Bonnin, A. C., & Villeneuve, E. (1999). Pain evaluation in preschool children and by their parents. *Acta Paediatrica, 88*, 422–427.

Sweet, S. D., & McGrath, P. J. (1998). Physiological measures of pain. In G. A. Finley (Ed.), *Measurement of pain in infants and children* (pp. 59–81). Seattle, WA: IASP Press.

Taddio, A., & Katz, J. (2005). The effects of early pain experience in neonates on pain responses in infancy and childhood. *Paediatric Drugs, 7*(4), 245–257.

Taddio, A., Nulman, I., Koren, B. S., Stevens, B., & Koren, G. (1995). A revised measure of acute pain in infants. *Journal of Pain and Symptom Management, 10*(6), 456–463.

Taddio, A., Shah, V., Gilbert-MacLeod, C., & Katz, J. (2002). Conditioning and hyperalgesia in newborns exposed to repeated heel lances. *Journal of the American Medical Association, 288*(7), 857–861.

Tarbell, S. E., Marsh, J. L., & Cohen, I. T. C. (1991). Reliability and validity of the Pain Assessment Scale: A scale for measuring postoperative pain in young children. *Journal of Pain and Symptom Management, 6*(3), 196–196.

Tesler, M. D., Savedra, M. C., Holzemer, W. L., Wilkie, D. J., Ward, J. A., & Paul, S. M. (1991). The Word–Graphic Rating Scale as a measure of children's and adolescents' pain intensity. *Research in Nursing and Health, 14*(5), 361–371.

Tucker, C. L., Slifer, K. J., & Dahlquist, L. M. (2001). Reliability and validity of the Brief Behavioral Distress Scale: A measure of children's distress during invasive medical procedures. *Journal of Pediatric Psychology, 26*(8), 513–523.

van Dijk, M., de Boer, J. B., Koot, H. M., Duivenvoorden, H. J., Passchier, J., Bouwmeester, N., et al. (2001). The association between physiological and behavioral pain measures in 0- to 3-year-old infants after major surgery. *Journal of Pain and Symptom Management*, 22(1), 600–609.

van Dijik, M., Peters, J. W., Bouwmeester, N. J., & Tibboel, D. (2002). Are postoperative pain instruments useful for specific groups of vulnerable infants? *Clinics in Perinatology*, 29(3), 469–491.

Varni, J. W., Seid, M., & Rode, C. A. (1999). The PedsQL: Measurement model for the Pediatric Quality of Life Inventory. *Medical Care*, 37(2), 126–139.

Varni, J. W., Seid, M., Smith Knight, T., Burwinkle, T., Brown, J., & Szer, I. S. (2002). The PedsQL in pediatric rheumatology: Reliability, validity, and responsiveness of the Pediatric Quality of Life Inventory Generic Core scales and Rheumatology module. *Arthritis and Rheumatism*, 46(3), 714–725.

Varni, J. W., Thompson, K. L., & Hanson, V. (1987). The Varni/Thompson Pediatric Pain Questionnaire: I. Chronic musculoskeletal pain in juvenile rheumatoid arthritis (Questionnaire attached). *Pain*, 28(1), 27–38.

Villarruel, A. M., & Denyes, M. J. (1991). Pain assessment in children: Theoretical and empirical validity. *ANS Advances in Nursing Science*, 14(2), 32–41.

von Baeyer, C. L., & Spagrud, L. J. (2007). Systematic review of observational (behavioral) measures of pain for children and adolescents aged 3 to 18 years. *Pain*, 127(1–2), 140–150.

von Baeyer, C. L., Spagrud, L. J., McCormick, J. C., Choo, E., Neville, K., & Connelly, M. A. (2009). Three new datasets supporting use of the Numerical Rating Scale (NRS-11) for children's self-reports of pain intensity. *Pain*, 143(3), 223–227.

Walco, G. A., Conte, P. M., Labay, L. E., Engel, R., & Zeltzer, L. K. (2005). Procedural distress in children with cancer: Self-report, behavioral observations, and physiological parameters. *Clinical Journal of Pain*, 21(6), 484–490.

Walker, L. S., & Greene, J. W. (1991). The functional disability inventory: Measuring a neglected dimension of child health status. *Journal of Pediatric Psychology*, 16(1), 39–58.

Walker, S. M. (2008). Pain in children: Recent advances and ongoing challenges. *British Journal of Anaesthesia*, 101(1), 101–110.

Warnock, F., & Sandrin, D. (2004). Comprehensive description of newborn distress behavior in response to acute pain (newborn male circumcision). *Pain*, 107(3), 242–255.

West, N., Oakes, L., Hinds, P. S., Sanders, L., Holden, R., Williams, S., et al. (1994). Measuring pain in pediatric oncology ICU patients. *Journal of Pediatric Oncology Nursing*, 11(2), 64–68; discussion 69–70.

Westerling, D. (1999). Postoperative recovery evaluated with a new tactile scale (TaS) in children undergoing ophthalmic surgery. *Pain*, 83(2), 297–301.

Whaley, L., & Wong, D. L. (1987). *Nursing care of infants and children*. St. Louis, MO: Mosby.

Wong, D. L., & Baker, C. M. (1988). Pain in children: Comparison of assessment scales. *Pediatric Nursing*, 14(1), 9–17.

CHAPTER 12

Assessment of Pain in Older Persons

LYNN R. GAUTHIER
LUCIA GAGLIESE

Pain is highly prevalent among older people. Up to 40% of older adults living independently (Thomas, Peat, Harris, Wilkie, & Croft, 2004) and 27–83% of those in institutional settings (Fox, Raina, & Jadad, 1999) report pain that interferes with daily function. This wide range is likely due to methodological or sample variation across studies (Fox et al., 1999). Approximately 40–80% of community-dwelling (Pahor et al., 1999; Woo, Ho, Lau, & Leung, 1994) and 16–27% of institutionalized older adults do not receive any treatment for their pain (Lichtenberg & McGrogan, 1987; Roy & Thomas, 1986).

Similar to other age groups, pain in older people has far-reaching negative impacts, including psychological distress, cognitive impairment, physical disability, social withdrawal, self-neglect, and suicidality (Gibson & Weiner, 2005; Juurlink, Herrmann, Szalai, Kopp, & Redelmeier, 2004). Despite this, older people are at risk for inadequate treatment. Multiple interacting factors contribute to inadequate pain management, with lack of proper assessment being primary among these (Gagliese & Melzack, 1997b). Fortunately, empirical attention to the development, refinement, and validation

of pain scales for use with older people has increased. In this chapter, we review evidence supporting the use of various scales for the assessment of pain in older people and across age groups. As well, we consider the special issues related to older people that should be considered in assessment, especially when one is interested in comparisons across age groups. Throughout this chapter, we focus on older people who are cognitively intact and capable of providing verbal or written self-reports of subjective states. Hadjistavropoulos, Breau, and Craig (Chapter 13, this volume) discuss pain assessment in older people who are not able to provide verbal reports of pain.

SPECIAL CONSIDERATIONS IN THE ASSESSMENT OF OLDER PEOPLE

The goal of pain assessment is to measure accurately a person's pain and its impact on important life domains. This is best achieved using a standardized protocol that comprises measurement tools validated for the population of interest. In addition, whether carried out for clinical or research purposes, a comprehensive assessment must consider the multiple, interacting biopsychosocial factors that may contribute to the experience of pain and inform the planning and implementation of care (Dworkin et al., 2005; see Turk & Robinson, Chapter 10, this volume). The age of the person being assessed is an important consideration, because it may impact not only the selection of tools and constructs to assess but also the goals and effects of treatment.

The older person may present some unique assessment challenges (Lichtenberg, 1999). The first is practical: how to maximize the older person's ability and willingness to engage in the pain assessment. One must accommodate normal age-related changes that may hinder completion of assessment protocols (Lichtenberg, 1999; Mody et al., 2008), including visual or auditory impairments. Mild cognitive impairment and normal age-related changes in cognitive processing also may interfere with comprehension of questions or instructions. As a result, older people may be less able than younger people to tolerate the burden of long assessment sessions. Modification of assessment protocols (e.g., adding breaks and allowing completion of some longer questionnaires over multiple sessions or at home) may be necessary to enhance compliance. There may be more flexibility for these types of adjustments within the clinical setting, but it is increasingly recognized that researchers should design protocols with the special practical needs of older patients in mind to maximize adherence and minimize attrition and data loss (Mody et al., 2008).

In addition to these practical concerns, older people's beliefs about pain and aging may be obstacles to effective assessment. These beliefs are important to interpreting symptoms, seeking health care, making treatment decisions, and adhering to management plans (Ferrell & Juarez, 2002). Many still believe that pain is a normal part of aging and not amenable to or worthy of care (Martin, Williams, Hadjistavropoulos, Hadjistavropoulos, & MacLean, 2005). In addition, they may believe that "good patients" do not report pain. These beliefs may make the older person reluctant to report symptoms. Age-related barriers to the use of analgesics may also impact people's willingness to report symptoms (Ross, Carswell, Hing, Hollingworth, & Dalziel, 2001). For

instance, older age has been associated with increased fears of opioid tolerance and addiction, as well as the belief that medication should be saved for "severe" pain (Ward et al., 1993). If older people mistakenly attribute manageable symptoms to normal aging or fear the use of analgesics, rather than seek health care they may try to adapt to their deteriorating condition by limiting physical and social activities (Goodwin, Black, & Satish, 1999). Therefore, it is important to address pain-related attitudes and knowledge as part of effective comprehensive assessment.

One of the fundamental challenges in the assessment of older people is the differentiation of the effects of normal aging from those of age-related illness. This is a formidable task given the heterogeneity of normal aging and the high prevalence of comorbidities (Lichtenberg, 1999). The heterogeneity evident within older populations makes chronological age a poor predictor of functional level. Heterogeneity may be greater across settings than within settings (Lichtenberg, 1999). For example, there is more heterogeneity between 80-year-olds seen in community, acute care, or long-term care settings than there is within the 80-year-olds seen in any one of these settings. Related to this, the basic question of how to define an "older" person remains. To date, no consensus exists, and there has been wide variability in the definition of "elderly" or "older person" in research, with ages ranging from the mid-50s to over 90 years old (Gagliese, 2009). This has contributed to discrepant research results and limited cross-study integration. In the end, it may be that meaningful, age-related cutoffs will vary across subgroups of older people based on their health and functional status.

Despite the heterogeneity noted earlier, it is well known that advancing age impacts on every aspect of health and illness, including risk, mechanisms, symptom experience, psychosocial adaptation, treatment efficacy, and survival (Cassel, 2003). In general, older people are more susceptible than younger people to poor outcomes, including increased disability, symptom burden, and mortality. This may be due in part to reduced physiological reserve, homeostenosis, and multisystem functional decline associated with normal aging (Cassel, 2003). Advancing age is marked by a high prevalence of comorbid conditions, including core geriatric syndromes, such as frailty, pressure ulcers, incontinence, falls, functional decline, and delirium (Inouye, Studenski, Tinetti, & Kuchel, 2007). Comorbidities are also associated with polypharmacy, which may impact on pain and function and also have implications for treatment planning (Fulton & Allen, 2005). Cumulative comorbidities also may be related to greater pain and mood disturbance in older people with chronic pain (Rosso, Gallagher, Luborsky, & Mossey, 2008). Therefore, it is evident that a comprehensive assessment of pain, not only in older people but also across the adult lifespan, should include measures of comorbidity. Among the most widely used measures is the *Charlson Comorbidity Index* (CCI; Charlson, Pompei, Ales, & MacKenzie, 1987), a weighted index of 19 conditions that can be adjusted for increasing age and has been well validated for use with older adults (see Extermann, 2000, for a review). It is usually based on chart review and patient interview, although a self-report version with promising psychometric properties is also available (Katz, Chang, Sangha, Fossel, & Bates, 1996).

Given these challenges, it is important that clinicians assessing older persons adopt a biopsychosocial approach standardized to include measures validated for elders. One such approach used in geriatric research and clinical practice is the *comprehensive geriatric assessment* (CGA), which advocates a multidisciplinary biopsychosocial orientation (Devons, 2002). In addition to current pain and pain history, the CGA includes evaluations of functional status; comorbidity; socioeconomic conditions; nutritional status; polypharmacy; and geriatric syndromes, such as depression, delirium and cognitive status, gait and falls, and neglect and abuse (Balducci, 2003). To date, standardized CGA protocols specifically for older people with chronic pain have not been developed. Nonetheless, the principles of CGA may present a useful framework for moving toward the standardization of pain assessment in older people and may, in fact, have relevance for patients of all ages. To this end, a recent consensus statement provides detailed recommendations for an interdisciplinary clinical assessment that is consistent with CGA (Hadjistavropoulos et al., 2007).

MEASUREMENT OF PAIN

The measurement of pain is the first step in pain assessment. Accordingly, one of the areas that has received the most empirical attention is the examination of the psychometric properties of various pain scales for use with older people. Self-reports of pain remain the "gold standard" for both clinical and research purposes. It is essential that all comprehensive pain assessments include pain tools that have been validated for older people and across the adult lifespan. Many aspects of the experience of pain can be measured, but the most common aspects are pain intensity, qualities, and location/distribution. Each of these is considered in turn.

Measures of Pain Intensity

The most frequently assessed component of pain is *intensity*: how much it hurts (Jensen & Karoly, Chapter 2, this volume). Commonly used measures of pain intensity include visual analogue scales (VASs), verbal descriptor scales (VDSs), facial pain scales, and numerical rating scales (NRSs) (see Jensen & Karoly, Chapter 2, this volume). Most of these scales were initially developed and validated for use with younger adults. It is not appropriate simply to assume that they also are valid for older people, especially those who may be frail or have mild cognitive difficulties.

At present, evidence regarding the validity and reliability of these scales when used with older people can guide tool choices for both research and clinical applications. Many studies have found that cognitively intact, older people can provide valid and reliable responses on most single-item pain intensity scales (Benesh, Szigeti, Ferraro, & Gullicks, 1997; Gagliese & Melzack, 1997a; Helme, Katz, Gibson, & Corran, 1989; Herr & Mobily, 1993). This has been shown in various clinical and research settings with a variety of subgroups of older people. An important question has been whether there are age differences in the ability to complete various pain tools. Because all scales are associated with some completion difficulties (Gagliese, Weizblit, Ellis, & Chan, 2005), age-related variation in these difficulties is of prime importance. Several studies have found that older people are as able as younger people to complete most pain intensity scales. The NRS and VDS generally have the highest rates of completion, with over 85% of older people able to provide scorable responses (Gagliese et al., 2005; Herr, Spratt, Mobily, & Richardson, 2004; Peters, Patijn, & Lame, 2007).

Preferences for various pain intensity scales have also been measured. This represents an aspect of face validity, because participants are asked which scale they prefer, which is easiest to complete, and which is the best representation of their pain. It is important to choose a scale with face validity to maximize compliance and minimize attrition in research settings (Mody et al., 2008). Generally, older people report that they prefer to complete the NRS and VDS, including variants such as thermometers or box scores (Benesh et al., 1997; Gagliese et al., 2005; Herr & Mobily, 1993; Herr et al., 2004; Peters et al., 2007; Rodriguez, McMillan, & Yarandi, 2004).

There also is growing evidence for the construct validity of most single-item pain intensity scales. Moderate to high intercorrelations among these measures have been reported in samples of older people (Gagliese et al., 2005; Helme et al., 1989; Herr & Mobily, 1993; Herr, Spratt, Garand, & Li, 2007), with the magnitude of the correlations not differing between younger and older adults (Gagliese et al., 2005). In factor analyses of these measures, one "pain intensity" factor emerges in both younger and older groups (Gagliese et al., 2005; Peters et al., 2007), indicating that the scales are measuring a single underlying construct in a highly comparable way across age groups. It is important to note, however, that the construct validity of facial pain scales has been questioned. The faces used in these scales can be difficult to interpret (Pesonen, Suojaranta-Ylinen, Tarkkila, & Rosenberg, 2008) or are interpreted as expressing negative emotions, such as sadness or affective distress, in addition to pain. For instance, while the majority of older cognitively intact adults agreed that a modified version of the facial pain scale represented pain (67.7%), a substantial proportion also indicated that the faces represented anger (54.8%) or sadness (41.9%) (Kim & Buschmann, 2006). Although this issue requires further investigation, it may limit the appropriateness of the facial pain scale.

Most clinical and research uses of pain scales involve repeated administration. To that end, it is important that pain tools demonstrate test–retest reliability, if one expects consistency of estimates over time, or sensitivity, if one expects change over time. Test–retest reliability is a measure of stability, whereas sensitivity to change is a measure of validity (Anastasi, 1988). Ideally, measures should be able to demonstrate both of these properties under different conditions (Wetherell, 1996). The NRS, VDS, and facial pain scale each has demonstrated adequate to good test–retest reliability over intervals spanning 2 weeks (Miro, Huguet, Nieto, Paredes, & Baos, 2005; Taylor, Harris, Epps, & Herr, 2005). Pain scale sensitivity has received less empirical attention. This is surprising given the centrality of this property of pain scales to the identification of effective pain management interventions. There is some evidence for sensitivity across age groups for the NRS and facial pain scale (Gagliese & Katz, 2003; Herr et al., 2004), although this requires replication. Data regarding the sensitivity of the VDS are mixed, with some studies supporting its sensitivity (Frank, Moll, & Hort, 1982; Gagliese & Katz, 2003; Herr et al., 2004) and others challenging it (Frank et al., 1982; Hadjistavropoulos et al., 2007). Clearly, studies designed to assess the sensitivity of various scales for older people and across the adult lifespan are urgently needed.

In addition to demonstrating sensitivity, it is important to establish the magnitude of change that is clinically meaningful or important. Provisional targets for clinically important change for measures of pain intensity have been proposed (Dworkin et al., 2008); however, age-related constancy in these targets remains to be demonstrated. It is also important to distinguish between internal and external responsiveness. *Internal responsiveness* is represented by the change in a measure over time or following an intervention, whereas *external responsiveness* is the degree to which changes in a measure relate to changes in some external standard, such as health status (Husted, Cook, Farewell, & Gladman, 2000). It has been recommended that clinical trials in chronic pain employ more than one method of evaluating clinically important change (Dworkin et al., 2008). Establishing the clinically important change for the various pain intensity scales when used for older people should be a research priority. These data would determine whether clinically significant change and the magnitude of response required to detect effects between treatment and control groups (Dworkin et al., 2008) differ for younger and older patients with pain.

Despite the many gaps in our knowledge, the available evidence appears to support the use of many well-established scales with older people. However, this may not be the case for the VAS. Beginning with Kremer, Atkinson, and Ignelzi (1981), evidence indicates that older people have more difficulty than younger people completing VASs, with between 7 and 30% of older people unable to provide scorable responses (Gagliese & Melzack, 1997a; Herr & Mobily, 1993). Predictors of these difficulties include increasing age and psychomotor and cognitive impairment, but not gender or education level (Gagliese et al., 2005; Herr et al., 2004; Peters et al., 2007). Interestingly, older adults also experience difficulties using VASs to rate constructs other than pain (Tiplady, Jackson, Maskrey, & Swift, 1998). The VAS may draw on different cognitive tasks than other measures of pain intensity, in particular, abstract reasoning required to transform a subjective experience into a length of line. Older people may have more difficulties than younger people judging proportions of line length (Barrett & Craver-Lemley, 2008), which also may contribute to their difficulties with the VAS. More research is needed to elucidate the cognitive demands of VASs and the ways in which performance may be impacted by age. Consistent with data regarding scale failure, older people report that the VAS is more difficult to complete, is a poorer description of pain, and is less preferred for future use than other scales (Benesh et al., 1997; Herr & Mobily, 1993). These data suggest that even among those who are able to complete the VAS, this scale is difficult and of questionable face validity. This raises concerns regarding compliance, especially if repeated or independent completion of the VAS is required. Finally, data regarding the sensitivity of the VAS are mixed (Gagliese & Katz, 2003; Svensson, 1998). Taken together, this research suggests that VASs should not be used to assess pain intensity in older

people or across age groups. Instead, the data support the use of NRS or VDS scales.

Measures of Pain Quality

Unidimensional single-item scales, such as those described earlier, indicate only one element of the pain experience: intensity. Multidimensional measures, on the other hand, provide a more comprehensive description of an individual's pain. The *McGill Pain Questionnaire* (MPQ; Melzack, 1975) is the most widely used multidimensional measure of pain qualities (Wilke, Savedra, Holzemer, Tesler, & Paul, 1990). It comprises 20 sets of adjectives that describe the sensory, affective, evaluative, and miscellaneous components of pain. Subjects endorse those words that describe their feelings and sensations at that moment. There is much evidence for the validity, reliability, sensitivity, and discriminative abilities of the MPQ when used with younger adults (see Katz & Melzack, Chapter 3, this volume). Recent evidence has also supported its use with older people. Ability to complete the MPQ, validity, factor structure, reliability, and sensitivity have each been demonstrated and do not differ across adults of different ages (Fuentes, Hart-Johnson, & Green, 2007; Gagliese & Katz, 2003; Gagliese & Melzack, 2003; Gagliese et al., 2005).

The Short-Form MPQ (SF-MPQ; Melzack, 1987; see Katz & Melzack, Chapter 3, this volume) also may be appropriate for older people (Gagliese & Melzack, 1997a). Although one small study found increasing age to be related to completion problems (Grafton, Foster, & Wright, 2005), another study did not find age differences (Gagliese & Melzack, 1997a). Acceptable test–retest reliability, high concurrent validity, and sensitivity have been reported for older adults (Gagliese & Melzack, 1997a; Grafton et al., 2005; Helme et al., 1989; Strand, Ljunggren, Bogen, Ask, & Johnsen, 2008). There is some evidence that, across age groups, the same MPQ and SF-MPQ descriptors are chosen most frequently to describe the same type of pain (e.g., arthritis pain) (Gagliese & Melzack, 1997a, 2003), supporting its construct and discriminative validity.

Taken together, these data provide strong preliminary evidence that the MPQ and SF-

MPQ may be appropriate for use with older people. However, it is important to note that these studies have not included especially vulnerable older people. Except for Fuentes and colleagues (2007), who considered ethnic minorities ranging in socioeconomic status, the studies have focused on cognitively intact, older people with chronic or postoperative pain who were living independently. Research is urgently needed to validate the MPQ and SF-MPQ for other subgroups of older people, including those with limited education, reading difficulties, the oldest-old, and those with poorer physical status in long-term care settings. Research validating the many translations of the MPQ for use with older people would also be most welcome.

Measures of Pain Location and Distribution

In addition to descriptors of pain qualities, the MPQ includes line drawings of the body (a *pain map*) on which to indicate the spatial distribution of pain (Melzack, 1975). Although the interpretation of pain maps remains unclear (Jensen & Karoly, Chapter 2, this volume), a valid and reliable scoring method has been developed for younger adults (Margolis, Tait, & Krause, 1986). This method has demonstrated good test–retest reliability, convergent validity, and predictive validity when used to score pain maps of nursing home residents (Weiner, Peterson, & Keefe, 1998). A comparison of the psychometric properties of this scoring method between younger and older pain patients has yet to be reported.

Escalante, Lichtenstein, White, Rios, and Hazuda (1995) have developed a scoring system specifically for assessing arthritis pain in older adults, with promising preliminary psychometric data. It is associated with good interrater, intrarater, and test–retest reliability, and acceptable levels of internal consistency (Escalante et al., 1995; Lichtenstein, Dhanda, Cornell, Escalante, & Hazuda, 1998). Interestingly, in these studies, participants point to the painful area on the drawing, and the interviewers make the markings, a scoring method originally developed for use with children (Savedra, Tesler, Holzemer, Wilkie, & Ward, 1989). It is not clear whether similar results would be obtained if older partici-

pants completed the pain maps independently. The relationship of this measure to MPQ and VDS scores has been inconsistent, with reports of weak (Lichtenstein et al., 1998) and strong (Escalante et al., 1995) correlations. This inconsistency should not be taken as a challenge to the usefulness of the pain map. There is no obvious a priori reason to expect a strong relationship between pain location and intensity or qualities. It is easy to imagine that one can experience highly localized severe pain, highly localized mild pain, diffuse severe pain, and diffuse mild pain. Each of these situations would lead to a different correlation between pain location and intensity. Although preliminary, these data suggest that older people are able to use pain maps to indicate the location of their pain. This method of scoring the pain map has not been tested in younger adults.

Summary

There is converging evidence that NRSs, VDSs, the MPQ, and the SF-MPQ are valid and reliable for use across the adult lifespan. These scales also would be the most appropriate for the assessment of age-related patterns in pain. Pain maps appear to provide useful data regarding the location and spatial distribution of pain, although the available scoring methods have not been tested across age groups. Importantly, these instruments also have been recommended as outcome measures by the Initiative on Methods, Measurement, and Pain Assessment in Clinical Trials (IMMPACT; Dworkin et al., 2005). There appear to be several problems with use of the VAS, including completion difficulties, low face validity, and unclear levels of reliability and sensitivity. Larger studies are needed to assess more adequately the psychometric properties of the previously discussed scales across the adult lifespan. It is important that the recommended scales be incorporated into both clinical and research settings to provide the best possible pain measurement, to increase confidence in study results, and to maximize our ability to integrate findings across studies. The growing consensus toward a "gold standard" of pain assessment instruments is fundamental to advancing the science of pain and aging (Gagliese, 2009).

ASSESSMENT OF PAIN-RELATED IMPACT AND FUNCTIONAL LIMITATIONS

Pain-Specific Measures

A comprehensive pain assessment must incorporate measures of the impact and associated features of pain. This can include, but is certainly not limited to, the assessment of physical disability, interference of pain in the performance of daily and desired activities, and psychological distress. Self-report measures of many of these constructs have been developed and are in frequent use in both the research and clinical setting.

Among the most commonly used scales to assess pain-related impairment are the *Pain Disability Index* (PDI; Pollard, 1984) and the Brief Pain Inventory (BPI; Cleeland & Ryan, 1994). Both of these scales use NRSs to measure the extent to which the performance of obligatory and voluntary daily activities is limited by pain. There is growing evidence that the PDI and BPI may be valid, reliable, and sensitive when used by older people (Ersek, Turner, Cain, & Kemp, 2008; Fuentes et al., 2007; McDonald et al., 2008; Tittle, McMillan, & Hagan, 2003; Williams, Smith, & Fehnel, 2006). Studies using modified and disease-specific versions of the BPI for older adults are also emerging (Auret et al., 2008; Schmader et al., 2007); however, further psychometric testing of these versions in older people and across age groups is needed.

Disease-specific impact measures, such as the *Western Ontario and McMaster Universities Osteoarthritis Index* (WOMAC; Bellamy, Buchanan, Goldsmith, Campbell, & Stitt, 1988), the *Arthritis Impact Measurement Scales* (AIMS; Meenan, Gertman, & Mason, 1980), the revised AIMS for older adults (GERI-AIMS; Hughes, Edelman, Chang, Singer, & Schuette, 1991), the *Pain Disability Questionnaire* (Anagnostis, Gatchel, & Mayer, 2004), and the *Oswestry Low Back Pain Disability Questionnaire* (Fairbank, Couper, Davies, & O'Brien, 1980) have been developed. Some of these may be appropriate for use with older populations (Hadjistavropoulos et al., 2007), but detailed, age-related psychometric properties have not been reported.

Measures of pain-related functional impairment have been designed and developed

specifically for use with older adults. The *Geriatric Pain Measure* (GPM; Ferrell, Stein, & Beck, 2000), a 24-item measure of pain severity and pain-related functioning, was designed for use with cognitively intact, ambulatory, older adults. It includes 22 dichotomous yes–no response options and two NRSs of current and average pain severity (Ferrell et al., 2000). It demonstrates acceptable validity, with a moderate to strong correlation with the MPQ, good test–retest reliability, and high completion rates (Clough-Gorr et al., 2008; Ferrell et al., 2000). A 12-item short form of the GPM measuring pain severity, pain with ambulation, and disengagement due to pain has been developed. This version correlates strongly with the original and demonstrates acceptable validity and reliability (Blozik et al., 2007). A different, 13-item version of the GPM administered in an interview format to nursing home residents demonstrated acceptable reliability (Simmons, Ferrell, & Schnelle, 2002). However, 35% of the residents were unable or unwilling to complete the scale (Simmons et al., 2002), suggesting poor feasibility. The *Functional Pain Scale* (FPS; Gloth, Scheve, Stober, Chow, & Prosser, 2001) is a brief measure of pain and its impact on function. While it has the advantage of brevity, the FPS has been criticized as including only a narrow listing of activities that may be impacted by pain (Hadjistavropoulos et al., 2007). Although these scales were developed for use with older people, they do not always differentiate limitations due to pain from those due to aging or chronic illness. Not surprisingly, psychometric analyses of responses from younger people with pain are not available, limiting their use in studies of age-related patterns.

Generic Measures

Several generic measures of impairment due to chronic illness have demonstrated good psychometric properties in samples of people with chronic pain. In addition, some preliminary work has focused on their use with older people. For our purposes in this chapter, only those measures that have been studied in samples of older people with chronic pain are briefly discussed. The most extensively studied measures are the *Sickness Im-*

pact Profile (SIP; Bergner, Bobbitt, Pollard, Martin, & Gilson, 1976), the *Human Activity Profile* (HAP; Fix & Daughton, 1988), and the *Physical Activity Scale for the Elderly* (PASE; Washburn, Smith, Jette, & Janney, 1993).

The SIP is a 136-item inventory of the extent to which health problems interfere with physical and psychosocial functioning (Bergner et al., 1976). It has demonstrated good psychometric properties across various samples, including younger adults with chronic pain and older people with a variety of health problems in community, acute care, and institutional settings (Morishita et al., 1995). Item scaling analysis has shown that younger and older people do not differ significantly in the perception of the severity of dysfunction assessed by each item (Marchionni et al., 1997). The SIP has been shown to have comparable properties whether completed in person or during a telephone interview (Morishita et al., 1995), although comparability with independent completion has not been assessed. Among older people with chronic hip and knee pain, the physical and psychosocial subscales have been found to be moderately correlated (Hopman-Rock, Odding, Hofman, Kraaimaat, & Bijlsma, 1996). One limitation is that the SIP may suffer from ceiling effects (Andresen, Rothenberg, Panzer, Katz, & McDermott, 1998).

Although not widely used, the HAP has also been validated for older people with chronic pain (Fix & Daughton, 1988). This questionnaire assesses the overall, current, and past performance of 94 activities. It has demonstrated good levels of internal consistency, high test–retest reliability over a 2-week interval, concurrent validity, and sensitivity to treatment effects when used with older people with chronic pain (Bennell et al., 2004; Farrell, Gibson, & Helme, 1996).

The PASE also has shown promising psychometric properties for older people (Washburn et al., 1993). This self-report or interview measure comprises 12 items that assess frequency, duration, and intensity of participation in leisure, household, and occupational physical activities over the previous week. A weighted scoring system that reflects the amount of energy required to perform each activity is available. Among healthy older people, this scale correlates with the SIP and self-assessed health status, and has moderate to good levels of test–retest reliability in intervals ranging from 3 to 7 weeks (Washburn et al., 1993). Among older people with daily knee pain secondary to osteoarthritis, PASE scores are significantly correlated with performance on a walking test and measures of knee strength, but not with measures of pain intensity or frequency (Martin et al., 1999). The PASE has not been validated for younger individuals. Unfortunately, studies that directly compare the PASE, HAP, and SIP across age groups could not be located.

Far more work is needed to determine which measure of activity or disability due to pain is the most appropriate for older people and for the assessment of age-related patterns. The SIP has the most empirical evidence favoring its use; however, it is a very long questionnaire and may represent considerable burden, especially if repeated administration is necessary. The BPI, a briefer measure that has been extensively validated for use with younger people, has promising preliminary data regarding its use with older people and is the recommended measure at this time.

ASSESSMENT OF HEALTH-RELATED QUALITY OF LIFE

Increasingly, it is recognized that functional limitations are only one aspect of perceived overall health, well-being, and quality of life. Several measures have been developed to assess quality of life in older people (Haywood, Garratt, & Fitzpatrick, 2005). The most widely used is the *Medical Outcome Study Short-Form 36 Health Survey* (SF-36), a generic, multidimensional measure of functioning and well-being (McHorney, Ware, & Raczek, 1993). The subscales include Physical Functioning, Role Limitations Due to Physical Problems, Social Functioning, Bodily Pain, General Mental Health, Role Limitations Due to Emotional Problems, Energy and Fatigue, and General Health Perceptions (McHorney et al., 1993).

The SF-36 has demonstrated acceptable psychometric properties for community-dwelling older people (Sherman & Reuben, 1998). However, people age 75 and older may have greater difficulty completing it than those ages 65–74 (Hayes, Morris, Wolfe, & Morgan, 1995). These difficulties have been associated with greater functional impairment; therefore, the SF-36 may underestimate functional status among older respondents (Parker, Bechinger-English, Jagger, Spiers, & Lindesay, 2006). There are also substantial floor and ceiling effects (Andresen, Gravitt, Aydelotte, & Podgorski, 1999; Stadnyk, Calder, & Rockwood, 1998), possibly limiting sensitivity.

A few studies have assessed the psychometric properties of the SF-36 for use with older people with chronic pain. One study in the community and long-term care setting found moderate to high levels of internal consistency and a gradient of scores reflecting increasingly poor health (Murray, LeFort, & Ribeiro, 1998). The Physical Functioning composite score of the SF-36 demonstrated strong discriminant properties between older adults with and without chronic low back pain (CLBP) (Rudy, Weiner, Lieber, Slaboda, & Boston, 2007). Nonetheless, the face validity of the SF-36 may be questionable, and caution is recommended in the interpretation of responses (Murray et al., 1998). Mangione and colleagues (1993) compared the SF-36 in middle-aged and older elective surgery patients. They found similar levels of subscale internal consistency across age groups but significant age differences in the magnitude of subscale correlations. Most importantly, the correlation of overall health perception and pain was almost twice as high in middle-aged than in older patients. These authors suggest that the determinants of health-related quality of life may differ by age, and that the SF-36 may not assess those determinants that are most important to older patients (Mangione et al., 1993). Taken together, data regarding the use of the SF-36 in older people with pain or across age groups are not very encouraging. A short version of the SF-36, the SF-12 (Ware, Kosinski, & Keller, 1996), is also available. This version may be less burdensome, particularly for long protocols or repeated testing. Age-related variations in the psychometric properties of the SF-12 require testing in people with chronic pain. Many other quality of life scales are available; however, we were unable to find studies assessing their psychometric properties for older people with chronic pain.

ASSESSMENT OF PSYCHOSOCIAL FACTORS AND DISTRESS

A plethora of cognitive and affective factors has been found to be relevant to pain experience, treatment response, and long-term adjustment (Gatchel, Peng, Peters, Fuchs, & Turk, 2007). Consistent with the growing evidence that the biopsychosocial model also applies to geriatric pain (Gagliese, 2009), a comprehensive assessment should include attention to the psychosocial context. However, to date, there is only limited information regarding the validity and reliability of most scales of psychological and cognitive factors for use with elders, making evidence-based recommendations difficult. Promising preliminary data supporting the psychometric properties of some measures, including the Pain Anxiety Symptoms Scale (Asmundson, Hadjistavropoulos, Bernstein, & Zvolensky, 2009) and the Falls Efficacy Scale (Tinetti, Richman, & Powell, 1990), when used with older people and/or across the lifespan, have been reported. However, more research is urgently needed to identify the best assessment battery for the older patient.

The assessment of psychological distress among older people, including those with pain, has received more empirical attention. Although the prevalence of major depressive disorder may decrease with age, there is growing evidence that subsyndromal, but clinically relevant, depression increases with age, especially among those over 80 years old (VanItallie, 2005). Similar to younger individuals, there is significant comorbidity of pain and depression in older adults (Gagliese & Melzack, 2003; Rosso et al., 2008), with up to 40% of older people with chronic pain obtaining scores on depression scales that indicate clinically relevant symptomatology (Lopez-Lopez, Montorio, Izal, & Velasco, 2008). There is evidence that the prevalence and intensity of depression among people with chronic noncancer (Gagliese & Melzack, 2003) and cancer pain (Gagliese, Gauthier, & Rodin, 2007) are similar across age groups, but see Weiner, Rudy, Morrow, Slaboda, and Lieber (2006) for an exception. Regardless of age-related patterns, it is evident that a significant proportion of older people with chronic pain experiences clinically relevant depression. Older people with moderate to severe pain, especially males with multiple medical comorbidities, may be at elevated risk for suicide (Juurlink et al., 2004). Therefore, screening for symptoms of depression, including suicidal ideation, is a priority in the assessment of older people with chronic pain.

Clinical differentiation of pain, depression, comorbid conditions, and normal aging may be difficult due to symptom overlap, especially somatic symptoms, such as sleep and appetite disturbance (Jeste, Blazer, & First, 2005). This may be further complicated because older people may be more likely to have atypical or unique presentations of both pain (Gagliese & Melzack, 2006) and depression (Blazer, 1990). In addition, comparable to pain, older people may be reluctant to report symptoms of depression, or they may believe that symptoms such as anhedonia or fatigue are part of normal aging (Butcher & McGonigal-Kenney, 2005). As a result, depression in older people may be underrecognized and undertreated (VanItallie, 2005).

To enhance the detection of depression among older people, completion of a well-validated, self-report scale is strongly recommended (Roman & Callen, 2008). To be useful, these scales must be able to identify clinically significant levels of depressive symptomatology with acceptable sensitivity and specificity (Papassotiropoulos & Heun, 1999). In other words, these scales must accurately identify cases of depression, while not misidentifying individuals (i.e., false positives and false negatives). It also is important to choose a scale that has been validated for older people or for use across the adult lifespan, if age-related patterns are of interest. In addition, the scale should have evidence supporting its use in people with pain. There are many depression scales available. We describe three of the most widely used in geriatric and pain research.

The *Geriatric Depression Scale* (GDS; Yesavage, 1988) was developed as a screening tool for older adults. Somatic items that may overestimate the prevalence of depression are excluded (Roman & Callen, 2008). Both the 30- and 15-item (Sheikh & Yesavage, 1986) versions of the GDS demonstrate good reliability and validity among older adults with chronic (Rudy et al., 2007) and postoperative pain (Zalon, 2004). There is some debate regarding the impact of pain on the performance of this scale. Marc, Raue, and Bruce (2008) found that the performance of the 15-item GDS was not influenced by pain. However, Karp, Rudy, and Weiner (2008) found that several of the 30 items from the full-length GDS were impacted by pain and proposed a 20-item version, the GDS-PAIN, which omits these items. Further research will be required to clarify the impact of pain on the properties of the GDS. Interestingly, there is some preliminary evidence supporting the use of the GDS for younger people, if the cutoffs for "caseness" are adjusted across age groups (Weintraub, Saboe, & Stern, 2007). To date, an analysis of the GDS' properties when completed by younger people with chronic pain is not available.

The *Center for Epidemiologic Studies—Depression Scale* (CES-D; Radloff, 1977) is a 20-item measure of depressive symptomatology. A 10-item short form has also been developed (Irwin, Artin, & Oxman, 1999). Both the full- and short-form CES-D have demonstrated high levels of reliability and validity, and the lack of somatic items makes them appropriate for medically ill populations (Irwin et al., 1999), including those with chronic pain (Tverskoy et al., 1994). Although this scale was not originally designed for older people, it has been validated for use across the adult lifespan (Radloff & Teri, 1986; Roman & Callen, 2008). Its sensitivity for detection of caseness among older people has been demonstrated (Irwin et al., 1999), but it is not clear whether it has similar (Gerety et al., 1994) or lower (Lyness et al., 1997) sensitivity than the GDS. Its psychometric properties for older people with chronic pain remain to be demonstrated.

The *Beck Depression Inventory* (Beck, 1978) is also a widely used measure with substantial evidence for its validity, reliability, and sensitivity for use with younger people with pain (Morley, Williams, & Black, 2002). There is some evidence supporting its use with older people (Gallagher, 1986). However, the inclusion of somatic symptoms may inflate scores among older people, especially those with comorbid physical conditions (Gallagher, 1986), making it a less preferable choice for use with this group.

Unfortunately, studies that specifically assess the reliability, validity, factor structure, sensitivity, and specificity of depression scales in people of various ages with chronic pain are not available. This is extremely important, because chronic pain, advancing age, and medical comorbidities may each necessitate a change in the application of these scales and reconsideration of the criteria by which symptoms are judged to be clinically significant (Jeste et al., 2005; Turk & Okifuji, 1994). Therefore, the extent to which these scales can be used with older adult patients with chronic pain remains to be determined. Given the very little evidence available at this time, it appears that the GDS and CES-D may be appropriate for the assessment of depression in older people with pain. The CES-D may also be the best choice to assess age-related variation. However, until further data are available, research findings based on these scales must be interpreted with caution.

ALTERNATE PAIN ASSESSMENT STRATEGIES

Pain Diaries

Pain diaries, which allow for multiple self-assessments of pain, analgesic use, mood, and functioning, may be valid and reliable instruments (Maunsell, Allard, Dorval, & Labbe, 2000). Pain scales incorporated into diaries include the NRS, VDS, and ordinal scales assessing pain impact (Maunsell et al., 2000; Schumacher et al., 2002). Paper-based pain diaries have been implemented in studies of nursing home patients (Hager & Brockopp, 2007), as well as community-dwelling older people with cancer (Storto et al., 2006) and osteoarthritis (Gaines, Metter, & Talbot, 2004). Methodological problems with traditional paper versions of pain diaries, such as noncompliance with instructions for completion, may influence the accuracy of reports and the quality of data. This noncompliance may introduce significant recall bias (Gendreau, Hufford, & Stone, 2003). Age-related patterns in these methodological issues have yet to be examined. Electronic pain diary methodology may mitigate some of the compliance issues (Gaertner, Elsner, Pollmann-Dahmen, Radbruch, & Sabatowski, 2004; Gendreau et al., 2003). While electronic diary methodology has been used in studies of older people (Kamarck et al., 2002), age-related patterns in their acceptability and validity are unknown. These data are needed to determine

the feasibility of this methodology with older people and to identify modifications needed to overcome any potential age-related limitations to the use of the equipment.

Electronic Assessments

Recent advances in the use of electronic pain assessment tools offer great clinical and research potential. Clinically, computerized assessments can provide immediate data capture and availability of data to clinic staff members, who may then easily compare current patient assessments with assessments from prior visits to determine change over time (Lee, Kavanaugh, & Lenert, 2007). Electronic versions of assessment tools may also be preferred over paper versions by patients (Cook et al., 2004). This assessment modality may also introduce data quality control, such as prevention of missing, incorrect, and out-of-range data and reduction of data entry errors by research staff (Gendreau et al., 2003). Recent studies have compared paper and electronic versions of the MPQ and SF-MPQ (Cook et al., 2004; Wilkie et al., 2003); however, few studies have examined age-related patterns in the feasibility, acceptability, and equivalency of paper and computerized versions of these and other pain measures. One study found no age differences in the time taken to complete PAIN*Report*It, which included an electronic version of the MPQ (Wilkie et al., 2003), but another study found that older adults took significantly longer than younger adults to complete computerized assessments (Koestler, Libby, Schofferman, & Redmond, 2005). Both studies have small sample sizes, limiting the conclusions that can be drawn.

Studies of the utility of electronic assessments of health-related quality of life (HRQoL) in older adults are emerging (Boissy, Jacobs, & Roy, 2006). Data regarding age-related acceptability of electronic HRQoL scales have been equivocal. Age was unrelated to preference or perceived difficulty of electronic assessments (Saleh et al., 2002; Williams, Templin, & Mosley-Williams, 2004). Another study found that a majority of older adults preferred an electronic version of the SF-36 to a paper version (Ryan, Corry, Attewell, & Smithson, 2002). However, Wilson and colleagues (2002) found that significantly more younger than older adults preferred a computerized version over a paper version of a HRQoL measure. Finally, Buxton, White, and Osoba (1998) found older age to be related to longer time to complete a touch screen HRQoL measure. Given the potential clinical and research utility of computerized assessment, future studies examining age-related patterns in the equivalency and psychometric properties of these assessment tools are needed to determine the utility of this mode of assessment across the adult lifespan.

CONCLUSIONS

The proportion of older people in our society is rapidly increasing. These people will require effective assessment and management of both acute and chronic pain. We have presented a framework for comprehensive assessment that reflects a biopsychosocial model of pain and its impact. Assessment of older people must be evidence-based and sensitive to the heterogeneity and special needs of this group. To that end, we have recommended various scales that have some promising data to support their use; however, these recommendations are preliminary and derived from an evidence base with significant gaps. There is an urgent need for systematic research designed to identify the most valid tools for assessing pain and its impact in the diverse subgroups of older people and across the adult lifespan. For example, despite the increased susceptibility to neuropathic pain with aging (Torrance, Smith, Bennett, & Lee, 2006), the recently developed neuropathic pain scales (e.g., Bennett et al., 2007) have not been subjected to detailed psychometric analyses across different age groups. Such gaps are a serious hindrance to the progress of the field of pain and aging. It is impossible to interpret studies regarding the mechanisms of age-related changes in pain, the effectiveness of pain management strategies, and the interaction of pain with other highly prevalent disorders of aging until these data are available. Further research focused on establishing the psychometric properties of the available scales will also allow us to refine our recommendations for comprehensive evidence-based assessment protocols for use with diverse subgroups of older people. As a result, we will be better able to meet the challenges of providing effective and safe pain management that maximizes function and quality of life for people of all ages.

ACKNOWLEDGMENTS

Lucia Gagliese is supported by a Canadian Institutes of Health Research New Investigator Award. Lynn R. Gauthier is a Research Student of the Canadian Cancer Society through an award from the National Cancer Institute of Canada. Our research in geriatric pain assessment is funded by grants from the Canadian Institutes of Health Research and the University of Toronto held by Lucia Gagliese, and the National Science and Engineering Research Council held by Ronald Melzack.

REFERENCES

Anagnostis, C., Gatchel, R. J., & Mayer, T. G. (2004). The Pain Disability Questionnaire: A new psychometrically sound measure for chronic musculoskeletal disorders. *Spine*, 29(20), 2290–2303.

Anastasi, A. (1988). *Psychological testing* (6th ed.). New York: Macmillan.

Andresen, E. M., Gravitt, G. W., Aydelotte, M. E., & Podgorski, C. A. (1999). Limitations of the SF-36 in a sample of nursing home residents. *Age and Ageing*, 28, 562–566.

Andresen, E. M., Rothenberg, B. M., Panzer, R., Katz, P., & McDermott, M. P. (1998). Selecting a generic measure of health-related quality of life for use among older adults: A comparison of candidate instruments. *Evaluation and the Health Professions*, 21(2), 244–264.

Asmundson, G. J. G., Hadjistavropoulos, T., Bernstein, A., & Zvolensky, M. J. (2009). Latent structure of fear of pain: An empirical test among a sample of community dwelling older adults. *European Journal of Pain*, 13(4), 419–425.

Auret, K. A., Toye, C., Goucke, R., Kristjanson, L. J., Bruce, D., & Schug, S. (2008). Development and testing of a modified version of the Brief Pain Inventory for use in residential aged care facilities. *Journal of the American Geriatrics Society*, 56(2), 301–306.

Balducci, L. (2003). New paradigms for treating elderly patients with cancer: The comprehensive geriatric assessment and guidelines for supportive care. *Journal of Supportive Oncology*, 1(4, Suppl. 2), 30–37.

Barrett, A. M., & Craver-Lemley, C. E. (2008).

Is it what you see, or how you say it?: Spatial bias in young and aged subjects. *Journal of the International Neuropsychological Society*, 14(4), 562–570.

Beck, A. T. (1978). *Depression Inventory*. Philadelphia: Center for Cognitive Therapy.

Bellamy, N., Buchanan, W. W., Goldsmith, C. H., Campbell, J., & Stitt, L. W. (1988). Validation study of WOMAC: A health status instrument for measuring clinically important patient relevant outcomes to antirheumatic drug therapy in patients with osteoarthritis of the hip or knee. *Journal of Rheumatology*, 15(12), 1833–1840.

Benesh, L. R., Szigeti, E., Ferraro, F. R., & Gullicks, J. N. (1997). Tools for assessing chronic pain in rural elderly women. *Home Healthcare Nurse*, 15, 207–211.

Bennell, K. L., Hinman, R. S., Crossley, K. M., Metcalf, B. R., Buchbinder, R., Green, S., et al. (2004). Is the Human Activity Profile a useful measure in people with knee osteoarthritis? *Journal of Rehabilitation Research and Development*, 41(4), 621–630.

Bennett, M. I., Attal, N., Backonja, M. M., Baron, R., Bouhassira, D., Freynhagen, R., et al. (2007). Using screening tools to identify neuropathic pain. *Pain*, 127(3), 199–203.

Bergner, M., Bobbitt, R. A., Pollard, W. E., Martin, D. P., & Gilson, B. S. (1976). The Sickness Impact Profile: Validation of a health status measure. *Medical Care*, 14(1), 57–67.

Blazer, D. (1990). Depression in late life: An update. In M. P. Lawton (Ed.), *Annual review of gerontology and geriatrics* (Vol. 10, pp. 197–215). New York: Springer.

Blozik, E., Stuck, A. E., Niemann, S., Ferrell, B. A., Harari, D., von Renteln-Kruse, W., et al. (2007). Geriatric Pain Measure Short Form: Development and initial evaluation. *Journal of the American Geriatrics Society*, 55(12), 2045–2050.

Boissy, P., Jacobs, K., & Roy, S. H. (2006). Usability of a barcode scanning system as a means of data entry on a PDA for self-report health outcome questionnaires: A pilot study in individuals over 60 years of age. *BMC Medical Informatics and Decision Making*, 6, 42.

Butcher, H. K., & McGonigal-Kenney, M. (2005). Depression and dispiritedness in later life: A "gray drizzle of horror" isn't inevitable. *American Journal of Nursing*, 105(12), 52–62.

Buxton, J., White, M., & Osoba, D. (1998). Patients' experiences using a computerized program with a touch-sensitive video monitor for the assessment of health-related quality of life. *Quality of Life Research*, 7(6), 513–519.

Cassel, C. K. (2003). *Geriatric medicine: An evidence-based approach*. New York: Springer.

Charlson, M. E., Pompei, P., Ales, K. L., & MacKenzie, C. R. (1987). A new method of classifying prognostic comorbidity in longitudinal studies: Development and validation. *Journal of Chronic Diseases*, 40(5), 373–383.

Cleeland, C. S., & Ryan, K. M. (1994). Pain assessment: Global use of the Brief Pain Inventory. *Annals of the Academy of Medicine Singapore*, 23(2), 129–138.

Clough-Gorr, K. M., Blozik, E., Gillmann, G., Beck, J. C., Ferrell, B. A., Anders, J., et al. (2008). The Self-Administered 24-item Geriatric Pain Measure (GPM-24-SA): Psychometric properties in three European populations of community-dwelling older adults. *Pain Medicine*, 9(6), 695–709.

Cook, A. J., Roberts, D. A., Henderson, M. D., Van Winkle, L. C., Chastain, D. C., & Hamill-Ruth, R. J. (2004). Electronic pain questionnaires: A randomized, crossover comparison with paper questionnaires for chronic pain assessment. *Pain*, 110(1–2), 310–317.

Devons, C. A. J. (2002). Comprehensive geriatric assessment: Making the most of the aging years. *Current Opinion in Clinical Nutrition and Metabolic Care*, 5(1), 19–24.

Dworkin, R. H., Turk, D. C., Farrar, J. T., Haythornthwaite, J. A., Jensen, M. P., Katz, N. P., et al. (2005). Core outcome measures for chronic pain clinical trials: IMMPACT recommendations. *Pain*, 113(1–2), 9–19.

Dworkin, R. H., Turk, D. C., Wyrwich, K. W., Beaton, D., Cleeland, C. S., Farrar, J. T., et al. (2008). Interpreting the clinical importance of treatment outcomes in chronic pain clinical trials: IMMPACT recommendations. *Journal of Pain*, 9(2), 105–121.

Ersek, M., Turner, J. A., Cain, K. C., & Kemp, C. A. (2008). Results of a randomized controlled trial to examine the efficacy of a chronic pain self-management group for older adults. *Pain*, 138(1), 29–40.

Escalante, A., Lichtenstein, M. J., White, K., Rios, N., & Hazuda, H. P. (1995). A method for scoring the pain map of the McGill Pain Questionnaire for use in epidemiologic studies. *Aging (Milano)*, 7(5), 358–366.

Extermann, M. (2000). Measuring comorbidity in older cancer patients. *European Journal of Cancer*, 36(4), 453–471.

Fairbank, J. C., Couper, J., Davies, J. B., & O'Brien, J. P. (1980). The Oswestry Low Back Pain Disability Questionnaire. *Physiotherapy*, 66(8), 271–273.

Farrell, M. J., Gibson, S. J., & Helme, R. D. (1996). Measuring the activity of older people with chronic pain. *Clinical Journal of Pain*, 12(1), 6–12.

Ferrell, B. A., Stein, W. M., & Beck, J. C. (2000). The Geriatric Pain Measure: Validity, reliability and factor analysis. *Journal of the American Geriatrics Society*, 48(12), 1669–1673.

Ferrell, B. R., & Juarez, G. (2002). Cancer pain education for patients and the public. *Journal of Pain and Symptom Management*, 23(4), 329–336.

Fix, A. J., & Daughton, D. M. (1988). *Human Activity Profile: Professional manual*. Odessa FL: Psychological Assessment Resources.

Fox, P. L., Raina, P., & Jadad, A. R. (1999). Prevalence and treatment of pain in older adults in nursing homes and other long-term care institutions: A systematic review. *Canadian Medical Association Journal*, 160(3), 329–333.

Frank, A. J., Moll, J. M., & Hort, J. F. (1982). A comparison of three ways of measuring pain. *Rheumatology and Rehabilitation*, 21(4), 211–217.

Fuentes, M., Hart-Johnson, T., & Green, C. R. (2007). The association among neighborhood socioeconomic status, race and chronic pain in black and white older adults. *Journal of the National Medical Association*, 99(10), 1160–1169.

Fulton, M. M., & Allen, E. R. (2005). Polypharmacy in the elderly: A literature review. *Journal of the American Academy of Nurse Practitioners*, 17(4), 123–132.

Gaertner, J., Elsner, F., Pollmann-Dahmen, K., Radbruch, L., & Sabatowski, R. (2004). Electronic pain diary: A randomized crossover study. *Journal of Pain and Symptom Management*, 28(3), 259–267.

Gagliese, L. (2009). Pain and aging: The emergence of a new subfield of pain research. *Journal of Pain*, 10(4), 343–353.

Gagliese, L., Gauthier, L. R., & Rodin, G. (2007). Cancer pain and depression: A systematic review of age-related patterns. *Pain Research and Management*, 12(3), 205–211.

Gagliese, L., & Katz, J. (2003). Age differences in postoperative pain are scale dependent: A comparison of measures of pain intensity and quality in younger and older surgical patients. *Pain*, 103(1–2), 11–20.

Gagliese, L., & Melzack, R. (1997a). Age differences in the quality of chronic pain: A preliminary study. *Pain Research and Management*, 2, 157–162.

Gagliese, L., & Melzack, R. (1997b). Chronic pain in elderly people. *Pain*, 70, 3–14.

Gagliese, L., & Melzack, R. (2003). Age-related differences in the qualities but not the intensity of chronic pain. *Pain*, 104, 597–608.

Gagliese, L., & Melzack, R. (2006). Pain in the elderly. In S. B. McMahon & M. Koltzenburg (Eds.), *Melzack and Wall's textbook of pain* (pp. 1169–1179). Edinburgh, UK: Elsevier.

Gagliese, L., Weizblit, N., Ellis, W., & Chan, V. W. (2005). The measurement of postoperative pain: A comparison of intensity scales in younger and older surgical patients. *Pain*, 117(3), 412–420.

Gaines, J. M., Metter, E. J., & Talbot, L. A. (2004). The effect of neuromuscular electrical stimulation on arthritis knee pain in older adults with osteoarthritis of the knee. *Applied Nursing Research*, 17(3), 201–206.

Gallagher, D. (1986). The Beck Depression Inventory and older adults: Review of its development and utility. In T. L. Brink (Ed.), *Clinical gerontology* (pp. 149–163). New York: Haworth Press.

Gatchel, R. J., Peng, Y. B., Peters, M. L., Fuchs, P. N., & Turk, D. C. (2007). The biopsychosocial approach to chronic pain: Scientific advances and future directions. *Psychological Bulletin*, 133(4), 581–624.

Gendreau, M., Hufford, M. R., & Stone, A. A. (2003). Measuring clinical pain in chronic widespread pain: Selected methodological issues. *Best Practice and Research in Clinical Rheumatology*, 17(4), 575–592.

Gerety, M. B., Williams, J. W., Jr., Mulrow, C. D., Cornell, J. E., Kadri, A. A., Rosenberg, J., et al. (1994). Performance of case-finding tools for depression in the nursing home: Influence of clinical and functional characteristics and selection of optimal threshold scores. *Journal of the American Geriatrics Society*, 42(10), 1103–1109.

Gibson, S. J., & Weiner, D. K. (2005). *Progress in pain research and management: Pain in the older person*. Seattle, WA: IASP Press.

Gloth, F. M., III, Scheve, A. A., Stober, C. V., Chow, S., & Prosser, J. (2001). The Functional Pain Scale: Reliability, validity, and responsiveness in an elderly population. *Journal of the American Medical Directors Association*, 2(3), 110–114.

Goodwin, S., Black, S. A., & Satish, S. (1999). Aging versus disease: The opinions of older black, Hispanic, and non-Hispanic white Americans about the causes and treatment of common medical conditions. *Journal of the American Geriatrics Society*, 47(8), 1–13.

Grafton, K. V., Foster, N. E., & Wright, C. C. (2005). Test–retest reliability of the Short-Form McGill Pain Questionnaire: Assessment of intraclass correlation coefficients and limits of agreement in patients with osteoarthritis. *Clinical Journal of Pain*, 21(1), 73–82.

Hadjistavropoulos, T., Herr, K., Turk, D. C., Fine, P. G., Dworkin, R. H., Helme, R., et al. (2007). An interdisciplinary expert consensus statement on assessment of pain in older persons. *Clinical Journal of Pain*, 23(Suppl. 1), S1–S43.

Hager, K. K., & Brockopp, D. (2007). Pilot project: The chronic pain diary—assessing chronic pain in the nursing home population. *Journal of Gerontological Nursing, 33*(9), 14–19.

Hayes, V., Morris, J., Wolfe, C., & Morgan, M. (1995). The SF-36 Health Survey Questionnaire: Is it suitable for use with older adults? *Age and Ageing, 24*(2), 120–125.

Haywood, K. L., Garratt, A. M., & Fitzpatrick, R. (2005). Quality of life in older people: A structured review of generic self-assessed health instruments. *Quality of Life Research, 14*(7), 1651–1668.

Helme, R. D., Katz, B., Gibson, S., & Corran, T. (1989). Can psychometric tools be used to analyse pain in a geriatric population? *Clinical and Experimental Neurology, 26*, 113–117.

Herr, K., Spratt, K. F., Garand, L., & Li, L. (2007). Evaluation of the Iowa Pain Thermometer and other selected pain intensity scales in younger and older adult cohorts using controlled clinical pain: A preliminary study. *Pain Medicine, 8*(7), 585–600.

Herr, K. A., & Mobily, P. R. (1993). Comparison of selected pain assessment tools for use with the elderly. *Applied Nursing Research, 6*, 39–46.

Herr, K. A., Spratt, K., Mobily, P. R., & Richardson, G. (2004). Pain intensity assessment in older adults: Use of experimental pain to compare psychometric properties and usability of selected pain scales with younger adults. *Clinical Journal of Pain, 20*(4), 207–219.

Hopman-Rock, M., Odding, E., Hofman, A., Kraaimaat, F. W., & Bijlsma, J. W. (1996). Physical and psychosocial disability in elderly subjects in relation to pain in the hip and/or knee. *Journal of Rheumatology, 23*(6), 1037–1044.

Hughes, S. L., Edelman, P., Chang, R. W., Singer, R. H., & Schuette, P. (1991). The GERI-AIMS: Reliability and validity of the Arthritis Impact Measurement scales adapted for elderly respondents. *Arthritis and Rheumatism, 34*(7), 856–865.

Husted, J. A., Cook, R. J., Farewell, V. T., & Gladman, D. D. (2000). Methods for assessing responsiveness: A critical review and recommendations. *Journal of Clinical Epidemiology, 53*(5), 459–468.

Inouye, S. K., Studenski, S., Tinetti, M. E., & Kuchel, G. A. (2007). Geriatric syndromes: Clinical, research, and policy implications of a core geriatric concept. *Journal of the American Geriatrics Society, 55*(5), 780–791.

Irwin, M., Artin, K. H., & Oxman, M. N. (1999). Screening for depression in the older adult: Criterion validity of the 10-item Center for Epidemiological Studies Depression Scale (CES-D). *Archives of Internal Medicine, 159*(15), 1701–1704.

Jeste, D. V., Blazer, D. G., & First, M. (2005). Aging-related diagnostic variations: Need for diagnostic criteria appropriate for elderly psychiatric patients. *Biological Psychiatry, 58*(4), 265–271.

Juurlink, D. N., Herrmann, N., Szalai, J. P., Kopp, A., & Redelmeier, D. A. (2004). Medical illness and the risk of suicide in the elderly. *Archives of Internal Medicine, 164*(11), 1179–1184.

Kamarck, T. W., Janicki, D. L., Shiffman, S., Polk, D. E., Muldoon, M. F., Liebenauer, L. L., et al. (2002). Psychosocial demands and ambulatory blood pressure: A field assessment approach. *Physiology and Behavior, 77*(4–5), 699–704.

Karp, J. F., Rudy, T., & Weiner, D. K. (2008). Persistent pain biases item response on the Geriatric Depression Scale (GDS): Preliminary evidence for validity of the GDS-PAIN. *Pain Medicine, 9*(1), 33–43.

Katz, J. N., Chang, L. C., Sangha, O., Fossel, A. H., & Bates, D. W. (1996). Can comorbidity be measured by questionnaire rather than medical record review? *Medical Care, 34*(1), 73–84.

Kim, E. J., & Buschmann, M. T. (2006). Reliability and validity of the Faces Pain Scale with older adults. *International Journal of Nursing Studies, 43*(4), 447–456.

Koestler, M. E., Libby, E., Schofferman, J., & Redmond, T. (2005). Web-based touch-screen computer assessment of chronic low back pain: A pilot study. *CIN: Computers Informatics Nursing, 23*(5), 275–284.

Kremer, E., Atkinson, J. H., & Ignelzi, R. J. (1981). Measurement of pain: Patient preference does not confound pain measurement. *Pain, 10*, 241–249.

Lee, S. J., Kavanaugh, A., & Lenert, L. (2007). Electronic and computer-generated patient questionnaires in standard care. *Best Practice and Research in Clinical Rheumatology, 21*(4), 637–647.

Lichtenberg, P. A. (1999). *Handbook of assessment in clinical gerontology.* Hoboken, NJ: Wiley.

Lichtenberg, P. A., & McGrogan, A. J. (1987). Chronic pain in elderly psychiatric inpatients. *Clinical Biofeedback and Health, 10*, 3–7.

Lichtenstein, M. J., Dhanda, R., Cornell, J. E., Escalante, A., & Hazuda, H. P. (1998). Disaggregating pain and its effect on physical functional limitations. *Journals of Gerontology A: Biological Sciences and Medical Sciences, 53*(5), M361–M371.

Lopez-Lopez, A., Montorio, I., Izal, M., & Velasco, L. (2008). The role of psychological variables in explaining depression in older people with chronic pain. *Aging and Mental Health, 12*(6), 735–745.

Lyness, J. M., Noel, T. K., Cox, C., King, D. A., Conwell, Y., & Caine, E. D. (1997). Screening for depression in elderly primary care patients: A comparison of the Center for Epidemiologic Studies—Depression Scale and the Geriatric Depression Scale. *Archives of Internal Medicine, 157*(4), 449–454.

Mangione, C. M., Marcantonio, E. R., Goldman, L., Cook, E. F., Donaldson, M. C., Sugarbaker, D. J., et al. (1993). Influence of age on measurement of health status in patients undergoing elective surgery. *Journal of the American Geriatrics Society, 41*(4), 377–383.

Marc, L. G., Raue, P. J., & Bruce, M. L. (2008). Screening performance of the 15-item Geriatric Depression Scale in a diverse elderly home care population. *American Journal of Geriatric Psychiatry, 16*(11), 914–921.

Marchionni, N., Ferrucci, L., Baldasseroni, S., Fumagalli, S., Guralnik, J. M., Bonazinga, M., et al. (1997). Item re-scaling of an Italian version of the Sickness Impact Profile: Effect of age and profession of the observers. *Journal of Clinical Epidemiology, 50*(2), 195–201.

Margolis, R. B., Tait, R. C., & Krause, S. J. (1986). A rating system for use with patient pain drawings. *Pain, 24*, 57–65.

Martin, K. A., Rejeski, W. J., Miller, M. E., James, M. K., Ettinger, W. H., Jr., & Messier, S. P. (1999). Validation of the PASE in older adults with knee pain and physical disability. *Medicine and Science in Sports and Exercise, 31*(5), 627–633.

Martin, R., Williams, J., Hadjistavropoulos, T., Hadjistavropoulos, H. D., & MacLean, M. (2005). A qualitative investigation of seniors' and caregivers' views on pain assessment and management. *Canadian Journal of Nursing Research, 37*(2), 142–164.

Maunsell, E., Allard, P., Dorval, M., & Labbe, J. (2000). A brief pain diary for ambulatory patients with advanced cancer: Acceptability and validity. *Cancer, 88*(10), 2387–2397.

McDonald, D. D., Shea, M., Fedo, J., Rose, L., Bacon, K., Noble, K., et al. (2008). Older adult pain communication and the Brief Pain Inventory Short Form. *Pain Management Nursing, 9*(4), 154–159.

McHorney, C. A., Ware, J. E., Jr., & Raczek, A. E. (1993). The MOS 36-Item Short-Form Health Survey (SF-36): II. Psychometric and clinical tests of validity in measuring physical and mental health constructs. *Medical Care, 31*(3), 247–263.

Meenan, R. F., Gertman, P. M., & Mason, J. H. (1980). Measuring health status in arthritis: The Arthritis Impact Measurement Scales. *Arthritis and Rheumatism, 23*(2), 146–152.

Melzack, R. (1975). The McGill Pain Questionnaire: Major properties and scoring methods. *Pain, 1*, 277–299.

Melzack, R. (1987). The short-form McGill Pain Questionnaire. *Pain, 30*, 191–197.

Miro, J., Huguet, A., Nieto, R., Paredes, S., & Baos, J. (2005). Evaluation of reliability, validity, and preference for a pain intensity scale for use with the elderly. *Journal of Pain, 6*(11), 727–735.

Mody, L., Miller, D. K., McGloin, J. M., Freeman, M., Marcantonio, E. R., Magaziner, J., et al. (2008). Recruitment and retention of older adults in aging research. *Journal of the American Geriatrics Society, 56*(12), 2340–2348.

Morishita, L., Boult, C., Ebbitt, B., Rambel, M., Fallstrom, K., & Gooden, T. (1995). Concurrent validity of administering the Geriatric Depression Scale and the Physical Functioning dimension of the SIP by telephone. *Journal of the American Geriatrics Society, 43*(6), 680–683.

Morley, S., Williams, A. C., & Black, S. (2002). A confirmatory factor analysis of the Beck Depression Inventory in chronic pain. *Pain, 99*(1–2), 289–298.

Murray, M., LeFort, S., & Ribeiro, V. (1998). The SF-36: Reliable and valid for the institutionalized elderly? *Aging and Mental Health, 2*(1), 24–27.

Pahor, M., Guralnik, J. M., Wan, J. Y., Ferrucci, L., Penninx, B. W., Lyles, A., et al. (1999). Lower body osteoarticular pain and dose of analgesic medications in older disabled women: The Women's Health and Aging Study. *American Journal of Public Health, 89*(6), 930–934.

Papassotiropoulos, A., & Heun, R. (1999). Screening for depression in the elderly: A study on misclassification by screening instruments and improvement of scale performance. *Progress in Neuro-Psychopharmacology and Biological Psychiatry, 23*(3), 431–446.

Parker, S. G., Bechinger-English, D., Jagger, C., Spiers, N., & Lindesay, J. (2006). Factors affecting completion of the SF-36 in older people. *Age and Ageing, 35*(4), 376–381.

Pesonen, A., Suojaranta-Ylinen, R., Tarkkila, P., & Rosenberg, P. H. (2008). Applicability of tools to assess pain in elderly patients after cardiac surgery. *Acta Anaesthesiologica Scandinavica, 52*(2), 267–273.

Peters, M. L., Patijn, J., & Lame, I. (2007). Pain assessment in younger and older pain patients: Psychometric properties and patient preference of five commonly used measures of pain intensity. *Pain Medicine, 8*(7), 601–610.

Pollard, C. A. (1984). Preliminary validity study of the Pain Disability Index. *Perceptual and Motor Skills, 59*(3), 974.

Radloff, L. S. (1977). The CES-D scale: A self-report depression scale for research in the general population. *Applied Psychological Measurement, 1*, 385–401.

Radloff, L. S., & Teri, L. (1986). Use of the Center for Epidemiological Studies—Depression Scale with older adults. *Clinical Gerontologist, 5*(1–2), 119–136.

Rodriguez, C. S., McMillan, S., & Yarandi, H. (2004). Pain measurement in older adults with head and neck cancer and communication impairments. *Cancer Nursing, 27*(6), 425–433.

Roman, M. W., & Callen, B. L. (2008). Screening instruments for older adult depressive disorders: Updating the evidence-based toolbox. *Issues in Mental Health Nursing, 29*(9), 924–941.

Ross, M. M., Carswell, A., Hing, M., Hollingworth, G., & Dalziel, W. B. (2001). Seniors' decision making about pain management. *Journal of Advanced Nursing, 35*(3), 442–451.

Rosso, A. L., Gallagher, R. M., Luborsky, M., & Mossey, J. M. (2008). Depression and self-rated health are proximal predictors of episodes of sustained change in pain in independently living, community dwelling elders. *Pain Medicine, 9*(8), 1035–1049.

Roy, R., & Thomas, M. (1986). A survey of chronic pain in an elderly population. *Canadian Family Physician, 32*, 513–516.

Rudy, T. E., Weiner, D. K., Lieber, S. J., Sláboda, J., & Boston, J. R. (2007). The impact of chronic low back pain on older adults: A comparative study of patients and controls. *Pain, 131*(3), 293–301.

Ryan, J. M., Corry, J. R., Attewell, R., & Smithson, M. J. (2002). A comparison of an electronic version of the SF-36 General Health Questionnaire to the standard paper version. *Quality of Life Research, 11*(1), 19–26.

Saleh, K. J., Radosevich, D. M., Kassim, R. A., Moussa, M., Dykes, D., Bottolfson, H., et al. (2002). Comparison of commonly used orthopaedic outcome measures using palm-top computers and paper surveys. *Journal of Orthopaedic Research, 20*(6), 1146–1151.

Savedra, M. C., Tesler, M. D., Holzemer, W. L., Wilkie, D. J., & Ward, J. A. (1989). Pain location: Validity and reliability of body outline markings by hospitalized children and adolescents. *Research in Nursing and Health, 12*(5), 307–314.

Schmader, K. E., Sloane, R., Pieper, C., Coplan, P. M., Nikas, A., Saddier, P., et al. (2007). The impact of acute herpes zoster pain and discomfort on functional status and quality of life in older adults. *Clinical Journal of Pain, 23*(6), 490–496.

Schumacher, K. L., Koresawa, S., West, C., Dodd,

M., Paul, S. M., Tripathy, D., et al. (2002). The usefulness of a daily pain management diary for outpatients with cancer-related pain [Online]. *Oncology Nursing Forum, 29*(9), 1304–1313.

Sheikh, J. I., & Yesavage, J. A. (1986). Geriatric Depression Scale (GDS): Recent evidence and development of a shorter version. *Clinical Gerontologist, 5*, 165–173.

Sherman, S. E., & Reuben, D. (1998). Measures of functional status in community-dwelling elders. *Journal of General Internal Medicine, 13*(12), 817–823.

Simmons, S. F., Ferrell, B. A., & Schnelle, J. F. (2002). Effects of a controlled exercise trial on pain in nursing home residents. *Clinical Journal of Pain, 18*(6), 380–385.

Stadnyk, K., Calder, J., & Rockwood, K. (1998). Testing the measurement properties of the Short Form-36 Health Survey in a frail elderly population. *Journal of Clinical Epidemiology, 51*(10), 827–835.

Storto, G., Klain, M., Paone, G., Liuzzi, R., Molino, L., Marinelli, A., et al. (2006). Combined therapy of Sr-89 and zoledronic acid in patients with painful bone metastases. *Bone, 39*(1), 35–41.

Strand, L. I., Ljunggren, A. E., Bogen, B., Ask, T., & Johnsen, T. B. (2008). The Short-Form McGill Pain Questionnaire as an outcome measure: Test–retest reliability and responsiveness to change. *European Journal of Pain, 12*(7), 917–925.

Svensson, E. (1998). Ordinal invariant measures for individual and group changes in ordered categorical data. *Statistics in Medicine, 17*(24), 2923–2936.

Taylor, L. J., Harris, J., Epps, C. D., & Herr, K. (2005). Psychometric evaluation of selected pain intensity scales for use with cognitively impaired and cognitively intact older adults. *Rehabilitation Nursing, 30*(2), 55–61.

Thomas, E., Peat, G., Harris, L., Wilkie, R., & Croft, P. R. (2004). The prevalence of pain and pain interference in a general population of older adults: Cross-sectional findings from the North Staffordshire Osteoarthritis Project (NorStOP). *Pain, 110*(1–2), 361–368.

Tinetti, M. E., Richman, D., & Powell, L. (1990). Falls efficacy as a measure of fear of falling. *Journal of Gerontology, 45*(6), P239–P243.

Tiplady, B., Jackson, S. H., Maskrey, V. M., & Swift, C. G. (1998). Validity and sensitivity of visual analogue scales in young and older healthy subjects. *Age and Ageing, 27*(1), 63–66.

Tittle, M. B., McMillan, S. C., & Hagan, S. (2003). Validating the Brief Pain Inventory for use with surgical patients with cancer [Online]. *Oncology Nursing Forum, 30*(2), 325–330.

Torrance, N., Smith, B. H., Bennett, M. I., & Lee, A. J. (2006). The epidemiology of chronic pain of predominantly neuropathic origin: Results from a general population survey. *Journal of Pain, 7*(4), 281–289.

Turk, D. C., & Okifuji, A. (1994). Detecting depression in chronic pain patients: Adequacy of self-reports. *Behaviour Research and Therapy, 32*(1), 9–16.

Tverskoy, M., Oz, Y., Isakson, A., Finger, J., Bradley, E. L., Jr., & Kissin, I. (1994). Preemptive effect of fentanyl and ketamine on postoperative pain and wound hyperalgesia. *Anesthesia and Analgesia, 78*(2), 205–209.

VanItallie, T. B. (2005). Subsyndromal depression in the elderly: Underdiagnosed and undertreated. *Metabolism: Clinical and Experimental, 54*(5, Suppl. 1), 39–44.

Ward, S. E., Goldberg, N., Miller-McCauley, V., Mueller, C., Nolan, A., Pawlik-Plank, D., et al. (1993). Patient-related barriers to management of cancer pain. *Pain, 52*(3), 319–324.

Ware, J., Jr., Kosinski, M., & Keller, S. D. (1996). A 12-Item Short-Form Health Survey: Construction of scales and preliminary tests of reliability and validity. *Medical Care, 34*(3), 220–233.

Washburn, R. A., Smith, K. W., Jette, A. M., & Janney, C. A. (1993). The Physical Activity Scale for the Elderly (PASE): Development and evaluation. *Journal of Clinical Epidemiology, 46*(2), 153–162.

Weiner, D., Peterson, B., & Keefe, F. (1998). Evaluating persistent pain in long term care residents: What role for pain maps? *Pain, 76*(1–2), 249–257.

Weiner, D. K., Rudy, T. E., Morrow, L., Slaboda, J., & Lieber, S. (2006). The relationship between pain, neuropsychological performance, and physical function in community-dwelling older adults with chronic low back pain. *Pain Medicine, 7*(1), 60–70.

Weintraub, D., Saboe, K., & Stern, M. B. (2007). Effect of age on Geriatric Depression Scale performance in Parkinson's disease. *Movement Disorders, 22*(9), 1331–1335.

Wetherell, A. (1996). Performance tests. *Environmental Health Perspectives, 104*(Suppl. 2), 247–273.

Wilke, D. J., Savedra, M. C., Holzemer, W. L., Tesler, M. D., & Paul, S. M. (1990). Use of the McGill Pain Questionnaire to measure pain: A meta-analysis. *Nursing Research, 39*, 36–41.

Wilkie, D. J., Judge, M. K. M., Berry, D. L., Dell, J., Zong, S., & Gilespie, R. (2003). Usability of a computerized PAINReportIt in the general public with pain and people with cancer pain. *Journal of Pain and Symptom Management, 25*(3), 213–224.

Williams, C. A., Templin, T., & Mosley-Williams, A. D. (2004). Usability of a computer-assisted interview system for the unaided self-entry of patient data in an urban rheumatology clinic. *Journal of the American Medical Informatics Association, 11*(4), 249–259.

Williams, V. S. L., Smith, M. Y., & Fehnel, S. E. (2006). The validity and utility of the BPI interference measures for evaluating the impact of osteoarthritic pain. *Journal of Pain and Symptom Management, 31*(1), 48–57.

Wilson, A. S., Kitas, G. D., Carruthers, D. M., Reay, C., Skan, J., Harris, S., et al. (2002). Computerized information-gathering in specialist rheumatology clinics: An initial evaluation of an electronic version of the Short Form 36. *Rheumatology, 41*(3), 268–273.

Woo, J., Ho, S. C., Lau, J., & Leung, P. C. (1994). Musculoskeletal complaints and associated consequences in elderly Chinese aged 70 and over. *Journal of Rheumatology, 21*, 1927–1931.

Yesavage, J. A. (1988). Geriatric Depression Scale. *Psychopharmacology Bulletin, 24*(4), 709–711.

Zalon, M. L. (2004). Correlates of recovery among older adults after major abdominal surgery. *Nursing Research, 53*(2), 99–106.

CHAPTER 13

Assessment of Pain in Adults and Children with Limited Ability to Communicate

THOMAS HADJISTAVROPOULOS
LYNN M. BREAU
KENNETH D. CRAIG

Pain in persons with communication difficulties due to intellectual disabilities (IDs), dementia, head injury, and related neurological conditions is often underassessed and undermanaged (Horgas & Tsai, 1998; Kaasalainen et al., 1998; Morrison & Sui, 2000; Sengstaken & King, 1993). The high prevalence of these conditions underscores the need to investigate pain in these populations. For example, dementia is estimated to occur in 1.4 to 1.6% of people between the ages of 65 and 69 years, with estimates increasing to 16–25% in those over age 85 (American Psychiatric Association, 2005). As well, the prevalence of developmental IDs is estimated to be at least 1% of the population (American Psychiatric Association, 2005). Estimates of the incidence of head injuries in the United States alone range from 500,000 to 1.9 million per year, with a large portion of these injuries resulting in cognitive disorders, of which 10% are considered severe (Berrol, 1989; Frankowski, Annegers, & Whitman, 1985; Gennarelli, 1983; Lezack, 1995). These numbers add up to millions of people in North America alone. Moreover, populations (e.g., patients recovering from anesthesia and others who

are intubated) also present with temporary limitations in ability to communicate.

In populations with limited ability to communicate, there is a high incidence of acute and chronic pain problems. They suffer pain arising from the same injuries and diseases that afflict those without communication limitations, as well as pain more specific to their conditions. For example, many children with IDs experience pain due to comorbid physical/medical problems (Breau, Camfield, McGrath, & Finley, 2007). Poor detection of common health problems in this population may also lead to untreated pain (Hunt, Mastroyannopoulou, Goldman, & Seers, 2003), as may injuries, which are frequent in this group (Braden, Swanson, & Di Scala, 2003). Comorbidities with physical injuries are also very common among adults who sustain head injuries, while the prevalence of pain problems among persons with dementia who reside in long-term care facilities is estimated to be as high as 80% (e.g., Charlton, 2005). In light of this, it is not surprising that a large-scale survey of members of the American Pain Society and of the American Academy of Pain Medicine indicates that the undertreatment of pain among persons with cognitive impairments represents one of the most pressing ethical concerns facing pain clinicians (Ferrell et al., 2001). It is widely believed that undertreatment of pain in these populations is due at least in part to the challenge caregivers face in evaluating pain and in distinguishing its signs from those of other distress (e.g., Martin, Williams, Hadjistavropoulos, Hadjistavropoulos, & MacLean, 2005).

A CONCEPTUAL MODEL OF PAIN COMMUNICATION

A social communications model of pain has been proposed (e.g., Craig, 2009; Hadjistavropoulos & Craig, 2002; Hadjistavropoulos, Craig, & Fuchs-Lacelle, 2004; Prkachin & Craig, 1995) in which the experience and communication of pain are viewed within the context of a three-step A-B-C process. The first step in the process (A) captures the subjective internal experience of pain, which is affected by a variety of both intrapersonal (biological and psychological) and interpersonal factors (Melzack & Katz, 2004; Melzack & Wall, 1965). The second step (B) involves encoding pain experience into expressive behavior that may be communicated to observers, with varying degrees of efficiency. This may take the form of verbal (i.e., self-report) and nonverbal pain behaviors (e.g., paralinguistic vocalizations, grimacing, limping, and body movements). The final step of the communications model (C) addresses the process whereby pain behaviors are decoded by observers seeking to provide help. The focus of this chapter is on the interface between Steps B and C of the model: the expressive pain behavior and the tools available to health professionals to decode it.

Hadjistavropoulos and Craig (2002) used the communications model of pain to understand pain expression in those with and without communication limitations. They observed that behavioral pain responses manifested as Step B in the communications model vary with respect to the dimension of reflexive automaticity and cognitive executive mediation. Self-report is heavily reliant on cognitive executive mediation (conscious deliberation, planning, language skills) whereas nonverbal behaviors (e.g., facial reactions) are primarily automatic and less subject to voluntary control. As severity of cognitive deficits increases, the focus of the assessment requires a shift away from self-report to automatic, nonverbal behaviors. Hadjistavropoulos and Craig (2002) note that while automatic pain behaviors have the advantage of typically being available among persons with diminished capacity, they tend to be more difficult to decode than self-report of pain and are often ignored; that is, signs of nonverbal distress are difficult to decode, because certain behaviors (e.g., agitation, difficulty sleeping) are ambiguous as signs of pain or other types of distress. In consequence, it is important to address the specificity of pain assessment tools, but research in this area often has failed to do so.

Another important theoretical question relates to the behavioral domains that need to be assessed when pain is evaluated using nonverbal expression. The American Geriatrics Society Panel on Persistent Pain in Older Persons (2002) suggested that a comprehensive nonverbal assessment should cover the following domains: facial expressions, verbalizations/vocalizations, body movements, changes in interpersonal interactions, changes in activity patterns or routines, and mental status changes. Examination of the extent to which clinical pain assessment tools cover these domains could be used to assess their comprehensiveness. We note, however, that the domains recommended by the American Geriatrics Society represent very broad categories, and clinicians must work with more specific and observable manifestations of pain within these categories.

THE EXPERIENCE OF PAIN AMONG PERSONS WITH COMMUNICATION IMPAIRMENTS

The diverse types of central nervous system damage that can lead to communication impairments could affect the way that pain is experienced and expressed. Certain conditions may produce pain insensitivity (diminished sensation), whereas others may cause pain indifference. Oberlander Gilbert, Chambers, O'Donnell, and Craig (1999) observed diminished pain reactivity in some adolescents with significant neurological impairment. Nevertheless, research has failed to identify differences in the pain threshold of patients with mild to moderate dementia despite the possibility of a small increase in pain tolerance when compared with age-matched controls (Benedetti et al., 1999, 2004; Gibson, Voukelatos, Ames, Flicker, & Helme, 2001).

Focusing on pain as a multidimensional construct rather than as a unidimensional sensation may prove more valuable. Deterioration in executive functions leads to a loss of ability to understand the meaning of pain or the ability to engage in self-management skills to control pain. Farrell, Gibson, and Helme (1996) have pointed out that Alzheimer's disease is a condition of the neocortex that leaves the somatosensory cortex relatively unaffected. Thus, we might expect sensory discrimininative aspects of pain to be preserved in patients with Alzheimer's disease, although distortions in perception (related to parietal lobe dysfunction) may take place. Farrell and colleagues also observed that emotional components of pain may be affected in Alzheimer's disease as a result of neuronal loss in the limbic system and prefrontal cortex. Similarly, people with frontal lobe dementia, and other conditions that involve frontal lobe damage, may exhibit disinhibited reactions to pain.

Research involving both older and younger adults has also shown that automatic, reflexive patterns of reaction to acute phasic pain, such as facial activity, do not correlate with intelligence quotients and do not vary as a function of cognitive status (e.g., Hadjistavropoulos et al., 1998; LaChapelle, Hadjistavropoulos, & Craig, 1999). In a related study, Hadjistavropoulos, LaChapelle, MacLeod, Snider, and Craig (2000) showed that reactions in response to discomforting physical activities are slightly increased among persons with dementia compared to their cognitively intact peers, possibly due to increased anxiety or fear that persons with cognitive impairments might experience because of difficulty in interpreting the context of pain. Thus, although a blunting of pain reactions may occur among certain individuals with significant neurological impairments, as reported by Oberlander and colleagues (1999), this cannot be assumed for large numbers of persons with limited ability to communicate.

ASSESSMENT PROCEDURES

Since the last edition of this text, tremendous progress has been made in the area of pain assessment in persons with limited ability to communicate. We describe the latest developments here.

Self-Report Measures

Children

When reliable self-report is available, it can be a valuable tool. However, self-reports are vulnerable to bias and situational influences, and they require substantial cognitive competence. Fanurik, Koh, Harrison, Conrad, and Tomerlin (1998) were the first to explore the self-report abilities of children with borderline to profound ID. Only half of the children in their study with borderline ID and less than 30% of children with mild ID were able to pass brief tests assessing whether they comprehended order and magnitude, two concepts important to understanding and using self-report scales of pain intensity. More recently, however, Benini and colleagues (2004) found that simplifying standard self-report scales, by reducing the number of options or increasing the size of the symbols, increased both the number of children capable of using the scales to rate pain after venipuncture and the number who chose a rating indicating pain. The scales used by Benini and colleagues included the *Eland Color Scale* (Eland, 1985), an adaptation of that scale, the *Facial Affective Scale* (McGrath, deVeber, & Hearn, 1985), and a modified version of this scale.

Zabalia, Jacquet, and Breau (2005) found higher rates of successful use of self-report pain rating scales than had either the Benini (2004) or Fanurik (1998) groups. In their study, 14 children (ages 8–18) with mild to moderate ID provided ratings based on vignettes depicting pain due to vaccination, falling off a bike, falling while roller blading, and a burn. The children used the *Faces Pain Scale—Revised* (Hicks, von Baeyer, Spafford, van Korlaar, & Goodenough, 2001) and a 10-cm visual analogue scale to indicate how much pain they believed the person in the vignette experienced, as well as how much pain they would experience personally in the same situation. All children were able to complete the ratings using the two scales, and mean ratings using the 10-cm visual analogue scale (8.4, $SD = 1.2$) and Faces Pain Scale—Revised (7.9, $SD = 1.3$) were appropriate for the events depicted. The children's responses suggested they could use both self-report scales, although they rated their personal pain as lower than that of the person depicted in the vignettes. They also provided verbal descriptors of the pain vignettes similar to those that typical children of a similar mental age would provide. This suggested that the child research participants could identify differences in the nature of the pain that could result from these different painful events. In contrast, only 21% of Fanurik's group (1998) were capable of using the 0- to 5-point numerical scale. Similarly, in the Benini group's (2004) study, rates of completion and pain ratings varied by scale. Using a series of wooden blocks to reflect no pain (1 cm) to most pain (5 cm), 99% of children indicated they had pain due to the venipuncture. However, this changed to 50–56% reporting any pain by choosing a sad face with the two versions of the Facial Affective Scale, and only 50–75% of children could indicate the site of the venipuncture. The discrepancy between these results and those of Fanurik and colleagues (1998) and Benini and colleagues (2004) suggested that children with ID were more capable of evaluating pain based on vignettes than based on real-life pain situations. This could occur as a result of reduced ability to concentrate during pain, or emotions such as fear may have distracted them or interfered with cognitive abilities. In fact, Benini and colleagues found that children reporting more fear were less capable of using self-report scales. Professionals should keep this in mind when asking children to "practice" using a scale by rating hypothetical events, such as scraping a knee. The child's ability in using a tool for these trials may not reflect his or her ability during actual pain.

Overall, there is little research to confirm that children with ID are capable of reliably using self-report tools designed for typically developing children in real-life situations. It may be that only those with milder impairments have the required skills and can implement these when in pain. There is a considerable need to understand linguistic capabilities of children and adults with cognitive and communication limitations. Craig, Stanford, Fairburn, and Chambers (2006) observed that children with Down's syndrome generally have a vocabulary of pain-specific words, but the number of words is smaller, and the words appear later in early child development than is the case with typical children. Until further research is available to inform the use of self-report tools for children, they should be used with caution.

Adults

Many persons with limited ability to communicate are capable of self-reporting pain despite the presence of cognitive impairment. Typically they are evaluated for their ability to use unidimensional pain intensity scales rather than multidimensional scales seeking details on various qualities of pain. For example, Chibnall and Tait (2001) found that older adults with moderate dementia and average *Modified Mini-Mental State Examination* (MMSE; Folstein, Folstein, & McHugh, 1975) scores of 18 (out of a possible 30), which fall in the mild to moderately impaired range, tended to provide valid responses on the 21-point Box Scale (Jensen, Miller, & Fisher, 1998). Scherder and Bouma (2000) demonstrated that the *Coloured Analogue Scale* (CAS; McGrath et al., 1996), originally developed for children with marginal self-report skills, was interpreted correctly by patients with early-stage Alzheimer's disease and by 80% of patients with moderate dementia. Similarly, Weiner, Peterson, Ladd, McConnell, and Keefe (1999) concluded that seniors with dementia who could respond to a numerical 0- to 10-point scale tended to have MMSE scores that ranged from 18 to 22, whereas those who could not respond tended to have MMSE scores in the neighborhood of 12–14 (severe dementia). Based on the findings of Chibnall and Tait (2001) and Weiner and colleagues (1999), it would be reasonable to suggest that, as a rule of thumb, older adults who can be described as presenting with moderate and mild dementia, with MMSE scores of 18 or higher, tend to be able to provide valid responses to simple self-report measures, such as a 1- to 10-point numerical scale, the CAS, and the 21-point Box Scale (Hadjistavropoulos, 2005). It is noted, however, that no cognitive measure can indicate with certainty whether or not self-report will be valid. Multidimensional pain scales, due to their greater degree of complexity, are less likely to be useful with patients who have dementia. We recommend that self-report assessment should be attempted (even if only simple questions, e.g., "Does this hurt?"), but with increasing caution as the severity of cognitive impairment increases. It also important to note that among older adults and other persons with diminished sensory abilities, adaptations (e.g., the use of a larger font) are often necessary. Observational assessment procedures should supplement self-report or be used exclusively, if self-report is unavailable.

Observational Assessment Procedures Primarily Suitable for Research

We briefly review two basic approaches to pain assessment that are primarily suitable for research. The first of these systems is the *Facial Action Coding System* (FACS; Ekman & Friesen, 1978; Ekman, Friesen, & Hager, 2002) and approaches based on it. The second system is *Pain Behavior Measurement* (PBM; Keefe & Block, 1982).

The FACS is an atheoretical, comprehensive, anatomically based system developed to provide objective descriptors of facial activity (see Craig, Prkachin, & Grunau, Chapter 6, this volume). Using slow-motion video, qualified coders identify specific facial reactions, referred to as *action units*, using explicit and rigorous behavioral criteria. The very detailed objective scoring criteria minimize subjective judgments. Studies involving patients with pain have demonstrated excellent interrater reliability (see Craig et al., Chapter 6, this volume). Given these strengths, the FACS is a suitable index of pain for research studies (e.g., clinical trials or investigations of basic mechanisms in pain) involving patients with limitations in ability to communicate. Its main disadvantage is the time-consuming nature of both the application of the system and the required training.

Another observational approach used to assess pain among persons with cognitive impairments is PBM. This approach was originally developed and validated by Keefe and Block (1982) and has been used by others (e.g., Fuchs-Lacelle et al., 2003; see Keefe, Somers, Williams, & Smith, Chapter 7, this volume). The procedure involves trained coders, who note the frequency of clearly defined pain behaviors (bracing, sighing, rubbing the affected area, grimacing, and guarding) while the patient undergoes a series of standardized structured activities, such as standing and walking. Although the PBM is less labor-intensive than the FACS, it can still be time-consuming to use in busy clinical settings because of its requirements for a standardized protocol of patient activity. It remains, however, a promising tool for research studies involving persons with cognitive impairments.

Children

Pain expression in newborn and young infants has been studied using a version of the FACS, the *Baby-FACS* (Oster, Hegley, & Nagel, 1992), developed because anatomical differences between very young children and older children and adults require adaptations of the basic system. More often however, study of the facial expression of pain in infants has been accomplished using the *Neonatal Facial Action Coding System* (NFCS) to focus only on facial actions identified when infants are in pain (Craig, Hadjistavropoulos, Grunau, & Whitfield, 1994; Lilley, Craig, & Grunau, 1997). Although the NFCS has been used clinically (Grunau, Oberlander, Holsti, & Whitfield, 1998), its primary application has been in research. A similar measure, the *Child Facial Coding System* (CFCS; Chambers, Cassidy, McGrath, Gilbert, & Craig, 1996) again focusing only on facial actions associated with pain (Breau et al., 2001; Gilbert et al., 1999) has been applied to the study of pain in children with communication limitations. Studies involving children with ID have reported mixed results. Oberlander and colleagues (1999) found no change in facial reaction to pain during a mock and real immunization for eight adolescents with considerable and significant neurological impairment. In contrast, Nader, Oberlander, Chambers, and Craig (2004), using the CFCS, found vigorous facial activity when 21 children with autism were observed during insertion of intravenous needles, with greater facial activity relative to typical control children during similar events. This contradicts widespread assumptions of pain insensitivity or indifference in these children. Mercer and Glenn (2004) also found facial response changes using the *Maximally Discriminative Facial Movement Coding System* (MAX) in eight infants with developmental delay (ages 4–9 months) who were receiving immunizations. While facial expression was not diminished, it was more diffuse than in a comparison group of 30 infants without ID. FACS-based systems are based on empirical evidence that specific independent facial movements are present during pain. However, MAX requires that sets of facial movements reflecting specific emotions, such as fear, anger, or pain, are observed in three facial areas (forehead and brow, eyes and nose, mouth and chin). Partial expressions are deemed to occur if the movements for a given expression are seen only in one of the three facial areas. These differences in how the systems work may differentially affect the ability of CFCS and MAX to capture the pain expression of children with ID.

Very few studies of the facial expression of pain in children with communication limitations have been undertaken, leading to the mixed observations noted here. It seems clear that they should not be treated as a homogenous group. With more study using the rigorous research tools that generally are too cumbersome for clinical use, clinically useful tools may emerge.

Adults

FACIAL ACTION CODING SYSTEM

LaChapelle and colleagues (1999) used FACS to assess pain in adults (mean age = 49.5 years) with IDs who were undergoing intramuscular injections. Thirty-five percent of these individuals were unable to self-report pain. The study supported the usefulness of facial activity in identifying pain in this population.

Most applications of the FACS in adults with cognitive impairments have focused on older adults with dementia. Generally, the findings on pain reactivity to invasive procedures show that the facial actions of both cognitively intact older adults and those with dementia increase with respect to frequency

and intensity (compared to a baseline period), even in response to very minor pain (Hadjistavropoulos, Craig, Martin, Hadjistavropoulos, & McMurtry, 1997; Hadjistavropoulos et al., 1998; Hadjistavropoulos, LaChapelle, Hadjistavropoulos, Green, & Asmundson, 2002; Kunz, Scharmann, Hemmeter, Schepelmann, & Lautenbacher, 2007; Lints-Martindale, Hadjistavropoulos, Barber, & Gibson, 2007). No substantial differences in facial responses seem to exist between older adults with and those without cognitive impairments, although there appears to be a tendency for older adults with dementia to be somewhat more responsive (Hadjistavropoulos et al., 2000). Moreover, Lints-Martindale and colleagues (2007) demonstrated that facial reactions to pain, assessed using FACS, increase as a function of stimulus intensity. This supports the usefulness of the system as a research tool in discriminating among different levels of pain in older adults with cognitive impairment.

PAIN BEHAVIOR MEASUREMENT

Weiner, Pieper, McConnell, Martinez, and Keefe (1996) found evidence in support of the validity of this system among older adults by showing that more physically discomforting activities (involving the axial skeleton and requiring movements that are often needed for the performance of activities of daily living) led to more pain behaviors than did less physically demanding activities. Hadjistavropoulos and colleagues (2000) used the PBM with older adults suffering from dementia and cognitively intact older adults, all of whom presented with a variety of musculoskeletal problems. The number of PBM behaviors increased during more physically demanding activities compared to more passive ones, regardless of patient cognitive status. These findings provided evidence that nonverbal behaviors can be used to determine whether pain is present or absent, as well as evaluate degree of pain severity in this population. Studies establishing the behaviors assessed with PBM as specific to pain, in contrast to non-noxious but aversive states, are needed. Nevertheless, the PBM has potential as a useful tool for research studies of pain in older persons with cognitive impairments.

Observational Assessment Procedures with Potential for Clinical Application

Children

With the exception of one study that examined the pain behavior of children following surgery (Reynell, 1965), early pain assessment research with children with disabilities used case study methodologies (Collignon, Guisiano, Porsmoguer, Jimeno, & Combe, 1995; Collignon, Porsmoguer, Behar, Combe, & Perrin, 1992; Mette & Abittan, 1988). In a departure from this approach, Giusiano, Jimeno, Collignon, and Chau (1995) recorded pain behaviors observed during a physical exam of 100 individuals ages 2–33 in a long-term care facility. This seminal study provided evidence that a set of common pain behaviors could be observed and aggregated into an observational assessment tool for children with ID. Since then, there has been considerable development of observational pain tools to be used with children with disabilities.

Psychometric evaluation of three of many observational tools now demonstrates their usefulness. The *Non-Communicating Children's Pain Checklist* (NCCPC; Breau, Finley, McGrath, & Camfield, 2002) has the most research to support clinical application at this time. However, preliminary evidence suggests that both the *Echelle Douleur Enfant San Salvador* (DESS) and *Paediatric Pain Profile* (PPP) are useful for some research applications and may, with further research, prove to be appropriate for clinical settings in the future.

ECHELLE DOULEUR ENFANT SAN SALVADOR

Since 1995, Collignon, Giusiano, and colleagues (1995) have continued development of the DESS. In a second study, they empirically reduced the initially identified 22 behaviors to the 10 most salient items and recommended cutoff scores for "pain is possible" and "definite pain needing treatment" (Collignon & Giusiano, 2001). An item was removed if, based on ratings by a physician or nurse for 8-hour periods for 31 residents in pain and 31 without pain, it was deemed difficult to detect, "nonpertinent," because it varied due to level of impairment or was thought to be redundant. Interrater reliability for the 10-item scale ranged from .39 to

.52, and the relation of scores to the three experts' ratings of pain were low (Cohen's kappa = .47 to .74). Standard psychometric tests of sensitivity and specificity were also not reported, and no comparison of mean scores for those who did and did not have pain were presented, so the validity of the tool is unclear. Because this scale was based on research with children and adults, it may be useful across age groups. However, items on the DESS are rated in relation to the individual's typical behavior, meaning that people who are unfamiliar with a child cannot use the tool as intended. Furthermore, because validation of the DESS was conducted in French, cutoff values may not be valid in English translation. Thus, this scale appears most useful for research purposes, especially with Francophone groups, with clinical application requiring more psychometric development.

THE PAEDIATRIC PAIN PROFILE

This 20-item PPP was developed through interviews with 121 caregivers of children with ID (Hunt et al., 2004). Interrater reliability between parents and a caregiver was reported to be good, and scores decreased after analgesics were given. A cutoff score of 14 was considered to reflect moderate pain rated 2 or more on a 0- to 4-point scale completed by the parent/caregiver at the same time. A second study, including 60 of the 121 children, examined behavior from 3-minute videotape clips of the child during daily activities, such as lying in bed, being dressed, being transferred (Hunt et al., 2007). Each videotaped activity was also rated by the parent and researchers using a 0- to 10-point numerical rating scale for pain and a 5-point verbal rating scale (*no pain* to *very severe pain*). A new method of computing scores was based on the percentage of maximum total score possible, accounting for missing items for that child. A new cutoff score of 24% was derived for moderate pain based on 10 episodes from seven children, and a cutoff score of 12.5% for mild pain based on 39 episodes for 15 children. One positive attribute of the scale is the opportunity to document baseline behavior when the child is pain-free, as well as when experiencing common pains. This might be particularly helpful in untangling the temporal patterns of specific pains in children who have multiple conditions that cause chronic or recurrent pain and in longitudinal research. However, with uncertainty about recommendations in cutoff values, limited investigation of various populations, and a need for data from hospital settings, the PPP needs more research support.

NON-COMMUNICATING CHILDREN'S PAIN CHECKLIST

In the mid-1990s, a series of studies reported the development, testing, and revision of the NCCPC. The items were generated from interviews with 20 caregivers of individuals ages 6–29 years with severe to profound IDs. Reliability of independent coders who generated the items was good. The first report described use of the scale by 33 caregivers in a home setting for "everyday pain" (Breau, McGrath, Camfield, Rosmus, & Finley, 2000). This original scale included yes–no responses to 30 items in seven categories: Vocal, Eating/Sleeping, Social/Personality, Facial Expression, Activity, Body and Limbs, and Physiological. The results indicated no significant difference in scores between two independent pain episodes, indicating reliability over time, but a significant difference in scores during episodes of pain and calm, suggesting that the scale was sensitive to pain. A variation, the NCCPC—Postoperative Version (NCCPC-PV), was investigated for use with postoperative pain (Breau et al., 2002). This excluded the Eating/Sleeping subscale, and observers rated each item as "not at all," just a little," "fairly often," or "very often" during 10-minute pre- and postoperative observations of 24 children. A cutoff score for moderate to severe pain was set at 11 and detected 88% of cases. Later, a score of 6–10 was developed to detect mild pain, with 75% accuracy. Caregiver (parents and primary care) and researcher total scores increased after surgery, providing criterion validity. Good interrater reliability between caregivers and researchers was also reported for the relations, indicating reliable scoring by observers less familiar with the child (researchers).

The original NCCPC was revised for the home setting, the NCCPC—Revised (NCCPC-R), adopting the continuous scoring of the NCCPC-PV. A study of a large sample (Breau et al., 2000) involved 2-hour observations of everyday types of pain events to develop a cutoff score of 7 on the 30-item NCCPC-R. Cutoff scores for clinically meaningful pain were developed, yielding 84% sensitivity when ratings were compared for observations during pain and observations when the children were pain-free. Because two incidents of pain were examined for each child, consistency in displayed pain behavior could be examined and was found to be substantial. This contradicted earlier suggestions that children with ID show pain in inconsistent ways. Similar scores on the NCCPC can be anticipated when the scale is used over time or for different types of pain.

The NCCPCs were designed for children with very limited verbal abilities due to their ID. Hadden and von Baeyer (2005) have used the NCCPC-R in children with cerebral palsy and varying levels of verbal skill. The presence of items that parents reported to be generally present during pain did not vary with the children's communication ability (Hadden & von Baeyer, 2002). In a subsequent study, children with cerebral palsy who had a wide range of verbal abilities were observed during home physiotherapy exercises (Hadden & von Baeyer, 2005). Scores on the NCCPC-PV were significantly higher during active stretching that was expected to be painful. These two studies provide evidence that the NCCPC scales may be valid for higher functioning children with developmental disabilities and comorbid physical problems. The NCCPC-R also appears valid for children who self-injure (Breau et al., 2003), despite some reports that they may be less sensitive to pain due to altered endogenous opioid levels (Gillberg, Terenius, & Lonnerholm, 1985; Sandman, Barron, Chicz-DeMet, & DeMet, 1990). There is also initial evidence that some patterns of self-injury may reflect the presence of chronic pain.

The NCCPCs have been translated in several languages. A recent study of 24 children in a rehabilitation hospital revealed good reliability and validity for the Swiss German version when completed by parents or caregivers (Kleinknecht, 2007). However, a cutoff score of 5 was more appropriate for this Swiss German version, highlighting the need for validating translated versions of scales, because interpretations of items may differ due to language constraints or cultural factors. Children may also display behavior differently depending on cultural norms regarding appropriate pain expression. A French translation of the NCCPC-PV was developed in Canada and France. Thorough translation and back-translation procedures were completed by a group that included the lead developer of the scale (LB) and medical and nursing professionals who work with individuals with IDs from both countries to ensure that the language used would be acceptable in both countries. The French version of the NCCPC-PV (called the "Grille d'Évaluation de la Douleur—déficience Intellectuelle"; GED-DI), at the time of this writing, was being validated in hospitals in Canada and France. A change in the observation time is also being tested, in an attempt to improve feasibility of the NCCPC-PV GED-DI in a clinical setting. Observations were reduced from the 10 minutes, as in previous research, to 5 minutes. Preliminary data for the GED-DI with 77 participants ages 3–57 suggest that scores increase after surgery and may be similar to those found with the English version (Breau et al., 2008). Mean preoperative scores were below 7.0, while mean postoperative scores were over 14.0. Further detailed analyses will reveal whether the scores differ due to age (child–adult) or culture, and whether new cutoffs will be needed.

The past 10 years have brought advances in pain assessment for children with ID. Self-report should not be abandoned in a child who has an ID or developmental disability, because it may be valid and reliable for a particular child. Other patterns of pain expression should be considered, with the NCCPC scales currently best supported by evidence either to supplement self-report or to replace self-report when it is not available. The scales do not require that children be moved or manipulated during observations; they are observed during natural events. The NCCPC-PV is recommended for chronic or acute pain (included in Appendix 13.1). It has fewer items than the NCCPC-R and requires a shorter observation time (10 minutes vs. 2 hours). It does not include items regarding eating and sleeping. These items are more difficult to assess, particularly by observers who are unfamiliar with a child, and cannot be judged over a short time frame. When chronic or recurrent pain is suspected, multiple applications of the NCCPC-PV can provide information regarding the temporal pattern of pain. Repeated observations may help to distinguish between behavior that is due to pain and behavior related to other common problems, such as nonpainful illness or sleep difficulties.

Although the NCCPC-PV may be sufficient to assist in management of acute pain due to procedures or injury, additional information may be helpful for cases of chronic pain. Any information regarding pain quality and location that can be collected assists with diagnosis. Some research suggests that self-injury may also be a cue of not only pain presence but also pain location and temporal pattern (Breau et al., 2003). Changes in a person's functioning may also signify that pain is present and should be investigated thoroughly (Breau, Camfield, McGrath, & Finley, 2007). The NCCPC-PV provides information regarding a person's facial reaction to pain, verbalizations, body movements, social behavior, and activity level. It also provides information about physical appearance (e.g., tears, change in skin color). Because the NCCPC-PV is meant to be used for isolated periods of time, it does not evaluate *change* in any of the areas assessed by the items on the scale. This is a strength, because the observer need not know the child's typical display in any of these areas to use the scale. The NCCPC-PV is also not intended to assess changes in activities of daily living or cognitive function, which also might inform about pain.

Younger Adults

Most research with observational pain assessment tools for adults with limited ability to communicate has focused on older adults with dementia. Nonetheless, recently the NCCPC-R has been used with adults with ID receiving vaccinations (Defrin, Lotan, & Pick, 2006). Scores increased significantly after vaccination regardless of level of ID. New data, using a further application of the NCCPC-R for episodes of chronic pain in adults (average age, 44 years), reveals mean total NCCPC-R scores of 4.8 ($SD = 5.2$) when pain is absent (Burkitt, Breau, Salsman, Sarfield-Turner, & Mullan, 2009). There were modifications to the NCCPC-R. Observation time was reduced to 5 minutes, and several items that were not sensitive to pain and did not relate well to total scores were removed. The resulting 24-item scale, named the *Chronic Pain Scale for Nonverbal Adults with Intellectual Disabilities* (CPS-NAID) yielded scores during pain (e.g., constipation, dysmenorrhea, hip displacement) of 28.2 (SD = 13.6) and when pain was absent of 4.7 (SD = 5.2). Further analysis of NCCPC-R items may be appropriate to improve psychometric sensitivity and specificity for chronic and acute pain.

Older Adults with Dementia

There has been a proliferation of research tools designed to assess pain among older adults with dementia (e.g., Abbey et al., 2004; Feldt, 2000; Fuchs-Lacelle & Hadjistavropoulos, 2004; Hurley, Volicer, Hanrahan, Houde, & Volicer, 1992; Simons & Malabar, 1995; Snow et al., 2004; Warden, Hurley, & Volicer, 2003; Wary & Collectif Doloplus, 1999). Some of these tools have promising psychometric properties, with recent evaluative literature reviews available (Aubin, Giguere, Hadjistavropoulos, & Verreault, 2007; Hadjistavropoulos, 2005; Zwakhalen, Hamers, Abu-Saad, & Berger, 2006). Several instruments consistently rated as being promising are the *Abbey Scale* (Abbey et al., 2004), the *Pain Assessment in Advanced Dementia* (PAINAD; Warden et al., 2003), the *Doloplus-2* (Wary & Collectif Doloplus, 1999), and the *Pain Assessment Checklist for Seniors with Limited Ability to Communicate* (PACSLAC; Fuchs-Lacelle & Hadjistavropoulos, 2004). We briefly review each of these tools here.

ABBEY SCALE

The Abbey Scale (Abbey et al., 2004) consists of six items (Facial Expression, Change in Body Language, Vocalization, Behavioral Change, Physiological Change, and Physical Change) scored along 4-point scales ranging from 0 = *absent* to 3 = *severe*. The items were derived from preexisting scales (Hurley et al., 1992; Simons & Malabar, 1995) and modified with the aid of a panel of experts using the Delphi procedure (e.g., Dalkey, 1969), a method of eliciting and refining group opinions. Relative to other scales with small numbers of items (e.g., Feldt, 2000), satisfactory internal consistency has been reported (alpha = .74–.81). Scores changed following pain interventions, but nurses who

completed the scale were not blinded as to whether an intervention had been administered. The scale requires knowledge of the patient, thereby limiting utility in acute care settings and by those unfamiliar with the patient. As well, the small number of items may miss idiosyncratic pain responses characteristic of some seniors with neurological damage, although this possibility needs to be studied.

PAIN ASSESSMENT IN ADVANCED DEMENTIA

The PAINAD (Warden et al., 2003) consists of five items (Breathing, Negative Vocalization, Facial Expression, Body Language, and Consolability), each rated along a scale ranging from 0 to 2. These items are accompanied by detailed descriptors. Warden and colleagues (2003) demonstrated that PAIN-AD scores decreased after the patients received pain medication, although raters may not have been "blind" with respect to whether a pain medication had been administered. The PAINAD has satisfactory interrater reliability but demonstrated low internal consistency under some administration conditions (Warden et al., 2003). Zwakhalen, Hamers, and Berger (2006) evaluated a Dutch translation and found that the PAINAD had good psychometric qualities in terms of reliability, validity (i.e., the scores varied as a function of potentially painful activity), and homogeneity (alpha range, .69–.74) (except for the Breathing item). Like the Abbey Scale, the PAINAD has a restricted number of items and does not comprehensively cover all of the behavioral domains of pain assessment recommended by the American Geriatrics Society Panel on Persistent Pain in Older Persons (2002).

DOLOPLUS-2

This instrument was developed in France but has been translated into English and used in English-speaking settings (Wary & Collectif Doloplus, 1999), with the English translation available, at the time of this writing, at *www.doloplus.com*. Two psychomotor, five somatic, and three psychosocial items are scored along 0- to 3-point scales. The ratings are clearly defined. For example, psychosocial item Social Life is rated as follows: 0, *participates normally in every activity* (meals, entertainment, therapy workshop);

1, *participates in activity when asked to do so only*; 2, *sometimes refuses to participate in any activity*; 3, *refuses to participate in anything*. Lefebvre-Chapiro and Collectif Doloplus (2001) reported that the scale had satisfactory interrater reliability and was significantly correlated with a self-report visual analogue scale (for patients who could complete the scale). Although the Doloplus-2 has satisfactory internal consistency, especially for the full scale (e.g., Zwakhalen, Hamers, & Berger, 2006), it has been criticized for its limited range of items (Gonthier, Vassal, Diana, Richard, & Navez, 1999). Based on nurses' ratings (Zwakhalen, Hamers, & Berger, 2006), the Doloplus-2 was considered to have less clinical usefulness than the PAINAD or the PACSLAC.

PAIN ASSESSMENT CHECKLIST FOR SENIORS WITH LIMITED ABILITY TO COMMUNICATE

Unlike most available pain assessment approaches developed for older adults with dementia, PACSLAC items cover all behavioral domains recommended for pain assessment by the American Geriatrics Society Panel on Pain in Older Persons (2002). (A copy of the PACSLAC has been included in the Appendix 13.2). The checklist examines 60 behaviors and requires less than 5 minutes to complete, because the behaviors are organized into conceptually derived categories (facial expression, body movement, social/personality characteristics, and other). Although a separate score can be derived for each conceptually derived category of items, developers of the scale have recommended use of the total score rather than subscale scores, because of better internal consistency of the overall scale. Initial development of the PACSLAC items was based on interviews with experienced nurses who worked with older adults with dementia (Fuchs-Lacelle & Hadjistavropoulos, 2004). These retrospective reports required nurses to recall patients when calm, while experiencing pain due to a fall or another painful event, and while they were distressed as a result of situational factors unrelated to pain. The selected pools of items are internally consistent and have been shown to discriminate among (retrospectively reported) pain-related events, calm events, and non-pain-related distress events (Fuchs-Lacelle & Hadjistavropoulos, 2004).

Further research demonstrating empirical correspondence of the list of PACSLAC behaviors to typical pain behaviors displayed by patients is warranted.

Since initial retrospective validation, prospective studies of PACSLAC as an assessment tool and an instrument to facilitate treatment have been undertaken. Fuchs-Lacelle, Hadjistavropoulos, and Lix (2008) reported excellent interrater reliability. This study also examined clinical utility. Nursing staff members were provided general guidelines about score interpretation and asked to complete the PACSLAC three times per week on a routine basis for each participating patient. Compared to a control group of patients, whose professional caregiver completed a checklist not designed to assess pain, patients with severe dementia for whom nursing staff routinely completed the PACSLAC were administered more PRN (*peri nata*—used on an as-needed basis) medications, partly addressing the undertreatment of pain in this population.[1] Interestingly, Fuchs-Lacelle and colleagues (2008) also found that nurses who completed the PACSLAC experienced reduced levels of nursing stress compared to the control group. Zwakhalen, Hamers, and Berger (2006), using a Dutch translation of the PACSLAC, also demonstrated that PACSLAC scores differentiate painful and nonpainful states. Moreover, based on a comparison of the PACSLAC with the PAINAD and the Doloplus-2, Zwakhalen, Hamers, and Berger reported that nurses found the PACSLAC to be more useful than the other two measures. It is worth noting that a French version of the PACSLAC is also available and has been investigated prospectively (Aubin et al., 2008).

A CLINICAL APPROACH TO ASSESSMENT

Hadjistavropoulos and colleagues (2007), Hadjistavropoulos (2005), and Herr and colleagues (2006) made clinical recommendations to facilitate the assessment of persons with severe dementia and limitations, and ability to communicate. The same assessment approaches may be appropriate for other populations with limited ability to communicate. Table 13.1 summarizes some of the key steps recommended for clinicians.

TABLE 13.1. Guidelines for the Pain Assessment of Older Adults with Dementia (e.g., Hadjistavropoulos et al., 2007; Hadjistavropoulos, 2005; Herr et al., 2006) and Modified to Be Relevant for a Wider Range of Persons with Cognitive Impairments

- Take into account patient history, physical examination results, and related information.
- Use both self-report and observational approaches, if possible.
- Older adults with mild to moderate dementia can typically use the CAS, NRS, and VDS. Children with borderline to mild mental retardation may be able to use the Faces Pain Scale—Revised in some situations with prior practice.
- Use a good, standardized nonverbal assessment scale (e.g., PACSLAC, NCCPC) but do so cautiously, taking into consideration that validation research is ongoing.
- It is generally assumed that pain assessment during a movement-based task is more likely to identify an underlying persistent pain problem, but research is needed to confirm this assumption among persons with limited ability to communicate.
- Examine whether use of analgesic medications results in a reduction of behavioral indicators of pain.
- A comprehensive pain assessment includes evaluation of other aspects of patient functioning (e.g., mood).
- Solicit assistance of knowledgeable informants.
- Use an individualized approach in collecting baseline scores for each patient.
- Solicit the assistance of caregivers who are familiar with the patients.
- If assessment tools are used to monitor pain levels over time, they must be used under consistent circumstances (e.g., during a structured program of physiotherapy, over the course of a typical evening).
- The PACSLAC, the NCCPC, and other related to tools are screening instruments and, as such, cannot be considered to represent definitive indicators of pain. In some instances, they may fail to identify pain, while in others they may suggest that pain is occurring when, in fact, it is not.
- Use an individualized approach and collect baseline scores for each patient. Deviations from typical baseline scores may be suggestive of changes in the pain status of the patient. Solicit the assistance of caregivers who are familiar with the patients.
- If assessment tools are used to monitor pain levels over time, they must be used under consistent circumstances (e.g., during a structured program of physiotherapy, over the course of a typical evening).

FUTURE DIRECTIONS

Although, over the past few years, we have seen the development and initial validation of a wide variety of tools designed to assess pain in persons with limited ability to communicate, more work is required. Translations and related psychometric investigations have begun to emerge (e.g., Kleinknecht, 2007; Zwakhalen, Hamers, & Berger, 2006), but validation in more languages is needed. Moreover, normative data on these assessments tools are limited, and information on their specificity is scarce in most cases. As such, fruitful directions for future research in this area include, but are not limited to (1) collection of systematic normative data for specific populations (e.g., patients with advanced Alzheimer's disease); (2) investigations involving the direct comparison of the psychometric properties of various assessment tools within a common patient sample; (3) translation and validation of assessment tools in more languages; and (4) more extensive investigations of the specificity of these pain assessment approaches (e.g., their ability to discriminate pain states from non-pain-related distress). Finally, in the case of older adults with dementia, most tools have been developed and validated in long-term care facilities. As such, it would be important to assess their psychometric properties and usefulness in acute care settings.

ACKNOWLEDGMENTS

This work was supported, in part, through funding from the Canadian Institutes of Health Research and the Social Sciences and Humanities Research Council of Canada. Disclosure: Thomas Hadjistavropoulos is a copyright holder of the Pain Assessment Checklist for Seniors with Limited Ability to Communicate. Lynn Breau is one of the developers of the Non-Communicating Children's Pain Checklist.

NOTE

1. It is important to note that although pain tends to be undertreated among older adults with dementia, mere increases in medications are not necessarily desirable. As such, ongoing evaluation of the clinical appropriateness of all medication regimens for older adult

patients, using the Beers criteria (Fick et al., 2003), is imperative.

REFERENCES

Abbey, J., Piller, N., De Bellis, A., Esterman, A., Parker, D., Giles, L., et al. (2004). The Abbey Pain Scale: A 1-minute numerical indicator for people with end-stage dementia. *International Journal of Palliative Nursing, 10,* 6–13.

American Geriatrics Society Panel on Persistent Pain in Older Persons. (2002). Clinical practice guidelines: The management of persistent pain in older persons. *Journal of the American Geriatrics Society, 50,* S205–S224.

American Psychiatric Association. (2005). *Diagnostic and statistical manual of mental disorders—IV (text revision)* (4th ed.). Washington, DC: Author.

Aubin, M., Giguere, A., Hadjistavropoulos, T., & Verreault, R. (2007). Evaluation systematique des instruments pour mesurer la douleur chez les personnes âgées ayant des capacités réduites a communiquer [Systematic evaluation of instruments designed to measure pain in older persons with limited ability to communicate]. *Pain Research and Management, 12,* 195–203.

Aubin, M., Verreault, R., Savoie, M., Lemay, S., Hadjistavropoulos, T., Fillion, L., et al. (2008). Validite et utilite clinique d'une grille d'observation (PACSLAC-F) pour evaluer la douleur chez des aines atteints de demence vivant en milieu de soins de longue duree [Validity and clinical utility of an observational scale (PACSLAC-F) designed for the evaluation of pain in older persons who have dementia and reside in long-term care facilities.] *Canadian Journal on Aging, 27,* 45–55.

Benedetti, F., Arduino, C., Vighetti, S., Asteggiano, G., Tarenzi, L., & Rainero, I. (2004). Pain reactivity in Alzheimer patients with different degrees of cognitive impairment and brain electrical activity deterioration. *Pain, 111,* 22–29.

Benedetti, F., Vighetti, S., Ricco, C., Lagna, E., Bergamasco, B., Pinessi, L., et al. (1999). Pain threshold and tolerance in Alzheimer's disease. *Pain, 80,* 377–382.

Benini, F., Trapanotto, M., Gobber, D., Agosto, C., Carli, G., Drigo, P., et al. (2004). Evaluating pain induced by venipuncture in pediatric patients with developmental delay. *Clinical Journal of Pain, 20,* 156–163.

Berrol, S. (1989). Moderate head injury. In P. Bach-y-Rita (Ed.), *Traumatic brain injury* (pp. 31–40). New York: Demos.

Braden, K., Swanson, S., & Di Scala, C. (2003). Injuries to children who had pre-injury cognitive impairment. *Archives of Pediatrics and Adolescent Medicine, 157,* 336–340.

Breau, L. M., Camfield, C. S., McGrath, P. J., & Finley, G. A. (2007). Pain's impact on adaptive functioning. *Journal of Intellectual Disability Research, 51*(Pt. 2), 125–134.

Breau, L. M., Camfield, C. S., Symons, F. J., Bodfish, J. W., Mackay, A., Finley, G. A., et al. (2003). Relation between pain and self-injurious behavior in nonverbal children with severe cognitive impairments. *Journal of Pediatrics, 142,* 498–503.

Breau, L. M., Finley, G. A., McGrath, P. J., & Camfield, C. S. (2002). Validation of the Non-Communicating Children's Pain Checklist—Postoperative Version. *Anesthesiology, 96,* 528–535.

Breau, L. M., Gregoire, M., Lévêque, C., Hannequin, M., Bureau, N., & Wood, C. (2008). Validation en français de la Grille d'évaluation de la douleur-déficience intellectuelle [Validation of the French Version of the Non-Communicating Children's Pain Checklist-Post Operative Version]. *Douleurs: Évaluation, Diagnostic, Traitment, 9*(54), A40.

Breau, L. M., McGrath, P. J., Camfield, C., Rosmus, C., & Finley, G. A. (2000). Preliminary validation of an observational pain checklist for persons with cognitive impairments and inability to communicate verbally. *Developmental Medicine and Child Neurology, 42,* 609–616.

Breau, L. M., McGrath, P. J., Craig, K. D., Santor, D., Cassidy, K. L., & Reid, G. J. (2001). Facial expression of children receiving immunizations: A principal components analysis of the child facial coding system. *Clinical Journal of Pain, 17,* 178–186.

Burkitt, C., Breau, L. M., Salsman, S., Sarfield-Turner, T., & Mullan, R. (2009). Pilot study of the feasibility of the Non-Communicating Children's Pain Checklist Revised for pain assessment for adults with intellectual disabilities. *Journal of Pain Management, 2,* 37–49.

Chambers, C. T., Cassidy, K. L., McGrath, P. J., Gilbert, C. A., & Craig, K. D. (1996). *Child Facial Coding System: A manual.* Halifax: Dalhousie University/Vancouver: University of British Columbia.

Charlton, J. E. (2005). *Core curriculum for professional education in pain* (3rd ed.). Seattle, WA: IASP Press.

Chibnall, J. T., & Tait, R. C. (2001). Pain assessment in cognitively impaired and unimpaired older adults: A comparison of four scales. *Pain, 92,* 173–186.

Collignon, P., & Giusiano, B. (2001). Validation of a pain evaluation scale for patients with severe cerebral palsy. *European Journal of Pain, 5,* 433–442.

Collignon, P., Guisiano, B., Porsmoguer, E., Jimeno, M. E., & Combe, J. C. (1995). Difficultes du diagnostic de la douleur chez l'enfant polyhandicape [Difficulties in the diagnosis of pain in the child with multiple handicaps]. *Annals of Pediatrics, 42,* 123–126.

Collignon, P., Porsmoguer, E., Behar, M., Combe, J. C., & Perrin, C. (1992). L'automutilation: expression de la douleur chez le sujet déficient mental profond [Self-mutilation: Expression of pain in the individual with profound mental retardation]. In *La douleur de l'enfant Quelles responses?* [Child pain: What are the answers?] (pp. 15–21). Paris: UNESCO.

Craig, K. D. (2009). The social communication model of pain. *Canadian Psychology, 50,* 22–32.

Craig, K. D., Hadjistavropoulos, H. D., Grunau, R. V., & Whitfield, M. F. (1994). A comparison of two measures of facial activity during pain in the newborn child. *Journal of Pediatric Psychology, 19,* 305–318.

Craig, K. D., Stanford, E. A., Fairburn, N. S., & Chambers, C. T. (2006). Emergent pain language competence in infants and children. *Enfance, 1,* 52–71.

Dalkey, N. C. (1969). *The Delphi method: An experimental study of group opinion.* Santa Monica, CA: RAND Corporation.

Defrin, R., Lotan, M., & Pick, C. G. (2006). The evaluation of acute pain in individuals with cognitive impairment: A differential effect of the level of impairment. *Pain, 124,* 312–320.

Ekman, P., & Friesen, W. V. (1978). *Investigator's guide to the Facial Action Coding System.* Palo Alto, CA: Consulting Psychologists Press.

Ekman, P., Friesen, W. V., & Hager, J. C. (2002). *Facial Action Coding System: The manual on CD ROM.* Salt Lake City, UT: A Human Face.

Eland, J. M. (1989). *Eland Color scale: Directions for use.* Retrieved May 28, 2010, from *www.painresearch.utah.edu/cancerpain/attachb6.html*

Fanurik, D., Koh, J. L., Harrison, R. D., Conrad, T. M., & Tomerlin, C. (1998). Pain assessment in children with cognitive impairment: An exploration of self-report skills. *Clinical Nursing Research, 7,* 103–119; discussion 120–124.

Farrell, M. J., Gibson, S. J., & Helme, R. D. (1996). Measuring the activity of older people with chronic pain. *Clinical Journal of Pain, 12,* 6–12.

Feldt, K. S. (2000). The Checklist of Nonverbal pain Indicators (CNPI). *Pain Management Nursing, 1,* 13–21.

Ferrell, B. R., Novy, D., Sullivan, M. D., Banja, J., Dubois, M. Y., Gitlin, M. C., et al. (2001). Ethical dilemmas in pain management. *Journal of Pain, 2,* 171–180.

Fick, D. M., Cooper, J. W., Wade, W. E., Waller, J. L., Maclean, J. R., & Beers, M. H. (2003). Updating the Beers criteria for potentially inappropriate medication use in older adults:

Results of a US consensus panel of experts. *Archives of Internal Medicine, 163,* 2716–2724.

Folstein, M. F., Folstein, S. E., & McHugh, P. R. (1975). "Mini-mental state": A practical method for grading the cognitive state of patients for the clinician. *Journal of Psychiatric Research, 12,* 189–198.

Frankowski, R. F., Annegers, J. F., & Whitman, S. (1985). The descriptive epidemiology of head trauma in the United States. In D. P. Becker & T. Povlishock (Eds.), *Central nervous system trauma: Status report 1985* (pp. 33–43). Bethesda, MD: National Institutes of Health.

Fuchs-Lacelle, S., & Hadjistavropoulos, T. (2004). Development and preliminary validation of the Pain Assessment Checklist for Seniors with Limited Ability to Communicate (PACSLAC). *Pain Management Nursing, 5,* 37–49.

Fuchs-Lacelle, S., Hadjistavropoulos, T., & Lix, L. (2008). Pain assessment as intervention: A study of older adults with severe dementia. *Clinical Journal of Pain, 24,* 697–707.

Fuchs-Lacelle, S., Hadjistavropoulos, T., Sharpe, D., Williams, J., Martin, R., & LaChapelle, D. (2003). Comparing two observational systems in the assessment of knee pain. *Pain Research and Management, 8,* 205–211.

Gennarelli, T. A. (1983). Head injury in man and experimental animals: Clinical aspects. *Acta Neurochirurgica Supplementum, 32,* 1–13.

Gibson, S. J., Voukelatos, X., Ames, D., Flicker, L., & Helme, R. D. (2001). An examination of pain perception and cerebral event-related potentials following carbon dioxide laser stimulation in patients with Alzheimer's disease and age-matched control volunteers. *Pain Research and Management, 6,* 126–132.

Gilbert, C. A., Lilley, C. M., Craig, K. D., McGrath, P. J., Court, C. A., Bennett, S. M., et al. (1999). Postoperative pain expression in preschool children: Validation of the Child Facial Coding System. *Clinical Journal of Pain, 15,* 192–200.

Gillberg, C., Terenius, L., & Lonnerholm, G. (1985). Endorphin activity in childhood psychosis: Spinal fluid levels in 24 cases. *Archives of General Psychiatry, 42,* 780–783.

Giusiano, B., Jimeno, M. T., Collignon, P., & Chau, Y. (1995). Utilization of neural network in the elaboration of an evaluation scale for pain in cerebral palsy. *Methods of Information in Medicine, 34,* 498–502.

Gonthier, R., Vassal, P., Diana, M. C., Richard, A., & Navez, M. L. (1999). Sémiologie et évaluation de la douleur chez le sujet dément ou non communicant [Semiology and the assessment of pain in the individual with dementia or inability to communicate]. *Info Kara, 53,* 12–12.

Grunau, R. E., Oberlander, T., Holsti, L., & Whitfield, M. F. (1998). Bedside application of the Neonatal Facial Coding System in pain assessment of premature neonates. *Pain, 76,* 277–286.

Hadden, K. L., & von Baeyer, C. L. (2002). Pain in children with cerebral palsy: Common triggers and expressive behaviors. *Pain, 99,* 281–288.

Hadden, K. L., & von Baeyer, C. L. (2005). Global and specific behavioral measures of pain in children with cerebral palsy. *Clinical Journal of Pain, 21,* 140–146.

Hadjistavropoulos, T. (2005). Assessing pain in older persons with severe limitations in ability to communicate. In S. J. Gibson & D. Weiner (Eds.), *Pain in the elderly* (pp. 135–151). Seattle, WA: IASP Press.

Hadjistavropoulos, T., & Craig, K. D. (2002). A theoretical framework for understanding self-report and observational measures of pain: A communications model. *Behaviour Research and Therapy, 40,* 551–570.

Hadjistavropoulos, T., Craig, K. D., & Fuchs-Lacelle, S. K. (2004). Social influences and the communication of pain. In T. Hadjistavropoulos & K. D. Craig (Eds.), *Pain: Psychological perspectives* (pp. 87–112). Mahwah, NJ: Erlbaum.

Hadjistavropoulos, T., Craig, K. D., Martin, N., Hadjistavropoulos, H., & McMurtry, B. (1997). Toward a research outcome measure of pain in frail elderly in chronic care. *Pain Clinic, 10,* 71–80.

Hadjistavropoulos, T., Herr, K., Turk, D. C., Fine, P. G., Dworkin, R. H., Helme, R., et al. (2007). An interdisciplinary expert consensus statement on assessment of pain in older persons. *Clinical Journal of Pain, 23*(Suppl. 1), S1–S43.

Hadjistavropoulos, T., LaChapelle, D., MacLeod, F., Hale, C., O'Rourke, N., & Craig, K. D. (1998). Cognitive functioning and pain reactions in hospitalized elders. *Pain Research and Management, 3,* 145–151.

Hadjistavropoulos, T., LaChapelle, D. L., Hadjistavropoulos, H. D., Green, S., & Asmundson, G. J. (2002). Using facial expressions to assess musculoskeletal pain in older persons. *European Journal of Pain, 6,* 179–187.

Hadjistavropoulos, T., LaChapelle, D. L., MacLeod, F. K., Snider, B., & Craig, K. D. (2000). Measuring movement-exacerbated pain in cognitively impaired frail elders. *Clinical Journal of Pain, 16,* 54–63.

Herr, K., Coyne, P. J., Key, T., Manworren, R., McCaffery, M., Merkel, S., et al. (2006). Pain assessment in the nonverbal patient: Position statement with clinical practice recommendations. *Pain Management Nursing, 7,* 44–52.

Hicks, C. L., von Baeyer, C. L., Spafford, P. A., van Korlaar, I., & Goodenough, B. (2001). The Faces Pain Scale—Revised: Toward a common

metric in pediatric pain measurement. *Pain, 93,* 173–183.

Horgas, A. L., & Tsai, P. F. (1998). Analgesic drug prescription and use in cognitively impaired nursing home residents. *Nursing Research, 47,* 235–242.

Hunt, A., Goldman, A., Seers, K., Crichton, N., Mastroyannopoulou, K., Moffat, V., et al. (2004). Clinical validation of the paediatric pain profile. *Developmental Medicine and Child Neurology, 46,* 9–18.

Hunt, A., Mastroyannopoulou, K., Golman, A., & Sears, K. (2003). Not knowing—the problem of pain in children with severe neurological impairment. *International Journal of Nursing Studies, 40,* 171–183.

Hunt, A., Wisbeach, A., Seers, K., Goldman, A., Crichton, N., Perry, L., et al. (2007). Development of the Paediatric Pain Profile: Role of video analysis and saliva cortisol in validating a tool to assess pain in children with severe neurological disability. *Journal of Pain and Symptom Management, 33,* 276–289.

Hurley, A. C., Volicer, B. J., Hanrahan, P. A., Houde, S., & Volicer, L. (1992). Assessment of discomfort in advanced Alzheimer patients. *Research in Nursing and Health, 15,* 369–377.

Jensen, M. P., Miller, L., & Fisher, L. D. (1998). Assessment of pain during medical procedures: A comparison of three scales. *Clinical Journal of Pain, 14,* 343–349.

Kaasalainen, S. J., Robinson, L. K., Hartley, T., Middleton, J., Knezacek, S., & Ife, C. (1998). The assessment of pain in the cognitively impaired elderly: A literature review. *Perspectives, 22,* 2–8.

Keefe, F. J., & Block, A. R. (1982). Development of an observational method for assessing pain behavior in chronic low back pain in pain patients. *Behavior Therapy, 12,* 363–375.

Kleinknecht, M. (2007). [Reliability and validity of the german language version of the "NCCPC-R"]. *Pflege, 20,* 93–102.

Kunz, M., Scharmann, S., Hemmeter, U., Schepelmann, K., & Lautenbacher, S. (2007). The facial expression of pain in patients with dementia. *Pain, 133,* 221–228.

LaChapelle, D. L., Hadjistavropoulos, T., & Craig, K. D. (1999). Pain measurement in persons with intellectual disabilities. *Clinical Journal of Pain, 15,* 13–23.

Lefebvre-Chapiro, S., & Collectif Doloplus. (2001). The Doloplus-2 Scale: Evaluating pain in the elderly. *European Journal of Palliative Care, 8,* 191–194.

Lezack, M. D. (1995). *Neuropsychological assessment* (3rd ed.). New York: Oxford University Press.

Lilley, C. M., Craig, K. D., & Grunau, R. E. (1997). The expression of pain in infants and toddlers: Developmental changes in facial action. *Pain, 72,* 161–170.

Lints-Martindale, A. C., Hadjistavropoulos, T., Barber, B., & Gibson, S. J. (2007). A psychophysical investigation of the Facial Action Coding System as an index of pain variability among older adults with and without Alzheimer's disease. *Pain Medicine, 8,* 678–689.

Martin, R., Williams, J., Hadjistavropoulos, T., Hadjistavropoulos, H. D., & MacLean, M. (2005). A qualitative investigation of seniors' and caregivers' views on pain assessment and management. *Canadian Journal of Nursing Research, 37,* 142–164.

McGrath, P. A., deVeber, L. L., & Hearn, M. J. (1985). Multidimensional pain assessment in children. In H. L. Fields, R. Dubner, & F. Cevero (Eds.), *Advances in pain research and therapy* (Vol. 9, pp. 387–393). New York: Raven Press.

McGrath, P. A., Seifert, C. E., Speechley, K. N., Booth, J. C., Stitt, L., & Gibson, M. C. (1996). A new analogue scale for assessing children's pain: An initial validation study. *Pain, 64,* 435–443.

Melzack, R., & Katz, J. (2004). The gate control theory: Reaching for the brain. In T. Hadjistavropoulos & K. D. Craig (Eds.), *Pain: Psychological perspectives* (pp. 13–34). Mahwah, NJ: Erlbaum.

Melzack, R., & Wall, P. D. (1965). Pain mechanisms: A new theory. *Science, 150,* 971–979.

Mercer, K., & Glenn, S. (2004). The expression of pain in infants with developmental delays. *Child: Care, Health and Development, 30,* 353–360.

Mette, F., & Abittan, J. (1988). Essais d'évaluation de la douleur chez le polyhandicoupe [Tests for the evaluation of pain in the individual with multiple handicaps.] *Annales Kinésithérapie, 15,* 101–104.

Morrison, R. S., & Sui, A. L. (2000). A comparison of pain and its treatment in advanced dementia and cognitively impaired patients with hip fracture. *Journal of Pain and Symptom Management, 19,* 240–248.

Nader, R., Oberlander, T. F., Chambers, C. T., & Craig, K. D. (2004). Expression of pain in children with autism. *Clinical Journal of Pain, 20,* 88–97.

Oberlander, T. F., Gilbert, C. A., Chambers, C. T., O'Donnell, M. E., & Craig, K. D. (1999). Biobehavioral responses to acute pain in adolescents with a significant neurologic impairment. *Clinical Journal of Pain, 15,* 201–209.

Oster, H., Hegley, D., & Nagel, L. (1992). Adult judgments and fine-grained analysis of infant facial expressions: Testing the validity of a priori coding formulas. *Developmental Psychology, 28,* 1115–1131.

Prkachin, K. M., & Craig, K. D. (1995). Expressing pain: The communication and interpretation of facial pain signals. *Journal of Nonverbal Behavior, 19,* 191–205.

Reynell, J. K. (1965). Post-operative disturbances observed in children with cerebral palsy. *Developmental Medicine and Child Neurology, 7,* 360–376.

Sandman, C. A., Barron, J. L., Chicz-DeMet, A., & DeMet, E. M. (1990). Plasma B-endorphin levels in patients with self-injurious behavior and stereotypy. *American Journal of Mental Retardation, 95,* 84–92.

Scherder, E. J., & Bouma, A. (2000). Visual analogue scales for pain assessment in Alzheimer's disease. *Gerontology, 46,* 47–53.

Sengstaken, E. A., & King, S. A. (1993). The problems of pain and its detection among geriatric nursing home residents. *Journal of the American Geriatrics Society, 41,* 541–544.

Simons, W., & Malabar, R. (1995). Assessing pain in elderly patients who cannot respond verbally. *Journal of Advanced Nursing, 22,* 663–669.

Snow, A. L., Weber, J. B., O'Malley, K. J., Cody, M., Beck, C., Bruera, E., et al. (2004). NOPPAIN: A nursing assistant-administered pain assessment instrument for use in dementia. *Dementia and Geriatric Cognitive Disorders, 17,* 240–246.

Warden, V., Hurley, A. C., & Volicer, L. (2003). Development and psychometric evaluation of the Pain Assessment in Advanced Dementia (PAINAD) scale. *Journal of the American Medical Directors Association, 4,* 9–15.

Wary, B., & Collectif Doloplus. (1999). [Doloplus-2, a scale for pain measurement]. *Soins Gerontologie, 19,* 25–27.

Weiner, D., Peterson, B., Ladd, K., McConnell, E., & Keefe, F. (1999). Pain in nursing home residents: An exploration of prevalence, staff perspectives, and practical aspects of measurement. *Clinical Journal of Pain, 15,* 92–101.

Weiner, D., Pieper, C., McConnell, E., Martinez, S., & Keefe, F. (1996). Pain measurement in elders with chronic low back pain: Tradtional and alternative approaches. *Pain, 67,* 461–467.

Zabalia, M., Jacquet, D., & Breau, L. M. (2005). Rôle du niveau verbal sur l'expression et l'évaluation de la douleur chez des sujets déficients intellectuals. *Douleur et Analgésie, 2,* 65–70.

Zwakhalen, S. M., Hamers, J. P., Abu-Saad, H. H., & Berger, M. P. (2006). Pain in elderly people with severe dementia: A systematic review of behavioural pain assessment tools. *BMC Geriatrics, 6,* 3.

Zwakhalen, S. M., Hamers, J. P., & Berger, M. P. (2006). The psychometric quality and clinical usefulness of three pain assessment tools for elderly people with dementia. *Pain, 126,* 210–220.

APPENDIX 13.1. Non-Communicating Children's Pain Checklist— Postoperative Version (NCCPC-PV)

NAME: _____ UNIT/FILE #: _____ DATE: _____ (dd/mm/yy)

OBSERVER: _____ START TIME: ____ AM/PM STOP TIME: ____ AM/PM

How often has this child shown these behaviors in the last 10 minutes? Please circle a number for each behavior. If an item does not apply to this child (e.g., this child cannot reach with his or her hands), then indicate "not applicable" for that item.

0 = NOT AT ALL	1 = JUST A LITTLE	2 = FAIRLY OFTEN	3 = VERY OFTEN	NA = NOT APPLICABLE

I. Vocal

1. Moaning, whining, whimpering (fairly soft).	0	1	2	3	NA
2. Crying (moderately loud).	0	1	2	3	NA
3. Screaming/yelling (very loud).	0	1	2	3	NA
4. A specific sound or word for pain (e.g., a word, cry or type of laugh).	0	1	2	3	NA

II. Social

5. Not cooperating, cranky, irritable, unhappy.	0	1	2	3	NA
6. Less interaction with others, withdrawn.	0	1	2	3	NA
7. Seeking comfort or physical closeness.	0	1	2	3	NA
8. Being difficult to distract, not able to satisfy or pacify.	0	1	2	3	NA

III. Facial

9. A furrowed brow.	0	1	2	3	NA
10. A change in eyes, including squinting of eyes, eyes opened wide, eyes frowning.	0	1	2	3	NA
11. Turning down of mouth, not smiling.	0	1	2	3	NA
12. Lips puckering up, tight, pouting, or quivering.	0	1	2	3	NA
13. Clenching or grinding teeth, chewing or thrusting tongue out.	0	1	2	3	NA

IV. Activity

14. Not moving, less active, quiet.	0	1	2	3	NA
15. Jumping around, agitated, fidgety.	0	1	2	3	NA

V. Body and Limbs

16. Floppy	0	1	2	3	NA
17. Stiff, spastic, tense, rigid	0	1	2	3	NA
18. Gesturing to or touching part of the body that hurts	0	1	2	3	NA
19. Protecting, favoring, or guarding part of the body that hurts	0	1	2	3	NA
20. Flinching or moving the body part away, being sensitive to touch	0	1	2	3	NA
21. Moving the body in a specific way to show pain (head back, arms down, curls up, etc.)	0	1	2	3	NA

VI. Physiological

22.	Shivering	0	1	2	3	NA
23.	Change in color, pallor	0	1	2	3	NA
24.	Sweating, perspiring	0	1	2	3	NA
25.	Tears	0	1	2	3	NA
26.	Sharp intake of breath, gasping	0	1	2	3	NA
27.	Breath holding	0	1	2	3	NA

SCORE SUMMARY:

Category:	I	II	III	IV	V	VI	TOTAL
Score:							

Using the NCCPC-PV

The NCCPC-PV was designed to be used for children, ages 3 to 18 years, who are unable to speak because of cognitive (mental/intellectual) impairments or disabilities. It can be used *whether or not* a child has physical impairments or disabilities. Descriptions of the types of children used to validate the NCCPC-PV can be found in Breau et al. (2002). The NCCPC-PV was designed to be used without training by parents and caregivers (carers), or by other adults who are not familiar with a specific child (do not know him or her well).

The NCCPC-PV may be freely copied for clinical use or use in research funded by not-for-profit agencies. For-profit agencies should contact Lynn Breau: Pediatric Pain Research, IWK Health Centre, 5850 University Avenue, Halifax, Nova Scotia, Canada B3J 3G9 (*lbreau@ns.sympatico. ca*).

The NCCPC-PV was intended to assess pain after surgery or due to other procedures conducted in hospital. If short or long-term pain is suspected for a child at home or in a long-term residential setting, the Non-Communicating Children's Pain Checklist—Revised may be used. It can be obtained by contacting Lynn Breau. Information regarding the NCCPC-R can be found in Breau, L. M., McGrath, P. J., Camfield, C. S., & Finley, G. A. (2002). Psychometric properties of the Non-Communicating Children's Pain Checklist—Revised. *Pain, 99,* 349–357.

Administration

To complete the NCCPC-R, base your observations on the child's behavior over *10 minutes. It is not necessary to watch the child continuously for this period.* However, it is recommended that the observer be in the child's presence for the majority of this time (e.g., be in the same room with the child). Although shorter observation periods may be used, the cutoff scores described below may not apply.

At the end of the observation time, indicate how frequently (how often) each item was seen or heard. This should not be based on the child's typical behavior or in relation to what he or she usually does. Below is a guide for deciding the frequency of items.

0 = Not present at all during the observation period. (Note that if the item is not present because the child is not capable of performing that act, it should be scored as "NA").

1 = Seen or heard rarely (hardly at all), but is present.

2 = Seen or heard a number of times, but not continuously (not all the time).

3 = Seen or heard often, almost continuously (almost all the time); anyone would easily notice this if he or she saw the child for a few moments during the observation time.

NA = Not applicable. This child is not capable of performing this action.

Scoring

1. Add up the scores for each subscale and enter below that subscale number in the Score Summary at the bottom of the sheet. Items marked "NA" are scored as "0" (zero).
2. Add up all subscale scores for Total Score.
3. Check to see whether the child's score is greater than the cutoff score.

Cutoff Score

Based on the scores of 24 children ages 3 to 18 (Breau et al., 2002), a Total Score of *11 or more* indicates that a child has *moderate to severe pain*. Based on unpublished data from this same sample, a *Total Score of 6–10* indicates that a child has *mild pain*. When parents and caregivers completed the NCCPC-PV in hospital for the study group, this was accurate 88% of the time. When other observers completed the NCCPC-PV, this was accurate 75% of the time.

Use of Cutoff Scores

As with all observational tools, caution should be taken in using cutoff scores, because they may not be 100% accurate. They should not be the only basis for deciding whether a child should be treated for pain. In some cases children may have lower scores when pain is present. For more detailed instructions on use of the NCCPC-PV in such situations, please refer to the full manual, available from Lynn Breau, Pediatric Pain Research, IWK Health Centre, 5850 University Avenue, Halifax, Nova Scotia, Canada B3J 3G9 (*lbreau@ns.sympatico.ca*).

APPENDIX 13.2. Pain Assessment Checklist for Seniors with Limited Ability to Communicate (PACSLAC)

DATE: _____   TIME ASSESSED: _____

NAME OF PATIENT/RESIDENT: _____

Purpose

This checklist is used to assess pain in patients/residents who have dementia and have limited ability to communicate verbally.

Instructions

Indicate with a checkmark, which of the items on the PACSLAC occurred during the period of interest.

Scoring the subscales is derived by counting the checkmarks in each column.
To generate a Total Pain Score sum all four subscale totals.

Comments:

_____
_____
_____
_____
_____
_____
_____
_____
_____
_____
_____
_____
_____
_____
_____
_____

Facial Expressions	Present
Grimacing	
Sad Look	
Tighter face	
Dirty look	
Change in eyes (squinting, dull, bright, increased movement)	
Frowning	

Pain expression	
Grim face	
Clenching teeth	
Wincing	
Opening mouth	
Creasing forehead	
Screwing up nose	

Activity/Body Movement	
Fidgeting	
Pulling away	
Flinching	
Restless	
Pacing	
Wandering	
Trying to leave	
Refusing to move	
Thrashing	
Decreased activity	
Refusing medications	
Moving slow	
Impulsive behavior (e.g., repetitive movements)	
Uncooperative/Resistant to care	
Guarding sore area	
Touching/holding sore area	
Limping	
Clenched fist	
Going into fetal position	
Stiff/rigid	
Social/Personality/Mood	
Physical aggression (e.g., pushing people and/or objects, scratching others, hitting others, striking, kicking)	
Verbal aggression	
Not wanting to be touched	
Not allowing people near	
Angry/mad	
Throwing things	
Increased confusion	
Anxious	

Social/Personality/Mood *(cont.)*	
Upset	
Agitated	
Cranky/irritable	
Frustrated	
Other*	
Pale face	
Flushed, red face	
Teary eyed	
Sweating	
Shaking/trembling	
Cold and clammy	
Changes in sleep (please circle):	
Decreased sleep or	
Increased sleep during day	
Changes in appetite (please circle):	
Decreased appetite or	
Increased appetite	
Screaming/yelling	
Calling out (i.e., for help)	
Crying	
A specific sound or vocalization	
For pain, "ow," "ouch"	
Moaning and groaning	
Mumbling	
Grunting	

Subscale Scores:

Facial Expressions _____

Activity/Body Movement _____

Social/Personality/Mood _____

Other _____

Total Checklist Score _____

*"Other" subscale includes physiological changes, eating and sleeping changes, and vocal behaviors.

This version of the scale does not include the items "sitting and rocking," "quiet/withdrawn," and "vacant blank stare," as these were not found to be useful in discriminating pain from nonpain states.

PART IV

ASSESSMENT OF SPECIFIC PAIN CONDITIONS AND SYNDROMES

CHAPTER 14

Assessment of Acute Pain, Pain Relief, and Patient Satisfaction

Shawn T. Mason
James A. Fauerbach
Jennifer A. Haythornthwaite

In February 1992, the Agency for Healthcare Policy and Research (AHCPR) issued their first clinical practice guideline called *Acute Pain Management: Operative or Medical Procedures and Trauma.* Incorporated into this guideline was earlier work conducted by the American Pain Society Committee on Quality Assurance Standards for Acute Pain and Cancer Pain, which developed and published its own set of standards, most recently in 2005 (Gordon et al., 2005). These standards include the following: (1) Identify and treat pain promptly, highlighting the importance of comprehensive assessment and preventive efforts; (2) involve patients and families in decisions and plans, with emphasis on tailored treatment plans; (3) improve multimodal intervention and eliminate inappropriate practices; (4) modify interventions as needed with attention to intensity, functional status, and side effects; and (5) monitor outcomes and treatment process according to quality standards. Specific strategies for implementing these guidelines have been in place since the first publication (Miaskowski & Donovan, 1992)

In 1996, the President of the American Pain Society, James Campbell, promoted "Pain as the Fifth Vital Sign" in his presidential address to increase awareness of pain assessment and treatment among health care professionals. The integration of pain as a vital sign became the theme for the U.S. Veterans Health Administration's (VHA) implementation of a nationwide program addressing the inconsistent and often inaccessible pain management services throughout the VHA system. The VHA issued a toolkit titled "Pain Assessment: The Fifth Vital Sign" that guides implementation of systematic pain assessment and its documentation, education for health care providers, and education for patients and families. In late July, 1999, the Joint Commission on the Accreditation of Healthcare Organizations (JCAHO) expanded existing standards to apply across the continuum of care. The standards, implemented in 2001, require accredited health care organizations to monitor and manage pain, and to educate staff and patients about the importance of effective pain management.

In performing an assessment of acute pain, either in a clinical trial or in routine clinical care, measurement considerations include feasibility, convenience, and speed of completion; responsivity to treatment effects; and clinical utility. Because no single measure of pain intensity can be considered universally valid across clinical settings, instrument features should be weighed in selection, since errors can occur in using almost every scale. Clinical factors to consider include the patient's age, educational level, level of consciousness, availability of the patient's writing hand, the frequency of assessment, and the burden of the assessment process relative to the amount of information obtained. For a discussion of special populations, the reader is referred to the other chapters in this volume.

A multitude of factors influence pain ratings. The clinician must consider the many factors that influence self-report, such as gender, social support, expectancies (e.g., placebo), and provider characteristics (Oken, 2008). Similar factors can influence the provider's judgment of pain, including not only the patient's report of pain but also his or her social and psychological presentation (Tait, Chibnall, & Kalauokalani, 2009). Any judgment of pain made by a provider based only on observation must be viewed with caution due to the known underestimation by both nurses and physicians asked to rate a patient's pain without benefit of the patient's self-report (Ahlers et al., 2008).

PAIN INTENSITY

Three pain intensity scales are most commonly used in clinical settings: visual analogue scales (VASs), numerical rating scales (NRSs), and verbal rating scales (VRSs). The psychometric properties and relative strengths of these scales are discussed in more detail elsewhere (Scott & McDonald, 2008; see Jensen & Karoly, Chapter 2, this volume). Pain intensity scales can refer to various periods of time, including pain right now, lowest pain during a period of time (e.g., since last medication dose), highest pain, and typical pain. Acute pain assessment needs to target resting or tonic pain, intermittent or phasic pain, and procedural pain.

The first type of scale, the VAS, provides a line, usually 100 mm long, that includes anchors from "no pain" to "the most intense pain sensation imaginable." The patient places a mark on the line that indicates the intensity of pain experienced during a period of time. The patient's rating is the distance (millimeters) from 0. These scales are useful,

simple, and have been widely validated in the pain literature. However, the VAS, by requiring a clear visuospatial estimation and a precise motoric response by the patient, may have limited use in some clinical settings. Although the additional step of measurement can deter use, a recent software program is designed to facilitate data collection and storage (Marsh-Richard, Hatzis, Mathias, Venditti, & Dougherty, 2009).

An NRS asks patients to rate their pain using numbers ranging from 0 ("no pain") to 10 or 100 ("the worst pain imaginable") and typically requires written or verbal ratings. Scales typically consist of 21 or 11 points, and both have fared well, but researchers generally recommend the 21-point scale. Clinical and experimental studies show that the verbal NRS has adequate psychometric properties when compared to the VAS (Bijur, Latimer, & Gallagher, 2003). The NRS is reliable and sensitive to changes in severity, satisfactory in detecting changes in pain across age groups, and is preferred by patients over most other acute pain instruments (Herr, Spratt, Mobily, & Richardson, 2004). Whether or not this scale has ratio properties (i.e., equal intervals between response categories) remains inconsistent (Hartrick, Kovan, & Shapiro, 2003). Conservatively, interpretation should generally be limited to relative changes in pain (e.g., increase or decrease) rather than percentage of increase or decrease.

A VRS includes a list of adjectives that reflect the extremes of pain (e.g., "none" to "severe"). These scales have demonstrated validity relative to other pain scales and are generally responsive to treatment effects. However, patients may have difficulty selecting an appropriate adjective to describe their pain, and these scales generally do not show ratio properties. For example, an early study comparing different pain scales demonstrated that the modal numerical rating was 0 for "none," 3 (ranging from 1 to 5) for "mild," 5 (ranging from 3 to 7) for "moderate," 10 (ranging from 7 to 10) for "severe" (Downie et al., 1978). Of the three types of scales, VRSs show the poorest measurement properties (Hartrick et al., 2003; Lund et al., 2005).

These three commonly used pain intensity rating scales place different demands on the patient and show different scaling properties.

No single method is superior across all clinical settings with all types of patients, and other scales might be more appropriate with special populations. Although, historically, VAS measures show the strongest scaling characteristics and the greatest responsivity to treatment, not all patients understand how to use this type of scale, and its utility may be severely limited with special populations (e.g., hand-injured, visually or cognitively impaired, or children). Recent work with oral surgery patients suggests that the VAS and the 11-item NRS (NRS-11) are very similar in their power to detect differences in pain, and choosing one over the other is a matter of preference. Comparatively, the VRS is consistently less responsive to change (Breivik, Bjornsson, & Skovlund, 2000).

These measures of pain intensity are mainly used in clinical settings due to their practical features. However, pain is widely understood as a multidimensional experience, including both sensory and affective dimensions (Melzack & Wall, 1965). Although less commonly used in routine clinical assessment, the *Short-Form McGill Pain Questionnaire* (Melzack, 1987) was developed in postsurgical and obstetrical samples and has recently demonstrated adequate psychometric properties in patients with acute burn pain (Mason et al., 2008). Measurement of acute pain may extend to include pain-related interference, as has been done with use of the Brief Pain Inventory (Cleeland & Ryan, 1994) in hospitalized cancer patients with acute pain (Wells, 2000).

required for patients to decline rescue medication averaged 33%, or an improvement of ≥ 2 in NRS units (Farrar, Berlin, & Strom, 2003; Farrar, Portenoy, Berlin, Kinman, & Strom, 2000). These findings, however, may not apply uniformly across individuals with varying degrees of pain.

Initial work using morphine analgesia demonstrated the relative importance of initial pain intensity as an important predictor of pain relief (Lasanga, 1962). Contemporary studies extend this finding and suggest that present pain is a reliable and strong predictor of pain relief during an episode of acute back pain. In a sample of patients with low back pain, the initial robust relationship between recall of pain relief and actual (calculated) relief diminished over a 12-month period, and present pain intensity remained as a strong and independent predictor of relief ratings (Haas, Nyiendo, & Aickin, 2002).

Unlike pain intensity, different types of pain relief measures—VRSs and VASs—show similar scaling characteristics. However, the discordance, at times, between ratings of pain relief and actual changes in pain intensity raises questions about which of these outcome measures is more accurate, and which should be used in determining the outcome of a pain treatment intervention. Research on these scales identifies multiple factors that influence the accuracy of pain reports, including both pain intensity and pain relief, following a therapeutic intervention.

PAIN RELIEF

The most common methods for assessing pain relief include VASs, typically anchored with descriptors of "no relief" to "complete relief," and VRSs that provide categories (e.g., "none," "slight," "moderate," "lots," "complete"). Some VRSs include "worse" as an additional anchor. The scaling characteristics of verbal ratings of pain relief are similar to VAS ratings of pain relief. In clinical studies, a rescue model is commonly used to operationalize the concept of adequate pain relief. In this model, patients can request additional pain medication if the initial dose did not provide adequate relief. According to a few large studies, the percentage of relief

FACTORS THAT INFLUENCE THE RECALL OF PAIN

Clinical assessment of pain often requires the patient to describe pain experienced during past episodes and relief obtained from past treatments. The accurate recall of painful episodes is of significant clinical import, since the decision to undergo potentially painful diagnostic, dental, or surgical procedures may depend on recall of pain experienced during prior episodes of the same or similar events. Furthermore, the treatment prescribed to a patient in pain often depends on the accurate retrospective ratings of previous acute pain episodes. Finally, if patients cannot accurately describe their previous acute pain episodes, then clinical trials that investigate the effectiveness of anesthetic agents need to include real-time measures of pain intensity and pain relief.

Pain Intensity Ratings

Data on the accuracy of pain recall remain somewhat inconsistent, but many recent studies identify circumstances associated with increased accuracy. Interestingly, the consistent sex differences observed in pain sensitivity (Paller, Campbell, Edwards, & Dobs, 2009) may also apply to the recall of pain. Although female and male adolescent cancer patients reported comparable current pain intensity, females' ratings of recalled pain were significantly higher than those of males (Rosseland & Stubhaug, 2004), suggesting the potential that sex influences the recall of pain.

The time period of recall is another dimension that may increase accuracy of recall. Shorter time periods increase accuracy of acute pain intensity ratings and many pain behaviors (Linton & Nordin, 2006; Singer, Kowalska, & Thode, 2001). Ratings of pain recall 24 hours following noncardiac surgery are highly correlated with the computed average of pain ratings (Jensen, Mardekian, Lakshminarayanan, & Boye, 2008), and experimental data from healthy males receiving injections of capsaicin suggest that pain intensity memories consolidate within the first 24 hours, then remain stable (Jantsch et al., 2009). Among individuals with chronic pain, daily recall of pain can be quite accurate (Broderick et al., 2008), and accuracy may occur over periods up 3 months (Linton & Nordin, 2006; Singer et al., 2001), but recall over 3 months may be primarily determined by patient memories of typical pain (Broderick et al., 2008). Time delay to recall may interact with other features of the clinical setting, particularly with extended periods of recall. For example, labor pain recall is less accurate over a 5-year period, but only for those with positive experiences during the event (Waldenstrom & Schytt, 2009). Variability of pain intensity is another factor that affects recall. Fluctuation in pain intensity during the time period being assessed is associated with less accurate recall, contributing to a bias toward overestimation for both intensity and duration (Niere & Jerak,

2004; Stone, Schwartz, Broderick, & Shiffman, 2005).

The method of assessment—VAS or VRS—may also influence the accuracy of pain recall. A VAS of pain intensity overestimates baseline pain, whereas a VRS yields both overestimates and underestimates of baseline pain (Linton & Gotestam, 1983). Retrospective ratings of pain intensity are somewhat influenced by present pain intensity, but factors such as elapsed time do not appear to have as large an effect as previously thought. When comparing pain diary data with weekly recall, patients with low back pain are fairly accurate (Jamison, Raymond, Slawsby, McHugo, & Baird, 2006), but this appears to be less true in headache samples, whose frequency recall is more accurate than intensity recall (Niere & Jerak, 2004).

When patients are asked to describe pain during a medical procedure or a over period of time, it is clear that they do not simply compute an arithmetic average of their pain experienced during the relevant period. In other words, all pain experiences are not equally weighted in patients' summary ratings. Phenomena studied in the memory literature, including recency, salience, and state-dependent effects, provide a basis for identifying factors that can influence constructions of pain memories.

Recency Effects

Evidence for these patterns in memory comes from studies that obtained serial pain ratings during painful medical procedures and compared these to summary ratings made after completion of the procedure. Participants' recall of their total pain during the procedure was highly related to the pain experienced during the last few moments of the painful episode (i.e., *recency effect*). For example, retrospective ratings of pain intensity made by patients undergoing colonoscopy procedures were strongly related to the pain intensity recorded in real time during the last 3 minutes of the procedure (called *end pain*; Redelmeier, Katz, & Kahneman, 2003). Because of the addition of 3 minutes of minimal pain to the procedure, patients reported the overall experience as less aversive. This condition had two important characteristics. First, time between peak pain and the end of the procedure was extended. Second, end pain was minimally painful by comparison. Evidence for this effect was recently demonstrated in labor pain, where mothers who selected epidural analgesia, compared to women who did not, recalled their pain as more intense. When women who received the epidural rated their recalled pain, end pain and peak pain were essentially the same experience, and their pain recall did not apparently include the period of no pain following analgesia administration (Waldenstrom & Schytt, 2009).

Salience Effects

These same studies provide support for the *salience effect*, which is the tendency to recall most accurately that part of a stimulus that has the strongest positive or negative valence. Retrospective ratings of pain intensity made by patients following painful colonoscopy procedures also strongly correlated with the peak pain intensity recorded during the procedure (Redelmeier et al., 2003). In experimental work, accurate recall of peak pain and pain duration up to 1 week later has been observed (Jantsch et al., 2009). In a large sample of postoperative surgical patients, peak pain showed a stronger effect on recall than end pain (Jensen et al., 2008).

State and Assimilation Effects

The accuracy and completeness of memory has been shown to be a function of state effects (e.g., pain or mood) present during memory acquisition across some studies. The valence of the emotional experience relates to labor pain ratings and memory recall. New mothers who rated the birthing experience as positive reported less intense labor pain than those with negative experiences. Positive valence correlated with poorer recall and forgetfulness of labor pain, whereas negative valence correlated with accurate recall (Waldenstrom & Schytt, 2009). Similar state-dependent effects of mood on recalled pain have also been observed during laboratory manipulations of stress in community volunteers. Mood ratings predicted recall in a group exposed to concurrent stress at the time of pain exposure, whereas no effect

of mood on recall of pain was observed in a control group not exposed to concurrent stress (Gedney & Logan, 2004).

Some investigators have demonstrated that a participant's current pain level affects the accuracy of recall for prior painful episodes. This effect has been termed an *assimilation* effect, in that recollections of pain are assimilated to current experiences of pain. In an early study demonstrating this phenomenon, high levels of present pain intensity were associated with retrospective *over*estimation of usual, maximum, and minimum pain during the past week, whereas low levels of present pain intensity were associated with retrospective *under*estimation of diary-rated pain (Eich, Reeves, Jaeger, & Graff-Radford, 1985). More work is needed in this area, because a recent, large-scale postoperative study found that the level of current pain had less influence than expected over a 24-hour recall period (Jensen et al., 2008).

Duration Effects

In constructing summary ratings of pain, it is perhaps intuitively appealing to suggest that the duration of acute pain contributes to one's remembered pain intensity; that is, longer duration of pain may contribute to higher ratings, and shorter duration may contribute to lower ratings. The data are not consistent on this issue.

Duration neglect is the phenomenon whereby subsequent recollections of acute pain are unrelated to the duration of the painful episode. In an influential study, laboratory manipulations demonstrated neglect for the duration of an aversive experience and documented the role of peak and end ratings (Fredrickson & Kahneman, 1993). The retrospective evaluations appeared to be determined by a weighted average of "snapshots" of the actual experience, as if duration did not matter. A later study of pain during colonoscopy revealed that retrospective ratings of pain were not related to the duration of the procedure (Redelmeier et al., 2003). In fact, the addition of time to the end of the procedure with low levels of pain lessened the intensity of pain recall ratings. Alternatively, postsurgical patients with breast cancer did show a *duration effect*, such that retrospective ratings of postoperative pain worsened as the duration of chronic pain continued through the year following surgery (Tasmuth, Estlanderb, & Kalso, 1996). The influence of mood may be particularly relevant during long periods of retrospective recall, since positive mood habituates (i.e., decreases) with continued exposure to a positive stimulus, whereas negative mood increases with continued exposure to a negative stimulus.

Summary

There are circumstances under which the recall of pain can be relatively accurate. Using a validated instrument to assess a specific episode of pain within a short period of recall (e.g., less than 30 days) maximizes accuracy. In addition, under certain circumstances, small changes in mood do not influence the accuracy of memory for either pain or pain behavior. On the other hand, some conditions are known to erode the accuracy of reports of recalled pain, including high levels of present pain intensity. Retrospective pain reports are subject to many of the same effects observed in all learning-based studies, including recency (i.e., end pain), salience (i.e., peak pain), and assimilation (i.e., past experience reconstructed to be consistent with present pain intensity); that is, pain remembered will be influenced by pain experienced near the end of an episode, peak pain during the episode, and the individual's present pain intensity.

Pain Relief Ratings

The rating of pain relief entails remembering an earlier pain state, evaluating the current pain state, comparing the current state to that remembered earlier state, and selecting a rating from the scale provided. Studies suggest that the process of rating relief involves different parameters or cognitive factors than does rating present pain intensity. The memory effects outlined earlier may explain the complicated relationship between changes in pain intensity and ratings of pain relief, which are imperfectly correlated

Baseline pain, present pain, remembered pain, and time since baseline are all factors that influence ratings of pain relief. Demonstration of the complexity of pain relief ratings has been shown in an extensive study

of patients with acute and chronic low back pain followed for up to 12 months (Haas et al., 2002). Over time, these investigators found that ratings of recalled pain relief were increasingly associated with pain at the time of the relief rating, and increasingly unrelated to the actual computed pain relief based on earlier ratings. This pattern was particularly pronounced in patients with acute low back pain, supporting the interpretation that patients' ratings of pain relief are complicated constructions that rely heavily on their present state, possibly more so than the change they have experienced with treatment or over time.

PATIENT SATISFACTION

Patient satisfaction with pain management is measured in an attempt to address the undertreatment of pain and to assist in the development and improvement of pain management services. To assist with quality assurance of pain services, the American Pain Society Quality of Care Committee disseminated a patient satisfaction measure in 1991, which was revised in 1995, resulting in a new tool, largely derived from existing scales. It includes an assessment of the impact of pain on function, satisfaction with pain management, perceived barriers to pain management, and clarity of guidelines for using medications for outpatients. This updated measure has shown acceptable levels of internal consistency with inpatients (McNeill, Sherwood, Starck, & Thompson, 1998) and with Hispanic patients (McNeill, Sherwood, & Starck, 2004), and the scale has been translated into Norwegian (Dihle, Helseth, & Christophersen, 2008). Factor analysis of similar satisfaction items revealed a single factor and convergent validity with other measures of patient satisfaction (Calvin, Becker, Biering, & Grobe, 1999).

Past efforts that focused on global measures of satisfaction demonstrated the potential complexity involved in interpreting patient satisfaction ratings. For example, high ratings of patient satisfaction (i.e., 75% satisfied or very satisfied) have been observed in the presence of moderate to high ratings of pain (Dawson et al., 2002). This finding, however, is not consistent across studies, since other studies show the expected relationship between high pain ratings and lower satisfaction ratings (e.g., Roth et al., 2005). Ratings of satisfaction can be biased in the positive direction, creating ceiling effects (Ward & Gordon, 1996), and global ratings appear to lack the specificity needed to evaluate fully the adequacy of pain management services. It has long been known that global patient satisfaction ratings are extremely difficult to change (Ward & Gordon, 1996). More recent studies mirror these findings, such that programmatic changes in a walk-in clinic did not increase ratings of pain relief, despite institutionwide documented improvements in recording patient histories, implementing pain treatment, using analgesics, and using a standardized assessment tool (Junod Perron, Piguet, & Bovier, 2007). Specifically, ratings of the adequacy of pain relief, efforts on the part of the staff, and adequacy of dosing were not improved as a result of this systemwide program (Junod Perron et al., 2007). Alternatively, systematic anesthesiology-managed postoperative pain management results in higher satisfaction ratings, concurrent with better pain control, compared to nonstandardized pain care (Roth et al., 2005).

Correlates of Patient Satisfaction

The imperfect relationship between pain ratings and satisfaction scores has led to the investigation of other factors that could influence ratings of satisfaction. Variables of interest have included characteristics of the patient, the provider, the pain, and the treatment. In the postoperative setting, female sex and younger age are patient characteristics associated with lower satisfaction scores (Svensson, Sjostrom, & Haljamae, 2001), which is not wholly surprising considering the established sex differences in pain sensitivity identified earlier. Other patient characteristics of relevance include pain-related cognitions (e.g., catastrophizing; Haythornthwaite, Lawrence, & Fauerbach, 2001) and beliefs about pain (Dawson et al., 2002). In particular, the presence of mood disorders in patients is associated with low satisfaction scores, but it may also reflect difficulties in establishing a therapeutic relationship (Bair et al., 2007). Patient and provider characteristics can be independent or interact to create a negative experience. For example, information sharing from the provider improves satisfaction ratings (Dawson et al., 2002). Although very little empirical research has investigated patient–provider interactions focused on pain management (Dawson et al., 2002), providers likely are more comfortable sharing information and setting appropriate expectations for pain when patients are receptive and engaged in the interaction. Pain variables include but are not limited to the following: maximum and average pain intensity ratings, recall of maximum pain, last recalled pain level, degree of pain interference, and efficacy of treatment for pain reduction. In the immediate postoperative period these variables demonstrate a significant relationship with global satisfaction scores (Jensen, Martin, & Cheung, 2005; Jensen, Mendoza, Hanna, Chen, & Cleeland, 2004) and fully mediate the effects of patient variables (e.g., demographics). Of note, ratings of *dis*satisfaction with pain relief management (from somewhat to very dissatisfied) during this acute period were associated with a VAS score > 40. Treatment-related variables, particularly side effects of treatment, can influence ratings of satisfaction (e.g., opioid-related side effects such as constipation and nausea (Jensen et al., 2004).

Pain and satisfaction assessments are quite complex and may interact with each other, as the studies discussed earlier suggest. The interaction among the patient, the provider, the pain, and the treatment should be considered when implementing pain management programs and measuring patient satisfaction. Altogether, these studies suggest that higher satisfaction scores are more likely when providers educate and interact with their patients, minimize peak pain experiences, provide adequate rescue or relief medications, and treat or minimize side effects.

SUMMARY

The measurement of satisfaction with pain management is a growing area and existing scales have evolved with experience; however, much work remains if this area is to make substantial contributions and guide innovation and quality improvement. Patient satisfaction is best regarded as a multidimensional construct of importance in its own right because ratings of pain intensity and relief are fairly unreliable as indicators of satisfaction. The determinants of satisfaction with pain management include an amalgam of patient characteristics, provider characteristics, interaction between patient and provider, and adequacy of pain treatment.

ADVERSE EFFECTS OF TREATMENT

Most acute pain treatments have adverse effects in a portion of patients treated, and adverse effects are recommended as an important domain for measurement in clinical trials (Turk et al., 2003). Thus, the assessment of adverse effects is recommended under most circumstances in which acute clinical pain is managed. There are few standardized measures of side effects, and clinical trials typically use a loosely structured interview to derive information about side effects and adverse events of study interventions. The experience of adverse effects is assessed and, if present, the patient typically is asked to rate the severity of each symptom (e.g., "mild," "moderate," "severe"; Raja et al., 2002). In many circumstances, the assessment of side effects might include specific symptoms known to occur frequently with a particular agent. For example, opioids, the most common analgesic agents used for acute pain care, frequently cause constipation or nausea. Thus, the assessment of these specific symptoms might occur systematically throughout treatment with opioids.

CONCLUSIONS AND RECOMMENDATIONS

The assessment of acute pain requires consideration of multiple factors, such as feasibility, convenience, and clinical utility. No single pain intensity scale is appropriate for all settings, and each scale has its strengths and weaknesses. When appropriate, VASs are recommended, since they show the strongest scaling properties and generally are more sensitive to treatment effects than the alternatives. However, in many clinical settings an 11- or 21-point NRS is adequate and easily implemented. The inclusion of pain relief scales, either categorical or VASs, may improve clinical decision making, since these scales often detect changes not detected by serial measures of pain intensity.

Many ratings of pain intensity and all ratings of pain relief require the patient to remember pain from a previous period of time. Retrospective ratings of pain intensity, even over as short a period as an hour, are strongly weighted by peak and end pain experience. Pain relief ratings may have greater immediate relevance in a busy clinical environment than do retrospective pain intensity ratings, since relief ratings provide a broader measure of outcome, especially when tied to the evaluation of a specific pain-reducing intervention. Furthermore, disparities between changes in pain intensity and ratings of pain relief are to be expected due to a complex interplay of factors such as response-shift bias, attentional limitations, and patient expectations.

The assessment of acute pain ideally includes consideration of patient satisfaction with pain management and the occurrence of side effects of treatment. These areas of assessment have received less attention but clearly play a role in evaluating pain care. Greater understanding of the factors that influence satisfaction ratings, particularly the influence of patient–provider interactions, may elucidate the seeming paradox of high satisfaction in the context of high pain. Scales to assess side effects systematically are needed if this domain is to be included in the evaluation of pain interventions (e.g., Turk et al., 2003).

The clinician conducting painful procedures is challenged by two conflicting goals—the accurate measurement of pain versus the optimal treatment of pain. The combined effects on memory from peak pain intensity, end-of-episode pain intensity, and duration neglect have clinical relevance. Clinicians wanting to optimally lower patients' subsequent memories for pain should focus on reducing the peak intensity experienced during the episode (Redelmeier & Kahneman, 1996). By making the peak anesthetic effect coincide with the end of the procedure, memory for pain is also minimized. However, these suggestions may counter the clinician's natural tendency to try to minimize the duration of exposure to pain, sometimes at the "price" of heightening peak pain. Similarly, interventions based on diverting attention away from pain (i.e., distraction) are less likely to be effective if the patient is required to attend to the pain to rate its intensity for the purposes of assessment. Therefore, clinicians need to consider the potentially deleterious impact of pain assessment itself when certain types of pain management interventions are used.

ACKNOWLEDGMENTS

The writing of this chapter was supported in part by grants from the National Institutes on Health (No. R24 AT004641) and the U.S. Department of Education (No. H133A070045).

REFERENCES

Agency for Health Care Policy and Research. (1992). *Acute pain management: Operative or medical procedures and trauma* (U.S. Department of Health and Human Services, AHCPR Pub. No. 92-0032). Rockville, MD: Author.

Ahlers, S. J. G. M., van Gulik, L., van der Veen, A. M., van Dongen, H. P. A., Bruins, P., Belitser, S. V., et al. (2008). Comparison of different pain scoring systems in critically ill patients in a general ICU. *Critical Care*, 12(1), 1–8.

American Pain Society Quality of Care Committee. (1995). Quality improvement guidelines for the treatment of acute pain and cancer pain. *Journal of the American Medical Association*, 274, 1874–1880.

Bair, M. J., Kroenke, K., Sutherland, J. M., McCoy, K. D., Harris, H., & McHorney, C. A. (2007). Effects of depression and pain severity on satisfaction in medical outpatients: Analysis of the medical outcomes study. *Journal of Rehabilitation Research and Development*, 44(2), 143–151.

Bijur, P. E., Latimer, C. T., & Gallagher, E. J. (2003). Validation of a verbally administered numerical rating scale of acute pain for use in the emergency department. *Academic Emergency Medicine*, 10(4), 390–392.

Breivik, E. K., Bjornsson, G. A., & Skovlund, E. (2000). A comparison of pain rating scales by sampling from clinical trial data. *Clinical Journal of Pain*, 16(1), 22–28.

Broderick, J. E., Schwartz, J. E., Vikingstad, G., Pribbernow, M., Grossman, S., & Stone, A. A. (2008). The accuracy of pain and fatigue items across different reporting periods. *Pain*, 139(1), 146–157.

Calvin, A., Becker, H., Biering, P., & Grobe, S. (1999). Measuring patient opinion of pain management. *Journal of Pain and Symptom Management*, 18, 17–26.

Cleeland, C. S., & Ryan, K. M. (1994). Pain assessment: Global use of the Brief Pain Inventory. *Annals of Academic Medicine*, 23, 129–138.

Dawson, R., Spross, J. A., Jablonski, E. S., Hoyer, D. R., Sellers, D. E., & Solomon, M. Z. (2002). Probing the paradox of patients' satisfaction with inadequate pain management. *Journal of Pain and Symptom Management*, 23(3), 211–220.

Dihle, A., Helseth, S., & Christophersen, K. A. (2008). The Norwegian version of the American Pain Society Patient Outcome Questionnaire: Reliability and validity of three subscales. *Journal of Clinical Nursing*, 17(15), 2070–2078.

Downie, W. W., Leatham, P. A., Rhind, V. M., Wright, V., Branco, J. A., & Anderson, J. A. (1978). Studies with pain rating scales. *Annals of the Rheumatic Diseases*, 37(4), 378–381.

Eich, E., Reeves, J. L., Jaeger, B., & Graff-Radford, S. B. (1985). Memory for pain: Relation between past and present pain intensity. *Pain*, 23(4), 375–380.

Farrar, J. T., Berlin, J. A., & Strom, B. L. (2003). Clinically important changes in acute pain outcome measures: A validation study. *Journal of Pain and Symptom Management*, 25(5), 406–411.

Farrar, J. T., Portenoy, R. K., Berlin, J. A., Kinman, J. L., & Strom, B. L. (2000). Defining the clinically important difference in pain outcome measures. *Pain*, 88(3), 287–294.

Fredrickson, B. L., & Kahneman, D. (1993). Duration neglect in retrospective evaluations of affective episodes. *Journal of Personality and Social Psychology*, 65(1), 45–55.

Gedney, J. J., & Logan, H. (2004). Memory for stress-associated acute pain. *Journal of Pain*, 5(2), 83–91.

Gordon, D. B., Dahl, J. L., Miaskowski, C., McCarberg, B., Todd, K. H., Paice, J. A., et al. (2005). American Pain Society recommendations for improving the quality of acute and cancer pain management: American Pain Society Quality of Care Task Force. *Archives of Internal Medicine*, 165(14), 1574–1580.

Haas, M., Nyiendo, J., & Aickin, M. (2002). One-year trend in pain and disability relief recall in acute and chronic ambulatory low back pain patients. *Pain*, 95(1–2), 83–91.

Hartrick, C. T., Kovan, J. P., & Shapiro, S. (2003). The numeric rating scale for clinical pain measurement: A ratio measure? *Pain Practice*, 3(4), 310–316.

Haythornthwaite, J. A., Lawrence, J. W., & Fauerbach, J. A. (2001). Brief cognitive interventions for burn pain. *Annals of Behavioral Medicine, 23*(1), 42–49.

Herr, K. A., Spratt, K., Mobily, P. R., & Richardson, G. (2004). Pain intensity assessment in older adults: Use of experimental pain to compare psychometric properties and usability of selected pain scales with younger adults. *Clinical Journal of Pain, 20*(4), 207–219.

Jamison, R. N., Raymond, S. A., Slawsby, E. A., McHugo, G. J., & Baird, J. C. (2006). Pain assessment in patients with low back pain: Comparison of weekly recall and momentary electronic data. *Journal of Pain, 7*(3), 192–199.

Jantsch, H. H. F., Gawlitza, M., Geber, C., Baumgärtner, U., Krämer, H. H., Magerl, W., et al. (2009). Explicit episodic memory for sensory-discriminative components of capsaicin-induced pain: Immediate and delayed ratings. *Pain, 143*(1–2), 97–105.

Jensen, M. P., Mardekian, J., Lakshminarayanan, M., & Boye, M. E. (2008). Validity of 24-h recall ratings of pain severity: Biasing effects of "peak" and "end" pain. *Pain, 137*(2), 422–427.

Jensen, M. P., Martin, S. A., & Cheung, R. (2005). The meaning of pain relief in a clinical trial. *Journal of Pain, 6*(6), 400–406.

Jensen, M. P., Mendoza, T., Hanna, D. B., Chen, C., & Cleeland, C. S. (2004). The analgesic effects that underlie patient satisfaction with treatment. *Pain, 110*(1–2), 480–487.

Junod Perron, N., Piguet, V., & Bovier, P. A. (2007). Long-term effectiveness of a multifaceted intervention on pain management in a walk-in clinic. *Quarterly Journal of Medicine, 100*(4), 225–232.

Lasanga, L. (1962). The psychophysics of clinical pain. *Lancet, 2,* 572–575.

Linton, S. J., & Gotestam, K. G. (1983). A clinical comparison of two pain scales: Correlation, remembering chronic pain, and a measure of compliance. *Pain, 17,* 57–65.

Linton, S. J., & Nordin, E. (2006). A 5-year follow-up evaluation of the health and economic consequences of an early cognitive behavioral intervention for back pain: A randomized, controlled trial. *Spine, 31*(8), 853–858.

Lund, I., Lundeberg, T., Sandberg, L., Budh, C., Kowalski, J., & Svensson, E. (2005). Lack of interchangeability between visual analogue and verbal rating pain scales: A cross sectional description of pain etiology groups. *BMC Medical Research Methodology, 5*(1), 31.

Marsh-Richard, D. M., Hatzis, E. S., Mathias, C. W., Venditti, N., & Dougherty, D. M. (2009). Adaptive visual analog scales (AVAS): A modifiable software program for the creation, administration, and scoring of visual analog scales. *Behavior Research Methods, 41*(1), 99.

Mason, S. T., Arceneaux, L. L., Abouhassan, W.,

Lauterbach, D., Seebach, C., & Fauerbach, J. A. (2008). Confirmatory factor analysis of the Short Form McGill Pain Questionnaire with burn patients. *Eplasty, 8,* e54.

McNeill, J. A., Sherwood, G. D., & Starck, P. L. (2004). The hidden error of mismanaged pain: A systems approach. *Journal of Pain and Symptom Management, 28*(1), 47–58.

McNeill, J. A., Sherwood, G. D., Starck, P. L., & Thompson, C. J. (1998). Assessing clinical outcomes: Patient satisfaction with pain management. *Journal of Pain and Symptom Management, 16*(1), 29–40.

Melzack, R. (1987). The Short-Form McGill Pain Questionnaire. *Pain, 30,* 191–197.

Melzack, R., & Wall, P. D. (1965). Pain mechanisms: A new theory. *Science, 150,* 971–979.

Miaskowski, C., & Donovan, M. (1992). Implementation of the American Pain Society quality assurance standards for relief of acute pain and cancer pain in oncology nursing practice. *Oncology Nursing Forum, 19*(3), 411–415.

Niere, K., & Jerak, A. (2004). Measurement of headache frequency, intensity and duration: Comparison of patient report by questionnaire and headache diary. *Physiotherapy Research International, 9*(4), 149–156.

Oken, B. S. (2008). Placebo effects: Clinical aspects and neurobiology. *Brain, 131*(11), 2812–2823.

Paller, C. J., Campbell, C. M., Edwards, R. R., & Dobs, A. S. (2009). Sex-based differences in pain perception and treatment. *Pain Medicine, 10*(2), 289–299.

Raja, S. N., Haythornthwaite, J. A., Pappagallo, M., Clark, M. R., Travison, T. G., Sabeen, S., et al. (2002). Opioids versus antidepressants in postherpetic neuralgia: A randomized, placebo-controlled trial. *Neurology, 59*(7), 1015–1021.

Redelmeier, D. A., & Kahneman, D. (1996). Patients' memories of painful medical treatments: Real-time and retrospective evaluations of two minimally invasive procedures. *Pain, 66,* 3–8.

Redelmeier, D. A., Katz, J., & Kahneman, D. (2003). Memories of colonoscopy: A randomized trial. *Pain, 104*(1–2), 187–194.

Rosseland, L. A., & Stubhaug, A. (2004). Gender is a confounding factor in pain trials: Women report more pain than men after arthroscopic surgery. *Pain, 112*(3), 248–253.

Roth, W., Kling, J., Gockel, I., Rümelin, A., Hessmann, M. H., Meurer, A., et al. (2005). Dissatisfaction with post-operative pain management—a prospective analysis of 1,071 patients. *Acute Pain, 7*(2), 75–83.

Scott, D., & McDonald, W. (2008). Assessment, measurement, and history. In P. E. Macintyre, S. Walker, & D. J. Rowbotham (Eds.), *Clini-*

cal pain management (2nd ed., pp. 131–135). London: Hodder & Stoughton.

Singer, A. J., Kowalska, A., & Thode H. C. (2001). Ability of patients to accurately recall the severity of acute painful events. *Academic Emergency Medicine, 8*(3), 292–295.

Stone, A. A., Schwartz, J. E., Broderick, J. E., & Shiffman, S. S. (2005). Variability of momentary pain predicts recall of weekly pain: A consequence of the peak (or salience) memory heuristic. *Personality and Social Psychology Bulletin, 31*(10), 1340–1346.

Svensson, I., Sjostrom, B., & Haljamae, H. (2001). Influence of expectations and actual pain experiences on satisfaction with postoperative pain management. *European Journal of Pain, 5*(2), 125–133.

Tait, R. C., Chibnall, J. T., & Kalauokalani, D. (2009). Provider judgments of patients in pain: Seeking symptom certainty. *Pain Medicine, 10*(1), 11–34.

Tasmuth, T., Estlanderb, A. M., & Kalso, E. (1996). Effect of present pain and mood on the memory of past postoperative pain in women treated surgically for breast cancer. *Pain, 68*(2–3), 343–347.

Turk, D. C., Dworkin, R. H., Allen, R. R., Bellamy, N., Brandenburg, N., Carr, D. B., et al. (2003). Core outcome domains for chronic pain clinical trials: IMMPACT recommendations. *Pain, 106*(3), 337–345.

Waldenstrom, U., & Schytt, E. (2009). A longitudinal study of women's memory of labour pain—from 2 months to 5 years after the birth. *BJOG: An International Journal of Obstetrics and Gynaecology, 116*(4), 577–583.

Ward, S. E., & Gordon, D. B. (1996). Patient satisfaction and pain severity as outcomes in pain management: A longitudinal view of one setting's experience. *Journal of Pain and Symptom Management, 11*(4), 242–251.

Wells, N. (2000). Pain intensity and pain interference in hospitalized patients with cancer. *Oncology Nursing Forum, 27*(6), 985–991.

CHAPTER 15

Clinical Assessment of Low Back Pain

PAUL J. WATSON

Despite decades of research and clinical experience, low back pain (LBP) continues to be one of the commonest reasons for seeking health care from a family physician. Most episodes of back pain do not result in significant disability. The assertions that LBP is self-limiting and of relatively short duration, in that most will recover in 4–6 weeks, is not borne out by the research. People often have repeated episodes of LBP, and those that consult are highly likely still to be reporting symptoms, even if they are only transient, a year later. Many people with LBP therefore do not consult and do not become significantly limited by the condition even if it persists.

The most significant failure of years of research is the inability of physiological and anatomical perspectives to explain the causes of back pain or the likely prognosis. The possible serious causes of LBP, or "red flags," have been identified, and once these are ruled out, physical findings help little in predicting outcome. Consequently, the clinical examination of LBP requires not only an assessment for serious pathology but also the need to identify and manage the predictors of poor outcome that are often related to the psychological and social domains.

EPIDEMIOLOGY OF LBP

According to convention, LBP is divided by its duration. Pain is classified as acute up to 6 weeks' duration, subacute from 6 to 12 weeks' duration, and thenceforth is deemed chronic. However, the nature of LBP is not a steady trajectory; the more typical pattern is periods of pain followed by remission with subsequent episodes. Even those patients who report pain for many years admit, when questioned, that the pain has not been continuous throughout that time (Croft, Macfarlane, Papageorgiou, Thomas, & Silman, 1998). Pain and disability usually improve most in the first 3 months, but improvement then slows, and many people remain in stasis.

Estimates of the prevalence of LBP vary according to the classification used. Estimates for the point prevalence indicate that about one-third of the population will report back pain; this rises to over two-thirds for the 1-year prevalence to between 80 and 90% for the lifetime prevalence (Walker, 2000). Previous reports suggest that the incidence of back pain increases in middle years and decreases slightly thereafter, but recently this association with age has been questioned (Airaksinen et al., 2006).

Only a relatively small number of people actually consult a physician with their back pain. In the United Kingdom, about 20% of people who report back pain actually consult their family physician (Macfarlane, Jones, & Hannaford, 2006). This still results in about 1 in 15 persons in the population consulting with back pain in any year.

LBP is a frequent reason for work loss. Work loss due to injury and illness is influenced by national social and economic influences, but LBP is the third commonest reason for certified work loss after common respiratory diseases and common mental illness in the United Kingdom (Watson, Bowey, Purcell-Jones, & Gales, 2008). In the United States (Wasiak, Kim, & Pransky, 2006) and Australia (Buchbinder & Jolley, 2005) it is one of the commonest, if not *the* commonest, reasons for work loss. Most people who report pain in any year still report symptoms a year later (Airaksinen et al., 2006; Croft et al., 1998). Many of those who are absent from work with back pain will be absent from work again with back pain in the following year (Wasiak, Pransky, Verma, & Webster, 2003). This second episode will not only last longer but will also accrue more health- and non-health-associated costs (Watson, Main, Waddell, Gales, & Purcell-Jones, 1998; Wasiak et al., 2006).

The greatest costs of LBP are societal, including wage replacement and other social benefit costs, and lost production. Data from the United Kingdom in 1998 demonstrated that the total cost of LBP was £1,632 million ($2,690 million US) of which societal costs were estimated at £10,668 million ($17,584 million US) (Maniadakis & Gray, 2000). To put these costs in context, a similar analysis of the costs of coronary heart disease based on data gathered in 1999 can be used as comparison. The health care cost of heart disease was £1.73 billion ($2.85 billion US), greater than the £1.63 billion spent on back pain in the previous year (Liu, Maniadakis, Gray, & Rayner, 2002). However, the total cost of heart disease was £7.06 billion ($12.53 billion US) compared with approximately the LBP cost given earlier (Liu et al., 2002). This magnitude of cost is typical for other countries and demonstrates that health care costs only represent 80–90% of the total costs of back pain (Waddell, 2004).

THE CONTEXT OF THE ASSESSMENT

Each patient attends an assessment with a certain expectation of what will occur. This is shaped by his or her understanding of back pain, previous experience of assessment and treatment for back pain, and perception of his or her role and the clinician's role in the management of the condition. It should also be understood that the patient's response to assessment, the information he or she gives, and how he or she behaves will be colored by perception of the likely outcome of the assessment. The way people present may differ depending on whom they see and why they think they are undergoing assessment. Their behavior in the assessment by a physical therapist for treatment is likely to be very different than their behavior during assessment by a physician for disability payments.

CLASSIFICATION

Most guidelines on the management of LBP suggest that patients be examined and classified according to three groups (Airaksinen et al., 2006; Staal et al., 2003):

- Those with nonspecific mechanical LBP
- Those with nerve root pain
- Those with signs suggestive of serious pathology

In the context of LBP, *mechanical* LBP refers to pain associated with movement and posture. *Serious pathology* refers to the likelihood of neoplasm, infection, trauma, or inflammation. It is essential to note here that this classification refers to those patients whose LBP may or may not radiate into one or both legs, and it does not include those who have obvious significant spinal deformity (e.g., kyphoscoliosis) or possible neurological conditions.

IDENTIFICATION OF "RED FLAGS"

The term "red flags" was first coined with respect to LBP in the Clinical Standards Advisory Group (CSAG; 1994) report for the management of LBP. This report emphasized the importance of a diagnostic triage for back pain on assessment. The aim of the assessment was to classify the pain as simple LBP needing no further medical investigations, possible nerve root pain for which a surgical opinion might be considered, and possible serious spinal pathology in which further specialist investigation is essential. It is the latter group which are defined by the presence of red flags.

Both the CSAG in the United Kingdom and the Agency for Healthcare Policy and Research (AHCPR; Bigos et al., 1994) in the United States produced lists of signs and symptoms suggestive of serious spinal pathology (given in Table 15.1). The majority of these concern the clinical history and presentation of the patient, with additional clinical examination findings.

Waddell has suggested that less than 1% of LBP involves a serious spinal disorder (Waddell, 2004). This depends on where and when patients are seen. In a case series of 900 patients with mainly chronic LBP in

a secondary care orthopedic clinic, Waddell (1982) identified 35 patients with tumor, 15 with infection, 25 with osteoporosis, and 23 with other pathologies (total 10.8%). In the primary care setting, the incidence of serious pathologies that cause back pain has been estimated as follows: cancer, 0.7%; osteoporotic fracture, 4%; ankylosing spondylitis, 0.3%; and spinal infections, 0.01% (Jarvik & Deyo, 2002). However, Jarvik and Deyo emphasize the importance of the clinical history in identifying serious pathology in particular cancers. Serious conditions are rare in primary care consulting settings in patients with LBP without a significant clinical history. Kendrick and colleagues (2001a) and Kerry, Hilton, Dundas, Rink, and Oakeshott (2002), for example, reported no examples of serious pathology in two large groups (total 1,080) of U.K. patients in primary care screened for clinical history, although the incidence is likely to be greater in those referred for treatment (McGuirk, King, Govind, Lowry, & Bogduk, 2001).

Red flags are still subject to clinical interpretation and depend on the importance of the clinical history and the number of findings. A previously fit and well male laborer, age 19 (red flag < 20), who sustains an onset of LBP following heavy lifting is unlikely to require an immediate specialist referral based on just one red flag. A 49-year-old woman with a previous history of breast cancer (red flag) and gradual-onset thoracic pain (red flag) should be investigated thoroughly.

It is unethical to perform clear-cut randomized controlled trials based on the efficacy of red flags or their worth in identifying serious pathology. Many of the suggested assessments for red flags give rise to a high number of false positives, but a combination of the red flags leads to a lower, false-negative rate (Deyo, 1986; Deyo & Diehl, 1988; Grubb, Bradford, Pritchard, & Ebersold, 1994). Hence, red flags are never intended to be diagnostic; they only indicate the need for further investigations, many of which may prove to have negative results.

There is still a considerable body of evidence indicating that clinicians' knowledge of the red flags is poor even so long after guidelines were developed. This is particularly so in primary care and, more specifically, in family physicians. Di Iorio, Henley,

TABLE 15.1. Red Flags Identified by the CSAG (1994)

- Age of onset < 20 or > 55 years
- Violent trauma (e.g., fall from a height, road traffic accident)
- Constant progressive, nonmechanical pain
- Thoracic pain
- Previous history of
  - Carcinoma
  - Systemic steroid use
  - Drug abuse
  - HIV
- Systemically unwell (e.g., unexplained weight loss)
- Persistent severe restriction of lumbar flexion
- Widespread neurological abnormality
- Structural deformity

Additional AHCPR indicators:

- Pain that worsens when supine
- Severe nighttime pain

In addition to the above, an intermediate group was also identified—signs and symptoms that are associated with cauda equina syndrome or serious ongoing neurological damage and require emergency referral to a spinal surgeon:

- Difficulty with micturition
- Loss of anal sphincter tone/fecal incontinence
- Saddle anesthesia over the perineum, genitals, and anus
- Widespread nerve root pain or progressive motor weakness
- Gait disturbance

and Doughty (2000) reported that 50% of primary care physicians failed to identify five out of seven red flags, a figure in agreement with Overmeer, Linton, Holmquist, Eriksson, and Engfeldt (2005) who found physiotherapists to be more aware. Confusion about red flags also leads to unnecessary referrals of nonurgent cases to secondary care and further investigations, particularly imaging studies (Negrini, Politano, Carabalona, & Mambrini, 2001). However, the correct application of red flags and guidelines for their use, if taught to and adhered to by triaging health care professionals, can lead to a reduction in the number of inappropriate referrals for surgical opinion and radiography. Evidence-based guidelines suggest that primary care practitioners reassure and encourage patients to resume activities if evaluation reveals no evidence of red flags. Research suggests that the majority of primary care practitioners do not adhere to these evidence-based practice guidelines (Feuerstein, Hartzell, Rogers, & Marcus, 2006). The reason why physicians do not adhere to guidelines is often due to lack of confidence in their own skills and fear of missing significant pathology (McGuirk et al., 2001; Schers, Wensing, Huijsmans, van Tulder, & Grol, 2001; Weatherley & Hourigan, 1998).

The results from a careful assessment, where no red flag is identified, can (and should) be used to reassure the patient that there is no evidence of serious pathology and further investigations are not warranted. This information is often of primary concern to patients (Petrie et al., 2005) and, if presented appropriately, can reduce distress and worry, and enhance treatment compliance (Gask & Usherwood, 2003; Main, Sullivan, & Watson, 2008).

NERVE ROOT PAIN

Leg pain is a regular feature associated with LBP. However, not all leg pain is indicative of nerve root pain. Pain in the muscles of the lower back can be associated with pain radiating into the legs. There is often confusion in the understanding of clinicians and patients that all leg pain is "sciatica" and caused by nerve root compression; this is not the case. Neither can the intensity of the pain be used as an indication of the presence of nerve root compression. Once again, the patient may well attribute severe pain to nerve root pain.

The prevalence of sciatica in LBP has been estimated at around 1.5% (Deyo & Tsui-Wu, 1987). In the acute situation, the pain usually differs from that of pain arising from other structures, in that it is sharp and shooting in nature and often corresponds to a dermatomal distribution. However, many people with chronic LBP may have poorly defined pain, in addition to sciatic-type pain.

Observation of the patient standing and dressed in only underwear often demonstrates a lateral lumbar shift or list away from the side of the pain; any attempt to correct the list will increase the pain (Geraci, Alleva, & McAdam, 2002). This alone is only suggestive of the possibility of nerve root involvement and can occur in its absence.

Patients with pain may report tingling, loss of sensation, or numbness in a roughly dermatomal distribution. Compression of the nerve root that interferes with the nerve conductivity will be present, depending on the severity and duration, sensory dysfunction, motor weakness, muscle wasting, and obtunded tendon reflexes. These tests will approximate the neurological innervation at each spinal nerve root. Assessment of muscle strength in each of the representative nerve roots (ankle dorsiflexion and plantar flexion, knee flexion and extension, hip flexion and extension) should be performed. An assessment for sensory impairment using light touch and pinprick over the dermatomal areas is also performed. The results of this examination are compared with that of the unaffected leg.

Neural tension tests are performed to substantiate the clinical picture. These include the straight leg raise (SLR), in which the patient's leg is elevated by the clinician until the radicular symptoms are reproduced. This can be refined by including dorsiflexion at the ankle or by the bow string test, in which the hip and knee are initially flexed and the knee is gradually extended by the clinician, with the foot in the dorsiflexed position, until a positive response is reported or the movement is limited by soft tissue extensibility. In the crossed straight leg test the clinician elevates the asymptomatic leg and pain is reported in the symptomatic leg. This has been reported to be a more sensitive but much less specific test than SLR, particularly in the presence of a prolapsed large disc. In the slumped sitting test, the patient sits on the edge of the couch with the neck flexed, and the thoracic and lumbar spines flexed, and the hands clasped behind the back. The symptomatic leg is straightened and the foot dorsiflexed; in a positive test the patient will report pain. The slump test has an advantage in that it may be able to discriminate more clearly between radicular and muscular pain. Any one of the preceding tests may be used.

Assessment of the upper lumbar nerve roots is performed by the femoral nerve stretch, in which the patient is in the supine position, or it can be adapted to the side lying position for those who find the former position difficult. The hip is drawn into slight extension and the knee is brought into flexion, until a positive result is elicited or the movement is limited by soft tissue extensibility. In all cases a comparison with the asymptomatic leg is made.

Integrating the findings gives the picture of nerve root involvement, including the pattern of the root pain, signs of nerve root irritation, signs of root compression, and confirmation of these with MRI findings. Radiology alone is insufficient to confirm nerve root involvement, because disc herniations are common and may be unconnected to the patient's symptoms.

DIFFERENTIAL DIAGNOSIS

Major structural deformities (kyphosis, scoliosis) should be apparent in an appropriately conducted assessment. Patients, following initial assessment, are often classified as having "nonspecific LBP." There are many professional attributions for the cause of LBP and some would challenge the idea that LBP is ever "nonspecific," citing pain arising from the disc, muscle activity, and facet joint involvement. A recent review suggested that pain arising from the facet joint cannot be reliably assessed by physical examination, patient report, localization, or pain on movement (Rubinstein & Van Tulder, 2008) but may with good reliability be identified by lumbar facet joint anesthetic block. However, there is only moderate to weak

evidence that interventions targeting these joints or the nerves supplying them lead to improvement; randomized controlled trials (RCTs) have proved equivocal.

A similar disappointing picture is presented with the identification of the lumbar disc as a possible cause of LBP; the only assessment finding associated with disc disease and pain was the phenomenon of centralization using the McKenzie diagnostic approach. No other assessment, including magnetic resonance imaging (MRI) or discography, could reliably identify the disc as cause of pain (Rubinstein & Van Tulder, 2008) and interventions to treat disc pain have proved disappointing.

Although movements and muscle activity of people with LBP often differ from those of pain-free controls (Ferreira, Ferreira, & Hodges, 2004), the relationship between these "abnormalities" and back pain have lacked specificity, and treatments to correct such movement impairments seem to be no more effective than general exercise approaches, making it difficult to attribute cause and effect (Ferreira et al., 2007; Koumantakis et al., 2005).

ASSESSING PHYSICAL IMPAIRMENT

The American Medical Association's (AMA) *Guides to the Evaluation of Permanent Impairment* defines impairment as "a loss, loss of use, or derangement of any body part, organ system, or organ function" (Cocchiarella & Andersson, 2001). The aim of an assessment of impairment is to gain objective information on the functioning of parts of the body that can be interpreted relatively independently of the behavior of the individual. Such impairments should also distinguish patients with back pain from asymptomatic individuals. In this respect, impairments are the medical component of disability. Pain itself cannot be incorporated into an assessment of impairment, because it is subjective and relies on patient report rather than independent validation. However, it is included in the AMA's *Guides* within specific chapters, and with an entire chapter on pain. Furthermore, pain can only be related to the whole person, not to the affected part, because assessment and examination often do not identify abnormalities that can account for the pain (Main, Robinson, & Watson, 2005).

It is very difficult to equate impairment with physical capacity, because it is inevitably influenced by multiple factors, including patients' interpretation of the test, their perception of the likely consequences of testing, and fear of movement, as well as the actual impairment itself. In this regard, such tests are an assessment of physical performance, not of actual physical capacity, and they should be seen as such. The fact that they are often reported to have good reliability and reproducibility demonstrates that they are stable psychophysiological phenomena.

It is important that the test environment be adequately controlled. Factors influencing test performance include standardization of the starting position; the instructions given; the level of feedback and encouragement; the presence of others; and the duration and timing of testing. All patients undergoing tests, such as range of motion, should be given the opportunity to "warm up" before testing.

Physical performance testing not only serves as an evaluation of the patients current performance, but it can also be recorded regularly to monitor progress and offer a form of feedback and encouragement. The reliability, reproducibility, and validity of most assessments of range of spinal motion are good provided that attention is paid to the details of the measurement. In the previous edition of this book, Waddell and Turk (2001) provided a good description of the procedure.

Lumbar motion is best measured in the clinic using an inclinometer. The anatomical landmarks are used to identify the lumbar spine levels at S2 and T12–L1, and at thoracic levels T12 and T9; horizontal marks are made on the skin. The starting position for all assessments is for the patient to stand with the heels as close together as possible, and to adopt as straight a posture as possible. The baseline measurements are made in this position at S2 and T12–L1. For flexion, patients are instructed to lean forward toward their toes as far as they are able to go, keeping the knees straight. At full flexion, the readings are repeated. True lumbar flexion can now be calculated from the total lumbopelvic movement.

For extension, patients are asked to lean as far backward as they can. Support from behind by the assessor will give the patient more confidence to perform the movement. Once again, the measurements are taken at the two marked positions and the true extension is calculated.

Lateral flexion is performed by leaning to the side, running the hand down the lateral aspect of the thigh. Care must be taken that the patient does not flex forward during this movement, as is often the case. Measurements are taken at T12 and T9.

FUNCTIONAL CAPACITY EVALUATIONS

Functional capacity evaluations (FCEs) are commonly conducted in people with LBP, often at the behest of insurance companies or third-party payers. They may range from simple timed tasks to the use of complex machines to test maximum force, range of motion, or endurance in various planes of motion. This is mainly to assess function in terms of the demands of their employment rather than to indicate clinical severity per se. However, FCEs are in common usage in many countries to identify treatment protocols and to monitor the progress of injured workers. The number of tests is too broad to address here. They are often aggressively marketed. Some have acceptable test–retest and interrater reliability, provided that those who administer them have been trained appropriately (Gross & Battié, 2002).

The relationship between FCE testing and the predictive ability to determine successful outcome with respect to return to work is poor, and performance on such testing explains only a small amount of variance in predicting ability to work (Gross & Battié, 2004, 2005).

IMAGING

Referral for urgent imaging (and appropriate medical or surgical referral) is required if there is a suspicion of significant pathology (see Table 15.1) or when cauda equina syndrome is identified.

No strong evidence supports the use of routine imaging in the assessment of LBP in the absence of clinical indications of nerve root pain or a suspicion of serious pathology. Imaging often reveals changes in structures that are mainly coincidental to the back pain (Jarvik, 2003) and better interpreted as normal, age-related changes.

If an assessment for red flags is performed adequately, the likelihood of a serious condition being overlooked is very rare. The prevalence of cancer in people with LBP has been estimated at < 1 in 1,000 (Hollingworth et al., 2003), and the cost of routine imaging would be prohibitive to detect a condition with such low prevalence. There is evidence that routine imaging does not change the clinical diagnosis or treatment decision and has only a marginal effect on patient outcome (Gillan et al., 2001).

Patients might feel slightly more reassured but there is conflicting evidence of whether there is any positive effect on disability, pain, or function (Gilbert et al., 2004; Kendrick et al., 2001b). Imaging in this situation is usually done for the benefit of the referring clinician. When it does change the treatment, this is usually in favor of increased surgical interventions (Jarvik, 2003).

Discography is purported to investigate the contribution of disc abnormalities seen on imaging to the patient's LBP. Currently there is little agreement on what constitutes a positive discogram or the treatment that should follow, so there appears to be little to recommend this procedure in clinical assessment (Carragee, Lincoln, Parmar, & Alamin, 2006; Scuderi et al., 2008).

ASSESSING PAIN AND DISABILITY

It has been well documented that not only is relationship between pain and disability weak but its importance may also vary according to the duration and where in the health care system the patient is seen. At best pain only explains about 25% of the variance associated with disability (Woby, Roach, Urmston, & Watson, 2007), and some studies have demonstrated that pain contributes as little as 8% of the variance for disability scores (Turner, Jensen, & Romano, 2000).

The traditional way of recording LBP by duration classifies it into acute, recurrent and chronic LBP. True acute LBP of recent onset, and without a previous history of back pain, is relatively uncommon in clinical practice. Few people with back pain consult a physician for their first episode. In the typical LBP picture, the patient has recovered from previous episodes of back pain without health care interventions. Many people are able to manage their symptoms themselves with over-the-counter medications and behavioral adaptations in work and activities of daily living. Only when patients perceive the symptoms to be more significant or when self-management strategies cease to be effective will they consult a physician. So many cases of back pain may be interpreted as recurrent problems. In these cases, and in those with early onset of back pain, the relationship between back pain and disability may be quite substantial.

Those who become chronically disabled by LBP demonstrate a different picture. The relationship between the report of pain and the level of disability is much less robust, as exemplified in the earlier study by Turner and colleagues (2000). Many of these patients will not have responded to previous treatments, and their lifestyles and social interactions demonstrate an adaptation to chronic incapacity.

Classically, pain is assessed for different domains, locations, overall intensity, and sensory and affective components. The assessment of pain is explored in detail in other chapters in this volume.

An assessment of the anatomical distribution assists in the identification of a clinical diagnosis. This is particularly useful when not only nerve root pain but also pain arising from other structures cannot be identified from the distribution of the pain alone (Rubinstein & Van Tulder, 2008). Nerve root pain from the sciatic nerve often is reported below the knee, but pain arising from other structures generally is not. The location of the pain is part of the clinical questioning and can be usefully recorded on a pain drawing by the patient. The patient draws on a mannequin, indicating the location and to some extent the nature of the pain. This may be scored according to the area completed (Margolis, Tait, & Krause, 1986). Pain drawings often can be rather florid and may not be associated with neuroanatomical patterns. Patients who are highly distressed often give widespread and detailed representations of their pain in pain drawings, and this has been suggested to be indicative of psychological distress (Ransford, Cairns, & Mooney, 1976). The pain drawing should not be used as a screening tool, because up to 50% of distressed pain patients present a "normal" pain drawing (Parker, Wood, & Main, 1995).

The simplest and perhaps most commonly used scales of intensity are the visual analogue scale (VAS) and the verbal report scale (VRS), which are understood by most patients with simple explanation and can be used readily in the clinic setting (see Jensen and Karoly, Chapter 2, this volume, for a detailed discussion). A measure of the sensory quality of the pain is assessed by presenting the patient with list of descriptors from which the patient chooses. The Short-Form McGill Pain Questionnaire, for example, has 11 sensory descriptive words from which the patient chooses, assigning an intensity rating to each (see Katz & Melzack, Chapter 3, this volume).

Chronic pain fluctuates greatly and clinicians are familiar with the situation of being told by their patients that this "is a good day," and that the pain was much worse yesterday, last week, and so forth. Composite measures, such as the Brief Pain Inventory (Cleeland & Ryan, 1994), ask patients about their pain now, in the last 24 hours, on an average day, and at its worst in an attempt to capture this information.

DISABILITY

The *International Classification of Function* distinguishes between impairments assessed on clinical assessment and through performance testing; activity limitation that represents what people perceive they can or cannot do, or what they are prepared to do or not do as a result of their back pain; and participation that relates to engagement in activities and behaviors considered normal for a person of the same age, sex, and culture. Disability relates more to personal factors, whereas participation may be affected by society, employers, and the physical environment. If people are unable to work because of their back pain, then it may be because of any or all three of the following: the impairment, patients' own perceptions of their ability, and attitudes held by their employers. For example, an employer may stipulate that a person must be fully fit and pain-free before returning to work.

Just as pain does not relate strongly to disability, disability is not strongly related to impairment, and the relationship among the three becomes less clear in people with chronic pain. In assessing disability, it is important to emphasize that one is not assessing whether an activity is painful but whether patients are restricted in their activity due to the pain. Many people find that their symptoms are more noticeable when they perform certain activities, but that they do not necessarily restrict them.

There are many assessments of disability. It is important that the instrument assess a broad range of activities that one might realistically expect to be affected by LBP. The items included should represent a range of different activities with differing demands. There should be some rating of the degree to which each item is compromised. Ideally, disability should be assessed in a number of domains encompassing all aspects of normal life, including physical activity, sleep, activities of daily living (ADLs; including work, where applicable), social activity, and psychological functioning. Commonly used instruments vary greatly in the representation of these domains. The majority of the items (about 80%) in the Roland–Morris Disability Questionnaire (RMDQ; Roland & Morris, 1983) concerns physical activities, with one item on sleep, one related to psychological functioning, and one on social functioning. A little under half of the items, out of 10, in the Oswestry Back Pain Questionnaire (Fairbank, Couper, Davies, & O'Brien, 1980) relate to physical activity and two items relate to ADLs, one to sleep, one to pain, and one to sex life. The Sickness Impact Profile (SIP; Bergner, Bobbitt, Carter, & Gilson, 1991) is more evenly distributed between physical activity and psychological functioning. Some measures have normative datasets that reflect the health of the population in general and allow comparisons with other health care conditions. The one with the most comprehensive data set is the Short Form–36 (SF-36; Ware & Sherbourne, 1992) and its derivatives.

It is difficult to recommend one questionnaire over another. The RMDQ is derived from the SIP but has considerably fewer items (RMDQ has 24; SIP has 136), and there seems little difference between the two as outcome measures, but the brevity of the RMDQ is preferred by patients. There is some evidence that the RMDQ suffers from a ceiling effect but is more sensitive than the Oswestry Back Pain Questionnaire at lower levels of disability (Roland & Fairbank, 2000).

PAIN BEHAVIOR

Pain behavior relates to all the behavioral expressions related to being in pain, including facial expression, vocalization, verbalization, change in posture and gait, seeking health care, avoidance of activity, and receipt of health-related compensation (see Keefe, Somers, Williams, & Smith, Chapter 7, this volume). Pain behavior occurs in a social context, and expression of the behavior will vary depending on the social context at the time. It can be seen as a form of social communication and is not only a product of the response to the sensory component but is also shaped by the social environment (Fordyce, 1976); Sullivan, 2008). For example, if bending increases back pain, the patient will restrict that movement, and this will be obvious to an observer. The patient may at the same time demonstrate a facial expression of pain. As the movement of bending becomes associated with pain, the onset of that movement is accompanied by the facial expression of a pain. If concern is expressed by another person, or if threatening information is presented about the risks of bending and the potential harm, the behavioral expression is likely to be greater.

Unfortunately for patients, there is often a misunderstanding about the very interactive nature of pain behavior and the influence of context and the social environment. The clinician's need to objectify the cause of pain can lead then to making judgments about the veracity of the patient's condition, and intense expressions of pain behavior can be misconstrued as willful exaggeration or even a willingness on the patient's part to deceive.

Waddell, Main, Morris, di Paola, and Gray (1984) suggested a system of assessing signs and symptoms, described as "nonorganic," that are unrelated to the back pain condition. These can be used as part of the clinical examination. The patient can be asked if he or she has experienced any of the following symptoms (Waddell et al., 1984):

Nonorganic symptoms

1. Pain at the tip of the tailbone—other than coccydinia
2. Whole-leg pain—nonanatomical stocking distribution pain
3. Whole-leg numbness—nonanatomical stocking distribution numbness
4. Whole-leg giving way—without specific localized weakness
5. Complete absence of any spells without pain—over a long period
6. Intolerance of and reactions to treatment—all or most treatments have aggravated the condition
7. Emergency admissions for LBP—pain so severe that an emergency admission must be made

These must be used with care. They must be viewed as a whole on a continuum. They are not "diagnostic," and an increased number of positive responses is an indication of increased likelihood of distress, and nothing more. The presence of one or more of these symptoms must be considered in light of the assessment as a whole.

A number of measures have been developed clinically to assess pain behavior. Some rely on the presence of a separate observer (Prkachin, Hughes, Schultz, Joy, & Hunt, 2002) (others can be rated by the assessor during the performance of standardized physical tests; Moores & Watson, 2004). These can provide a score to identify those who are demonstrating considerable behavioral responses. Waddell and colleagues (1984) developed a series of standardized tests as part of the clinical assessment, and these have been used in clinical practice for some years.

- Increased tenderness.
  - Superficial tenderness in the skin on gentle pinching.
  - Nonanatomical tenderness—deep tenderness over a widespread area that is nonanatomical.
- Response to simulated movement/loading of the spine.
  - Axial compression—pressure downward on the skull produces pain in the lumbar spine.
  - Simulated rotation—whole-body rotation while keeping the spine still produces pain in the lumbar spine.

- Distraction testing—a response to one test when conducted in another, nonthreatening condition produces a completely different response; one example Waddell gives is the distracted SLR test, whereby a patient reports pain on the SLR but can sit upright with the legs at 90° when relaxed or distracted.
- Regional disturbances—widespread loss of sensation or weakness in the lower limbs on formal testing that does not approximate accepted neuroanatomy.
- Overreaction to assessment—whereby the patient demonstrates disproportionate verbalizing, vocalizing, and grimacing throughout the examination even during innocuous tests.

One must remember that the responses to examination are a product of patients' previous experience of examinations, their perception of the possible outcome of the assessment (access to treatment or benefit), and their perception of what is likely to make their pain worse (movement, palpation). An increased number of positive responses on these type of examinations is a sign of psychological distress, not an indication of malingering, and should not influence the clinician's interpretation of the clinical examination. Likewise, it should not result in labeling the patient as "exaggerating" or that his or her pain is "psychological." Put simply, increased responses are a sign that psychosocial factors need to be examined and addressed if treatment is to be optimized.

PSYCHOSOCIAL ASSESSMENT

The biomedical component of the assessment outlined earlier assists in determining the possible cause of the pain, the degree of impairment, and reported disability. This cannot be artificially separated from those factors that influence the expression of the pain and disability (see Turk & Robinson, Chapter 10, this volume).

The influence of psychosocial factors on the presentation of back pain, their relationship to the severity of disability reported, and their influence on the outcome from a wide variety of treatments has been understood for some time. Kendall, Linton, and Main (1997) coined the term "yellow flags," sug-

gesting that they are analogous to red flags, in that red flags draw attention to the possibility of serious pathology; yellow flags required the clinician to look for the presence of factors likely to lead to a poor outcome, if not addressed. At that time the attention was on returning people with an episode of acute LBP to work. Since then, the term "yellow flags" has expanded to cover LBP of all durations and comprises largely individual psychological factors associated with unfavorable clinical outcomes and the transition to persistent pain and disability. The original "yellow flags" considered perceptions regarding the work environment, but these have more recently been incorporated into a second level of assessment specifically about work, the "blue flags."

Since the original yellow flags, there has been considerable research and a number of reviews supporting the important role of psychological factors in outcome. There remain problems with the "yellow flags" approach. First, the importance of each factor might vary due to the duration of the problem. The predictive ability of a factor may vary according to the outcome or interest (return to work, pain, disability). There is no "one-size-fits-all" method for assessing yellow flags, which makes screening to determine specific treatment difficult. We are still in the early stages of recommending specific questionnaires for use in clinical practice.

In addition to the "yellow flags," other authors have suggested other obstacles to recovery. These include the perceptions about work (where return to work is the outcome of interest), or "blue flags," and the context within which the person lives, the social and environmental setting, or "black flags." This chapter does not address either of these; the reader is directed to more specialist publications (Kendall, Burton, Watson, & Main, 2009).

Despite these shortcomings there is consensus on the more important factors, and it has been argued by some that it is better to use a broad range of assessment tools and be overinclusive rather than miss cases that will go on to develop long-term incapacity and prolonged health care seeking.

Although there is much discussion about the relative importance of factors, the consensus is that the key factors identified are beliefs about back pain and its prognosis, emotional reactions to the pain and its interference with daily activity, fear of further injury, psychological distress, self-efficacy, depression, and catastrophizing.

A wide variety of questionnaires is available for the assessment of these variables, because it is unlikely that a "gold standard" screening questionnaire will be developed soon. Using a limited number of instruments to assess the main areas and integrate this information into the patient interview seems the most pragmatic solution at present (Main & Watson, 2002).

Beliefs, Expectancies, and Appraisal

It is very difficult to separate out these three components clearly, but beliefs relate to our preexisting understanding of back pain shaped by our culture and learning in the social environment. This does not mean that people come to the consultation already molded in their beliefs. Beliefs may change in light of new experience and information provided. However, information that reinforces previously existing beliefs is more likely to be integrated than that which challenges it radically. Expectancies are the patient's perception of the course of the condition and the treatment that is most likely to be appropriate. In addition to this is patients' own expectations of their role and their own ability to influence events or self-efficacy beliefs. Appraisal relates to patients' judgment about events, including their own efforts to manage their problem. A negative appraisal that the condition is beyond their control does not favor a positive outcome. A person who has received threatening information about back pain, who believes back pain is harmful and that treatment by a skilled professional is the most important route, and who does not believe he or she can personally influence the outcome of the condition is unlikely to do well.

Depression may not necessarily mean full clinical depression, although this is not uncommon in chronic LBP, but is instead described as a feeling of sadness or being down. It may also manifest as helplessness or agitation. Depression may also result in poor sleep and altered eating, and often it is accompanied by an increased report of pain. Depressed people engage in more negative appraisals of themselves and their condition, which exacerbates their perception of their inability to manage their problem. The onset of depression is most likely when the pain limits participation in valued activities and roles; the greater the interference, the more likely depression is. The onset of depression might therefore not be directly related to the observation of functional limitation, what one can do physically in comparison to others, but may interfere with what one wants to do or feels it is his or her duty to do (Morley & Sutherland, 2008; Rudy, Kerns, & Turk, 1988).

Catastrophizing has been identified as a major influence on the behavioral presentation of LBP, the severity of reported disability, the intensity of pain, and the outcome from treatment. It is characterized as negative perceptions and ruminations about one's ability to cope with pain and a propensity to identify selectively with negative information. Such patients are also more likely to see an increase in their pain as a sign of a worsening condition. Although it is often included in instruments that assess coping, catastrophizing is probably better considered as a form of negative appraisal.

Over the past 15 years there has been interest in the influence of specific fears about hurting and harming, and how these might influence the development of disability. Vlaeyen, Kole-Snijders, Boeren, and van Eek (1995; Vlaeyen & Linton, 2000) proposed a fear–avoidance model of pain related disability. It builds on the concept of avoidance learning, in that successful avoidance of pain develops into a long-term strategy that increases disability. The model proposes that, following injury or the onset of symptoms, a person might remain active despite the pain, and this will result in recovery. Those who engage in avoidance are more likely to do this if they successfully avoid pain. Avoidance is more likely in persons with a tendency to catastrophize in the presence of threatening information about back pain. The model suggests that avoidance leads not only to disability but also to secondary physical deconditioning. Repeated avoidance of activity and, in particular, avoidance of valued activity results in depression and increased perception of pain. Although there is some disagreement about the model and the predictive ability of fear–avoidance, there is general agreement that fears about injury and damage, and avoidance are both important and need to be assessed and addressed.

The two most used instruments to assess fear–avoidance in LBP are the Tampa Scale of Kinesiophobia (Kori, Miller, & Todd, 1990) and the Fear–Avoidance Beliefs Questionnaire (Waddell, Newton, Henderson, Somerville, & Main, 1993). Both can be criticized because they may assess beliefs about fear of movement and activity, but neither gives an adequate assessment of avoidance of activity. The Pain Anxiety Symptoms Scale (McCracken, Zayfert, & Gross, 1992) has tried to address this in order to inform clinical assessment and treatment but still lacks specificity for the types of activities that patients avoid. To help inform about specific activities that are feared and to incorporate this into treatment, a series of photographs of daily activities were developed by Kugler, Wijn, Geilen, de Jong, and Vlaeyen (1999). These help to identify feared activities and ask patients to place the photographs in a hierarchy according to their fears that the activity will do harm to their backs.

SUMMARY

The initial aim of the assessment is to separate significant pathology that requires further investigation and/or urgent treatment from other causes of LBP. The latter are grouped together as nonspecific LBP. There is some evidence that, even within this group, subclassifications or causes may be determined, but evidence that this leads to improved treatment outcome is currently weak and requires further study.

Assessment of physical incapacity must be done carefully and accurately, because the outcome of such assessment often has implications for the patient beyond the diagnosis and measurement of current ability.

Chronic LBP is a multifactorial problem that becomes more complex with the passage of time and the development of disability. A physical examination alone is insufficient to assess accurately the condition's impact on the patient. A comprehensive and careful assessment of psychological and behavioral factors is required, using appropriate and established psychological assessment instruments. Such an assessment will enlighten the

clinician as to the barriers to treatment that need to be overcome for optimal recovery. The clinician must keep in mind that these factors, and not pain intensity, have much more influence on the level of disability. Further training in the application and interpretation of these tests is likely to be required in the development of treatment plans.

REFERENCES

Airaksinen, O., Brox, J. I., Cedraschi, C., Hildebrandt, J., Klaber Moffett, J., Kovacs, F., et al. (2006). European Guidelines for the management of chronic non-specific low back pain. *European Spine Journal, 15*(Suppl. 2), S192–S300.
Bergner, M., Bobbitt, R. A., Carter, W. B., & Gilson, B. S. (1991). The Sickness Impact Profile: Validation of a health status measure. *Medical Care, 19,* 561–571.
Bigos, S., Bowyer, O., Braen, G., Brown, K., Deyo, R., Haldeman, S., et al. (1994). *Acute back pain problems in adults.* (Clinical Practice Guideline No. 14, ACHPR Publication No. 95-0642). Rockville, MD: Agency for Healthcare Policy and Research, Public Health Service, U.S. Department of Health and Human Services.
Buchbinder, R., & Jolley, D. (2005). Effects of a media campaign on back beliefs is sustained 3 years after its cessation. *Spine, 30,* 1323–1330.
Carragee, E. J., Lincoln, T., Parmar, V. S., & Alamin, T. (2006). A gold standard evaluation of the "discogenic pain" diagnosis as determined by provocative discography. *Spine, 31,* 2115–2123.
Cleeland, C. S., & Ryan, K. M. (1994). Pain assessment: Global use of the Brief Pain Inventory. *Annals of the Academy of Medicine (Singapore), 23,* 129–138.
Clinical Standards Advisory Group. (1994). *Report of a CSAG Committee on Back Pain.* London: Her Majesty's Stationery Office.
Cocchiarella, L., & Andersson, G. B. J. (2001). *Guides to the evaluation of permanent impairment.* Chicago: AMA Press.
Croft, P. R., Macfarlane, G. J., Papageorgiou, A. C., Thomas, E., & Silman, A. J. (1998). Outcome of low back pain in general practice: A prospective study. *British Medical Journal, 316,* 1356–1359.
Deyo, R. A. (1986). Early diagnostic evaluation of low back pain. *Journal of Internal Medicine, 1,* 328–338.
Deyo, R. A., & Diehl, A. (1988). Cancer as a cause of low back pain: Frequency, clinical

presentation and diagnostic strategies. *Journal of General Internal Medicine, 3,* 330–338.

Deyo, R. A., & Tsui-Wu, Y. (1987). Descriptive epidemiology of low back pain and its related medical care in the United States. *Spine, 12,* 264–268.

Di Iorio, D., Henley, E., & Doughty, A. (2000). A survey of primary care physician practice patterns and adherence to acute low back problem guidelines. *Archives of Family Medicine, 9,* 1015–1021.

Fairbank, J. C., Couper, J., Davies, J. B., & O'Brien, J. P. (1980). The Oswestry Low Back Pain Disability Questionnaire. *Physiotherapy, 66,* 271–273.

Ferreira, M., Ferreira, P., Latimer, J., Herbert, R., Hodges, P. W., Jennings, M., et al. (2007). Comparison of general exercise, motor control exercise and spinal manipulative therapy for chronic low back pain: A randomized trial. *Pain, 131,* 31–37.

Ferreira, P., Ferreira, M., & Hodges, P. W. (2004). Changes in recruitment of the abdominal muscles in people with low back pain: Ultrasound measurement of muscle activity. *Spine, 29,* 2560–2566.

Feuerstein, M., Hartzell, M., Rogers, H., & Marcus, S. (2006). Evidence-based practice for acute low back pain in primary care: Patient outcomes and cost of care. *Pain, 124,* 140–149.

Fordyce, W. E. (1976). *Behavioural methods for chronic pain and illness.* St Louis, MO: Mosby.

Gask, L., & Usherwood, T. (2003). The consultation. In R. Mayou, M. Sharpe, & A. Carson (Eds.), *ABC of psychological medicine* (pp. 1–3). London: BMJ Books.

Geraci, M. C., Alleva, J. T., & McAdam, F. B. (2002). The physical examination of the spine and its functional kinetic chain. In A. J. Cole & S. Herring (Eds.), *Low pack pain handbook* (2nd ed., pp. 69–93). Philadelphia: Hanley & Belfus.

Gilbert, F. J., Grant, A. M., Gillan, M. G. C., Vale, L., Scott, N. W., Campbell, M. K., et al. (2004). Does early imaging influence management and improve outcomes in patients with low back pain?: A pragmatic randomised controlled trial. *Health Technology Assessment, 8,* 1–131.

Gillan, M. G. C., Gilbert, F. J., Andrew, J. E., Grant, A. M., Wardlaw, D., Valentine, N. W., et al. (2001). Influence of imaging on clinical decision making in the treatment of lower back pain. *Radiology, 220,* 393–399.

Gross, D. P., & Battié, M. C. (2002). Reliability of safe maximum lifting determinations of a functional capacity evaluation. *Physical Therapy, 82,* 364–371.

Gross, D. P., & Battié, M. C. (2004). The prognostic value of functional capacity evaluation in patients with chronic low back pain: Part 2. Sustained recovery. *Spine, 29,* 920–924.

Gross, D. P., & Battié, M. C. (2005). Functional capacity evaluation performance does not predict sustained return to work in claimants with chronic back pain. *Journal of Occupational Rehabilitation, 15,* 285–294.

Grubb, M., Bradford, L., Pritchard, D., & Ebersold, M. (1994). Primary Ewing's sarcoma of the spine. *Spine, 19,* 309–313.

Hollingworth, W., Gray, D. T., Martin, B. I., Sullivan, S. D., Deyo, R. A., & Jarvik, J. G. (2003). Rapid magnetic resonance imaging for diagnosing cancer-related pain. *Journal of General Internal Medicine, 18,* 303–312.

Jarvik, J. G., & Deyo, R. A. (2002). Diagnostic evaluation of low back pain with emphasis on imaging. *Annals of Internal Medicine, 137,* 586–597.

Kendall, N., Linton, S. J., & Main, C. J. (1997). *Guide to assessing psychosocial yellow flags in acute low back pain: Risk factors for long-term disability and work loss.* Wellington: Accident Rehabilitation and Compensation Insurance Corporation of New Zealand and the National Health Committee, Ministry of Health.

Kendall, N. A. S., Burton, A. K., Watson, P., & Main, C. J. (2009). *Tackling musculoskeletal problems: The psychosocial flags framework—a guide for the clinic and workplace.* London: The Stationery Office.

Kendrick, D., Fielding, K., Bentley, E., Kerslake, R., Miller, P., & Pringle, M. (2001a). Radiography of the lumber spine in primary care patients with low back pain: A randomised controlled trial. *British Medical Journal, 322,* 400–405.

Kendrick, D., Fielding, K., Bentley, E., Miller, P., Kerslake, R., & Pringle, M. (2001b). The role of radiography in primary care patients with low back pain of at least 6 weeks duration: A randomised (unblinded) controlled trial. *Health Technology Assessment, 5,* 1–69.

Kerry, S., Hilton, S., Dundas, D., Rink, E., & Oakeshott, P. (2002). Radiography for low back pain: A randomised controlled trial and observational study in primary care. *British Journal of General Practice, 52,* 469–474.

Kori, S. H., Miller, R. P., & Todd, D. D. (1990, January/February). Kinesiophobia, a new view of chronic pain behavior. *Pain Management,* pp. 35–43.

Kugler, K., Wijn, J., Geilen, M., de Jong, J., & Vlaeyen, J. (1999). *The photographic series of daily activities (PHODA)* [CD ROM version 1.0].

Liu, J. L. Y., Maniadakis, N., Gray, A., & Rayner,

D. (2002). The economic burden of coronary heart disease in the UK. *Heart, 88,* 597–603.

Macfarlane, G. J., Jones, G. T., & Hannaford, P. C. (2006). Managing low back pain presenting to primary care: Where do we go from here? *Pain, 122,* 219–222.

Main, C., Sullivan, M. J. L., & Watson, P. J. (2008). *Pain management: Practical applications of the biopsychosocial perspective in clinical and occupational settings.* Edinburgh, UK: Churchill Livingstone.

Main, C. J., Robinson, J. P., & Watson, P. J. (2005). Disability, incapacity and rehabilitation for pain patients. In D. M. Justins (Ed.), *Pain 2005—an updated review* (pp. 331–340). Seattle, WA: IASP Press.

Main, C. J., & Watson, P. J. (2002). The distressed and angry low back pain (LBP) patient. In L. Gifford (Ed.), *Topical issues in pain* (pp. 175–200). Falmouth, UK: CNS Press.

Maniadakis, N., & Gray, A. (2000). The economic burden of back pain in the UK. *Pain, 84,* 95–103.

Margolis, R. B., Tait, R. C., & Krause, S. J. (1986). A rating system for use with patient pain drawings. *Pain, 24,* 57–65.

McCracken, L., Zayfert, C., & Gross, R. T. (1992). The Pain Anxiety Symptoms Scale: Development and validation of a scale to measure fear of pain. *Pain, 50,* 67–73.

McGuirk, B., King, W., Govind, J., Lowry, J., & Bogduk, N. (2001). Safety, efficacy, and cost effectiveness of evidence-based guidelines for the management of acute low back pain in primary care. *Spine, 26,* 2615–2622.

Moores, L. L., & Watson, P. J. (2004). The development of a measurement tool for the assessment of pain behaviour in real time. *Physiotherapy, 90,* 12–18.

Morley, S., & Sutherland, R. (2008). Self-pain enmeshment: Future possible selves, sociotropy, autonomy and adjustment to chronic pain. *Pain, 137,* 366–377.

Negrini, S., Politano, E., Carabalona, R., & Mambrini, A. (2001). General practitioners' management of low back pain: Impact of clinical guidelines in a non-English-speaking country. *Spine, 26,* 2727–2733.

Overmeer, T., Linton, S. J., Holmquist, L., Eriksson, M., & Engfeldt, P. (2005). Do evidence-based guidelines have an impact in primary care?: A cross-sectional study of Swedish physicians and physiotherapists. *Spine, 30,* 146–151.

Parker, H., Wood, P. L. R., & Main, C. J. (1995). The use of the pain drawing as a screening measure to predict psychological distress in chronic low back pain. *Spine, 20,* 236–243.

Petrie, K. J., Frampton, T., Large, R. G., Moss-Morris, R., Johnson, M., & Meechan, G.

(2005). What do patients expect from their first visit to a pain clinic? *Clinical Journal of Pain, 21,* 297–301.

Prkachin, K., Hughes, E., Schultz, I., Joy, P., & Hunt, D. (2002). Real-time assessment of pain behavior during clinical assessment of low back pain patients. *Pain, 95,* 23–30.

Ransford, A. O., Cairns, D., & Mooney, V. (1976). The pain drawing as an aid to the psychological evaluation of patients with low back pain. *Spine, 1,* 127–134.

Roland, M., & Fairbank, J. C. (2000). The Roland–Morris Disability Questionnaire and the Oswestry Disability Questionnaire. *Spine, 25,* 3115–3124.

Roland, M., & Morris, R. (1983). A study in the natural history of back pain: Part 1. The development of a reliable and sensitive measure of disability in low back pain. *Spine, 8,* 141–144.

Rubinstein, S. M., & Van Tulder, M. (2008). A best evidence review of diagnostic procedures for neck and low back pain. *Baillieres Best Practice and Research Clinical Rheumatology, 22,* 471–482.

Rudy, T., Kerns, R. D., & Turk, D. C. (1985). Chronic pain and depression: Towards a cognitive behavioural mediation model. *Pain, 35,* 129–140.

Schers, H., Wensing, M., Huijsmans, Z., van Tulder, M., & Grol, R. (2001). Implementation barriers for general practice guidelines on low back pain a qualitative study. *Spine, 26,* E348–E353.

Scuderi, G. J., Brusovanik, G. V., Golish, S. R., Demeo, R., Hyde, J., Hallab, N., et al. (2008). A critical evaluation of discography in patients with lumbar intervertebral disc disease. *Spine Journal, 8,* 624–629.

Staal, J. B., Hlobil, H., van Tulder, M. W., Waddell, G., Burton, A. K., Koes, B. W., et al. (2003). Occupational health guidelines for the management of low back pain: An international comparison. *Occupational and Environmental Medicine, 60,* 618–626.

Sullivan, M. J. L. (2008). Toward a biopsychomotor conceptualization of pain: Implications for research and intervention. *Clinical Journal of Pain, 24,* 281–290.

Turner, J. A., Jensen, M. P., & Romano, J. M. (2000). Do beliefs, coping and catastrophising independently predict functioning in patients with chronic pain? *Pain, 85,* 115–125.

Vlaeyen, J. W., Kole-Snijders, A. M., Boeren, R. G., & van Eek, H. (1995). Fear of movement/(re)injury in chronic low back pain and its relation to behavioral performance. *Pain, 62,* 363–372.

Vlaeyen, J. W., & Linton, S. J. (2000). Fear–avoidance and its consequences in chronic musculoskeletal pain: A state of the art. *Pain, 85*, 317–332.

Waddell, G. (1982). An approach to backache. *British Journal of Hospital Medicine, 23*, 187–219.

Waddell, G. (2004). *The back pain revolution*. Edinburgh, UK: Churchill Livingstone.

Waddell, G., Main, C., Morris, E. W., di Paola, M. P., & Gray, I. C. (1984). Chronic low back pain, psychological distress and illness behaviour. *Spine, 9*, 209–213.

Waddell, G., Newton, M., Henderson, I., Somerville, D., & Main, C. J. (1993). A Fear–Avoidance Beliefs Questionnaire (FABQ) and the role of fear-avoidance beliefs in chronic low back pain and disability. *Pain, 52*, 157–168.

Waddell, G., & Turk, D. C. (2001). Clinical assessment of low back pain. In D. C. Turk & R. Melzack (Eds.), *Handbook of pain assessment* (2nd ed., pp. 431–453). New York: Guilford Press.

Walker, B. F. (2000). The prevalence of low back pain: A systematic review of the literature from 1966 to 1998. *Journal of Spinal Disorders, 13*, 205–217.

Ware, J. E., & Sherbourne, C. D. (1992). The MOS 36-Item Short Form Health Survey (SF-36): I. Conceptual framework and item selection. *Medical Care, 30*, 473–483.

Wasiak, R., Kim, J., & Pransky, G. (2006). Work disability and costs caused by recurrence of low back pain: Longer and more costly than in first episodes. *Spine, 31*, 219–225.

Wasiak, R., Pransky, G., Verma, S., & Webster, B. (2003). Recurrence of low back pain: Definition–sensitivity analysis using administrative data. *Spine, 28*, 2283–2291.

Watson, P. J., Bowey, J., Purcell-Jones, G., & Gales, T. (2008). General practitioner sickness absence certification for low back pain is not directly associated with beliefs about back pain. *European Journal of Pain, 12*, 314–320.

Watson, P. J., Main, C. J., Waddell, G., Gales, T. F., & Purcell-Jones, G. (1998). Medically certified work loss, recurrence and costs of wage compensation for back pain: A follow-up study of the working population of Jersey. *British Journal of Rheumatology, 37*, 82–86.

Weatherley, C. R., & Hourigan, P. G. (1998). Triage of back pain by physiotherapists in orthopaedic clinics. *Journal of the Royal Society of Medicine, 91*, 377–379.

Woby, S. R., Roach, N. K., Urmston, M., & Watson, P. J. (2007). The relation between cognitive factors and levels of pain and disability in chronic low back pain patients presenting for physiotherapy. *European Journal of Pain, 11*, 869–877.

CHAPTER 16

Assessment of Fibromyalgia Syndrome, Myofascial Pain Syndromes, and Whiplash-Associated Disorders

A Comprehensive Approach

JAMES P. ROBINSON
DENNIS C. TURK

Muscle pain is common among patients with clinically significant musculoskeletal pain. A large number of patients present with the following symptoms and findings: (1) the pain is not well localized but is prominent in areas of muscle; (2) the pain has an aching quality and is described as muscular soreness; (3) the patients demonstrate tenderness in areas where they report "aching" pain. We use these three simple criteria in this chapter as descriptive of muscle pain.

There are marked differences in the opinions of physicians regarding the pathophysiology underlying the symptoms of muscle pain, as well as the importance physicians place on such symptoms. Even the terminology to describe muscle pain has become a potential battleground. For example, as a first approximation, we can say that regional muscle pain has a great deal of overlap with the term *myofascial pain* (MFP) that some physicians use. Moreover, fibromyalgia syndrome (FM) is typically diagnosed when patients report widespread pain that typically has the features of muscle pain. This chapter describes methods for diagnosing MFP and FM, and examines some of the controversies surrounding these clinical entities. Also,

we discuss the contribution that muscle pain makes to one common musculoskeletal disorder—whiplash.

PATIENT EVALUATION

The evaluation of any medical patient is designed to accomplish several goals. These include establishing a diagnosis and identifying concomitant problems that might affect the patient's prognosis and response to treatment. The overall purpose of the evaluation is to gain information that will optimize treatment of the patient. In the context of muscular pain, a clinician has to address three general issues:

1. Does the patient have muscular pain that is affecting him or her significantly? If so, does the patient meet diagnostic criteria for FM, MFP, or whiplash-associated disorder (WAD)?
2. What other medical information is needed to characterize the patient's pain better and formulate a treatment plan?
3. What psychosocial factors may be influencing the patient's presentation?

In this chapter, we discuss methods for addressing questions 1 and 2. Methods for addressing question 3 are described by Turk and Robinson (Chapter 10, this volume).

FIBROMYALGIA SYNDROME

Physicians dating back to the 19th century have pondered the significance and etiology of widespread aching, muscular pain, and muscular tenderness. They used a number of terms to describe muscular pain, and developed a variety of theories to explain it (Reynolds, 1983; Simons, 2001). In 1904, Gowers introduced the term *fibrositis*, which was used sporadically during the early part of the 20th century but during the 1960s and 1970s came to be used with increasing frequency by rheumatologists.

In the 1960s, rheumatology was a relatively new specialty. Patients with widespread pain were often referred for rheumatological evaluation to determine whether their symptoms were the result of a systemic inflammatory process, such as rheumatoid arthritis. Some rheumatologists became interested in patients who presented with widespread, seemingly muscular pain, but did not evidence a well-defined rheumatological disorder. During the 1970s and 1980s, authors began to publish articles describing these patients in the rheumatological literature (Smythe, 1986, 1989). Rheumatologists typically used the label *fibrositis* to describe a syndrome characterized by widespread, seemingly muscular pain, tenderness to palpation of certain muscles, and the absence of markers of a well-defined rheumatological syndrome. The first attempt to provide specific clinical criteria for the diagnosis of fibrositis was made by Smythe and Moldofsky (1977). In 1981, Yunus, Masi, Calabro, Miller, and Feigenbaum recommended the term *fibromyalgia* as preferable to *fibrositis*, because the inflammatory process suggested by the term *fibrositis* was not found.

During the 1980s, research on fibrositis/fibromyalgia increased sharply. Rheumatologists gradually adopted FM as the preferable term. A key advance came in 1990, in a multicenter study undertaken by rheumatologists to identify optimal criteria for identifying FM, at least for purposes of research (Wolfe et al., 1990). After considering several different diagnostic criteria, the researchers concluded that only two were needed to create maximal sensitivity and specificity: a history of widespread musculoskeletal pain, and a report of pain in at least 11 of 18 designated sites during deep palpation of the sites. The 18 sites were called *active sites*.

At a descriptive level, FM has similarities and differences from MFP syndrome. The two are similar in that patients with both kinds of problems report aching pain that, to an evaluating physician, appears to be muscular in origin. But there are several differences. First, the rheumatologists who first studied FM in the 1970s and 1980s took an empirical approach to the disorder: They observed patients with common clinical features and worked to develop a measurable case definition for FM. Clinicians who use the American College of Rheumatology (ACR) criteria today can agree about whether patients have FM, even if they are uncertain about the pathophysiology underlying it. As an example of this empirical approach, FM specialists have had no trouble giving up the idea that FM reflects abnormalities in muscle to embrace recent research suggesting that FM may fundamentally reflect altered nervous system functioning (Staud, 2004; Staud & Rodriguez, 2006). In contrast, the pioneers of MFP research developed elaborate theories about the pathophysiology underlying the trigger points (TrPs) that played such a central role in the theory. This emphasis on theory persists. Thus, although it is possible in principle to have a case definition of MFP analogous to the ACR criteria for FM, in reality, the assertion that a patient has MFP entails assumptions about the pathophysiology underlying the patient's symptoms.

Another difference is that the tender points that define FM do not necessarily have all the characteristics (e.g., taut bands and referred pain) of myofascial TrPs (Wolfe et al., 1992). Finally, FM is, by definition, a widespread pain syndrome, whereas MFP is usually thought of as a regional pain syndrome.

At this time consensus is that FM is distinctly different from MFP syndrome (Mense & Simons, 2001). It is worth noting, however, that during the 1980s, when little was known about FM, careful consideration was given to the hypothesis that the widespread muscular tenderness reported by patients with FM actually reflected the fact that they had multiple myofascial TrPs (Simons, 1986).

It is beyond the scope of this chapter to review the voluminous research on FM, or to consider the multiple pathophysiological hypotheses advanced to explain it. It is interesting to note, however, that much of the FM research during the 1980s addressed the possibility that the disorder is fundamentally a disorder of muscle (Bennett, 1989). This seemed like a plausible hypothesis, since patients with FM reported significant pain during deep palpation of muscles.

During the past 15 years, FM researchers have shifted away from explaining the disorder on the basis of peripheral pathology (i.e., abnormalities in muscles), and have instead reached the conclusion that the fundamental problem in the disorder is a disturbance in central nervous system (CNS) processing of sensory information. Recent formulations of the pathophysiology of FM have relied heavily on basic neurobiological findings regarding CNS sensitization (Staud, 2004; Staud & Rodriguez, 2006). In a similar vein, recently published reviews of treatments for FM highlight the fact that the best supported treatments address FM as a systemic problem rather than as a local or multifocal disorder of muscles (Carville et al., 2008; Goldenberg, Burckhardt, & Crofford, 2004).

The history of concepts regarding FM over the past 25 years forms a cautionary tale. Early researchers took the seemingly obvious perspective that since patients with FM report muscular tenderness, they must have some abnormality in their muscles (Bennett, 1989). In contrast, current thinking emphasizes that the muscular tenderness of patients with FM is essentially an epiphenomenon of a disturbance in CNS function. The same type of analysis might turn out to be appropriate for myofascial TrPs.

DIAGNOSING FM

The ACR study mentioned earlier (Wolfe et al., 1990) provides a simple and reproducible method for diagnosing FM. Although the authors of the study made it clear that they were attempting to develop criteria for research on FM, the criteria they developed

can serve clinicians well. Essentially, a clinician examining a patient for possible FM has to address three issues:

1. Does the patient have widespread pain? ACR criteria indicate that to meet this criterion, the patient must "frequently or usually" have spinal pain, pain above and below the waist, and on the left and right sides of the body. The easiest way to determine whether a patient meets the widespread pain criterion is to have him or her fill out a pain drawing, and then ask follow-up questions to clarify factors the patient considered in completing the drawing.

2. Is the pain chronic? ACR criteria did not specify the duration of symptoms necessary for a diagnosis of FM, but others (e.g., Hauser, Bernardy, Arnold, Offenbacher, & Schiltenwolf, 2009) have noted that symptoms should be present for at least 3 months.

3. During palpation at a force of up to 4 kg, does the patient report at least mild pain in at least 11 of 18 active sites designated by the ACR?

ADDITIONAL MEDICAL EVALUATION FOR FM

A clinician who decides that a patient meets diagnostic criteria for FM should not terminate his or her evaluation at that point. Instead, he or she should determine whether the patient has an accompanying medical condition that is clinically important. In some instances (e.g., hypothyroidism in a patient with FM), the accompanying condition might plausibly be viewed as the cause of the patient's muscular pain; in others, the accompanying condition might have implications for treatment, even if it does not provide an alternative explanation of the patient's symptoms (Boissevain & McCain, 1991).

Different authors have proposed various lists of conditions that should be considered in patients with FM; our list is given in Table 16.1. With these possibilities in mind, it is appropriate for an examiner to do a screening laboratory assessment on patients with FM. A minimal list recommended by Clauw (2009) includes a complete blood count, serum chemistries, and tests for

TABLE 16.1. Medical Conditions That Can Mimic Fibromyalgia

1. Rheumatological
   a. Early inflammatory arthritis—for example, systemic lupus erythematosus, rheumatoid arthritis
   b. Polymyalgia rheumatica
2. Endocrine—hypothyroidism
3. Neurological—postpolio syndrome; multiple sclerosis
4. Miscellaneous—hepatitis C

thyroid-stimulating hormone, erythrocyte sedimentation rate, and C-reactive protein. Although many clinicians routinely order serological studies, such as antinuclear antibody or rheumatoid factor on patients with FM, Clauw suggested that these be reserved for patients whose physical findings suggest inflammatory arthritis, or who have a history that is atypical of FM.

Also, since FM is, by definition, a chronic pain syndrome, it is important for an examiner to assess patients with regard to factors that have a high prevalence among patients with chronic pain in general. General strategies for assessing patients with chronic pain are described by Turk and Robinson (Chapter 10, this volume).

DIAGNOSING MFP

It is far more challenging to diagnose MFP than to diagnose FM. One reason for this is that MFP theorists have proposed complex, arduous physical examination procedures in the diagnosis of MFP. Another complicating factor is that muscles exist throughout the body, and MFP has been proposed to explain a bewildering array of medical conditions. Thus, for example, MFP has been discussed by neurologists (for headaches), dentists (for temporomandibular joint dysfunction) and gynecologists (for pelvic pain). For simplicity, our discussion focuses on pain involving the spine or extremities.

The starting point for evaluating a patient for possible MFP is a history regarding the location(s) of the patient's pain. As in the diagnosis of FM, a pain diagram is very helpful in eliciting relevant information. Obviously, a physician should only use a pain diagram as a starting point in assessing a patient's

musculoskeletal symptoms. The drawing should be supplemented by detailed questioning of the patient. This permits the physician to determine better the distribution of the patient's pain, as well as its quality and associated symptoms, including numbness, paresthesias, and focal weakness.

Myofascial pain should be considered if a patient reports diffuse pain in some region of his or her body, especially if the pain pattern fits one of the patterns described in textbooks on MFP (Travell & Simons, 1983, 1992).

Supporters of MFP theory emphasize that a primary goal of the physical examination of a person with suspected MFP is the identification of TrPs. The conceptual definition of a TrP was given earlier. Simons (2001) lists the following as physical findings indicative of TrPs:

1. A taut band in an affected muscle.
2. A tender nodule somewhere along the course of a taut band—this is the TrP.
3. Patient recognition. When pressure is applied to the tender nodule, the patient reports pain and indicates that the maneuver reproduces his or her typical pain.
4. Pressure on the tender nodule causes not only local pain, but also pain and sometimes sensory disturbances in a characteristic referral pattern.
5. Snapping palpation of the TrP evokes a transient twitch of muscle fibers in the taut band.
6. The patient demonstrates limited range of motion of the muscle that contains TrPs.
7. When the affected muscle is contracted strongly, the patient experiences pain and demonstrates weakness.

Given this list, an obvious question arises: Which of these criteria should be met before a diagnosis of MFP is given? Simons (2001) notes that there is no generally accepted answer to this question. He proposes that the minimal criteria for identifying MFP is that a patient meet criteria 1, 2, and 3.

As far as practical aspects of an examination for muscle pain/MFP/TrPs are concerned, several points are important. First, the text by Travell and Simons (1983, 1992) gives detailed information about techniques for identifying TrPs in specific muscles. The examiner should review this material to obtain hints about patient positioning and specific examination techniques. Second, the examiner should be prepared for situations in which only some of the findings associated with TrPs are obtained. For example, the examiner will frequently encounter patients with tenderness over muscles, but without local twitch responses, taut bands, or other findings thought to markers of TrPs. Third, the examiner needs to be careful about the amount of force exerted during an examination for TrPs. As the abundant literature on pressure pain threshold demonstrates, any person will report pain when an examiner pushes very forcefully on his or her muscles. It is probably best to use the criterion proposed by the ACR for the diagnosis of FM. In their landmark paper on research criteria for the diagnosis of FM, rheumatologists with expertise in FM recommended that an examiner push on a muscle with a force of up to 4 kilograms (Wolfe et al., 1990). If a patient does not report localized or referred pain by then, the site should be considered negative for muscle tenderness or TrP.

ADDITIONAL MEDICAL EVALUATION FOR MFP

As with FM, a key issue in the medical evaluation of a patient with MFP is to determine whether the MFP is an important cause of the patient's symptoms and activity limitations or an epiphenomenon of some other problem. Proponents of MFP theory emphasize that MFP is the cause of significant pain and functional limitation. As noted earlier, skeptics tend to ignore MFP entirely. However, to the extent that one can infer their opinions, it appears that they view MFP as a secondary phenomenon that does not warrant direct treatment. It is impossible to say whether the proponents of MFP or the skeptics are correct in their appraisals. The truth probably lies in the middle; therefore, MFP is probably an important and independent determinant of pain and functional limitation for some patients who appear to have muscular pain, but not as many as proponents of MFP theory suggest.

A practical implication of the uncertainty regarding the causal role of MFP is that clinicians should look carefully for other musculoskeletal pathology in any patient who has been diagnosed with MFP. Careful evaluation of a patient's pain diagram can facilitate this evaluation. In the simplest case, a patient will describe an area of pain that is classic for MFP—one that closely matches one of the patterns described by Travell and Simons (1983, 1992). See Figure 16.1. This type of pain diagram would increase the probability that the patient actually has MFP. It should be noted, though, that pain patterns reported by healthy volunteers following cervical facet joint injections with hypertonic saline can be very similar to pain patterns in patients suspected to have MFP from certain neck and shoulder girdle muscles (Dwyer, Aprill, & Bogduk, 1990). Thus, a pain pattern that is consistent with MFP is by no means diagnostic of MFP.

Several other patterns of pain are frequently revealed in pain diagrams. Some patients describe very localized pain (e.g., slightly off center in the lower cervical region; see Figure 16.2). This type of drawing is more suggestive of joint pain (such as a C5–6 facet arthropathy) than of MFP. Other patients indicate pain in a pattern that is classic for a radiculopathy (Figure 16.3). The presence of a radiculopathy does not rule out concurrent MFP. Indeed, some experts in muscular pain argue that MFP is common in radiculopathies, and at least one (Gunn, 1996) argues that MFP is essentially always a by-product of a radiculopathy or neuropathy. A pain diagram in a classic radicular pattern, however, should alert an examiner to the strong possibility that the patient has something going on other than straightforward MFP. It implies that even if the patient has physical findings consistent with MFP, it is probably more appropriate to direct treatment toward the radiculopathy than toward the MFP. Another common pattern is very widespread pain (Figure 16.4). This pattern is suggestive of FM rather than regional MFP. Finally, some patients' drawings indicate pain that is limited to one body region but is diffuse within that region, and does not correspond in any obvious way to a classic MPS (Figure 16.5). It is possible that the pain of such patients reflects MFP but is complex because it is a product of multiple TrPs. However, it is equally likely that these patients have muscle pain that is not readily construed as MFP.

Beyond examining pain diagrams, physicians should employ the full range of di-

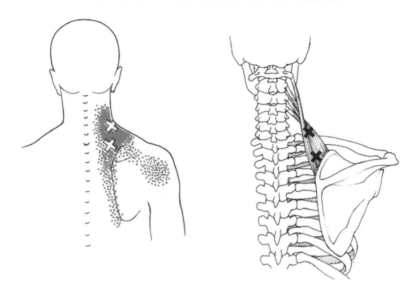

FIGURE 16.1. Consolidated referred pain pattern of the two trigger point locations (*X*'s) for the right levator scapulae muscle. The essential pain pattern is *solid*, and the spillover pattern is *stippled*. From Travell and Simons (1992). Copyright by Lippincott Williams and Wilkins. Reprinted by permission.

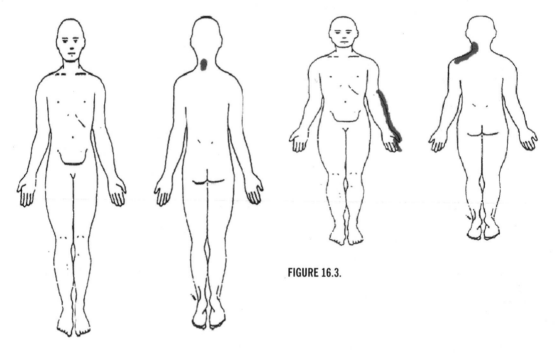

FIGURE 16.3.

FIGURE 16.2.

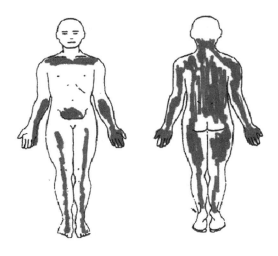

FIGURE 16.4.

agnostic methods to determine whether a patient has musculoskeletal or neurological problems associated with his or her MFP. These might include a variety of imaging studies, diagnostic blocks, and electrodiagnostic evaluations.

The most important evaluations for a patient with MFP involve the joints, periarticular structures, and nerves in the region where the patient has symptoms. This contrasts with the medical evaluation of a patient with FM, where systemic factors

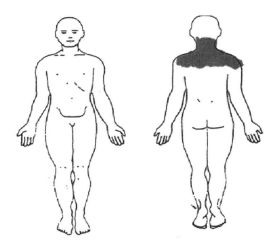

FIGURE 16.5.

become the focus of attention. It should be noted, though, that proponents of MFP theory have said that some metabolic/nutritional factors act as risk or perpetuating factors for MFP. For example, Dommerholt and Shah (2010) state:

> Any nutritional or metabolic condition that interferes with the energy supply of muscle tissue can contribute to the development of myofascial trigger points. . . . Laboratory levels can be within the "normal" range, yet be insufficient for a given individual, which makes it more difficult to diagnose, but no less important. Common nutritional and metabolic deficiencies or insufficiencies include vitamins B1, B6, B12, and D insufficiency states, iron, magnesium, and zinc insufficiency states, and thyroid deficiency states, among others. . . . The importance of metabolic and nutritional perpetuating factors is illustrated for vitamin D. (p. 462)

Obviously, this sweeping statement does not provide specific guidance to clinicians as they evaluate patients with MFP. However, it suggests that a thorough workup of a patient with MFP should include a chemistry panel, thyroid function tests, and perhaps an assessment of vitamin D level.

Finally, a comprehensive evaluation of a patient with MFP should include the assessment strategies described by Turk and Robinson (Chapter 10, this volume) for chronic pain in general. The rationale for this recommendation is that MFP pain rarely becomes clinically important except in patients with chronic musculoskeletal pain.

DIAGNOSIS OF OTHER TYPES OF MUSCLE PAIN

In a patient with widespread pain, a diagnosis of FM is an obvious choice. The patient with regional pain that appears to be muscular in nature and meets criteria for a diagnosis of MFP would also be an obvious choice. But as noted earlier, in some patients with regional pain, it is difficult to identify all or even most of the findings purported to be characteristic of MFP. Proponents of MFP theory emphasize that skilled examiners can identify most or all of items 1–7 (discussed earlier) and say essentially nothing about the practical problems that routinely arise during examinations for TrPs. These include palpating deep muscles that are relatively inaccessible, palpating muscles in obese patients, and palpating muscles in patients who report severe pain and do not tolerate a manual examination of their muscles. Also, proponents say nothing about how patients with apparent muscular pain but without myofascial TrPs should be treated, or how their conditions should be conceptualized. We believe that many of these patients can probably benefit from treatment for myofascial pain, even though they do not have all of the classic findings for TrPs. The one exception is that they might not be good candidates for TrP injections, since proponents of MFP theory recommend that these be given in myofascial TrPs.

WHIPLASH-ASSOCIATED DISORDERS

Neck disorders that develop in the context of acceleration–deceleration injuries are often called whiplash injuries. Often these occur in motor vehicle collisions (MVCs). The term *whiplash* (WL) has been used variously to describes a process (the head of the passenger or driver is subject to acceleration and deceleration forces that hyperextend and hyperflex the neck; Gay & Abbot, 1953), the resulting injury (i.e., WL injury), and the syndrome of symptoms following such an injury (WL syndrome) (Barnsley, Lord, & Bogduk, 1994; Mayou & Radanov, 1996).

The Quebec Task Force (Spitzer et al., 1995) defined a WL as an acceleration–deceleration mechanism of energy transfer to the neck. It may result from a rear-end or side-impact MVC, but it can also occur during diving or other mishaps. The impact may result in bony or soft-tissue injuries (WL) that may in turn lead to a variety of clinical manifestations (whiplash-associated disorders [WADs]). The Quebec Task Force on Whiplash-Associated Disorders created a grading system of WADs caused by MVCs. This distinguishes individuals with neck pain but no physical findings (Grade I) from ones with pain plus musculoskeletal findings, such as reduced cervical range of motion (Grade II), neurological injury (Grade III), or major skeletal injury (e.g., a fracture; Grade IV; see Table 16.2). Grade I and II WADs comprise more than 90% of all WADs (Spitzer et al., 1995).

TABLE 16.2. Quebec Task Force Clinical Classification of WAD

Grade	Clinical features
I	Complaint of neck pain, stiffness or tenderness; no physical signs
II	Complaint of neck pain, stiffness or tenderness; musculoskeletal signs present (e.g., reduced range of motion)
III	Complain of neck pain; signs of neurological injury present
IV	Complaint of neck pain; evidence of fracture or dislocation

The signs and symptoms of WADs have been described in numerous studies (e.g., Barnsley et al., 1993; Mayou & Radanov, 1996). Onset of symptoms after the injury may be delayed for several hours, and symptoms worsen within 24–48 hours. The percentage of people with WADs who go on to develop chronic symptoms has been reported to range from 13 to 64% (Barnsley et al., 1993; Pennie & Agambar, 1991). The wide variation is likely due to the method of recruiting participants in studies (e.g., emergency department, newspapers, referred to specialist), time since MVC (hours to months), and criteria used to define WADs. Once WADs become chronic, they are extremely resistant to treatment.

Whereas it has generally seemed obvious to many physicians (though not necessarily true) that MFP and FM involve muscle pain, the role of muscle pain in WAD is not at all obvious. WAD is defined on the basis of the location of a patient's pain, and the circumstances surrounding its onset. There is nothing in the case definition of WAD that has any necessary connection to muscles or muscular pain. In fact, multiple structures other than muscles have been implicated in the neck pain that patients with WAD I and II injuries report. Bogduk and colleagues (Bogduk, 2002; Gibson, Bogduk, MacPherson, & McIntosh, 2000) have pioneered techniques for identifying the structural basis of patients' reports of symptoms by careful application of injection procedures designed to provoke or palliate pain. Using these techniques, they have reported that approximately 70% of individuals with persistent neck pain following MVCs have pain mediated by one or more of the cervical facet joints. Moreover, in a carefully designed randomized controlled trial, they have demonstrated that among individuals who have been diagnosed with facet joint–mediated pain, approximately 70% will experience prolonged symptom relief in response to injections (facet neurotomies) designed to denervate the affected facet joint (Lord, Barnsley, Wallis, McDonald, & Bogduk, 1996; McDonald, Lord, & Bogduk, 1999).

Although attempts to replicate these provocative results have met with only partial success (Manchikanti, Singh, Rivera, & Pampati, 2002), the research by Bogduk and others strongly supports the conclusion that at least some individuals with persistent WAD do have facet arthropathies. Other investigators have implicated injury to the intervertebral discs (Clemens & Burrow, 1972; Watkinson, Gargan, & Bannister, 1991) as a factor in persistent WAD. Still others have reported that ligamentous injuries play a significant role in WAD (e.g., Stemper, Yoganandan, Pintar, & Rao, 2006; Tominaga et al., 2006) and that the severity of self-reported disability among people with WADs correlates with the severity of ligamentous injuries found on magnetic resonance imaging (MRI) scans.

In the aggregate, this research points to multiple anatomical structures that can act as pain generators in patients with persistent WAD I or WAD II. However, the studies to date raise more questions than they answer. Consider, for example, research supporting the significance of ligamentous injuries to WAD. One important limitation in this research is that most of it has involved rats (Lee, Davis, Mejilla, & Winkelstein, 2004), computer simulations (Stemper et al., 2006), or cadavers (Stemper, Yoganandan, Gennarelli, & Pintar, 2005) rather than patients with persistent WAD. Moreover, research on asymptomatic people (Roy, Hol, Laerum, & Tillung, 2004; Wilmink & Patijn, 2001) and ones with neck pain secondary to cervical spondylosis rather than injury (Saifuddin, Green, & White, 2003) suggest that the MRI signals that some investigators have interpreted as indicators of ligamentous injuries should actually be considered normal variants or indicators of cervical degenerative disc disease.

In addition to intervertebral disc pathology, facet joint injury, and ligamentous injury, it is certainly possible that muscle dysfunction and muscle hypersensitivity contribute to WL pain in some patients. The role of myofascial problems in patients with neck pain, though not necessarily ones with WL, has received a great deal of attention from Simons (2001) and other proponents of MFP theory. But other investigators have generally not focused on the possibility that a substantial proportion of patients with WAD might have muscular pain. However, it is striking that many patients with WL report poorly localized pain that is aching in quality, and demonstrate tenderness in muscles of the neck and shoulder girdle. For example, unpublished data from our laboratory indicate that 18% of patients with symptoms of WAD report diffuse pain that is sufficiently widespread to suggest a diagnosis of FM. Moreover, widespread tenderness to palpation of muscles is also prevalent in patients with WL injuries. For example, Turk, Robinson, and Burwinkle (2006) found that 46% of a cohort of people with WADs, with no other known injuries, met the tender point criterion for a diagnosis of FM (i.e., they reported tenderness in at least 11 of the 18 sites designated by the ACR for the diagnosis (Wolfe et al., 1990). The significance of this widespread hyperalgesia strongly suggests that muscular pain is important for many patients with WL injuries.

DIAGNOSING MUSCULAR PAIN IN PATIENTS WITH WAD

In the previous discussion regarding the evaluation of patients with suspected MFP or FM, we emphasized that physicians need to consider a variety of explanations for patients' symptoms. The same logic applies to patients with WAD. In fact, since the role of muscle pain in WAD has received relatively little attention in research, our discussion below focuses on the overall evaluation of a patient with WAD, and places the evaluation of muscle pain as a cause of symptoms within the context of a comprehensive evaluation. The appropriate procedures for the medical evaluation of WADs depend to some extent on the point in time when the evaluation is performed. This discussion assumes that the patient being evaluated was involved in an MVC 3 months earlier, and was presumed to have a WAD I or II. It should be noted at the outset that there is no uniformly accepted algorithm for evaluating such a patient. In fact, as we discuss below, physicians differ sharply about some aspects of the medical evaluation of a presumed WAD I or II. It is helpful to organize the task of medical evaluation by considering questions that a physician essentially always wants to address. These are shown in Figure 16.6.

Are There "Red Flags"?

Although the assumption in this section is that the patient is undergoing evaluation for residuals of an MVC approximately 3 months earlier, occasionally the physician will find that the patient has misattributed his or her symptoms, and is actually symp-

tomatic because of a disease rather than because of the MVC. A general medical history that addresses issues such as weight loss or fevers should alert the physician to focus on the possibility of neoplasm or infection (Bigos et al., 1994).

If Symptoms Appear to Be the Result of Injury in the MVC, What Is the Nature of the Injury?

Neurological Disorders

The physician needs to be alert to clinical evidence of a cervical radiculopathy or a cervical myelopathy. Evidence for these possibilities comes from the patient's history (e.g., pain and paresthesias into an upper extremity in a segmental distribution) and a careful neurological examination. A cervical MRI scan is an important ancillary test, since it can demonstrate constriction of nerve roots or the spinal cord.

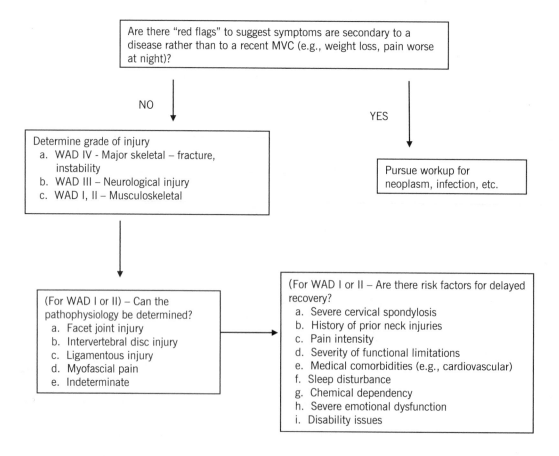

FIGURE 16.6. Issues to address in the medical evaluation of patients with WAD.

Major Skeletal Injuries

Radiological studies are needed to rule out the possibility that a patient has suffered a cervical spine fracture, or a ligamentous injury severe enough to yield instability. X-rays that include flexion and extension views are usually sufficient.

Musculoskeletal Pain Apparently Emanating from Joints of the Spine

Pain that is well localized to the neck or that spreads from the neck in a well-known referral pattern (Dwyer et al., 1990; Slipman et al., 2005) suggests that a patient is symptomatic as a result of an injury to a cervical disc or facet joint. In principle, a ligament injury could also be postulated as the cause of a patient's WAD symptoms. This possibility is difficult to rule in or to rule out, because the clinical symptoms associated with various ligament injuries are unknown, and there is uncertainty about the appropriate interpretation of MRI findings proposed by some investigators as indicators of ligament injury.

Myofascial Pain

MFP should be suspected if the pain diagram of a patient with WAD indicates fairly widespread pain in the neck and shoulder girdle region, especially if the pain approximates one of the myofascial patterns described by MFP proponents (Travell & Simons, 1983, 1992). If MFP is suspected, an examiner should use the procedures described earlier to determine whether a patient meets criteria for diagnosing MFP.

WIDESPREAD "NONANATOMIC" PAIN

Physicians who practice musculoskeletal medicine try to explain symptoms following an injury in terms of well-defined, objectively measurable structural lesion in joints, periarticular tissues, muscles, and nerves in the body region where the patient is symptomatic (Robinson, Ricketts, & Hanscom, 2005). Although this approach often yields enormous dividends, the symptoms of many patients with WADs do not fit a pattern that suggests some discrete injury to a musculoskeletal structure. In this setting, a few pos-

sibilities should be considered. One is that the patient has muscular pain—for example, one of the many cervical MFP syndromes discussed by Travell and Simons (1983, 1992). A second possibility is irritation of a cervical disc or cervical facet joint with referred pain (Dwyer et al., 1990; Slipman et al., 2005). A final possibility is that a patient's pain might be "nonanatomic" because it is largely a reflection of altered CNS functioning rather than of ongoing nociception from a peripheral source (Robinson & Apkarian, 2009). It should be noted that this option may well encompass the other two.

Specific Procedures

History

It is beyond the scope of this chapter to discuss the elements of a thorough history. It is worth noting, though, that in evaluating a patient with WAD, the physician should pay careful attention to certain historical items that are considered only cursorily in other clinical settings. In particular, the physician should be careful to assess the patient's history with respect to chemical dependency, his or her reported level of incapacitation, and his or her status with respect to litigation and compensation.

Physical Examination

A neurological examination should be performed on all patients with a WAD. In the context of WAD I or II injuries, this will be negative. A musculoskeletal examination of WAD I and II patients often is not especially revealing with respect to determining the role that pathology in intervertebral discs, facet joints, or ligaments play in a patient's symptoms (Bogduk & McGuirk, 2006). But some useful information can be gleaned from a physical examination. First, the examiner can determined the severity of the patient's functional limitations—especially restricted motion of the neck and pain-inhibited weakness of neck and upper extremity muscles. Second, the physician can determine whether the patient demonstrates significant apprehension and "nonorganic signs" (Main & Waddell, 1998; Waddell, McCulloch, Kummel, & Venner, 1980). Research indicates that patients with nonorganic signs usually have significant somatic anxiety. This emotional distress may impair their recoveries, and may be a focus of treatment.

Finally, the physical examination is crucial to the determination of whether MFP is an important contributor to a patient's pain. At the very least, the physician should examine for muscular tenderness, both in muscles of the neck/shoulder girdle and in remote sites. Although examination of muscle tenderness in remote sites may not seem particularly germane to the evaluation of a patient with a WAD, there is growing evidence that patients with WAD often have widespread tenderness (Banic et al., 2004; Turk et al., 2006). The presence of widespread muscular tenderness would greatly strengthen the hypothesis that muscular pain/dysfunction is contributing to a patient's symptoms. Physicians familiar with examination procedures for myofasical TrPs should strongly consider looking for them.

Ancillary Studies

Although laboratory studies and electrodiagnostic evaluations are occasionally helpful in the assessment of patients with WAD, imaging modalities are the procedures that are done most frequently. There is significant controversy about how and when imaging should be done on patients with WAD. Without attempting to resolve these controversies in any systematic way, we suggest the following:

1. Since WL involves trauma, it is reasonable to check for the possibility of a cervical spine fracture or significant spinal instability using plain X-rays of the cervical spine.
2. Additional imaging is generally not needed for a patient with a WAD I or II injury. However, if there is some clinical evidence of a neurological injury, an MRI scan is generally indicated.
3. Computed tomography (CT) scans and bone scans usually have a limited role; they can be obtained to identify an occult fracture or an inflamed facet joint.

A great deal of controversy surrounds the use of discography and injections to diagnose facet joint–mediated pain (medial branch blocks or intra-articular facet joint injections). Although these procedures utilize imaging, they rely on pain provocation and pain palliation in response to injections to determine the anatomic basis of patients' pain. Some experts in spine care recommend cervical spine fusions following positive discography, or denervation of the sensory fibers to facet joints via radiofrequency medial branch ablations following positive medial branch blocks. It is beyond the scope of this chapter to review the controversies surrounding treatment based on discography or medial branch blocks. Instead, we offer a few opinions that are consistent with those of leaders in the area of spine care. First, patients with WAD with obvious concomitant psychological dysfunction or obvious markers of altered CNS function should not be referred for diagnostic procedures that rely on pain provocation and palpation (Carragee, Lincoln, Parmar, & Alamin, 2006). Second, the interpretation of discography is so uncertain that we do not recommend it in any circumstance. Third, there is research support for the use of medial branch blocks to detect cervical facet arthropathies, combined with treatment of facet joint–mediated pain by means of radiofrequency ablations of the appropriate medial branches (Lord et al., 1996; McDonald et al., 1999). We believe referral for medial branch blocks is appropriate for patients with WAD who continue to report symptoms despite conservative treatment, and who have no evidence of either altered CNS function or significant psychological dysfunction.

It should be noted that all of these ancillary tests are directed toward identifying major skeletal injuries, neurological injuries, or pathology in intervertebral discs or facet joints as causes of a patient's WAD. The role of muscle pain is determined by the history and physical examination; no ancillary tests are diagnostic of muscle dysfunction or muscle hypersensitivity in patients with WAD.

MUSCLE PAIN: BASIC CONCEPTS AND CONTROVERSIES

Terminology: Muscle Pain versus MPP

As noted earlier, we use muscle pain in a descriptive sense—to denote poorly localized, aching pain that appears to emanate from muscles, together with tenderness over the muscles. MFP is a more complex term, however, that has meaning only in relation to a complex theory. Simons (2001), a leading proponent of MFP, states:

> The myofascial pain syndrome, in its strict sense, is a regional pain syndrome characterized by the presence of myofascial trigger points (TrPs). . . . The most distinctive clinical characteristics of TrPs include circumscribed spot tenderness in a nodule that is part of a palpably tense band of muscle fibers, patient recognition of the pain that is evoked by pressure on the tender spot as being familiar, pain referred in the pattern characteristic of TrPs in that muscle, a local twitch response, painful limitation of stretch range of motion, and some weakness of that muscle. (p. 205)

It is plausible to surmise from this that MFP is essentially equivalent to muscle pain, and that TrPs are more or less equivalent to tender areas in muscle. In fact, many authors have used the term *myofascial pain syndrome* in a loose sense to describe a syndrome in which a patient presents with muscle tenderness and complaints of muscular pain (Bennett, 2007). Simons (2001) describes this situation as follows:

> [The term myofascial pain syndrome] has acquired both a general and a specific meaning, which need to be distinguished. . . . The general meaning includes a regional muscle pain syndrome of any soft tissue origin that is associated with muscle tenderness, . . . and it is commonly used in this sense by dentists. . . . The other meaning is specifically a MPS caused by TrPs. (p. 211)

However, there are several considerations that challenge the equation of MFP with muscle pain, and TrPs with tender areas in muscle:

1. The descriptive criteria given earlier for designating pain as muscle pain are fairly simple. In contrast, the clinical phenomena used to identify TrPs are more complex and difficult for clinicians to master. Although these criteria are nominally objective, research has demonstrated that the actual situation is more complex. A necessary condition for a clinical finding to be considered objective is that different observers are able to agree about when it is present (i.e., that there be acceptable interrater reliability). Re-

search has shown that interrater reliability is good for the identification of tender sites in muscles, as is done in examinations for FM (Aloush, Ablin, Reitblat, Caspi, & Elkayam, 2007; Khostanteen, Tunks, Goldsmith, & Ennis, 2000; Weiner, Sakamoto, Perera, & Breuer, 2006). To diagnose myofascial TrPs, examiners must be able to identify not only tenderness over certain areas of muscles but also other abnormalities, as described earlier by Simons (2001). The ability of physicians to identify these other features of TrPs reliably is questionable (Hsieh et al., 2000; Wolfe et al., 1992).

Another issue that bears on the objectivity of TrPs is that clinicians appear to have markedly different thresholds for deciding that a TrP exists, or that a patient has significant MFP. We are not aware of any published literature on this issue, but informal observation supports the view that some clinicians diagnose MFP in a very high proportion of patients with musculoskeletal pain, whereas others use the diagnosis much less frequently (and still others essentially do not consider MFP to be a legitimate medical diagnosis).

2. Although muscle pain can in principle be discussed without any hypotheses about its pathophysiology, "TrPs" and "MFP" are embedded in a complex theory about muscle dysfunction and related muscular pain. A recent formulation of this theory has been named "the integrated TrP hypothesis" (Simons, 2001). It is beyond the scope of this chapter to describe this hypothesis in detail, but broadly speaking, it postulates that TrPs are consequences of muscle overload and abnormal muscle metabolism.

3. A key assumption of MFP theory is that TrPs represent "upstream" biological abnormalities that put an individual at risk for pain but are not synonymous with pain. In a seminal text on MFP, Travell and Simons (1983, 1992) make it clear that they view a TrP as an indicator of deranged function in a muscle that predisposes an individual to muscular pain. The relation between TrPs and muscular pain could be seen as analogous to the relation between coronary artery stenosis and angina. The distinction that Travell and Simons make between TrPs and muscular pain permits them to introduce the concept of latent TrPs. These are points that meet the criteria for TrPs when they are ex-

amined but are not associated with clinically significant pain.

One might conceptualize relations between TrPs and muscle pain by the Venn diagram in Figure 16.7. As this diagram suggests, a substantial overlap between TrPs and muscle pain can be postulated. It is possible for individuals to have TrPs, however, but not have clinically significant muscle pain (i.e., latent TrPs). Another logical possibility shown in the diagram is that there might be individuals who have clinically significant muscle pain but not TrPs. Although Simons (2001) mentions this possibility, we are not aware of any detailed discussions of nonmyofascial muscular pain by MFP theory proponents.

Confusion between muscle pain as a descriptive term and MFP as a theory-laden term is aggravated by the fact that many researchers use the term *myofascial pain*, even though they have not followed the evaluation procedures necessary to determine whether patients have TrPs. Consequently, at the present time, it is difficult, if not impossible, to determine whether studies on "myofascial pain" address the construct defined by Travell and Simons (1983, 1992).

Divergent Perspectives on MFP

Proponents of MFP theory assert that MFP exists, and that it plays a major role in chronic musculoskeletal pain. Some research indicates a high prevalence of MFP among various patient populations, with rates ranging from 30% among patients in a general medical clinic (Skootsky, Jaeger, & Oye, 1989) to 85% among patients treated at a pain center (Fishbain, Goldberg, Meagher, Steele, & Rosomoff, 1986). As is the case with other forms of chronic pain, women seem to be more often afflicted than men. The sex difference, however, is not very large when it concerns MFP syndrome (Fricton, 1990). Even among young adults with no clinical muscle pain, the prevalence of latent TrPs (manifested by physical examination findings indicative of TrPs) has been reported to be approximately 50% (Sola, Rodenberger, & Gettys, 1955). These data suggest that MFP syndrome is a major cause of musculoskeletal pain.

At the opposite extreme, many physicians ignore MFP entirely. For example, the term *myofascial pain* does not appear in the index of *Essentials of Musculoskeletal Medicine* (Greene, 2001) or *Campbell's Operative Orthopaedics* (Canale, 2003). Still others criticize the concept of MFP, suggesting that patients diagnosed with MFP actually have chronic pain syndromes with somatoform features (Bohr, 1995).

Informal observation suggests that only a minority of physicians who specialize in the management of musculoskeletal disorders subscribe to the principles outlined by Simons (2001) and other proponents of myofascial theory. If this observation is valid, it raises an obvious question: Why do so many specialists in musculoskeletal medicine not

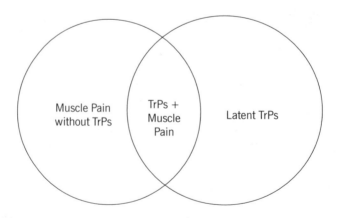

FIGURE 16.7. Venn diagram showing relations among myofascial pain (TrPs + muscle pain), latent TrPs, and muscle pain without TrPs.

follow the tenets proposed by Simons? The question is difficult to answer, because many physicians simply ignore MFP theory, without elaborating their reasons for doing so.

We assume that physicians who do not subscribe to the tenets of MFP theory notice that muscular pain is present in some of their patients (i.e., they notice that some patients report pain in muscles and demonstrate tenderness to palpation of muscles). We believe that they reject the MFP model for one of two reasons. Some follow what has been called the *structural lesion model of musculoskeletal pain* (Robinson et al., 2005). This model, which dominates in orthopedics, holds that musculoskeletal pain typically follows injury or dysfunction in joints, periarticular tissues, or nerves. From the standpoint of the structural lesion model, muscular pain would be construed as a secondary phenomenon that is not an appropriate target for treatment. Just as an infectious disease specialist addresses the pathogen causing an infection rather than directly treating the fever that occurs during an infection, so an orthopedist is likely to direct attention to joints, periarticular tissues, or nerves rather than to the muscle pain that might result from dysfunction in these tissues.

Other physicians argue that patients who present with muscular pain are actually demonstrating abnormal pain behavior (Pilowsky, 1995) that reflects psychiatric dysfunction (e.g., a somatoform disorder) rather than a genuine musculoskeletal disorder.

CONCLUSIONS

Despite the fact that muscle pain occurs commonly in everyone's life, clinicians and researchers have had great difficulty determining the significance of muscle pain and dysfunction in patients with chronic musculoskeletal symptoms. Extensive research has been done on two syndromes that ostensibly involve muscular pain—FM and MFP. In this chapter, we have discussed diagnostic criteria for these two disorders, and the evaluation of muscular pain that does not fit either diagnostic category. Also, we have discussed the role of muscle pain in one common regional pain syndrome—WAD.

We note that the medical evaluation of FM and MFP should not be limited to making a diagnosis; rather, it should include a broad search for comorbid conditions, some of which might be viewed as causes of patients' muscular pain. Also, since patients with FM or MFP typically have chronic symptoms, we believe their pain and functional limitations result from a complex interplay of factors. Thus, the assessment strategies described in this chapter should be supplemented by the ones described by Turk and Robinson (Chapter 10, this volume) for the evaluation of chronic pain.

ACKNOWLEDGMENT

Preparation of this chapter was supported by Grant No. AR44724 from the National Institutes of Health/National Institute of Arthritis and Musculoskeletal and Skin Disorders.

REFERENCES

Aloush, V., Ablin, J. N., Reitblat, T., Caspi, D., & Elkayam, O. (2007). Fibromyalgia in women with ankylosing spondylitis. *Rheumatology International, 27,* 865–868.

Banic, B., Petersen-Felix, S., Andersen, O. K., et al. (2004). Evidence for spinal cord hypersensitivity in chronic pain after whiplash injury and in fibromyalgia. *Pain, 107,* 7–15.

Barnsley, L., Lord, S., & Bogduk, N. (1994). Comparative local anaesthetic blocks in the diagnosis of cervical zygapophysial joint pain. *Pain, 55,* 99–106.

Bennett, R. (2007). Myofascial pain syndromes and their evaluation. *Best Practices in Research in Clinical Rheumatology, 21,* 427–445.

Bennett, R. M. (1989). Beyond fibromyalgia: Ideas on etiology and treatment. *Journal of Rheumatology, 16*(Suppl. 19), 185–191.

Bigos, S., Bowyer, O., Braen, G., et al. (1994). *Acute low back problems in adults* (Clinical Practice Guideline No. 14, AHCPR Publication No. 95-0642). Rockville, MD: Agency for Health Care Policy and Research, Public Health Service, U.S. Department of Health and Human Services.

Bogduk, N. (2002). Diagnostic nerve blocks in chronic pain. *Best Practices and Research in Clinical Anaesthesiology, 16,* 565–578.

Bogduk, N., & McGuirk, B. (2006). *Management of acute and chronic neck pain: An evidence-based approach.* New York: Elsevier.

Bohr, T. W. (1995). Fibromyalgia syndrome and

myofascial pain syndrome: Do they exist? *Neurological Clinics, 13*, 365–384.

Boissevain, M. D., & McCain, G. A. (1991). Toward an integrated understanding of fibromyalgia syndrome: I. Medical and pathophysiological aspects. *Pain, 45,* 227–238.

Canale, S. T. (Ed.). (2003*). Campbell's operative orthopaedics* (10th ed.). St. Louis, MO: Mosby.

Carragee, E. J., Lincoln, T., Parmar, V. K. S., & Alamin, T. (2006). A gold standard evaluation of the "discogneic pain" diagnosis as determine by provocative discography. *Spine, 31,* 2115–2123.

Carville, S. F., Arendt-Nielsen, L., Bliddal, H., et al. (2008). EULAR evidence-based recommendations for the management of fibromyalgia syndrome. *Annals of the Rheumatic Diseases, 67,* 536–541.

Clauw, D. J. (2010). Fibromyalgia. In J. C. Ballantyne, J. P. Rathmell, & S. M. Fishman (Eds.), *Bonica's management of pain* (4th ed., p. 710). Philadelphia: Lippincott Williams & Wilkins.

Clemens, H. J., & Burrow, K. (1972). Experimental investigation on injury mechanisms of cervical spine at frontal and rear-frontal vehicle impacts. In *Proceedings of the 16th STAPP Care Crash Conference* (pp. 76–104). Warrendale, PA: Society of Automotive Engineers.

Dommerholt, J., & Shah, J. P. (2010). Myofascial pain syndrome. In J. C. Ballantyne, J. P. Rathmell, & S. M. Fishman (Eds.), *Bonica's management of pain* (4th ed., pp. 450–471). Philadelphia: Lippincott Williams & Wilkins.

Dwyer, A., April, C., & Bogduk, N. (1990). Cervical zygapophyseal joint pain patterns: I. A study in normal volunteers. *Spine, 15,* 453–457.

Fishbain, D. A., Goldberg, M., Meagher, B. R., Steele, R., & Rosomoff, H. (1986). Male and female chronic pain patients categorized by DSM-III psychiatric diagnostic criteria. *Pain, 26,* 181–197.

Fricton, J. R. (1990). Musculoskeletal measures of orofacial pain. *Anesthesia Progress, 37,* 136–143.

Gay, J., & Abbot, K. (1953). Common whiplash injuries of the neck. *Journal of the American Medical Association, 152,* 1698–1704.

Gibson, T., Bogduk, N., MacPherson, J., & McIntosh, A. (2000). Crash characteristics of whiplash associated chronic neck pain. *Journal of Musculoskeletal Pain, 8,* 87–95.

Goldenberg, D. L., Burckhardt, C., & Crofford, L. (2004). Management of fibromyalgia syndrome. *Journal of the American Medical Association, 17,* 2388–2395.

Gowers, W. R. (1904). Lumbago: Its lessons and analogues. *British Medical Journal, 1,* 117–121.

Greene, W. B. (Ed.). (2001). *Essentials of musculoskeletal medicine* (2nd ed.). Rosemont, IL: American Academy of Orthopaedic Surgeons.

Gunn, C. C. (1996). *Gunn approach to the treatment of chronic pain: Intramuscular stimulation for myofascial pain of radiculopathic origin* (3rd ed.). Philadelphia: Churchill Livingstone.

Hauser, W., Bernardy, K., Arnold, B., Offenbacher, M., & Schiltenwolf, M. (2009). Efficacy of multicomponent treatment in fibromyalgia syndrome: A meta-analysis of randomized controlled clinical trials. *Arthritis Care and Research, 61,* 216–224.

Hsieh, C. Y., Hong, C. Z., Adams, A. H., Platt, K. J., Danielson, C. D., Hoehler, F. K., et al. (2000). Interexaminer reliability of the palpation of trigger points in the trunk and lower limb muscles. *Archives of Physical Medicine and Rehabilitation, 81,* 258–264.

Khostanteen, I., Tunks, E. R., Goldsmith, C. H., & Ennis, J. (2000). Fibromyalgia: Can one distinguish it from simulation?: An observer-blind controlled study. *Journal of Rheumatology, 27,* 2671–2676.

Lee, K. E., Davis, M. B., Mejilla, R. M., & Winkelstein, B. A. (2004). In vivo cervical facet capsule distraction: Mechanical implications for whiplash and neck pain. *STAPP Car Crash Journal, 48,* 373–395.

Lord, S. M., Barnsley, L., Wallis, B. J., McDonald, G. J., & Bogduk, N. (1996). Percutaneous radio-frequency neurotomy for chronic zygapophysial-joint pain. *New England Journal of Medicine, 335,* 1721–1726.

Main, C. J., & Waddell, G. (1998). Behavioral responses to examination: A reappraisal of the interpretation of "nonorganic signs." *Spine, 23,* 2367–2371.

Manchikanti, L., Singh, V., Rivera, J., & Pampati, V. (2002). Prevalence of cervical facet joint pain in chronic neck pain. *Pain Physician, 5,* 243–249.

Mayou, R., & Radanov, B. P. (1996). Whiplash neck injury. *Journal of Psychosomatic Research, 40,* 461–474.

McDonald, G., Lord, S. M., & Bogduk, N. (1999). Long-term follow-up of patients treated with cervical radiofrequency neurotomy for chronic neck pain. *Neurosurgery, 45,* 61–68.

Mense, S., & Simons, D. G. (2001). *Muscle pain: Understanding its nature, diagnosis, and treatment.* Philadelphia: Lippincott Williams & Wilkins.

Pennie, B., & Agambar, L. (1991). Patterns of injury and recovery in whiplash. *Injury, 22,* 57–59.

Pilowsky, I. (1995). Low back pain and illness behavior (inappropriate, maladaptive, or abnormal). *Spine, 20,* 1522–1524.

Reynolds, M. D. (1983). The development of the

concept of fibrositis. *Journal of History of Medical and Allied Science, 38,* 5–35.

Robinson, J. P., & Apkarian, A. V. (2009). Low back pain. In E. A. Mayer & M. C. Bushnell (Eds.), *Functional pain syndromes: Presentation and pathophysiology* (pp. 128–142). Seattle, WA: IASP Press.

Robinson, J. P., Ricketts, D., & Hanscom, D. A. (2005). Musculoskeletal pain. In H. Merskey, J. D. Loeser, & R. Dubner (Eds.), *The paths of pain 1975–2005* (pp. 114–129). Seattle, WA: IASP Press.

Roy, S., Hol, P. K., Laerum, L. T., & Tillung, T. (2004). Pitfalls of magnetic resonance imaging of alar ligament. *Neuroradiology, 46,* 392–398.

Saifuddin, A., Green, R., & White, J. (2003). Magnetic resonance imaging of the cervical ligaments in the absence of trauma. *Spine, 28,* 1686–1691; discussion 1691–1692.

Simons, D. G. (1986). Fibrositis/fibromyalgia: A form of myofascial trigger points? *American Journal of Medicine, 81*(Suppl. 3A), 93–98.

Simons, D. G. (2001). Myofascial pain caused by trigger points. In S. Mense & D. G. Simons (Eds.), *Muscle pain: Understanding its nature, diagnosis, and treatment* (pp. 205–288). Philadelphia: Lippincott Williams & Wilkins.

Skootsky, S. A., Jaeger, B., & Oye, R. K. (1989). Prevalence of myofascial pain in general internal medicine practice. *Western Journal of Medicine, 151,* 157–160.

Slipman, C. W., Plastaras, C., Patel, R., et al. (2005). Provocative cervical discography symptom mapping. *Spine Journal, 5,* 381–388.

Smythe, H. (1986). Tender points: Evolution of concepts of the fibrositis/fibromyalgia syndrome. *American Journal of Medicine, 81*(Suppl. 3A), 2–6.

Smythe, H. (1989). Fibrositis syndrome: A historical perspective. *Journal of Rheumatology, 16*(Suppl. 19), 2–6.

Smythe, H. A., & Moldofsky, H. (1977). Two contributions to understanding of the "fibrositis" syndrome. *Bulletin of the Rheumatic Diseases, 28,* 928–931.

Sola, A. E., Rodenberger, M. L., & Gettys, B. B. (1955). Incidence of hypersensitive areas in posterior shoulder muscles. *American Journal of Physical Medicine, 34,* 585–590.

Spitzer, W. O., Skovron, M. L., Salmi, L. R., et al. (1995). Scientific monograph of the Quebec Task Force on Whiplash-Associated Disorders: Redefining "whiplash" and its management. *Spine, 20*(Suppl.8), 1S–73S.

Staud, R. (2004). New evidence for central sensitization in patients with fibromyalgia. *Current Rheumatology Reports, 6,* 259–281.

Staud, R., & Rodriguez, M. E. (2006). Mechanisms of disease: Pain in fibromyalgia syndrome. *Nature Clinics Practice of Rheumatology, 2,* 90–98.

Stemper, B. D., Yoganandan, N., Gennarelli, T. A., & Pintar, F. A. (2005). Localized cervical facet joint kinematics under physiological and whiplash loading. *Journal of Neurosurgery: Spine, 3,* 471–476.

Stemper, B. D., Yoganandan, N., Pintar, F. A., & Rao, R. D. (2006). Anterior longitudinal ligament injuries in whiplash may lead to cervical instability. *Medical Engineering and Physics, 28,* 515–524.

Tominaga, Y., Ndu, A. B., Coe, M. P., et al. (2006). Neck ligament strength is decreased following whiplash trauma. *BMC Musculoskeletal Disorders, 7,* 103.

Travell, J. G., & Simons, D. G. (1983). *Myofascial pain and dysfunction* (Vol. 1). Baltimore: Williams & Wilkins.

Travell, J. G., & Simons, D. G. (1992). *Myofascial pain and dysfunction* (Vol. 2). Baltimore: Williams & Wilkins.

Turk, D. C., Robinson, J. P., & Burwinkle, T. M. (2006). Prevalence of fibromyalgia tender points following whiplash injury. *Journal of Pain, 7*(Suppl. 2), S27.

Waddell, G., McCulloch, J. A., Kummel, E., & Venner, R. M. (1980). Nonorganic physical signs in low-back pain. *Spine, 5,* 117–125.

Watkinson, A., Gargan, M. G., & Bannister, G. C. (1991). Prognostic factors in soft tissue injuries of the cervical spine. *Injury, 22,* 307–309.

Weiner, D. K., Sakamoto, S., Perera, S., & Breuer, P. (2006). Chronic low back pain in older adults: Prevalence, reliability, and validity of physical examination findings. *Journal of the American Geriatric Society, 54,* 11–20.

Wilmink, J. T., & Patijn, J. (2001). MR imaging of alar ligament in whiplash-associated disorders: An observer study. *Neuroradiology, 43,* 859–863.

Wolfe, F., Simons, D. G., Fricton, J., Bennett, R. M., Goldenberg, D. L., Gerwin, R., et al. (1992). The fibromyalgia and myofascial pain syndromes: A preliminary study of tender points and trigger points in persons with fibromyalgia, myofascial pain syndrome and no disease. *Journal of Rheumatology, 19,* 944–951.

Wolfe, F., Smythe, H. A., Yunus, M. B., Bennett, R. M., Bombardier, C., Goldenberg, D. L., et al. (1990). The American College of Rheumatology 1990 criteria for the classification of fibromyalgia [Report of the Multicenter Criteria Committee]. *Arthritis and Rheumatism, 33,* 160–172.

Yunus, M., Masi, A. T., Calabro, J. J., Miller, K. A., & Feigenbaum, S. L. (1981). Primary fibromyalgia (fibrositis): Clinical study of 50 patients with matched normal controls. *Seminars in Arthritis and Rheumatism, 11,* 151–171.

CHAPTER 17

Assessment of Neuropathic Pain

IAN GILRON
NADINE ATTAL
DIDIER BOUHASSIRA
ROBERT H. DWORKIN

Neuropathic pain (NP) was defined in 1994 by the International Association for the Study of Pain (IASP), as "pain initiated or caused by a primary lesion or dysfunction in the nervous system" (Merskey & Bogduk, 1994, p. 212). NP may result from a wide variety of metabolic, toxic, infectious, traumatic, and mechanical disorders that affect the brain, spinal cord, or peripheral nerves. Examples of common and well-characterized NP conditions include cervical/lumbar radiculopathy, painful diabetic neuropathy, postsurgical/posttraumatic neuralgia, postherpetic neuralgia (PHN), chemotherapy-induced painful neuropathy, HIV neuropathy, spinal cord injury pain, multiple sclerosis–related pain, complex regional pain syndrome, and trigeminal neuralgia (Jensen, Gottrup, Sindrup, & Bach, 2001). Although more epidemiological studies are needed, the community prevalence of pain of neuropathic origin has been estimated to range between 7 and 8% (Bouhassira, Lantéri-Minet, Attal, Laurent, & Touboul, 2008; Torrance, Smith, Bennett, & Lee, 2006) of the general population, suggesting that this is a significant health problem with a substantial impact on quality of life and health care utilization (Atlas et al., 1996; Coplan et al., 2004; O'Connor, 2009; Zelman, Gore, Dukes, Tai, & Brandenburg, 2005).

In the setting of individual patient care, optimal assessment of NP may serve to (1) aid in formulating a differential diagnosis of, and prognosis for, the presenting problem; (2) guide appropriate treatment selection; and (3) evaluate individual responses to treatment (Backonja & Galer, 1998; Baron & Tölle, 2008; Hansson, 2002). On a larger, population scale or in the setting of clinical research, detailed assessment of NP is crucial for (1) the study of NP incidence, prevalence, and natural history; (2) the continued investigation into treatment-susceptible mechanisms of NP; and (3) the design and conduct of clinical trials (Cruccu et al., 2004). Over the past century or so, the assessment of NP has evolved immensely from early crude evaluations of pain (vs. no pain) as a dichotomous outcome (Fowler, 1886) to subsequent distinctions between spontaneous and evoked pain (Bigelow, Harrison, Goodell, Wolff, 1945) to multifaceted sensory and affective characteristics of pain intensity, pain quality, and pain unpleasantness (Melzack, 1975) to technologically detailed assessment of sensory function (Rolke et al., 2006a).

Since publication of the IASP definition of NP in 1994, consideration of its assessment is affected by as yet unresolved controversy over whether this definition is overly broad and may lead to the inclusion of conditions that are not truly due to organic nerve disease or injury (Backonja, 2003; Bennett, 2003; Max, 2002; Merskey, 2002; Treede et al., 2008). Whether or not a clearly demonstrable nerve lesion has been proven, several potential advantages of carefully and thoroughly assessing the person with suspected NP have been proposed. As a very fundamental clinical example, assessment of pain in a person with bilateral leg pain that allows for the differentiation between NP (e.g., due to diabetic neuropathy) and nociceptive ischemic pain (e.g., due to intermittent claudication associated with arterial occlusive disease) will have an immense impact on formulating a treatment strategy for that person's underlying problem, as well as his or her pain. From a research perspective, focused assessment of various features of NP may serve to link putative treatments (e.g., novel pharmacological targets), pain signs and symptoms (e.g., hyperalgesia, allodynia, shock–like or burning pains), and susceptible pain mechanisms (e.g., central sensitization, descending inhibition, and facilitation), with a view toward developing "mechanism-based" NP treatment strategies (Finnerup & Jensen, 2006; Woolf et al., 1998; Woolf & Max, 2001).

Although not the focus of this chapter, it should be noted that comprehensive clinical assessment of the *patient* with a NP problem must address a multitude of factors, including diagnosis of the underlying disease (e.g., neoplastic tumor compressing a nerve), impact of the current pain problem on physical function (e.g., occupational disability), mood (e.g., related depression) and sleep, a history of previously tried treatments and responses, and an evaluation of the patient's current coping strategies and support systems (see Turk & Robinson, Chapter 10, this volume). Thus, our objectives in this chapter are to describe current approaches to and investigative efforts for the advancement of the assessment of pain itself in human neuropathic conditions. As will be reviewed in detail, the development of methodology to better assess

NP has very much been a research endeavor. However, the role of NP assessment in routine clinical care is also discussed.

PAINFUL VERSUS NONPAINFUL SENSORY ABNORMALITIES

In addition to "positive" symptoms such as pain (reviewed in detail below), itching (Binder, Koroschetz, & Baron, 2008; Jacome, 1978), and other paresthesias (i.e., abnormal sensations that are not unpleasant) (Merskey & Bogduk, 1994) described as "tingling" (Tinel, 1915), "pins and needles" (Bennett, 2001), or "numbness," nerve injury or disease may also result in "negative" signs of sensory loss (Noordenbos, 1959; Rowbotham & Fields, 1989). If perceived as unpleasant, "tingling" or "pins and needles" sensations are instead referred to as *dysesthesias* (Merskey & Bogduk, 1994). Other nonpainful responses to external stimuli include *analgesia* ("absence of pain in response to a stimulus which is normally painful"), *hypoesthesia* ("decreased sensitivity to stimulation excluding the special senses"), and *hyperesthesia* ("increased sensitivity to stimulation excluding the special senses") (Merskey & Bogduk, 1994). As discussed in the later section on quantitative sensory testing, semiobjective measures of non-nociceptive detection thresholds during cutaneous mechanical and cold and heat stimulation may serve to evaluate functional abnormalities of A-β, A-δ, and C sensory nerve fibers (Yarnitsky, 1997) (see Figure 17.1).

Although a seemingly singular entity, pain due to nerve injury or disease has many different features that should be assessed. First, NP can exhibit "spontaneous" (or stimulus-independent) versus "evoked" (or stimulus-dependent) components, both of which may coexist at the same time (Bennett, 1994). There may be no predictable escape from spontaneous NP, whereas evoked pain may be minimized through avoidance of the pain-evoking stimulus (e.g., removal of a shirt in thoracic PHN or avoidance of walking in diabetic neuropathy). However, avoidance of stimulus-evoked NP may have an obvious negative impact on sleep, as well as physical and social function (Coplan et al., 2004; Zelman et al., 2005).

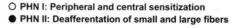

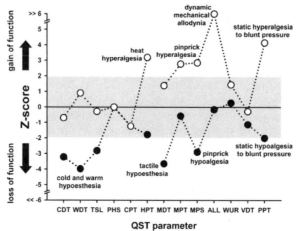

FIGURE 17.1. *z*-Score sensory profiles of two patients with postherpetic neuralgia (PHN). Patient PHN I (open circles) presents the QST profile of a 70-year-old woman suffering from PHN for 8 years. Ongoing pain was 80 on a 0–100 numerical rating scale. The profile shows a predominant gain of sensory function in terms of heat pain hyperalgesia (HPT), pinprick mechanical hyperalgesia (MPS), dynamic mechanical allodynia (ALL), and static hyperalgesia to blunt pressure (PPT) outside the 95% confidence interval of the distribution of healthy subjects (= gray zone). This profile is consistent with a combination of peripheral and central sensitization. Patient PHN II (filled circles) shows the QST profile of a 71-year-old woman with pain for 8 months. Ongoing pain was 70 on a 0–100 numerical rating scale. The QST profile shows predominant loss of sensory function. Note the cold (CDT) and warm detection thresholds (WDT), thermal sensory limen (TSL), tactile detection thresholds (MDT), mechanical pain thresholds to pinprick stimuli (MPT), and pressure pain thresholds (PPT) outside the normal range as presented by the gray zone. This profile is consistent with a combined small and large fiber sensory deafferentation. *z*-Score: numbers of standard deviations between patient data and group-specific mean value. From Rolke, Baron, et al. (2006). This figure has been reproduced with permission of the International Association for the Study of Pain. The figure may not be reproduced for any other purpose without permission.

SPONTANEOUS (STIMULUS-INDEPENDENT) VERSUS EVOKED (STIMULUS-DEPENDENT) NP

In the absence of external physical stimulation, *spontaneous* NP may be continuous (e.g., foot pain in diabetic neuropathy) or intermittent (e.g., spontaneous pain paroxysms in trigeminal neuralgia). Continuous pain is generally always present, although it may vary in intensity over time. For example, pain intensity ratings in patients with painful diabetic neuropathy and PHN have been reported to increase steadily throughout the course of a day (Odrcich, Bailey, Cahill, & Gilron, 2006). In addition to temporal variations in pain intensity, individuals with NP often also report variable pain *qualities*, such as burning, cold, sharpness, and squeezing (Attal et al., 2008; Galer & Jensen, 1997). Intermittent NPs, often referred to as pain *paroxysms*, are often described as "shooting," "stabbing," or "electric shock–like" in quality and may vary over time in intensity, duration, and frequency (Attal et al., 2008; Gilron, Booher, Rowan, Smoller, & Max, 2000).

Evoked or *stimulus-dependent* NP is generally defined with reference to the evoking stimulus. Whereas *hyperalgesia* denotes "an increased response to a stimulus which is normally painful," *allodynia* denotes "pain due to a stimulus which does not normally provoked pain" (Merskey & Bogduk, 1994, pp. 210–211). Other painful responses to evoking stimuli include *hyperpathia* ("an abnormally painful reaction to a stimulus, especially a repetitive stimulus, as well as an increased threshold") and *hypoalgesia* ("diminished pain in response to a normally painful stimulus") (Merskey & Bogduk, 1994, p. 212). Since normal activities and situations present evoking stimuli, evoked NP can substantially increase the overall severity of a patient's daily pain experience, as well as impede physical and social function. Quantitative evaluation of hyperalgesia and allodynia (discussed below) with respect to the required intensity of the evoking stimulus and/or the magnitude of the pain response may serve to characterize better the nature of NP in research, and possibly even patient care settings (Rolke, Baron, et al., 2006).

RESEARCH ON THE ASSESSMENT OF HUMAN NP

Measurement of Pain Quality Descriptors

Careful description and measurement of NP symptoms can serve to fulfill two broad goals: (1) diagnostic screening of NP versus non-neuropathic pain conditions and (2) detailed characterization of specific symptoms for use in research on natural history, pathophysiology, and treatment response.

Following early human investigations that highlighted various different pain qualities (e.g., "burning" vs. "pricking") (Bigelow et al., 1945; Weddell, Sinclair, & Feindel, 1948), more focused efforts toward expanding the nomenclature of verbal descriptors for the sensory, affective, and evaluative aspects of the pain experience represented major milestones in pain assessment (Gracely, McGrath, & Dubner, 1978; Melzack, 1975). In particular, development of the self-report McGill Pain Questionnaire (MPQ) by Ronald Melzack (1975) revealed that pain quality descriptors vary across different pain conditions (see also Katz & Melzack, Chapter 3, this volume). Subsequent studies showed that various descriptors from the MPQ could be useful in distinguishing between NP and non-neuropathic pain conditions (Boureau, Doubrère, & Luu, 1990; Dubuisson & Melzack, 1976; Masson, Hunt, Gem, & Boulton, 1989; Melzack, Terrence, Fromm, & Amsel, 1986) (see Table 17.1A), although negative data have been reported with use of the Short-Form MPQ (SF-MPQ; Rasmussen, Sindrup, Jensen, & Bach, 2004). Furthermore, the recognition of other limitations

of the MPQ, including the lack of specificity of its descriptors for NP, has since led to a multitude of more recent studies describing the role of self-report measures in the assessment of various NP qualities (Bennett, 2001; Bouhassira et al., 2004, 2005; Dworkin et al., 2009; Freynhagen, Baron, Gockel, & Tölle, 2006; Galer & Jensen, 1997; Krause & Backonja, 2003; Portenoy et al., 2005; Scholz et al., 2009) (see Table 17.1A). Short-form versions have been published for two of these (Backonja & Krause, 2003; Bennett, Smith, Torrance, & Potter, 2005), and some have been replicated in several different languages. As a rather inclusive (although not exhaustive) list, the studies shown in Tables 17.1A, 17.1B, and 17.1C are quite heterogeneous, with substantial differences in study purpose, methodology, validation strategy, target population, and sample size. It should be noted that Tables 17.1A, 17.1B, and 17.1C do not include studies of single, specific NP conditions, such as those of diabetic neuropathy (Bastyr, Price, Bril, & the MBBQ Study Group, 2005; Dyck et al., 1991; Feldman et al., 1994; Masson et al., 1989), carpal tunnel syndrome (Jensen, Gammaitoni, et al., 2006), trigeminal neuralgia (Melzack et al., 1986), and postthoracotomy NP (Maguire, Ravenscroft, Beggs, & Duffy, 2006). Although all studies involved subject- or patient-reported pain quality measures, four included also a physical examination component (Bennett, 2001; Bouhassira et al., 2005; Rasmussen et al., 2004; Scholz et al., 2009). For the purpose of using pain quality descriptors to discriminate between NP and non-neuropathic pain, some, but not all, studies involved populations with NP, as well as those with non-neuropathic pain (Bennett, 2001; Bouhassira et al., 2005; Dubuisson & Melzack, 1976; Dworkin et al., 2009; Freynhagen et al., 2006; Krause & Backonja, 2003; Portenoy et al., 2005; Scholz et al., 2009).

Across the studies shown in Table 17.1A, self-report measures of the severity of each rated pain quality varied from being dichotomous (i.e., "yes" or "no") (Bennett, 2001; Bouhassira et al., 2005; Boureau et al., 1990; Dubuisson & Melzack, 1976; Portenoy et al., 2005; Rasmussen et al., 2004), categorical (Freynhagen et al., 2006), ordinal (numerical scales) (Bouhassira et al., 2004; Dworkin et al., 2009; Galer &

TABLE 17.1A. Studies of Neuropathic Pain Assessment: Patient Report Descriptors

Descriptor	Instrument										
	MPQ	QDSA	NPS	LANSS	NPQ	NPSI	DN4	pain DETECT	IDpain	SF-MPQ-2	StEP
Hot/burning	•	•	•	•	•	•	•	•	•	•	
Pins and needles/prickling/tingling		•		•	•	•	•	•	•	•	•
Electrical shocks/lancinating/shooting		•		•	•	•	•	•	•	•	
Worse with touch/allodynia/sensitive		•	•	•	•	•		•	•	•	
Numb					•		•	•	•	•	
Cold			•		•		•			•	
Cramping/squeezing	•					•				•	
Sharp/stabbing	•	•	•		•	•				•	
Aching	•									•	
Itchy		•	•				•			•	
Dull		•	•								
Tender	•									•	
Throbbing	•									•	
Heavy	•									•	
Tiring–exhausting	•	•								•	
Fearful	•	•								•	
Radiating						•		•			
Temporal pain course pattern								•			
Gnawing	•									•	
Sickening	•									•	
Punishing–cruel	•									•	
Unpleasant			•		•						
Pressure						•					
Splitting										•	
Intense	•		•								
Annoying	•										

330

TABLE 17.1B. Studies of Neuropathic Pain Assessment: Physical Examination Features

Descriptor	LANSS	SSNP	DN4	StEP
		Instrument		
Pin prick–hyperalgesia	•	•	•	•
Pin prick–hypoesthesia		•	•	•
Vibration perception				•
Skin changes				•
Light touch–allodynia	•	•	•	
Light touch–hypoesthesia		•	•	
Brushing–allodynia		•	•	
Response to warm/cold stimulation		•	•	•
Proprioception				•
Movement-evoked pain				•
Deep tissue pressure				•
Straight leg raising				•
Temporal summation			•	•

Note. SSNP, signs and symptoms of neuropathic pain; StEP, standardized evaluation of pain.

Jensen, 1997; Scholz et al., 2009), and continuous (visual analogue scales) (Krause & Backonja, 2003). Despite these various differences, most studies evaluated the pain quality descriptors: "hot," "burning," "pins and needles," "prickling," "tingling," "electrical shock–like," "shooting," "worse with touch" (or "sensitive"), "numb," and "cold." When comparing patients with diagnosed NP to those with nociceptive pain, Bennett (2001) reported that descriptors significantly associated with NP included "hot–burning," "cutting–lacerating," "pins and needles," "pricking," "tingling," "tight–stretched," "numb," "electrical shock–like," "jumping–bursting," "radiating," and "stabbing–shooting." Using similar such comparisons, Bouhassira and colleagues (2005) reported that descriptors significantly associated with NP included "burning," "painful cold," "electrical shock–like," "tingling," "pins and needles," "itching," and "numb." However, it should be recognized that pain descriptors reported in NP versus nociceptive pain conditions have exhibited considerable overlap, and that no single pain quality descriptor is pathognomonic of NP (Hansson, Backonja, & Bouhassira, 2007).

It is crucial also to point out that the ability of any of the cited studies to identify any features that discriminate between NP and nociceptive pain rests upon the "gold standard" for making the diagnosis in each study participant. In most studies, this "gold standard" is a clinician-formulated diagnosis following patient history, physical examination, and completed laboratory investigations. Thus, the results of such studies must be interpreted in the context that the outcome of any diagnostic workup does not necessarily result in a discrete diagnosis of NP but rather a diagnosis with varying degrees of certainty (e.g., "definite," "probable," or "suspected" NP) (Rasmussen et al., 2004; Treede et al., 2008). With these caveats in mind, the expanding body of knowledge about NP quality descriptors resulting from these and other investigations has served not only to enhance the diagnostic precision of clinical NP assessment (Baron & Tölle, 2008) but also to facilitate badly needed epidemiology studies in NP (Bouhassira et al., 2008; Torrance et al., 2006), and to promote further the pursuit of mechanism-based NP classification and treatment (Baron, Tölle, Gockel, Brosz, & Freynhagen, 2009; Finnerup & Jensen, 2006).

Of the several tools specifically designed and validated to assess NP qualities, all contain several descriptors rated quantitatively in numerical pain scales. These include the Neuropathic Pain Scale (NPS; Galer & Jensen, 1997), the Neuropathic Pain Symptom

TABLE 17.1C. Studies of Neuropathic Pain Assessment: Study Purpose and Methodology

Instrument	Study purpose	Methodology
MPQ	Evaluate the discriminant value of pain descriptors across different pain syndromes	Study (by Dubuisson & Melzack, 1976) of 95 patients with phantom limb pain, postherpetic neuralgia, degenerative disc disease, and 5 other non-neuropathic pain conditions
QDSA	Evaluate diagnostic value of verbal descriptors in neuropathic pain	Study of 100 patients with neuropathic pain and 97 with non-neuropathic pain
NPS	Measurement of pain in neuropathic pain syndromes	Study 1: 78 patients with PHN, RSD, PNI and DN; study 2: response to treatment with IV lidocaine and phentolamine
LANSS	Screening and identification of patients with pain of predominantly neuropathic origin	Study 1: 30 neuropathic versus 30 nociceptive pain patients; study 2:20 neuropathic versus 20 nociceptive pain patients
NPQ	Measurement of neuropathic pain	Study of 149 patients with neuropathic and 233 non-neuropathic pain
NPSI	Evaluate symptoms of neuropathic pain	Study of 176 patients with central or peripheral neuropathic pain
SSNP	Determine if signs and symptoms vary with increasing evidence of neuropathic pain	Study of patients: 91 with "definite," 71 "possible," and 52 "unlikely" neuropathic pain
DN4	Development of a tool to diagnose neuropathic pain	Study of 89 patients with pain due to a nerve lesion and 71 patients with a non-neurological lesion
painDETECT	Evaluate neuropathic components in chronic low back pain	Study 1: validation study of 228 neuropathic and 164 nociceptive pain patients; study 2: epidemiological survey of 7,772 low back pain patients
IDpain	Differentiate between nociceptive and neuropathic pain	Study of 586 patients with nociceptive or neuropathic "non-headache" chronic pain
SF-MPQ-2	Measure major symptoms of both neuropathic and non-neuropathic pain	Study 1: 882 respondents to the American Chronic Pain Association website survey; study 2: analysis of data from an RCT of topical amitriptyline/ketamine in 226 DN patients
StEP	Standardized assessment of pain	Study of 130 patients with neuropathic pain and 57 patients with non-neuropathic low back pain

Note. QDSA, Questionnaire Douleur de Saint Antoine; NPQ, Neuropathic Pain Questionnaire; SSNP, signs and symptoms of neuropathic pain; StEP, standardized evaluation of pain.

Inventory (NPSI; Bouhassira et al., 2005), the SF-MPQ-2 (derived from the SF-MPQ; Dworkin et al., 2009), and the Pain Quality Assessment Scale (PQAS; derived from the NPS) (Jensen, Gammaitoni, et al., 2006).

The NPS (Galer & Jensen, 1997) includes 10 pain quality items (e.g., "sharp," "hot," "dull") rated on Likert scales and a temporal assessment of pain. In the NPS, each item is rated separately, but in further studies, various composite scores using selected items were proposed, although not formally validated (Galer, Jensen, Ma, Davies, & Rowbotham, 2002). A recent validation study of the NPS in multiple sclerosis showed that the NPS items could be grouped into three factors (Rog, Nurmikko, Friede, & Young, 2007). The NPSI contains 10 descriptors that can be grouped into five distinct dimensions on the basis of factor analysis, thus allowing evaluation of distinctive aspects of NP. It also contains two temporal items. The descriptors used to assess evoked pain have also been validated against quantitative sensory testing (Attal et al., 2008). Thus, it has been shown that self-reported pain evoked by brush, pressure, and cold stimuli correlated with allodynia/hyperalgesia (applied by the investigator) to brush, von Frey hairs, and cold stimuli. This suggests their relevance to assess evoked pain in clinical studies. A derived version from the NPS, the PQAS, has been developed by the same group to address some of the limitations of the NPS, which does not include several pain qualities commonly seen in neuropathic conditions (Jensen, Gammaitoni, et al., 2006). However, this scale has only been validated in carpal tunnel syndrome thus far (Jensen, Gammaitoni, et al., 2006; Victor et al., 2008). More recently, the SF-MPQ-2 was developed to overcome the limitations of the SF-MPQ, particularly in NP (Dworkin et al., 2009). This new questionnaire contains seven additional items more specifically related to NP, and the scoring of each symptom is based on 0- to 10-point numerical rating scales. Factor analysis identified four subscales. However further studies are necessary to confirm the psychometric properties of the SF-MPQ-2 in patients with neuropathic, non-neuropathic, and mixed pain conditions (Attal & Bouhassira, 2009; Dworkin et al., 2009).

Physical Examination

Because pain is a symptom associated with a multitude of serious and potentially life-threatening illnesses, physical examination is considered mandatory in anyone who initially presents with pain as their cardinal symptom to rule out such problems quickly (e.g., deep venous thrombosis and impending pulmonary embolism in a patient presenting with leg pain). Even in less acute situations (e.g., a person with long-standing pain who has already undergone a thorough primary care workup), physical examination is crucial in order to (1) demonstrate a serious interest in this distressing somatic symptom, (2) determine whether any changes have occurred since previous documented

examinations, and (3) acquire more insights into the inciting and perpetuating causes of the pain. Various aspects of physical examination might be indicated depending on the putative etiology of NP (e.g., cardiorespiratory examination in thoracic PHN; musculoskeletal and neurological examination in lumbar radiculopathy; neurological and dermatological examination in diabetic neuropathy). Inasmuch as NP is associated with a functional disturbance in sensory processing, perhaps the most informative aspect of physical examination in this setting is the sensory component of the neurological examination (Backonja & Galer, 1998). In light of this, a "bedside" physical examination has been recommended for the assessment of NP (Cruccu et al., 2004), including skin testing of light touch and vibration stimulation for the assessment of Aβ sensory nerve fiber function, and pinprick and thermal stimulation for the assessment of Aδ sensory nerve fiber function and thermal heat stimulation for the assessment of C sensory fiber function (see Table 17.2).

Following earlier human investigations demonstrating NP-related hyperalgesia and allodynia with simple physical examination methods (Baron, 2000; Fields, Rowbotham, & Baron, 1998; Treede, Meyer, Raja, & Campbell, 1992), the diagnostic value of such methods has been evaluated in more recent studies (Table 17.1) (Bennett, 2001; Bouhassira et al., 2005; Rasmussen et al., 2004; Scholz et al., 2009). In a study of patients grouped into NP versus nociceptive etiologies, Bennett (2001) evaluated dynamic allodynia to cotton wool and altered pinprick sensation (compared to a comparable nonpainful area) and reported that abnormalities in these measures were statistically significantly more frequent in NP. Rasmussen and colleagues (2004) studied three groups of patients with "definite," "possible," or "unlikely" NP, in which light touch and pinprick sensation were evaluated, as well as allodynia to brushing, responses to warm and cold thermal stimulation, and temporal summation to pinprick. In that investigation, only brush-evoked allodynia demonstrated statistically significant separation between the three classified groups. Light touch, pinprick, brush, and thermal stimulation were similarly evaluated by Bouhassira and colleagues (2005) in a study of

TABLE 17.2. Summary of Information Related to Assessment of Different Peripheral and Central Somatosensory Channels

Type of stimulus	Peripheral sensory channel	Central pathway	Bedside examination	QST
Thermal				
Cold	Aδ	Spinothalamic	Cold reflex hammer, cold and warm thermorollers or test-tubes device	Computer-controlled thermal testing device
Warmth	C	Spinothalamic		
Heat pain	C, Aδ	Spinothalamic		
Cold pain	C, Aδ	Spinothalamic		
Mechanical				
Static light touch	Aβ	Lemniscal	Q-tip	Calibrated von Frey hairs
Vibration	Aβ	Lemniscal	Tuning fork	Vibrameter
Brushing	Aβ	Lemniscal	Brush/cotton swab	Brush
Pinprick	Aδ, C	Spinothalamic	Pin	Calibrated pins
Blunt pressure	Aδ, C	Spinothalamic	Examiner's thumb	Algometer

Note. From Hansson, Backonja, and Bouhassira (2007). This table has been reproduced with permission of the International Association for the Study of Pain. The table may not be reproduced for any other purpose without permission.

NP versus nociceptive pain groups. Their results indicated, not surprisingly, significantly higher frequencies of sensory abnormalities in the NP group; however, hypoesthesia to touch, pinprick, and brush allodynia were estimated optimally to maximize the sensitivity and specificity of the resulting Neuropathic Pain Diagnostic Questionnaire (DN4) in combination with self-rated pain descriptors. Finally, Scholz and colleagues (2009) evaluated pinprick, thermal, and vibration perception; skin changes; proprioception; movement-evoked pain; deep tissue pressure; straight leg raising; and temporal summation in patients with mixed NP versus non-neuropathic low back pain. Results from this study, which employed a classification tree analysis, suggested that components of the physical examination identified as key determinants of "clustering" patient subtypes included pinprick and cold responses, skin changes and proprioception. Taken together, these results suggest that the relatively simple clinical examination methods just described are extremely valuable and informative for the assessment of NP.

Quantitative Sensory Testing

To date, the traditional etiology-based categorization of NP still prevails for clinical, experimental (Jensen & Baron, 2003), and pharmacological studies (Attal et al., 2006; Dworkin et al., 2007; Finnerup, Otto, McQuay, Jensen, & Sindrup, 2005). Therapeutic studies have generally evaluated NP as a global and uniform symptom. This empirical approach may be one main cause of therapeutic failure in these patients. This has raised the question of whether a different strategy, in which pain would be analyzed according to underlying mechanisms, could provide a more suitable approach for examining and classifying patients, with the ultimate goal of obtaining a better treatment approach (Baron, 2006). Such a mechanism-based approach to NP derives from the assumption that a precise phenotypic profile of patients with NP should help to improve selection of drugs targeting particular mechanisms (Attal et al., 2008; Baron, 2006; Woolf et al., 1998; Woolf & Mannion, 1999). Specific NP questionnaires (described earlier) and quantitative sensory testing (QST) may be relevant tools in the clinic to characterize better the multiple neuropathic phenotypes. Such phenotypic mapping is probably an important step to establish a future mechanism-based classification and therapy of NP.

General Principles and Normative Data of QST

QST may be defined as the analysis of perception in response to external stimuli of controlled intensity. QST is considered a semiobjective method, because whereas the stimulus is controlled, the response depends on subjective ratings by the individual being assessed. Thermal and mechanical stimuli may assess the different sensory modalities corresponding to different types of receptors, peripheral nerve fibers or central nervous system (CNS) pathways, without allowing the exact level of impairment to be determined. Mechanical sensitivity for tactile stimuli is generally measured using Von Frey hairs (Semmes–Weinstein filaments) (Waylett-Rendall, 1988), paintbrushes, pinprick sensation with weighted needles (Rolke, Baron, et al., 2006), and vibration sensitivity with an electronic vibrameter (Goldberg & Lindblom, 1979). Thermal perception and thermal pain are measured using a probe that operates on the Peltier principle (Claus, Hilz, Hummer, & Neundörfer, 1987; Fruhstorfer, Lindblom, & Schmidt, 1976; Yarnitsky, Sprechter, Zaslansky, & Hemli, 1995).

QST allows an assessment of sensory detection thresholds for innocuous stimuli and pain thresholds, generally using the method of limits, and less commonly the methods of levels (Shy et al., 2003). Such determination allows a more precise assessment of the magnitude of sensory deficits and a quantification of thermal and mechanical allodynia, which may be defined as an abnormal reduction of pain thresholds. Generally the contralateral homologous side is used as the control, but normative data for thermal and mechanical detection and pain thresholds for the hand, foot, and face have been recently proposed, based on a large group of healthy volunteers (Rolke et al., 2006a), and repeatability of these measures has also been assessed (Agostinho et al., 2008; Granot, Granovsky, Sprecher, Nir, & Yarnitsky, 2006). However, the range of thermal pain thresholds is very large within individuals, and the repeatability is lower than that of detection thresholds, which illustrates the difficulty of interpreting results regarding pain thresholds in individual patients and makes QST more appropriate for comparison of group data (Hansson & Haanpää, 2007). QST also includes the assessment of sensations induced by suprathreshold stimuli (Hansson & Lindblom, 1992). Determination of stimulus–response function contributes to identification and quantification of hyperalgesia. However, there is no widely accepted consensus regarding a specific algorithm for the assessment of thermal or mechanical allodynia and hyperalgesia.

The sensitivity and specificity of QST compared to standard clinical examination has been poorly assessed (Kelly, Cook, & Backonja, 2005; Rolke, Baron, et al., 2006a; Rolke, Margerl, et al., 2006b; Devigili et al., 2008), and the outcomes of QST and bedside testing do not necessarily coincide (Devigili et al., 2008; Hansson & Haanpää, 2007). One reason may be that measurements using QST are taken out from a restricted part of the painful area, whereas a more qualitative bedside examination allows testing of a large part of the innervation territory of the injured nervous structure (Devigili et al., 2008; Hansson & Haanpää, 2007). However, QST has also been found to be more sensitive than standard clinical examination or subjective symptoms in detecting thermal (cold) hyperalgesia in patients receiving chemotherapy with oxaliplatin (Attal et al., 2009).

Clinical Applications of QST for NP Evaluation and Diagnosis

Thermal QST has largely been used for the early diagnosis and follow-up of small fiber neuropathies that cannot be assessed by standard nerve conduction studies (Shy et al., 2003) and is recommended for the diagnosis and follow-up of diabetic neuropathies (Chong & Cros, 2004; Consensus Statement, 1988; Shy et al., 2003). Vibration thresholds may also be useful in assessing large-fiber neuropathies, such as chemotherapy-induced neuropathies (Shy et al., 2003). QST may also detect subclinical somatosensory deficits in patients with various chronic pain conditions. Thus, moderate thermal deficits have been identified using a thermotest in atypical facial pain (55% of the patients in a recent study) (Forssell, Tenovuo, Silvoniemi, & Jääskeläinen, 2007), idiopathic restless leg syndrome (Schattschneider et al., 2004), burning mouth syndrome (Granot & Nagler, 2005), and chronic ischemic pain of the lower limbs (Lang et al., 2006), suggesting a possible infraclinical small fiber neuropathy in some of these painful conditions.

QST in the Research Setting

Combined standardized QST profiling and specific questionnaires have been used in the research setting to detect phenotype subgroups in patients with NP to learn more about pathophysiological mechanisms (Baron, 2006). Such precise phenotypic mapping with QST is useful to distinguish between subtypes of patients with PHN and distinct sensory symptom profiles that are probably triggered by different mechanisms (Fields et al., 1998; Petersen, Fields, Brennum, Sandroni, & Rowbotham, 2000). The use of QST in patients with NP, often combined with complementary approaches (i.e., functional magnetic resonance imaging [fMRI], capsaicin, or menthol tests), has also largely contributed to analysis of some pathophysiological mechanisms involved in the genesis of pain and hyperalgesia in these patients (e.g., Defrin, Ohry, Blumen, & Urca, 2001; Ducreux, Attal, Parker, & Bouhassira, 2006; Finnerup, Johannesen, Fuglsang-Frederiksen, Bach, & Jensen, 2003; Krämer, Rolke, Bickel, & Birklein, 2004; Wasner, Lee, Engel, & McLachlan, 2008).

QST has shown, in particular, that spinothalamic tract impairment reflected by thermoalgesic deficits is a necessary but not sufficient condition for the development of central pain, and may discriminate among several subtypes of patients with central pain (based on the severity and characteristics of allodynia and somatosensory deficits), which may reflect distinct pathophysiological mechanisms. Whether this mechanism-based classification of patients with NP may have direct therapeutic implications remains to be confirmed in large studies (further discussion below). This knowledge should ultimately lead to an optimal polypharmacy, with pharmacological agents targeting specific molecular mechanisms in individual patients, thus forming the basis of a genuine mechanism-based therapeutic approach to NP (Baron, 2006; Woolf, 2004).

Special Laboratory Tests

Standard Electrodiagnostic Studies

Standard neurophysiological responses to electrical stimuli, such as nerve conduction studies and somatosensory evoked potentials, may demonstrate, locate, and quantify damage along the large-size non-nociceptive afferents, but they are unable to assess the function of nociceptive pathways (Cruccu et al., 2004). These techniques are essentially useful to determine the etiology of the nerve lesion or to complete exploration of the nerve lesion. For example, somatosensory evoked potentials may be helpful to predict the outcome of specific analgesic techniques for NP, such as spinal cord stimulation, that necessitates the relative integrity of lemniscal pathways (Sindou, Mertens, Bendavid, Garcia-Larréa, & Mauguière, 2003).

Microneurography

Microneurography is a minimally invasive technique allowing single-fiber recordings from nerve fibers in awake individuals (Jorum & Schmelz, 2006; Torebjörk, 1993). It is time-consuming and difficult, necessitating an expert investigator and a consenting patient. For this reason, the technique is unsuitable for the clinical setting. Microneurography has essentially been performed in healthy volunteers and has provided useful information about the physiology of nociceptors. A few studies in patients with NP have facilitated the detection of different forms of hyperexcitability of polymodal and mechanically insensitive C nociceptors, which might account for the somatosensory abnormalities, such as reduced receptor thresholds or spontaneous C nociceptor discharge (Campero, Serra, Marchettini, & Ochoa, 1998; Torebjörk, 1993) and temperature-dependent double spikes in patients with heat hyperalgesia (Bostock, Campero, Serra, & Ochoa, 2005). However, it has not been determined with certainty whether recorded abnormalities of nociceptors are essentially a reflection of the nerve lesion or whether they may be directly responsible for spontaneous pain or hyperalgesia. Thus, a recent study of patients with diabetic painful and nonpainful neuropathies was not able to discriminate between the two groups of patients on the basis of spontaneous activity and sensitization of nociceptors (Orstavik et al., 2006).

Nociceptive Reflexes

The nociceptive flexion reflex (RIII) recorded in the biceps femoris is mediated by nociceptive afferents and is modulated by various analgesic drugs, allowing analysis of their mechanisms of action (Cruccu, Ferracuti, Leardi, Fabbri, & Manfredi, 1991; Willer, 1985). There are very few studies of the RIII reflex in NP. In a study of 10 patients presenting with a traumatic peripheral nerve injury associated with brush-induced allodynia or static mechanoallodynia, the RIII reflex and concomitant painful sensation elicited by electrical stimulation of the sural nerve were analyzed; this allowed the investigation of counterirritation mechanisms in these patients (i.e., pain inhibits pain effect), probably depending on diffuse noxious inhibitory controls (DNICs) that modulate the spinal transmission of nociceptive signals. This study found that the two subtypes of mechanical allodynia had similar inhibiting effects on the concomitant painful sensation, but differential effects on the electrophysiological reflexes, showing that they do not have the same effect on DNICs (Bouhassira, Danziger, Attal, & Guirimand, 2003). Trigeminal reflexes (blink and masseter inhibitory reflex) that evaluate myelinated Aβ afferents are essentially used for diagnostic purposes to differentiate classical from symptomatic trigeminal neuralgia (Cruccu et al., 2004) and may also have some pathophysiological relevance. Thus, in a recent study of patients with ophthalmic PHN, the blink reflex was found to correlate with the intensity of paroxysmal pain, suggesting that this type of pain is related to Aβ fiber demyelination (Truini et al., 2008).

Laser-Evoked Potentials

For a number of years, several techniques have been proposed for the selective activation of pain afferents (Garcia-Larréa, 2006). To date, the most reliable neurophysiological method to activate pain afferents selectively appears to be provided by radiant heat pulse stimuli delivered by laser stimulators, which selectively excite the free nerve endings (A-δ and C) in the superficial skin layers (Bromm, Frieling, & Lankers, 1991; Bromm & Treede, 1991; Magerl, Zahid, Ellrich, Meyer, & Treede, 1999; Plaghki & Mouraux, 2003; Treede, Lorenz, & Baumgärtner, 2003). It is now widely agreed that laser-evoked potentials (LEPs) are nociceptive responses. Laser stimulation is coupled to the detection of

cortical evoked potentials, which are therefore called "laser-evoked potentials." Late LEPs reflect activity of A-δ fibers and their latency is 200–500 msec. Ultralate LEPs reflect activity of the unmyelinated nociceptive pathway and may be recorded with a very long latency of nearly 1 sec (Bragard, Chen, & Plaghki, 1996; Magerl et al., 1999). However due to technical difficulties, few studies have used ultralate LEPs in patients. Late LEPs have been used in numerous experimental studies in healthy volunteers (Bromm & Lorenz, 1998; Garcia-Larréa, Peyron, Laurent, & Mauguière, 1997). These studies have shown, in particular, that the vertex response LEPs were correlated with the intensity of stimulation and of painful sensation. Several studies have also used LEPs in patients with various types of peripheral or central NP (e.g., painful neuropathies, trigeminal neuralgia, PHN, radiculopathy, central lesions) (Agostino et al., 2000; Casey et al., 1996; Cruccu et al., 2003; Garcia-Larréa et al., 2002; Kakigi et al., 1991; Kanda et al., 1996; Ragazzoni et al., 1993; Treede et al., 1991; Treede, Meier, Kunze, & Bromm, 1988; Truini et al., 2003, 2008; Wu et al., 1999).

The studies noted earlier evidenced an attenuation or suppression of LEPs (reduction in amplitude, increased latency), sometimes accompanied by a lack of clinical abnormalities, generally contrasting with normal or subnormal somatosensory evoked potentials. In one study, the reduction in amplitude was correlated with the severity of constant pain in PHN (Truin et al., 2008). Significant, although more moderate, alterations of LEPs have also been detected in patients with superimposed hyperalgesia, suggesting that LEPs reflect not the severity of hyperalgesia, but rather the impairment of nociceptive pathways (Garcia-Larréa et al., 2002; Truini et al., 2008). Interestingly, LEP suppression or attenuation in NP sharply contrasts with findings of facilitation in chronic "dysfunctional" pain syndromes, such as fibromyalgia (Garcia-Larréa et al., 2002; Granot et al., 2001). On the basis of these studies, LEPs appear to be particularly sensitive compared to other neurophysiological tests to detect damage to nociceptive pathways. However, the specificity and sensitivity of LEPs for the study of nociceptive pathways has not been adequately assessed, and the specificity of the alterations observed with LEPs in patients with pain compared to patients without pain has yet to be determined. For these reasons, LEPs are essentially recommended in the research setting for NP and should not be used for medicolegal purposes.

Functional Neuroimaging

PRINCIPLES OF HEMODYNAMIC IMAGING

Positron emission tomography (PET) and fMRI estimate the cerebral blood flow or metabolic changes that reflect local synaptic activity in defined brain regions. PET is a nuclear medicine technique for the three-dimensional detection of an emitting isotope in a certain region of the body. It can also be used to assess physiological processes, such as mapping of neurotransmitter systems and drug uptake *in vivo*, for example, depending on the probe molecule chosen. fMRI can be used to detect variations in regional tissue oxygenation due to changes in oxygen uptake and blood supply to various areas of the brain. It offers a better temporal and spatial resolution than PET. Because no radioactivity is used, scans may be repeated an unlimited number of times in a given individual. The drawbacks of this technique include the presence of pulsation artifacts and the need for strict timing of stimulus induction and image acquisition (Kupers & Kehlet, 2006).

THE PAIN MATRIX

Most fMRI and PET studies have investigated the brain correlates of experimental pain in normal volunteers. It is now acknowledged that experimental painful stimuli activate a network of brain structures frequently referred to as the *physiological pain matrix*, which includes the primary and secondary somatosensory cortex (S1 and S2); lateral thalamus (Th) and insular cortex (IC), which are part of the lateral system and preferentially associated with the sensory-discriminative component of pain; and the anterior cingulate cortex (ACC) and prefrontal cortex (PFC), which are part of the medial system and more specifically linked to the emotional–affective aspect of pain (Casey, 1999; Kupers & Kehlet, 2006; Mois-

set & Bouhassira, 2007; Peyron, Laurent, & Garcia-Larréa, 2000). The PFC in particular is a major integration center that may be involved in the cognitive–motivational aspect of pain.

Other brain regions shown to be activated in several studies include the motor/premotor cortex, the supplementary motor area, the inferior/posterior parietal cortex, the basal ganglia, the cerebellum, and many brainstem nuclei, particularly the periaqueductal gray matter. The activation of these areas is often considered to reflect attentional processes and the preparation, selection, and inhibition of motor responses associated with the painful stimulus.

BRAIN IMAGING OF SPONTANEOUS NP

Several groups have reported that spontaneous NP was associated with decreased resting regional cerebral blood flow (rCBF) in the contralateral Th, and that such decrease can be reversed by analgesic procedures (Di Piero et al., 1991; Garcia-Larréa et al., 1999; Hsieh, Belfrage, Stone-Elander, Hansson, & Ingvar, 1995; Iadarola et al., 1995). However, the patients included in these studies were highly heterogeneous. In some studies, it was not entirely clear whether they had true NP, whereas in others, the presence of continuous, spontaneous pain during the scan was not fully assessed (Moisset & Bouhassira, 2007). Despite these limitations, these data suggest that the lateral pain system—particularly S1, S2, and the posterior insula, all of which are major components of the pain matrix—may not play a major role in spontaneous NP.

BRAIN IMAGING OF EVOKED NP

Most studies in NP focused on dynamic mechanical allodynia (Kupers & Kehlet, 2006; Moisset & Bouhassira, 2007). Despite some limitations (a small number of patients with heterogeneous etiologies of pain was analyzed), these studies consistently found that mechanical allodynia was associated with increased activation in the main components of the lateral pain system (S1, S2, and lateral Th) (Cesaro et al., 1991; Ducreux et al., 2006; Petrovic, Ingvar, Stone-Elander, Petersson, & Hansson, 1999; Peyron et al.,

1998, 2004; Schweinhardt et al., 2006). Another region consistently activated is the PFC (orbitofrontal, medial, and dorsolateral), which is the most frequently activated region in chronic pain studies (Apkarian, Bushnell, Treede, & Zubieta, 2005). This structure may be involved in not only the cognitive–evaluative aspect of pain but also pain modulation through its connection with the diencephalon and brainstem, as highlighted by its role in the placebo effect (Wager, 2004). In contrast, most studies reported an absence of activation of the ACC and IC (Ducreux et al., 2006; Petrovic et al., 1999). However, one cannot exclude that this apparent lack of activation may be due to the presence of continuous pain (e.g., these structures were activated during the "painful rest" condition and could not be further activated during the allodynic stimulation). In any case, mechanical allodynia seems to involve not the physiological pain matrix but a preferential activation of the sensory-discriminative lateral pain system and the PFC.

The sharp contrast between this pattern of activation and that associated with spontaneous pain is consistent with the involvement of different mechanisms in specific components of NP syndromes. Very few studies have assessed the changes in brain activity associated with cold allodynia (Ducreux et al., 2006; Peyron et al., 1998, 2004). The only direct comparison of brain activation associated with cold and dynamic allodynia, in a small group of patients with syringomyelia, suggests that these two subtypes of allodynia induce distinct changes in brain activity (Ducreux et al., 2006). However, further studies with a larger number of patients are required to determine whether this reflects true differences in the mechanisms of these subtypes of allodynia.

Skin and Nerve Biopsies

NERVE BIOPSY

Nerve biopsy is relatively invasive and may occasionally be associated with complications (pain, infection, permanent sensory loss). It remains essentially useful for the etiological diagnosis of some painful neuropathies (amyloidosis, vasculitis) but not for the

early detection and monitoring of small fiber neuropathies (Llewelyn et al., 1991) that are best assessed now using skin punch biopsy (Cruccu et al., 2004).

SKIN PUNCH BIOPSY

Skin punch biopsy is a minimally invasive technique that makes it possible to analyze Aδ and C intraepidermal nerve fiber (IENF) density, but it does not evaluate large myelinated fibers (Lauria et al., 2005; Sommer & Lauria, 2007). This technique is easy and relevant for patient follow-up. To date the clinical applications of skin punch biopsy have essentially concerned the diagnosis and follow-up of small fiber neuropathies (Cruccu et al., 2004). Thus, a loss in IENF density has been found in a large variety of painful small fiber neuropathies (Holland et al., 1998; Lauria et al., 2005). Skin biopsy appears to have very good sensitivity and specificity compared to clinical examination and QST in these conditions (Devigili et al., 2008). It has also been able to detect small fiber impairment in posttraumatic complex regional pain syndrome (CRPS) type I (Oaklander et al., 2006); thus, a reduction by 29% in epidermal neurite density was found in the CRPS-affected area compared to unaffected control sides and to symptom-matched controls, suggesting that patients with CRPS type I might have some infraclinical, persistent, minimal distal axonal injury accounting for their pain and autonomic dysfunction.

Skin punch biopsy has been less commonly used for the exploration of NP mechanisms. In studies comparing skin punch biopsy in patients with painful and nonpainful diabetic neuropathy, the loss in IENF only accounted for pain in a small subgroup of patients (Sorensen, Molyneux, & Yue, 2006a, 2006b). Similarly in PHN, one study found a loss in IENF density (Oaklander et al., 1998; Oaklander 2001; see Figure 17.2), whereas, conversely, another found that IENF was inversely correlated to mechanical allodynia, suggesting the role of the preservation of remaining nociceptive fibers in these patients (Rowbotham et al., 1996). These data suggest that the mechanisms of allodynia in these patients are diverse, as also emphasized by QST studies.

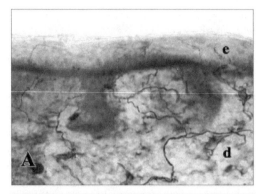

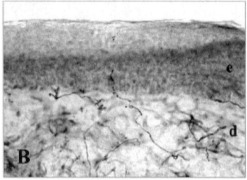

FIGURE 17.2. Representative labeled vertical skin-biopsy sections from subjects with and without PHN. (A) A biopsy from the previously shingles-affected site on the back of a 75-year-old woman without PHN. She had 1,672 epidermal neurites/mm². (B) A biopsy from the previously shingles-affected site on top of the shoulders of a 72-year-old woman with PHN who had 145 epidermal neurites/mm2. The epidermis (e) is uppermost, and the dermis (d) is at bottom. Individual neurites are visible, and neurite bundles are visible in the superficial dermis. From Oaklander (2001). This figure has been reproduced with permission of the International Association for the Study of Pain. The figure may not be reproduced for any other purpose without permission.

ASSESSMENT OF NP IN THE SETTING OF INTERVENTION TRIALS

Pain Intensity

Pain intensity, including average pain, pain at its worst, and at pain its best, is the most common primary outcome measure used to assess efficacy of treatments for chronic pain (Dworkin et al., 2005). If different pain components involve different territories, this can be documented on a body map. The 11-point numerical rating scales (NRSs) or visual analogue scales (VASs) appear similarly sensitive to change in NP. However, the NRS may have fewer failures than the VAS in older adult patients (Dworkin et al., 2005; Jensen, Karoly, & Braver, 1986) and is currently considered the most reliable to assess treatment effect (Dworkin et al., 2005). An additional measure of pain intensity using a categorical pain scale (in which patients choose one of the given verbal descriptors of the intensity of pain they feel) may be recommended as a secondary outcome (Dworkin et al., 2005), although it is sometimes less sensitive to change than NRSs (e.g., Boureau, Legallicier, & Kabir-Ahmadi, 2003; Karst et al., 2003).

Pain Quality and Temporal Aspects of Pain

The MPQ (Melzack, 1975), and the 15-item SF-MPQ (Melzack, 1987), the most frequently used self-rating multidimensional instruments to assess pain quality, have largely been used to evaluate the efficacy of treatments in NP (e.g., Goldstein, Lu, Detke, Lee, & Iyengar, 2005; Lesser, Sharma, LaMoreaux, & Poole, 2004). These scales are not specific for NP (see earlier discussion), and the SF-MPQ has occasionally been found to be only weakly sensitive to treatments in NP trials (Backonja et al., 2008; Berman, Symonds, & Birch, 2004; Gilron et al., 2009; Simpson et al., 2003; see, however, Gilron et al., 2005). The main purpose of the MPQ and the SF-MPQ is to discriminate between the sensory and affective dimensions of pain (see Katz & Melzack, Chapter 3, this volume). Contrary to the sensory components, the affective aspects of pain are not assessed by other pain questionnaires. It remains to be determined whether such differentiation may be relevant in NP assessment, particularly with regard to therapeutic outcome. In fact, therapeutic trials using this questionnaire in NP have invariably found similar impact of drugs on both sensory and affective pain components (see, e.g., Dworkin et al., 2003).

The lack of specificity of the MPQ and SF-MPQ for NP has led to the development of various different NP assessment scales discussed earlier and described in Table 17.1. Some of these scales have been used in treatment intervention trials such as the NPS

(Jensen, Friedman, Bonzo, & Richards, 2006), the Leeds Assessment of Neuropathic Symptoms and Signs (LANSS; Solak et al., 2007), the NPSI (e.g., Baron, Mayoral, et al., 2009), the SF-MPQ-2 (Dworkin et al., 2009), and the PQAS (Jensen, Gammaitoni, et al., 2006). The advantage of specific NP scales over more conventional assessment is they may capture distinct dimensions of NP experience that may be differentially sensitive to treatments (e.g., Jensen, Gammaitoni, et al., 2006; Levendoglu, Ogün, Ozerbil, Ogün, & Ugurlu, 2004; Lynch, Clark, & Sawynok, 2003; Ranoux, Attal, Morain, & Bouhassira, 2008; Rog et al., 2005). They may also be used to determine profiles of patients who are susceptible to therapeutic interventions based on specific symptoms or their combinations.

Temporal aspects represent a distinct dimension of NP (Dworkin et al., 2005). However few trials in NP except those dealing with trigeminal neuralgia (Attal, Cruccu, et al., 2006; Finnerup, Otto, et al., 2005) have assessed them specifically, although these aspects may be highly sensitive to change in NP (e.g., time to onset of pain relief, proportion of pain-free days, and number of pain paroxysms) (Gilron et al., 2000; Gimbel, Richards, & Portenoy, 2003; Ranoux et al., 2008; Rauck, Shaibani, Biton, Simpson, & Koch, 2007; Simpson, Messina, Xie, & Hale, 2007). Secondary analyses of a previous NP trial of gabapentin, morphine, and their combination (Gilron et al., 2005) showed that in comparison with placebo, none of these three active treatments had any effect on circadian increases in pain intensity from 8:00 A.M. to 8:00 P.M. (Odrcich et al., 2006).

Other Measures Designed to Assess Treatment Efficacy

Several additional methods have been conceived specifically to assess treatment efficacy (Dworkin et al., 2005). The numerical (VAS, NRS; 0–100%) or categorical pain relief scales are very sensitive to change in several NP trials. Thus, in a comparative placebo controlled trial of imipramine and venlafaxine in patients with diabetic PN, both active drugs were equally effective in relieving pain intensity, but imipramine had a much better effect on categorical pain relief

(Sindrup, Bach, Madsen, Gram, & Jensen, 2003). In two trials that used gabapentin or topiramate with negative or marginal effect on pain intensity, pain relief was significant with the active drugs (Gordh et al., 2008; Khoromi, Cui, Nackers, & Max, 2007).

The Global Impression of Change (GIC), which consists of seven verbal descriptors from "very much improved" to "very much worse," either reported by the patient (PGIC) or evaluated by the clinician (CGIC), is sensitive to a large variety of treatments in NP (e.g., Dworkin et al., 2003; Raskin et al., 2005; Serpell, 2002; Wernicke et al., 2006). It has occasionally been found to be more sensitive to treatments than pain intensity, probably because it may assess various aspects related to quality of life beyond pain (Gordh et al., 2008; Serpell, 2002). Other global outcome measures of efficacy include patient preference for treatment, satisfaction with treatment or with pain relief, or composite measures of treatment efficacy (e.g., André-Obadia, Mertens, Gueguen, Peyron, & Garcia-Larréa, 2008; Dogra, Beydoun, Mazzola, Hopwood, & Wan, 2005; Fregni et al., 2006; Gimbel et al., 2003; Raja et al., 2002; Raskin et al., 2004; Watson, Moulin, Watt-Watson, Gordon, & Eisenhoffer, 2003).

The proportion of responders is widely used in NP studies (e.g., Gordh et al., 2008; Lesser et al., 2004; Richter et al., 2005; Rowbotham, Goli, Kunz, & Lei, 2004). *Responders* are generally defined on the basis of a 50% pain relief. This has been the "gold standard" used in meta-analyses to calculate the "number needed to treat" (NNT; McQuay & Moore, 1998). However, it has been shown that a reduction ≥ 30% in NRS of pain intensity was also clinically important (Farrar, Young, LaMoreaux, Werth, & Poole, 2001) and may provide important complementary information (e.g., Abrams et al., 2007; Freynhagen, Strojek, Griesing, Whalen, & Balkenohl, 2005; Gordh et al., 2008; Kumar et al., 2007; Siddall et al., 2006). Importantly the NNT may vary depending on the method of calculation. Thus, in a trial of the effect of gabapentin on traumatic nerve injury pain, the NNT for marked improvement using categorical pain relief was 7.7, whereas the NNT for 50% improvement in average pain intensity from pain diaries was 28.0 (Gordh et al., 2008).

Several trials of NP have assessed the use of rescue medication (generally with weak analgesics, sometimes with opioids) as a secondary outcome of the efficacy of treatments. Discrepant findings have been observed with the use of this measure in NP, with good sensitivity (e.g., Boureau et al., 2003; Goldstein et al., 2005; Sindrup et al., 2003; Wernicke et al., 2006) or no sensitivity to change (e.g., Kumar et al., 2007; Sindrup, Graf, & Sfikas, 2006; Svendsen, Jensen, & Bach, 2004), probably because NP shows poor sensitivity to weak analgesics.

QST in the Context of Treatment Interventions

QST has been used in several therapeutic trials to measure the effects of treatments on evoked pains. Whereas most studies failed to detect treatment effects on pain thresholds in response to mechanical or thermal stimuli, treatments did significantly modulate brush-induced allodynia (intensity or area) (Kikuchi et al., 1999; Wallace, Dyck, Rossi, & Yaksh, 1996), hyperalgesia to static mechanical or cold stimuli (Nurmikko et al., 2007; Ranoux et al., 2008), and other less common components of NP (temporal summation, aftersensation, and radiating pain; e.g., Gottrup, Bach, Juhl, & Jensen, 2006). Some researchers have suggested that drugs such as morphine, lidocaine, or N-methyl-D-aspartate (NMDA) antagonists may not act uniformly on the different components of NP (e.g., Attal et al., 2000, 2002; Attal, Rouaud, Brasseur, Chauvin, & Bouhassira, 2004; Gottrup et al., 2006; Leung, Wallace, Ridgeway, & Yaksh, 2001; Ranoux et al., 2008; Wallace, Ridgeway, Leung, Gerayli, & Yaksh, 2000). In particular, the clinical profile of these agents might relate to their preferential antihyperalgesic and antiallodynic action. These techniques have also been used to predict the response to treatment interventions. Thus, it has been shown that a selected sensory abnormality (i.e., impaired thermal detection in the affected dermatomes) may predict the outcome of motor cortex stimulation in central pain (Drouot, Nguyen, Peschanski, & Lefaucheur, 2002) or of epidural steroid injection in patients with sciatica (Schiff & Eisenberg, 2003). One study showed that higher heat pain thresholds at baseline in the affected area might predict opioid response in PHN

(Edwards, Haythornthwaite, Tella, Max, & Raja, 2006). Finally it has also been reported that the presence of mechanical allodynia might predict treatment outcome with the sodium channel blockers lamotrigine or intravenous (IV) lidocaine (Attal et al., 2004; Finnerup, Sindrup, Bach, Johannesen, & Jensen, 2002), although one study using IV lidocaine in patients with central pain, stratified on the basis of the presence or absence of mechanical allodynia, failed to confirm these results (Finnerup, Biering-Sorensen, et al., 2005). Similarly QST was not helpful in predicting which patients with peripheral neuropathy or PHN would benefit from lidocaine patches (Herrmann, Pannoni, Barbano, Pennella-Vaughan, & Dworkin, 2006) and yielded unexpected results with the same treatment in patients with PHN classified on the basis of their putative underlying mechanisms (discussed earlier) (Wasner, Kleinert, Binder, Schattschneider, & Baron, 2005).

In conclusion, QST is very helpful for quantifying the effects of treatments on allodynia and hyperalgesia, and may sometimes reveal differential effects of treatments. However, the expected role of QST in the definition of a mechanism-based treatment of NP, although promising (Baron, 2006), has not yet been fully met (Finnerup & Jensen, 2006). One problem relates to the fact that most therapeutic studies using QST were in a single center, used small sample sizes, and did not use standardized assessment. Studies using standardized assessment (Rolke, Baron, et al., 2006) on large cohorts with adequate sample sizes are therefore recommended (see, e.g., Nurmikko et al., 2007).

ASSESSMENT OF NP IN THE CLINICAL SETTING OF PRIMARY CARE

Assessment of the patient with suspected NP should focus on (1) ruling out treatable conditions (e.g., acute spinal cord compression, occult neoplasm), (2) confirming the diagnosis of NP, and (3) identifying clinical features (e.g., insomnia, autonomic neuropathy) that might help to individualize treatment.

History

Initial assessment involves a description of pain onset, location, temporal variability, severity, aggravating–relieving factors, and prior treatments. Certain pain quality descriptors are characteristic of NP (discussed earlier), and some of the most characteristic sensory descriptors of NP include "hot," "burning," "sharp," "stabbing," "cold," and pain caused by touch. Other common nonpainful sensations include "tingling," "prickling," "itching," "numbness," and "pins and needles." NP typically gets worse toward the end of the day (Odrcich et al., 2006); pain during sleeping hours may warrant sedating analgesics (e.g., tricyclic antidepressants), and pain progression over recent months may prompt the search for an underlying neoplasm.

Evaluation of functional impact (e.g., activities of daily living, work) is critical for setting treatment goals. Evaluation of sleep hygiene (Smith & Haythornthwaite, 2004), mood disturbances (Dworkin & Gitlin, 1991; Haythornthwaite & Benrud-Larsen, 2000) as well as assessment of suicidal risk are very important (Fisher, Haythornthwaite, Heinberg, Clark, & Reed, 2001; Smith, Edwards, Robinson, & Dworkin, 2004). Recording previous treatments, particularly those that were poorly tolerated or ineffective, may prevent unnecessary treatment trials. However, many patients are not appropriately titrated (Richeimer, Bajwa, Kahraman, Ransil, & Warfield, 1997), and it is therefore necessary to ensure that an adequate dose and duration is attempted. Finally, screening for previous and ongoing alcohol or substance abuse may affect the decision to prescribe opioids, cannabinoids, or other sedating drugs, and may prompt earlier consultation with a psychologist and/or psychiatrist (Frank, Graham, Zyzanski, & White, 1992; Michna et al., 2004).

Physical Examination and Special Tests

Neurological examination is crucial, since the presence of true weakness (sometimes difficult to differentiate from pain-related or antalgic gait), absent or reduced reflexes, hyperalgesia, and allodynia all favor a diagnosis of NP (Backonja & Galer, 1998; Cruccu et al., 2004). Tactile allodynia can be elicited by lightly moving a piece of Kleenex tissue across the skin. Thermal allodynia can be demonstrated by applying an ice cube to the affected area; the paradoxical sensa-

tion of heat or burning is pathognomonic of nerve dysfunction. A hyperalgesic response to pinprick on the affected side compared to the unaffected side may radiate beyond the area of stimulation, and repeated pain pricks at the same site may build into an explosive pain. These features illustrate aberrant spatial and temporal summation of the painful stimulus, which sometimes is referred to as *hyperpathia*. Superimposed autonomic features, such as alterations in temperature, color, and sweating, and the development of trophic changes (e.g., shiny skin, hair loss) yield a diagnosis of CRPS (previously "reflex sympathetic dystrophy" or "causalgia"; Wilson, Stanton-Hicks, & Harden, 2005). Other tests may be useful (e.g., pain on straight leg raising is highly suggestive of lumbar nerve root irritation); the elicitation of trigger points favor a diagnosis of myofascial pain over NP.

CT and MRI scans can confirm the presence of a CNS lesion (e.g., herniated disc, spinal tumor, or neurofibroma) that may guide treatment of the underlying condition. For example, discal nerve root impingement may be amenable to surgical decompression, and tumor infiltration of nerve often responds to targeted radiation therapy. Electromyography (EMG) and nerve conduction studies (NCSs) may provide objective evidence of nerve injury (Mendell & Sahenk, 2003). However, since EMG and NCSs evaluate large nerve fiber function, a normal EMG or NCS does not rule out a painful small fiber neuropathy. A three-phase nuclear medicine bone scan may help to diagnose CRPS (Kozin, Soin, Ryan, Carrera, & Wortmann, 1981). Specific blood tests (e.g., glucose tolerance testing, thyroid function, CD4+ T-lymphocyte count) may be useful in certain situations.

CONCLUSION

Recent advancement in the methodology to assess NP has greatly facilitated research on natural history, pathophysiology, treatment response, and diagnosis of NP, and has likely also led to improvements in the clinical evaluation of individuals with possible NP. The distinct pain symptomatology (e.g., "burning" or "shooting" pain) associated predominantly with nerve lesions (e.g., as opposed to nociceptive pain conditions) has led to the comprehensive characterization of self-reported pain quality descriptors that are frequently associated with NP, and that may respond differentially to various therapeutic interventions. Since many NP conditions are associated with sensory dysfunction and exhibit hyperalgesia, allodynia, and other alterations in normal sensation, further development of QST may provide improved indicators of underlying pathophysiological mechanisms, as well as better assessments of treatment response. It is our hope that future improvement and application of the assessment methods described in this chapter will best serve to match patients with particular NP conditions, or even pain qualities, to specific treatments that lead to an optimal outcome.

REFERENCES

Abrams, D. I., Jay, C. A., Shade, S. B., Vizoso, H., Reda, H., Press, S., et al. (2007). Cannabis in painful HIV-associated sensory neuropathy: A randomized placebo-controlled trial. *Neurology, 68,* 515–521.

Agostinho, C. M., Scherens, A., Richter, H., Schaub, C., Rolke, R., Treede, R.-D., et al. (2008). Habituation and short-term repeatability of thermal testing in healthy human subjects and patients with chronic non-neuropathic pain. *European Journal of Pain, 13*(8), 779–785.

Agostino, R., Cruccu, G., Iannetti, G. D., Innocenti, P., Romaniello, A., Truini, A., et al. (2000). Trigeminal small-fibre dysfunction in patients with diabetes mellitus: A study with laser evoked potentials and corneal reflex. *Clinical Neurophysiology, 111,* 2264–2267.

André-Obadia, N., Mertens, P., Gueguen, A., Peyron, R., & Garcia-Larréa, L. (2008). Pain relief by rTMS: Differential effect of current flow but no specific action on pain subtypes. *Neurology, 71,* 833–840.

Apkarian, A. V., Bushnell, M. C., Treede, R. D., & Zubieta, J. K. (2005). Human brain mechanisms of pain perception and regulation in health and disease. *European Journal of Pain, 9*(4), 463–484.

Atlas, S. J., Deyo, R. A., Patrick, D. L., Convery, K., Keller, R. B., & Singer, D. E. (1996). The Quebec Task Force Classification for Spinal Disorders and the severity, treatment, and outcomes of sciatica and lumbar spinal stenosis. *Spine, 21,* 2885–2892.

Attal, N., Bouhassira, D., Gautron, M., Vaillant, J. N., Mitry, E., Lepère, C., et al. (2009). Thermal hyperalgesia as a marker of oxaliplatin neurotoxicity: A prospective quantified sensory assessment study. *Pain, 144,* 245–252.

Attal, N., Cruccu, G., Haanpää, M., Hansson, P., Jensen, T. S., Nurmikko, T., et al. (2006). EFNS guidelines on pharmacological treatment of neuropathic pain. *European Journal of Neurology, 13,* 1153–1169.

Attal, N., Fermanian, C., Fermanian, J., Lanteri-Minet, M., Alchaar, H., & Bouhassira, D. (2008). Neuropathic pain: Are there distinct subtypes depending on the aetiology or anatomical lesion? *Pain, 138,* 343–353.

Attal, N., Gaude, V., Brasseur, L., Dupuy, M., Guirimand, F., Parker, F., et al. (2000). Intravenous lidocaine in central pain: A double-blind placebo-controlled psycho-physical study. *Neurology, 544,* 564–574.

Attal, N., Guirimand, F., Brasseur, L., Gaude, V., Chauvin, M., & Bouhassira, D. (2002). Effects of IV morphine in central pain: A randomized placebo-controlled study. *Neurology, 58,* 554–563.

Attal, N., Rouaud, J., Brasseur, L., Chauvin, M., & Bouhassira, D. (2004). Systemic lidocaine in pain due to peripheral nerve injury and predictors of response. *Neurology, 62,* 218–225.

Backonja, M., Wallace, M. S., Blonsky, E. R., Cutler, B. J., Malan, P., Jr., Rauck, R., et al. (2008). NGX-4010, a high-concentration capsaicin patch, for the treatment of postherpetic neuralgia: A randomised, double-blind study. *Lancet Neurology, 7,* 1106–1112.

Backonja, M. M. (2003). Defining neuropathic pain. *Anesthesia and Analgesia, 97,* 785–790.

Backonja, M. M., & Galer, B. S. (1998). Pain assessment and evaluation of patients who have neuropathic pain. *Neurological Clinics, 16,* 775–790.

Backonja, M. M., & Krause, S. J. (2003). Neuropathic Pain Questionnaire—Short Form. *Clinical Journal of Pain, 19,* 315–316.

Baron, R. (2000). Peripheral neuropathic pain: From mechanisms to symptoms. *Clinical Journal of Pain, 16*(Suppl. 2), S12–S20.

Baron, R. (2006). Mechanisms of disease: Neuropathic pain—a clinical perspective. *Nature Clinical Practice Neurology, 2,* 95–106.

Baron, R., Mayoral, V., Leijon, G., Binder, A., Steigerwald, I., & Serpell, M. (2009). Efficacy and safety of 5% lidocaine (lignocaine) medicated plaster in comparison with pregabalin in patients with postherpetic neuralgia and diabetic polyneuropathy: Interim analysis from an open-label, two-stage adaptive, randomized, controlled trial. *Clinical Drug Investigation, 29*(4), 231–241.

Baron, R., & Tölle, T. R. (2008). Assessment and

diagnosis of neuropathic pain. *Current Opinion in Supportive and Palliative Care, 2*, 1–8.

Baron, R., Tölle, T. R., Gockel, U., Brosz, M., & Freynhagen, R. (2009). A cross-sectional cohort survey in 2100 patients with painful diabetic neuropathy and postherpetic neuralgia: Differences in demographic data and sensory symptoms. *Pain, 146*(1), 34–40.

Bastyr, E. J., III, Price, K. L., Bril, V., & the MBBQ Study Group. (2005). Development and validity testing of the neuropathy total symptom score-6: Questionnaire for the study of sensory symptoms of diabetic peripheral neuropathy. *Clinical Therapeutics, 27*, 1278–1294.

Bennett, G. J. (1994). Neuropathic pain. In P. D. Wall & R. Melzack (Eds.), *Textbook of pain* (pp. 201–224). Edinburgh, UK: Churchill Livingstone.

Bennett, G. J. (2003). Neuropathic pain: A crisis of definition? *Anesthesia and Analgesia, 97*, 619–620.

Bennett, M. (2001). The LANSS pain scale: The Leeds Assessment of Neuropathic Symptoms and Signs. *Pain, 92*, 147–157.

Bennett, M. I., Smith, B. H., Torrance, N., & Potter, J. (2005). The S-LANSS score for identifying pain of predominantly neuropathic origin: Validation for use in clinical and postal research. *Journal of Pain, 6*, 149–158.

Berman, J. S., Symonds, C., & Birch, R. (2004). Efficacy of two cannabis based medicinal extracts for relief of central neuropathic pain from brachial plexus avulsion: Results of a randomized controlled trial. *Pain, 112*, 299–306.

Bigelow, N., Harrison, I., Goodell, H., & Wolff, H. G. (1945). Studies on pain: Quantitative measurements of two pain sensations of the skin, with reference to the nature of the "hyperalgesia of peripheral neuritis." *Journal of Clinical Investigation, 24*, 503–512.

Binder, A., Koroschetz, J., & Baron, R. (2008). Disease mechanisms in neuropathic itch. *Nature Clinics in the Practice of Neurology, 4*, 329–337.

Bostock, H., Campero, M., Serra, J., & Ochoa, J. L. (2005). Temperature-dependent double spikes in C-nociceptors of neuropathic pain patients. *Brain, 128*(Pt. 9), 2154–2163.

Bouhassira, D., & Attal, N. (2009). All in one: Is it possible to assess all dimensions of any pain with a simple questionnaire? *Pain, 144*, 7–8.

Bouhassira, D., Attal, N., Alchaar, H., Boureau, F., Brochet, B., Bruxelle, J., et al. (2005). Comparison of pain syndromes associated with nervous or somatic lesions and development of a new neuropathic pain diagnostic questionnaire (DN4). *Pain, 114*, 29–36.

Bouhassira, D., Attal, N., Fermanian, J., Alchaar, H., Gautron, M., Masquelier, E., et al. (2004). Development and validation of the neuropathic pain symptom inventory. *Pain, 108*, 248–257.

Bouhassira, D., Danziger, N., Attal, N., & Guirimand, F. (2003). Comparison of the pain suppressive effects of clinical and experimental painful conditioning stimuli. *Brain, 126*, 1068–1078.

Bouhassira, D., Lantéri-Minet, M., Attal, N., Laurent, B., & Touboul, C. (2008). Prevalence of chronic pain with neuropathic characteristics in the general population. *Pain, 136*, 380–387.

Boureau, F., Doubrère, J. F., & Luu, M. (1990). Study of verbal description in neuropathic pain. *Pain, 42*, 145–152.

Boureau, F., Legallicier, P., & Kabir-Ahmadi, M. (2003). Tramadol in post-herpetic neuralgia: A randomized, double-blind, placebo-controlled trial. *Pain, 104*, 323–331.

Bragard, D., Chen, A. C., & Plaghki, L. (1996). Direct isolation of ultra-late (C-fibre) evoked brain potentials by CO_2 laser stimulation of tiny cutaneous surface areas in man. *Neuroscience Letters, 209*, 81–84.

Bromm, B., Frieling, A., & Lankers, J. (1991). Laser-evoked brain potentials in patients with dissociated loss of pain and temperature sensibility. *Electroencephalography and Clinical Neurophysiology, 80*, 284–291.

Bromm, B., & Lorenz, J. (1998). Neurophysiological evaluation of pain. *Electroencephalography and Clinical Neurophysiology, 107*, 227–253

Bromm, B., & Treede, R.-D. (1991). Laser-evoked cerebral potentials in the assessment of cutaneous pain sensitivity in normal subjects and patients. *Review of Neurology, 147*, 625–643

Campero, M., Serra, J., Marchettini, P., & Ochoa, J. L. (1998). Ectopic impulse generation and auto excitation in single myelinated afferent fibers in patients with peripheral neuropathy and positive sensory symptoms. *Muscle and Nerves, 21*, 1661–1667.

Casey, K. L. (1999). Forebrain mechanisms of nociception and pain: Analysis through imaging. *Proceedings of the National Academy of Sciences USA, 96*, 7668–7674.

Casey, K. L., Beydoun, A., Boivie, J., Sjolund, B., Holmgren, H., Leijon, G., et al. (1996). Laser-evoked cerebral potentials and sensory function in patients with central pain. *Pain, 64*, 485–491.

Cesaro, P., Mann, M. W., Moretti, J. L., Defer, G., Roualdés, B., Nguyen, J. P., et al. (1991). Central pain and thalamic hyperactivity: A single photon emission computerized tomographic study. *Pain, 47*, 329–336.

Chong, P. S., & Cros, D. P. (2004). Technology literature review: Quantitative sensory testing. *Muscle and Nerves, 29,* 734–747.

Claus, D., Hilz, M. J., Hummer, I., & Neundörfer, B. (1987). Methods of measurement of thermal thresholds. *Acta Neurologica Scandinavica, 76,* 288–296.

Consensus Statement. (1988). Report and recommendations of the San Antonio Conference on Diabetic Neuropathy. *Diabetes, 37,* 1000–1004.

Coplan, P. M., Schmader, K., Nikas, A., Chan, I. S., Choo, P., Levin, M. J., et al. (2004). Development of a measure of the burden of pain due to herpes zoster and postherpetic neuralgia for prevention trials: Adaptation of the brief pain inventory. *Journal of Pain, 5,* 344–356.

Cruccu, G., Anand, P., Attal, N., Garcia-Larréa, L., Haanpää, M., Jørum, E., et al. (2004). EFNS guidelines on neuropathic pain assessment. *European Journal of Neurology, 11,* 153–162.

Cruccu, G., Ferracuti, S., Leardi, M. G., Fabbri, A., & Manfredi, M. (1991). Nociceptive quality of the orbicularis oculi reflexes as evaluated by distinct opiate- and benzodiazepine-induced changes in man. *Brain Research, 556,* 209–217.

Cruccu, G., Pennisi, E., Truini, A., Iannetti, G. D., Romaniello, A., Le Pera, D., et al. (2003). Unmyelinated trigeminal pathways as assessed by laser stimuli in humans. *Brain, 126,* 2246–2256.

Defrin, R., Ohry, A., Blumen, N., & Urca, G. (2001). Characterization of chronic pain and somatosensory function in spinal cord injury subjects. *Pain, 89,* 253–263.

Devigili, G., Tugnoli, V., Penza, P., Camozzi, F., Lombardi, R., Melli, G., et al. (2008). The diagnostic criteria for small fibre neuropathy: From symptoms to neuropathology. *Brain, 131*(Pt. 7), 1912–1825.

Di Piero, V., Jones, A. K., Iannotti, F., Powell, M., Perani, D., Lenzi, G. L., et al. (1991). Chronic pain: A PET study of the central effects of percutaneous high cervical cordotomy. *Pain, 46,* 9–12.

Dogra, S., Beydoun, S., Mazzola, J., Hopwood, M., & Wan, Y. (2005). Oxcarbazepine in painful diabetic neuropathy: A randomized, placebo-controlled study. *European Journal of Pain, 9,* 543–554.

Drouot, X., Nguyen, J. P., Peschanski, M., & Lefaucheur, J. P. (2002). The antalgic efficacy of chronic motor cortex stimulation is related to sensory changes in the painful zone. *Brain, 125,* 1660–1664.

Dubuisson, D., & Melzack, R. (1976). Classification of clinical pain descriptions by multiple group discriminant analysis. *Experimental Neurology, 51,* 480–487.

Ducreux, D., Attal, N., Parker, F., & Bouhassira, D. (2006). Mechanisms of central neuropathic pain: A combined psychophysical and fMRI study in syringomyelia. *Brain, 129,* 963–976.

Dworkin, R. H., Corbin, A. E., Young, J. P., Jr., Sharma, U., LaMoreaux, L., Bockbrader, H., et al. (2003). Pregabalin for the treatment of postherpetic neuralgia: A randomized, placebo-controlled trial. *Neurology, 60,* 1274–1283.

Dworkin, R. H., & Gitlin, M. J. (1991). Clinical aspects of depression in chronic pain patients. *Clinical Journal of Pain, 7,* 79–94.

Dworkin, R. H., O'Connor, A. B., Backonja, M., Farrar, J. T., Finnerup, N. B., Jensen, T. S., et al. (2007). Pharmacologic management of neuropathic pain: Evidence-based recommendations. *Pain, 132,* 237–251.

Dworkin, R. H., Turk, D. C., Farrar, J. T., Haythornthwaite, J. A., Jensen, M. P., Katz, N. P., et al. (2005). Core outcome measures for chronic pain clinical trials: IMMPACT recommendations. *Pain, 113,* 9–19.

Dworkin, R. H., Turk, D. C., Revicki, D. A., Harding, G., Coyne, K. S., Peirce-Sandner, S., et al. (2009). Development and initial validation of an expanded and revised version of the Short-Form McGill Pain Questionnaire (SF-MPQ-2). *Pain, 144,* 35–42.

Dyck, P. J., Kratz, K. M., Lehman, K. A., Karnes, J. L., Melton, L. J., III, O'Brien, P. C., et al. (1991). The Rochester Diabetic Neuropathy Study: Design, criteria for types of neuropathy, selection bias, and reproducibility of neuropathic tests. *Neurology, 41,* 799–807.

Edwards, R. R., Haythornthwaite, J. A., Tella, P., Max, M. B., & Raja, S. (2006). Basal heat pain thresholds predict opioid analgesia in patients with postherpetic neuralgia. *Anesthesiology, 104,* 1243–1248.

Farrar, J. T., Young, J. P., Jr., LaMoreaux, L., Werth, J. L., & Poole, R. M. (2001). Clinical importance of changes in chronic pain intensity measured on an 11-point numerical pain rating scale. *Pain, 94,* 149–158.

Feldman, E. L., Stevens, M. J., Thomas, P. K., Brown, M. B., Canal, N., & Greene, D. A. (1994). A practical two-step quantitative clinical and electrophysiological assessment for the diagnosis and staging of diabetic neuropathy. *Diabetes Care, 17,* 1281–1289.

Fields, H. L., Rowbotham, M., & Baron, R. (1998). Postherpetic neuralgia: Irritable nociceptors and deafferentation. *Neurobiological Diseases, 5,* 209–227.

Finnerup, N. B., Biering-Sorensen, F., Johannesen, I. L., Terkelsen, A. J., Juhl, G. I., Kristensen, A. D., et al. (2005). Intravenous lidocaine relieves spinal cord injury pain: A randomized controlled trial. *Anesthesiology, 102,* 1023–1030.

Finnerup, N. B., & Jensen, T. S. (2006). Mechanisms of disease: Mechanism-based classification of neuropathic pain—a critical analysis. *Nature Clinical Practice Neurology, 2,* 107–115.

Finnerup, N. B., Johannesen, I. L., Fuglsang-Frederiksen, A., Bach, F. W., & Jensen, T. S. (2003). Sensory function in spinal cord injury patients with and without central pain. *Brain, 126,* 57–70.

Finnerup, N. B., Otto, M., McQuay, H. J., Jensen, T. S., & Sindrup, S. H. (2005). Algorithm for neuropathic pain treatment: An evidence based proposal. *Pain, 118,* 289–305.

Finnerup, N. B., Sindrup, S. H., Bach, F. W., Johannesen, I. L., & Jensen, T. S. (2002). Lamotrigine in spinal cord injury pain: A randomized controlled trial. *Pain, 96,* 375–383.

Fisher, B. J., Haythornthwaite, J. A., Heinberg, L. J., Clark, M., & Reed, J. (2001). Suicidal intent in patients with chronic pain. *Pain, 89,* 199–206.

Forssell, H., Tenovuo, O., Silvoniemi, P., & Jääskeläinen, S. K. (2007). Differences and similarities between atypical facial pain and trigeminal neuropathic pain. *Neurology, 69,* 1451–1459.

Fowler, G. R. (1886). The operative treatment of facial neuralgia—a comparison of methods and results. *Annals of Surgery, 3,* 269–320.

Frank, S. H., Graham, A. V., Zyzanski, S. J., & White, S. (1992). Use of the Family CAGE in screening for alcohol problems in primary care. *Archives of Family Medicine, 1,* 209–216.

Fregni, F., Boggio, P. S., Lima, M. C., Ferreira, M. J., Wagner, T., Rigonatti, S. P., et al. (2006). A sham-controlled, phase II trial of transcranial direct current stimulation for the treatment of central pain in traumatic spinal cord injury. *Pain, 122,* 197–209.

Freynhagen, R., Baron, R., Gockel, U., & Tölle, T. R. (2006). painDETECT: A new screening questionnaire to identify neuropathic components in patients with back pain. *Current Medical Research and Opinion, 22,* 1911–1920.

Freynhagen, R., Strojek, K., Griesing, T., Whalen, E., & Balkenohl, M. (2005). Efficacy of pregabalin in neuropathic pain evaluated in a 12-week, randomised, double-blind, multicentre, placebo-controlled trial of flexible- and fixed-dose regimens. *Pain, 115,* 254–263.

Fruhstorfer, H., Lindblom, U., & Schmidt, W. G. (1976). Method for quantitative estimation of thermal threshold in patients. *Journal of Neurology, Neurosurgery, and Psychiatry, 39,* 1071–1075.

Galer, B., & Jensen, M. (1997). Development and preliminary validation of a pain measure specific to neuropathic pain: The Neuropathic Pain Scale. *Neurology, 48,* 332–338.

Galer, B. S., Jensen, M. P., Ma, T., Davies, P. S., & Rowbotham, M. C. (2002). The lidocaine patch 5% effectively treats all neuropathic pain qualities: Results of a randomized, double-blind, vehicle-controlled, 3-week efficacy study with use of the neuropathic pain scale. *Clinical Journal of Pain, 18,* 297–301.

Garcia-Larréa, L. (2006). Evoked potentials in the assessment of pain. In F. Cervero & T. S. Jensen (Eds.), *Handbook of clinical neurology: Vol. 81. Pain* (pp. 437–461). Amsterdam: Elsevier.

Garcia-Larréa, L., Convers, P., Magnin, M., André-Obadia, N., Peyron, R., Laurent, B., et al. (2002). Laser-evoked potential abnormalities in central pain patients: The influence of spontaneous and provoked pain. *Brain, 125,* 2766–2781.

Garcia-Larréa, L., Peyron, R., Laurent, B., & Mauguière, F. (1997). Association and dissociation between laser-evoked potentials and pain perception. *NeuroReport, 17,* 3785–3789.

Garcia-Larréa, L., Peyron, R., Mertens, P., Gregoire, M. C., Lavenne, F., Le Bars, D., et al. (1999). Electrical stimulation of motor cortex for pain control: A combined PET-scan and electrophysiological study. *Pain, 83,* 259–273.

Gilron, I., Bailey, J. M., Tu, D., Holden, R. R., Jackson, A. C., & Houlden, R. L. (2009). Nortriptyline and gabapentin, alone and in combination for neuropathic pain: A double-blind, randomised controlled crossover trial. *Lancet, 374,* 1252–1261.

Gilron, I., Bailey, J. M., Tu, D., Holden, R. R., Weaver, D. F., & Houlden, R. L. (2005). Morphine, gabapentin, or their combination for neuropathic pain. *New England Journal of Medicine, 352,* 1324–1334.

Gilron, I., Booher, S. L., Rowan, M. S., Smoller, M. S., & Max, M. B. (2000). A randomized, controlled trial of high-dose dextromethorphan in facial neuralgias. *Neurology, 55,* 964–971.

Gimbel, J. S., Richards, P., & Portenoy, R. K. (2003). Controlled-release oxycodone for pain in diabetic neuropathy: A randomized controlled trial. *Neurology, 60,* 927–934.

Goldberg, J. M., & Lindblom, U. (1979). Standardised method of determining vibratory perception thresholds for diagnosis and screening in neurological investigation. *Journal of Neurology, Neurosurgery, and Psychiatry, 42,* 793–803.

Goldstein, D. J., Lu, Y., Detke, M. J., Lee, T. C., & Iyengar, S. (2005). Duloxetine vs. placebo in patients with painful diabetic neuropathy. *Pain*, *116*, 109–118.

Gordh, T. E., Stubhaug, A., Jensen, T. S., Arnèr, S., Biber, B., Boivie, J., et al. (2008). Gabapentin in traumatic nerve injury pain: A randomized, double-blind, placebo-controlled, crossover, multi-center study. *Pain*, *138*, 255–266.

Gottrup, H., Bach, F. W., Juhl, G., & Jensen, T. S. (2006). Differential effect of ketamine and lidocaine on spontaneous and mechanical evoked pain in patients with nerve injury pain. *Anesthesiology*, *104*, 527–536.

Gracely, R. H., McGrath, P., & Dubner, R. (1978). Validity and sensitivity of ratio scales of sensory and affective verbal pain descriptors: Manipulation of affect by diazepam. *Pain*, *5*, 19–29.

Granot, M., Buskila, D., Granovsky, Y., Sprecher, E., Neumann, L., & Yarnitsky, D. (2001). Simultaneous recording of late and ultra-late pain evoked potentials in fibromyalgia. *Clinical Neurophysiology*, *112*, 1881–1887.

Granot, M., Granovsky, Y., Sprecher, E., Nir, R. R., & Yarnitsky, D. (2006). Contact heat-evoked temporal summation: Tonic versus repetitive-phasic stimulation. *Pain*, *122*, 295–305.

Granot, M., & Nagler, R. M. (2005). Association between regional idiopathic neuropathy and salivary involvement as the possible mechanism for oral sensory complaints. *Journal of Pain*, *6*, 581–587.

Hansson, P. (2002). Neuropathic pain: Clinical characteristics and diagnostic workup. *European Journal of Pain*, *6*(Suppl. A), 47–50.

Hansson, P., Backonja, M., & Bouhassira, D. (2007). Usefulness and limitations of quantitative sensory testing: Clinical and research application in neuropathic pain states. *Pain*, *129*, 256–259.

Hansson, P., & Haanpää, M. (2007). Diagnostic work-up of neuropathic pain: Computing, using questionnaires or examining the patient? *European Journal of Pain*, *11*, 367–369.

Hansson, P., & Lindblom, U. (1992). Hyperalgesia assessed with quantitative sensory testing in patients with neurogenic pain. In W. D. Willis (Ed.), *Hyperalgesia and allodynia* (pp. 335–343). New York: Raven Press.

Haythornthwaite, J. A., & Benrud-Larsen, L. M. (2000). Psychological aspects of neuropathic pain. *Clinical Journal of Pain*, *16*, S-01–S105.

Herrmann, D. N., Pannoni, V., Barbano, R. L., Pennella-Vaughan, J., & Dworkin, R. H. (2006). Skin biopsy and quantitative sensory testing do not predict response to lidocaine patch in painful neuropathies. *Muscle Nerve*, *33*, 42–48.

Holland, N. R., Crawford, T. O., Hauer, P., Cornblath, D. R., Griffin, J. W., & McArthur, J. C. (1998). Small fiber sensory neuropathies: Clinical course and neuropathology of idiopathic cases. *Annals of Neurology*, *44*, 47–59.

Hsieh, J. C., Belfrage, M., Stone-Elander, S., Hansson, P., & Ingvar, M. (1995). Central representation of chronic ongoing neuropathic pain studied by positron emission tomography. *Pain*, *63*, 225–236.

Iadarola, M. J., Max, M. B., Berman, K. F., Byas-Smith, M. G., Coghill, R. C., Gracely, R. H., et al. (1995). Unilateral decrease in thalamic activity observed with positron emission tomography in patients with chronic neuropathic pain. *Pain*, *63*, 55–64.

Jacome, D. (1978). Phantom itching relieved by scratching phantom feet. *Journal of the American Medical Association*, *240*, 2432.

Jensen, M. P., Friedman, M., Bonzo, D., & Richards, P. (2006). The validity of the Neuropathic Pain Scale for assessing diabetic neuropathic pain in a clinical trial. *Clinical Journal of Pain*, *22*(1), 97–103.

Jensen, M. P., Gammaitoni, A. R., Olaleye, D. O., Oleka, N., Nalamachu, S. R., & Galer, B. S. (2006). The Pain Quality Assessment Scale: Assessment of pain quality in carpal tunnel syndrome. *Journal of Pain*, *7*, 823–832.

Jensen, M. P., Karoly, P., & Braver, S. (1986). The measurement of clinical pain intensity: A comparison of six methods. *Pain*, *27*, 117–126.

Jensen, T. S., & Baron, R. (2003). Translation of symptoms and signs into mechanisms in neuropathic pain. *Pain*, *102*, 1–8.

Jensen, T. S., Gottrup, H., Sindrup, S. H., & Bach, F. W. (2001). The clinical picture of neuropathic pain. *European Journal of Pharmacology*, *429*, 1–11.

Jorum, E., & Schmelz, M. (2006). Microneurography in the assessment of neuropathic pain. *Handbook of Clinical Neurology*, *81*, 427–438.

Kakigi, R., Shibasaki, H., Kuroda, Y., Neshige, R., Endo, C., Tabuchi, K., et al. (1991). Pain-related somatosensory potentials in syringomyelia. *Brain*, *114*(Pt. 4), 1971–1889.

Kanda, M., Mima, T., Xu, X., Fujiwara, N., Shindo, K., Nagamine, T., et al. (1996). Pain-related somatosensory evoked potentials can quantitatively evaluate hypalgesia in Wallenberg's syndrome. *Acta Neurologica Scandinavica*, *94*, 131–136.

Karst, M., Salim, K., Burstein, S., Conrad, I., Hoy, L., & Schneider, U. (2003). Analgesic effect of the synthetic cannabinoid CT-3 on chronic neuropathic pain: A randomized controlled trial. *Journal of the American Medical Association, 290,* 1757–1762.

Kelly, K. G., Cook, T., & Backonja, M. M. (2005). Pain ratings at the thresholds are necessary for interpretation of quantitative sensory testing. *Muscle Nerve, 32,* 179–184.

Khoromi, S., Cui, L., Nackers, L., & Max, M. B. (2007). Morphine, nortriptyline and their combination vs. placebo in patients with chronic lumbar root pain. *Pain, 130,* 66–75.

Kikuchi, A., Kotani, N., Sato, T., Takamura, K., Sakai, I., & Matsuki, A. (1999). Comparative therapeutic evaluation of intrathecal versus epidural methylprednisolone for long-term analgesia in patients with intractable postherpetic neuralgia. *Regional Anesthesia and Pain Medicine, 24,* 287–293.

Kozin, F., Soin, J. S., Ryan, L. M., Carrera, G. F., & Wortmann, R. L. (1981). Bone scintigraphy in the reflex sympathetic dystrophy syndrome. *Radiology, 138,* 437–443.

Krämer, H. H., Rolke, R., Bickel, A., & Birklein, F. (2004). Thermal thresholds predict painfulness of diabetic neuropathies. *Diabetes Care, 27,* 2386–2391.

Krause, S. J., & Backonja, M. M. (2003). Development of a neuropathic pain questionnaire. *Clinical Journal of Pain, 19,* 306–314.

Kumar, K., Taylor, R. S., Jacques, L., Eldabe, S., Meglio, M., Molet, J., et al. (2007). Spinal cord stimulation versus conventional medical management for neuropathic pain: A multi-centre randomised controlled trial in patients with failed back surgery syndrome. *Pain, 132,* 179–188.

Kupers, R., & Kehlet, H. (2006). Brain imaging of clinical pain states: A critical review and strategies for future studies. *Lancet Neurology, 5,* 1033–1044.

Lang, P. M., Schober, G. M., Rolke, R., Wagner, S., Hilge, R., Offenbächer, M., et al. (2006). Sensory neuropathy and signs of central sensitization in patients with peripheral arterial disease. *Pain, 124,* 190–200.

Lauria, G., Cornblath, D. R., Johansson, O., McArthur, J. C., Mellgren, S. I., Nolano, M., et al. (2005). EFNS guidelines on the use of skin biopsy in the diagnosis of peripheral neuropathy. *European Journal of Neurology, 12,* 747–758.

Lesser, H., Sharma, U., LaMoreaux, L., & Poole, R. M. (2004). Pregabalin relieves symptoms of painful diabetic neuropathy: A randomized controlled trial. *Neurology, 63,* 2104–2110.

Leung, A., Wallace, M. S., Ridgeway, B., & Yaksh, T. (2001). Concentration–effect relationship of intravenous alfentanil and ketamine on peripheral neurosensory thresholds, allodynia and hyperalgesia of neuropathic pain. *Pain, 91,* 177–187.

Levendoglu, F., Ogün, C. O., Ozerbil, O., Ogün, T. C., & Ugurlu, H. (2004). Gabapentin is a first line drug for the treatment of neuropathic pain in spinal cord injury. *Spine, 29,* 743–751.

Llewelyn, J. G., Gilbey, S. G., Thomas, P. K., King, R. H. M., Muddle, J. R., & Watkins, P. J. (1991). Sural nerve morphometry in diabetic autonomic and painful sensory neuropathy: A clinicopathological study. *Brain, 114,* 867–892.

Lynch, M. E., Clark, A. J., & Sawynok, J. (2003). A pilot study examining topical amitriptyline, ketamine, and a combination of both in the treatment of neuropathic pain. *Clinical Journal of Pain, 19,* 323–328.

Magerl, W., Zahid, A., Ellrich, J., Meyer, R. A., & Treede, R.-D. (1999). C and Aδ-fiber components of heat-evoked cerebral potentials in healthy human subjects. *Pain, 82,* 127–137.

Maguire, M. F., Ravenscroft, A., Beggs, D., & Duffy, J. P. (2006). A questionnaire study investigating the prevalence of the neuropathic component of chronic pain after thoracic surgery. *European Journal of Cardiothoracic Surgery, 29,* 800–805.

Masson, E. A., Hunt, L., Gem, J. M., & Boulton, A. J. (1989). A novel approach to the diagnosis and assessment of symptomatic diabetic neuropathy. *Pain, 38,* 25–28.

Max, M. B. (2002). Clarifying the definition of neuropathic pain. *Pain, 96,* 406–407.

McQuay, H., & Moore, A. (1998). *An evidence based resource for pain relief.* Oxford, UK: Oxford University Press.

Melzack, R. (1975). The McGill Pain Questionnaire: Major properties and scoring methods. *Pain, 1,* 275–299.

Melzack, R. (1987). The Short-Form McGill Pain Questionnaire. *Pain, 30,* 191–197.

Melzack, R., Terrence, C., Fromm, G., & Amsel, R. (1986). Trigeminal neuralgia and atypical facial pain: Use of the McGill Pain Questionnaire for discrimination and diagnosis. *Pain, 27,* 297–302.

Mendell, J. R., & Sahenk, Z. (2003). Clinical practice: Painful sensory neuropathy. *New England Journal of Medicine, 348,* 1243–1255.

Merskey, H. (2002). Clarifying definition of neuropathic pain. *Pain, 96,* 408–409.

Merskey, H., & Bogduk, N. (Eds.). (1994). *Classification of chronic pain: Descriptions of chronic pain syndromes and definitions of pain terms* [Task Force on the Taxonomy of the IASP] (2nd ed., pp. 209–214). Seattle, WA: IASP Press.

Michna, E., Ross, E. L., Hynes, W. L., Nedeljkovic, S. S., Soumekh, S., Janfaza, D., et al. (2004). Predicting aberrant drug behavior in patients treated for chronic pain: Importance of abuse history. *Journal of Pain and Symptom Management, 28*, 250–258.

Moisset, X., & Bouhassira, D. (2007). Brain imaging of neuropathic pain. *NeuroImage, 37*(Suppl. 1), S80–S88.

Noordenbos, W. (1959). *Pain.* Amsterdam: Elsevier.

Nurmikko, T. J., Serpell, M. G., Hoggart, B., Toomey, P. J., Morlion, B. J., & Haines, D. (2007). Sativex successfully treats neuropathic pain characterised by allodynia: A randomised, double-blind, placebo-controlled clinical trial. *Pain, 133*, 210–220.

Oaklander, A.-L. (2001). The density of remaining nerve endings in human skin with and without postherpetic neuralgia after shingles. *Pain, 92*(1–2), 139–145.

Oaklander, A.-L., Rissmiller, J. G., Gelman, L. B., Zheng, L., Chang, Y., & Gott, R. (2006). Evidence of focal small-fiber axonal degeneration in complex regional pain syndrome–I (reflex sympathetic dystrophy). *Pain, 120*, 235–243.

Oaklander, A.-L., Romans, K., Horasek, S., Stocks, A., Hauer, P., & Meyer, R. A. (1998). Unilateral postherpetic neuralgia is associated with bilateral sensory neuron damage. *Annals of Neurology, 44*, 789–795.

O'Connor, A. B. (2009). Neuropathic pain: Quality-of-life impact, costs and cost effectiveness of therapy. *Pharmacoeconomics, 27*, 95–112.

Odrcich, M., Bailey, J. M., Cahill, C. M., & Gilron, I. (2006). Chronobiological characteristics of painful diabetic neuropathy and postherpetic neuralgia: Diurnal pain variation and effects of analgesic therapy. *Pain, 120*, 207–212.

Orstavik, K., Namer, B., Schmidt, R., Schmelz, M., Hilliges, M., Weidner, C., et al. (2006). Abnormal function of C-fibers in patients with diabetic neuropathy. *Journal of Neuroscience, 26*, 11287–11294.

Petersen, K. L., Fields, H. L., Brennum, J., Sandroni, P., & Rowbotham, M. C. (2000). Capsaicin evoked pain and allodynia in postherpetic neuralgia. *Pain, 88*, 125–133.

Petrovic, P., Ingvar, M., Stone-Elander, S., Petersson, K. M., & Hansson, P. (1999). A PET activation study of dynamic mechanical allodynia in patients with mononeuropathy. *Pain, 83*, 459–470.

Peyron, R., Garcia-Larréa, L., Gregoire, M. C., Convers, P., Lavenne, F., Veyre, L., et al. (1998). Allodynia after lateral-medullary (Wallenberg) infarct: A PET study. *Brain, 121*, 345–356.

Peyron, R., Laurent, B., & Garcia-Larréa, L. (2000). Functional imaging of brain responses to pain: A review and meta-analysis. *Neurophysiology Clinics, 30*, 263–288.

Peyron, R., Schneider, F., Faillenot, I., Convers, P., Barral, F. G., Garcia-Larréa, L., et al. (2004). An fMRI study of cortical representation of mechanical allodynia in patients with neuropathic pain. *Neurology, 63*, 1838–1846.

Plaghki, L., & Mouraux, A. (2003). How do we selectively activate skin nociceptors with a high power infrared laser?: Physiology and biophysics of laser stimulation. *Neurophysiology Clinics, 33*, 269–277.

Portenoy, R., Cleeland, C., Backonja, M., Moskowitz, R., Parsons, B., McLeod, L., et al. (2005). A new validated patient-completed neuropathic pain screening tool for use in the primary care setting. *Journal of Pain, 6*(3), S27.

Ragazzoni, A., Amantini, A., Lombardi, M., Macucci, M., Mascalchi, M., & Pinto, F. (1993). Electric and CO_2 laser SEPs in a patient with syringomyelia. *Electroencephalography and Clinical Neurophysiology, 88*, 335–338.

Raja, S. N., Haythornthwaite, J. A., Pappagallo, M., Clark, M. R., Travison, T. G., Sabeen, S., et al. (2002). Opioids versus antidepressants in postherpetic neuralgia: A randomized, placebo-controlled trial. *Neurology, 59*, 1015–1021.

Ranoux, D., Attal, N., Morain, F., & Bouhassira, D. (2008). Botulinum toxin a induces direct analgesic effects in neuropathic pain: A double blind placebo controlled study. *Annals of Neurology, 64*, 274–283.

Raskin, J., Pritchett, Y. L., Wang, F., D'Souza, D. N., Waninger, A. L., Iyengar, S., et al. (2005). A double-blind, randomized multicentre trial comparing duloxetine with placebo in the management of diabetic peripheral neuropathic pain. *Pain, 6*, 346–356.

Raskin, P., Donofrio, P. D., Rosenthal, N. R., Hewitt, D. J., Jordan, D. M., Xiang, J., et al. (2004). Topiramate vs placebo in painful diabetic neuropathy: Analgesic and metabolic effects. *Neurology, 63*, 865–873.

Rasmussen, P. V., Sindrup, S. H., Jensen, T. S., & Bach, F. W. (2004). Symptoms and signs in patients with suspected neuropathic pain. *Pain, 110*, 461–469.

Rauck, R. L., Shaibani, A., Biton, V., Simpson, J., & Koch, B. (2007). Lacosamide in painful diabetic peripheral neuropathy: A phase 2 double-blind placebo-controlled study. *Clinical Journal of Pain, 23*, 150–158.

Richeimer, S. H., Bajwa, Z. H., Kahraman, S. S.,

Ransil, B. J., & Warfield, C. A. (1997). Utilization patterns of tricyclic antidepressants in a multidisciplinary pain clinic: A survey. *Clinical Journal of Pain*, 13, 324–329.

Richter, R. W., Portenoy, R., Sharma, U., Lamoreaux, L., Bockbrader, H., & Knapp, L. E. (2005). Relief of painful diabetic peripheral neuropathy with pregabalin: A randomized, placebo-controlled trial. *Journal of Pain*, 6, 253–260.

Rog, D. J., Nurmikko, T. J., Friede, T., & Young, C. A. (2005). Randomized, controlled trial of cannabis-based medicine in central pain in multiple sclerosis. *Neurology*, 65, 812–819.

Rog, D. J., Nurmikko, T. J., Friede, T., & Young, C. A. (2007). Validation and reliability of the Neuropathic Pain Scale (NPS) in multiple sclerosis. *Clinical Journal of Pain*, 23, 473–481.

Rolke, R., Baron, R., Maier, C., Toll, T. R., Treed, R.-D., Beyer, A., et al. (2006). Quantitative sensory testing in the German research network on neuropathic pain (DFNS): Standardized protocol and reference values. *Pain*, 123(3), 231–243.

Rolke, R., Magerl, W., Campbell, K. A., Schalber, C., Caspari, S., Birklein, F., et al. (2006). Quantitative sensory testing: A comprehensive protocol for clinical trials. *European Journal of Pain*, 10, 77–88.

Rowbotham, M. C., & Fields, H. L. (1989). Postherpetic neuralgia: The relation of pain complaint, sensory disturbance, and skin temperature. *Pain*, 39, 129–144.

Rowbotham, M. C., Goli, V., Kunz, N. R., & Lei, D. (2004). Venlafaxine extended release in the treatment of painful diabetic neuropathy: A double-blind, placebo-controlled study. *Pain*, 110, 697–706.

Rowbotham, M. C., Yosipovitch, G., Connolly, M. K., Finlay, D., Forde, G., & Fields, H. L. (1996). Cutaneous innervation density in the allodynic form of postherpetic neuralgia. *Neurobiological Diseases*, 3, 205–214.

Schattschneider, J., Bode, A., Wasner, G., Binder, A., Deuschl, G., & Baron, R. (2004). Idiopathic restless legs syndrome: Abnormalities in central somatosensory processing. *Journal of Neurology*, 251, 977–982.

Schiff, E., & Eisenberg, E. (2003). Can quantitative sensory testing predict the outcome of epidural steroid injections in sciatica?: A preliminary study. *Anesthesia and Analgesia*, 97, 828–832.

Scholz, J., Mannion, R. J., Hord, D. E., Griffin, R. S., Rawal, B., Zheng, H., et al. (2009). A novel tool for the assessment of pain: Validation in low back pain. *PLoS Medicine*, 6, e1000047.

Schweinhardt, P., Glynn, C., Brooks, J., McQuay, H., Jack, T., Chessell, I., et al. (2006). An fMRI study of cerebral processing of brush-evoked allodynia in neuropathic pain patients. *NeuroImage*, 32, 256–265.

Serpell, M. G. (2002). Gabapentin in neuropathic pain syndromes: A randomised, double-blind, placebo-controlled trial. *Pain*, 99, 557–566.

Shy, M. E., Frohman, E. M., So, Y. T., Arezzo, J. C., Cornblath, D. R., Giuliani, M. J., et al. (2003). Therapeutics and Technology Assessment Subcommittee of the American Academy of Neurology: Quantitative sensory testing: Report of the Therapeutics and Technology Assessment Subcommittee of the American Academy of Neurology. *Neurology*, 60, 898–904.

Siddall, P. J., Cousins, M. J., Otte, A., Griesing, T., Chambers, R., & Murphy, T. K. (2006). Pregabalin in central neuropathic pain associated with spinal cord injury: A placebo-controlled trial. *Neurology*, 67, 1792–800.

Simpson, D. M., McArthur, J. C., Olney, R., Clifford, D., So, Y., Ross, D., et al. (2003). Lamotrigine for HIV-associated painful sensory neuropathies: A placebo-controlled trial. *Neurology*, 60, 1508–1514.

Simpson, D. M., Messina, J., Xie, F., & Hale, M. (2007). Fentanyl buccal tablet for the relief of breakthrough pain in opioid-tolerant adult patients with chronic neuropathic pain: A multicenter, randomized, double-blind, placebo-controlled study. *Clinical Therapeutics*, 29, 588–601.

Sindou, M., Mertens, P., Bendavid, U., Garcia-Larréa, L., & Mauguière, F. (2003). Predictive value of somatosensory evoked potentials for long-lasting pain relief after spinal cord stimulation. *Neurosurgery*, 53, 1374–1384.

Sindrup, S. H., Bach, F. W., Madsen, C., Gram, L. F., & Jensen, T. S. (2003). Venlafaxine versus imipramine in painful polyneuropathy: A randomized, controlled trial. *Neurology*, 60, 1284–1289.

Sindrup, S. H., Graf, A., & Sfikas, N. (2006). The NK1-receptor antagonist TKA731 in painful diabetic neuropathy: A randomised, controlled trial. *European Journal of Pain*, 10, 567–571.

Smith, M. T., Edwards, R. R., Robinson, R. C., & Dworkin, R. H. (2004). Suicidal ideation, plans, and attempts in chronic pain patients: Factors associated with increased risk. *Pain*, 111, 201–208.

Smith, M. T., & Haythornthwaite, J. A. (2004). How do sleep disturbance and chronic pain inter-relate?: Insights from the longitudinal and cognitive-behavioral clinical trials literature. *Sleep Medicine Review*, 8, 119–132.

Solak, O., Metin, M., Esme, H., Solak, O.,

Yaman, M., Pekcolaklar, A., et al. (2007). Effectiveness of gabapentin in the treatment of chronic post-thoracotomy pain. *European Journal of Cardiothoracic Surgery, 32*(1), 9–12.

Sommer, C., & Lauria, G. (2007). Skin biopsy in the management of peripheral neuropathy. *Lancet Neurology, 6*, 632–642.

Sorensen, L., Molyneaux, L., & Yue, D. K. (2006a). The level of small nerve fiber dysfunction does not predict pain in diabetic neuropathy: A study using quantitative sensory testing. *Clinical Journal of Pain, 22*, 261–265.

Sorensen, L., Molyneaux, L., & Yue, D. K. (2006b). The relationship among pain, sensory loss, and small nerve fibers in diabetes. *Diabetes Care, 29*, 883–887.

Svendsen, K. B., Jensen, T. S., & Bach, F. W. (2004). The cannabinoid dronabinol reduces central pain in multiple sclerosis: A randomized double-blind placebo-controlled crossover trial. *British Medical Journal, 329*, 253–261.

Tinel, J. (1915). "Tingling" signs with peripheral nerve injuries. *Journal of Hand Surgery (British), 30*, 87–99.

Torebjörk, E. (1993). Human microneurography and intraneural microstimulation in the study of neuropathic pain. *Muscle and Nerve, 16*, 1063–1065.

Torrance, N., Smith, B. H., Bennett, M. I., & Lee, A. J. (2006). The epidemiology of chronic pain of predominantly neuropathic origin: Results from a general population survey. *Journal of Pain, 7*, 281–289.

Treede, R.-D., Jensen, T. S., Campbell, J. N., Cruccu, G., Dostrovsky, J. O., Griffin, J. W., et al. (2008). Neuropathic pain: Redefinition and a grading system for clinical and research purposes. *Neurology, 70*, 1630–1635.

Treede, R.-D., Lankers, J., Frieling, A., Zangemeister, W. H., Kunze, K., & Bromm, B. (1991). Cerebral potentials evoked by painful laser stimuli in patients with syringogmyelia. *Brain, 114*, 1595–1607.

Treede, R.-D., Lorenz, J., & Baumgärtner, U. (2003). Clinical usefulness of laser-evoked potentials. *Neurophysiology Clinics, 33*, 303–314.

Treede, R.-D., Meier, W., Kunze, K., & Bromm, B. (1988). Ultralate cerebral potentials as correlates of pain perception: Observation in a case of neurosyphilis. *Journal of Neurology, Neurosurgery, and Psychiatry, 51*, 1330–1333.

Treede, R. D., Meyer, R. A., Raja, S. N., & Campbell, J. N. (1992). Peripheral and central mechanisms of cutaneous hyperalgesia. *Progress in Neurobiology, 38*, 397–421.

Truini, A., Galeotti, F., Haanpää, M., Zucchi, R., Albanesi, A., Biasiotta, A., et al. (2008). Pathophysiology of pain in postherpetic neuralgia: A clinical and neurophysiological study. *Pain, 140*, 405–410.

Truini, A., Haanpää, M., Zucchi, R., Galeotti, F., Iannetti, G. D., Romaniello, A., et al. (2003). Laser-evoked potentials in postherpetic neuralgia. *Clinical Neurophysiology, 114*, 702–709.

Victor, T. W., Jensen, M. P., Gammaitoni, A. R., Gould, E. M., White, R. E., & Galer, B. S. (2008). The dimensions of pain quality: Factor analysis of the Pain Quality Assessment Scale. *Clinical Journal of Pain, 24*, 550–555.

Wager, T. D., Rilling, J. K., Smith, E. E., Sokolik, A., Casey, K. L., Davidson, R. J., et al. (20040. Placebo-induced changes in FMRI in the anticipation and experience of pain. *Science, 303*, 1162–1167.

Wallace, M. S., Dyck, J. B., Rossi, S. S., & Yaksh, T. L. (1996). Computer-controlled lidocaine infusion for the evaluation of neuropathic pain after peripheral nerve injury. *Pain, 66*, 69–77.

Wallace, M. S., Ridgeway, B. M., Leung, A. Y., Gerayli, A., & Yaksh, T. L. (2000). Concentration–effect relationship of intravenous lidocaine on the allodynia of complex regional pain syndrome types I and II. *Anesthesiology, 92*, 75–83.

Wasner, G., Kleinert, A., Binder, A., Schattschneider, J., & Baron, R. (2005). Postherpetic neuralgia: Topical lidocaine is effective in nociceptor-deprived skin. *Journal of Neurology, 252*, 677–686.

Wasner, G., Lee, B. B., Engel, S., & McLachlan, E. (2008). Residual spinothalamic tract pathways predict development of central pain after spinal cord injury. *Brain, 131*, 2387–2400.

Watson, C. P., Moulin, D., Watt-Watson, J., Gordon, A., & Eisenhoffer, J. (2003). Controlled-release oxycodone relieves neuropathic pain: A randomized controlled trial in painful diabetic neuropathy. *Pain, 105*, 71–78.

Waylett-Rendall, J. (1988). Sensibility evaluation and rehabilitation. *Orthopedic Clinics of North America, 19*, 43–56.

Weddell, G., Sinclair, D. C., & Feindel, W. H. (1948). An anatomical basis for alterations in quality of pain sensibility. *Journal of Neurophysiology, 11*, 99–109.

Wernicke, J. F., Pritchett, Y. L., D'Souza, D. N., Waninger, A., Tran, P., Iyengar, S., et al. (2006). A randomized controlled trial of duloxetine in diabetic peripheral neuropathic pain. *Neurology, 67*, 1411–1420.

Willer, J. C. (1985). Studies on pain: Effects of morphine on a spinal nociceptive flexion reflex and related pain sensation in man. *Brain Research, 331*, 105–114.

Wilson, P., Stanton-Hicks, M., & Harden, R. N (Eds.). (2005). *CRPS: current diagnosis and therapy* (Vol. 32 in the Progress in Pain Research and Management Series). Seattle, WA: IASP Press.

Woolf, C. J. (2004). Dissecting out mechanisms responsible for peripheral neuropathic pain: Implications for diagnosis and therapy. *Life Science, 74,* 2605–2610.

Woolf, C. J., Bennett, G. J., Doherty, M., Dubner, R., Kidd, B., Koltzenburg, M., et al. (1998). Towards a mechanism-based classification of pain? *Pain, 77,* 227–229.

Woolf, C. J., & Mannion, R. J. (1999). Neuropathic pain: Aetiology, symptoms, mechanisms, and management. *Lancet, 353,* 1959–1564.

Woolf, C. J., & Max, M. B. (2001). Mechanism-based pain diagnosis: Issues for analgesic drug development. *Anesthesiology, 95,* 241–249.

Wu, Q., Garcia-Larréa, L., Mertens, P., Beschet, A., Sindou, M., & Mauguière, F. (1999). Hyperalgesia with reduced laser evoked potentials in neuropathic pain. *Pain, 80,* 209–214.

Yarnitsky, D. (1997). Quantitative sensory testing. *Muscle and Nerve, 20,* 198–204.

Yarnitsky, D., Sprecher, E., Zaslansky, R., & Hemli, J. A. (1995). Heat pain thresholds: Normative data and repeatability. *Pain, 60,* 329–332.

Zelman, D. C., Gore, M., Dukes, E., Tai, K. S., & Brandenburg, N. (2005). Validation of a modified version of the Brief Pain Inventory for painful diabetic peripheral neuropathy. *Journal of Pain and Symptom Management, 29,* 401–410.

CHAPTER 18

Assessment of Headaches

FRANK ANDRASIK
DAWN C. BUSE
ALYSSA LETTICH

Headache is an extremely common condition that affects the majority of individuals at some point during their lifetime. Most headaches are benign; however, headache disorders can have a significant negative impact on functioning, productivity, and quality of life. Despite the number of individuals affected worldwide and the well-demonstrated significant burden that it causes, primary headache (e.g., migraine) remains underestimated, underdiagnosed, and undertreated (Lipton, Bigal, et al., 2007). Even with a diagnosis such as migraine, health care professionals may not fully assess the degree and scope of functional impairment and effect it has on a patient's quality of life and psychological well-being (Holmes, MacGregor, Sawyer, & Lipton, 2001). Yet this information is imperative in order to design the most effective and comprehensive treatment plan utilizing the available acute and preventive pharmacological treatments and biobehavioral interventions.

Headache, like many other pain disorders covered in this volume, is multifactorial and subjective, without reliable objective markers. Therefore, complete assessment requires a through evaluation and understanding of the headache disorder in the context of the patient's life. Headache is best conceptualized in a biopsychosocial framework (Andrasik, Flor, & Turk, 2005) and best treated with a coordinated multimodal approach (Lemstra, Stewart, & Olszynski, 2002). In this chapter we address the following aspects of assessment of patients with headache disorders: application of the biopsychosocial model to headache; headache classification and diagnostic considerations; and evaluation and treatment of related medical, psychological, and quality-of-life issues. We additionally review headache- and migraine-specific outcome measures, as well as other tools that are useful in a clinical headache practice or headache-related research. These outcome measures can be divided into the following categories: (1) headache diagnosis and symptomatology; (2) headache-related functional impairment, burden, and disability; (3) health-related quality of life; (4) treatment planning, optimization, and satisfaction; (5) cognitive and psychological aspects of headache; and (6) psychiatric comorbidities. The majority of instruments reviewed were developed and validated for adults; however, we also briefly discuss instruments appropriate for assessment of pediatric patients.

The following psychometric terms will be used. *Reliability* refers to how consistently a measure assesses a given variable, with test–retest and internal consistency being the two general ways that reliability is measured. *Intraclass correlation coefficient* (ICC) is a test–retest measure of reliability for quantitative (interval or ratio scale) variables and consists of the ratio of two variances. It yields the proportion of variance attributable to between-class differences. Another test–retest measure of reliability, Cohen's kappa, is a chance-corrected measure of agreement between pairs of variables (dichotomous or polychotomous variables). Kappa is always equal to or less than one, wherein a value of 1.0 implies perfect agreement. The interclass correlation coefficient Pearson's *r* is also a test–retest measure of reliability. It reflects the degree of linear relationship between two variables not of a common class. Pearson's *r* assumes a normal distribution, with values ranging from +1 to –1. A correlation of +1 means that there is a perfect positive linear relationship between variables, while a correlation of –1 means that there is a perfect negative linear relationship between variables. A correlation of 0 means that there is no linear relationship between the two variables. Spearman's rank correlation coefficient is a measure of interclass correlation for nonparametric data. Cronbach's alpha is a measure of internal consistency also used to determine reliability. It reflects how well each individual item in a scale correlates with the remaining items.

HEADACHE CLASSIFICATION AND DIAGNOSIS

Prior to the 1980s, there was little consensus about headache classification and diagnosis. In 1985 the International Headache Society (IHS) assembled headache experts from around the world to enumerate the various types and subtypes of headache, and to develop explicit and comprehensive diagnostic criteria. The resultant International Classification of Headache Disorders (ICHD) criteria was instrumental in standardizing headache diagnosis in clinical practice and research worldwide (Headache Classification Committee of the International Headache Society, 1988). This system has been endorsed by all national headache societies

within the IHS, the World Federation of Neurology, and the World Health Organization (WHO), and accepted for inclusion in the *International Classification of Diseases* (ICD), the international standard diagnostic classification for epidemiological, health management purposes, and clinical use. In 2004, the classification system was updated and revised, resulting in the ICHD-II (Silberstein et al., 2004). The ICHD-II classification system is divided into three sections: (1) primary headache disorders (i.e., headaches not attributable to another medical condition), which has four major categories and 57 subtypes; (2) secondary headaches (i.e., headaches attributable to another medical condition), of which there are eight major categories and 152 subtypes and subforms; and (3) cranial neuralgias, facial pain, and "other headaches yet to be defined."

This chapter focuses on primary headache disorders, or those that cannot be attributed to another medical condition, although we touch briefly on a secondary headache type that is increasingly being seen in practice— medication overuse headache (MOH). This headache type is singled out because it has been found to be particularly difficult to treat, and allowing the overuse to continue can compromise an otherwise effective intervention (see Andrasik, Grazzi, Usai, Buse, & Bussone, 2009; Grazzi, Andrasik, Usai, & Bussone, 2009). Primary headache disorders can be subdivided into migraine, tension-type headache (TTH), cluster headache (CH), other trigeminal autonomic cephalalgias, and other primary headaches. (See Silberstein et al., 2004, for a review of the International Headache Diagnostic Criteria [ICHD-II], and Lipton, Bigal, Steiner, Silberstein, & Olesen, 2004, for a useful clinical algorithm for the diagnosis of primary headache disorders.)

TTH is the most common type of primary headache. TTH can be subdivided into (1) infrequent episodic (headaches occurring less frequently than 1 day per month), (2) frequent episodic (headaches on 1–14 days per month), and (3) chronic daily headache (headaches on 15 or more days per month). The primary features of TTH are bilateral location (pain on both sides of the head), nonpulsating quality, and mild to moderate pain intensity, although features may vary across persons and across attacks.

Migraine has five major subtypes and may occur with aura (MA) or without aura (MO). Aura symptoms may include seeing flickering lights, spots or lines, loss of vision, feelings of "pins and needles" or numbness, and other symptoms. Migraine can also be subdivided by frequency into episodic migraine (EM; headache on 14 or fewer days per month) and chronic migraine (CM; headache on 15 or more days per month, of which at least 8 are migraine attacks) (Headache Classification Committee of the International Headache Society et al., 2006). Migraine attacks tend to be moderate to severe pain that lasts at least 4 hours. The pain is often unilateral, or one-sided, may have a pulsating quality, and may be aggravated by movement and activity. Migraineurs may experience nausea or vomiting, photophobia (sensitivity to light), and phonophobia (sensitivity to sound). Approximately 20% of migraineurs experience aura, characterized by focal neurological features that usually occur in the hour preceding the headache. Aura may not occur with every attack. It is not uncommon for migraine and TTH to "coexist" within the same individual and to warrant separate diagnoses (which in the past was variously termed mixed headache, tension–vascular headache, or combination headache).

CH is less common but extremely debilitating. CHs are a group of headache disorders characterized by trigeminal nerve and parasympathetic nervous system activation. A CH is often described as an excruciating, sharp pain in or around the eye. Cluster headaches last approximately 1 hour (although length varies) and most often occur in "clusters" of multiple episodes over 2 weeks to 3 months; however, it is possible to experience more chronic forms of CH.

EPIDEMIOLOGY, BURDEN, AND COMORBIDITY OF HEADACHE

Headache affects 91% of males and 96% of females at some point during their lifetime (Rasmussen, 1995). The majority of headaches are benign, and less than 0.1% of the lifetime prevalence of headache is associated with life-threatening conditions (Silberstein & Lipton, 1993). TTH is the most common type in the general population, with a 1-year-period prevalence ranging from 31 to 73% (Schwartz, Stewart, Simon, & Lipton, 1998). Migraine is less common, but it takes a sizable toll, with an estimated international annual prevalence of 12–13% (18.2% for women and 6.5% for men). There are an estimated 31 million migraine sufferers in the United States (Lipton, Stewart, Diamond, Diamond, & Reed, 2001). CH is less common, but extremely painful and debilitating (Finkel, 2003). Limited epidemiological studies suggest a prevalence rate of 56 to 326 people per 100,000, and CH is experienced by men four times more often than women (Torelli et al., 2006).

Primary headaches, such as migraine, can have a significant impact on all aspects of life, including daily functioning, productivity, and health-related quality of life (HRQoL) (e.g., Andrasik, 2001, 2006; Buse, Rupnow, & Lipton, 2009). The Global Burden of Disease Study by the WHO identified migraine in the top 20 causes of disability worldwide (out of 135 health conditions; Leonardi, Steiner, Scher, & Lipton, 2005). The study demonstrated that 30.8% of all years of healthy life lost to disability (YLD) were to mental and neurological disorders, including migraine. Migraine alone accounted for 1.4% of YLD.

The impact of headache disorders increases as frequency and severity of attacks increase (Bigal, Rapoport, Lipton, Tepper, & Sheftell, 2003, Bigal, Serrano, Reed, & Lipton, 2008; Buse, Manack, Serrano, Turkel, & Lipton, 2010). Approximately 31% of migraine sufferers miss work, and between 58 and 76% cannot participate in household responsibilities, family, or social activities due to headache (Lipton et al., 2001; Lipton, Bigal, 2003).

Migraine can place a significant burden on individuals' lives, both during attacks (ictally) and between attacks (i.e., interictally) (Dahlof & Dimenäs, 1995). Interictal burden may include worry about the next attack and change or avoidance of commitments in the occupational, social, and personal arenas. For example, a patient may decide that she cannot coach her child's soccer team due to worry that she would have to miss too many practices and games due to headache. Patients with high levels of interictal headache-related burden have been demonstrated to experience higher rates of psychological disorders than those with lower levels of interictal burden. In a population-based study of interictal headache burden, of respondents with "severe" levels of interictal burden, 44% met criteria for an anxiety disorder, 47% for panic disorder, and 46% for a depressive disorder, compared with 20, 23, and 25%, respectively, of headache sufferers with low or no interictal burden (Buse et al., 2007). Results were controlled for frequency and severity of headache, demonstrating that interictal burden is not solely related to the severity of the disease, but rather to a more complex interaction of disease severity with cognitions (e.g., expectations), mood (e.g., anxiety or depression), and behaviors.

Migraine is also associated with increased rates of comorbidity with many common medical and psychiatric disorders (Buse et al., 2010; Scher, Bigal, & Lipton, 2005). Medical comorbidities of migraine have been well established in the literature and include neurological disorders (e.g., stroke and epilepsy) (Dayno, Silberstein, & Lipton, 1996; Ottman & Lipton, 1994), chronic pain disorders (Scher, Stewart, & Lipton, 2006), asthma (Aamodt, Stovner, Langhammer, Hagen, & Zwart, 2007), and coronary artery disease (Cook et al., 2002), among other conditions.

Migraine is also associated with increased rates of comorbidity with many psychiatric disorders, including depression, anxiety, panic disorder, bipolar disorder, obsessive–compulsive disorder, and suicide attempts (Hamelsky & Lipton, 2006; Jette, Patten, Williams, Becker, & Wiebe, 2008). Migraine and depression have been shown to be bi-directional, so that no matter which occurs first, an individual who experiences one has a higher rate of risk for the other (Breslau & Davis, 1993). Anxiety and depression are correlated with greater impairment in functional ability and HRQoL in migraineurs, and lowered HRQoL is associated with increased migraine-related disability (Lanteri-Minet, Radat, Chautard, & Lucas, 2005). Forms of chronic daily headache, such as CM, have been found to be associated with even greater levels of functional impairment, health service utilization, and psychiatric and medical comorbidities than episodic and lower-frequency headaches (Bigal et al., 2008; Buse et al., 2010; Juang, Wang, Fuh, Lu, & Su, 2000; Lipton, Bigal, et al., 2007; Zwart et al., 2003).

THE BIOPSYCHOSOCIAL MODEL

The biopsychosocial model of headache proposes that biological, psychological, social factors, and their interactions all play significant roles in the experience and outcomes of headache disorders (Andrasik, Flor, & Turk, 2005). In the case of headache, biological and pathophysiological predispositions and mechanisms may be "triggered" by the interplay of the individual's physiological status (e.g., level of autonomic arousal), environmental factors (e.g., stressful circumstances, certain foods, alcohol, toxins, hormonal fluctuations), ability to cope with these factors (both cognitively and behaviorally), and consequential factors that may serve to reinforce, and thus increase, the person's chances of reporting head pain (Waggoner & Andrasik, 1990). Psychological factors do not play a causal role per se. Rather, psychological factors contribute to headache as (1) triggering factors, (2) maintaining factors, (3) exacerbating factors, or (4) sequelae to continued head pain and subsequent life disruption.

Models based on the biopsychosocial paradigm, such as "patient-centered care" (Platt et al., 2001), stress the importance of attention to the patient's physical and psychological well-being; involve and empower the patient in decision making and responsibility for participation and success of the treatment plan; and place attention and value on the relationship and interactions between the health care provider (HCP) and patient. These models incorporate elements of effective communication (American Academy on Communication in Healthcare, 2009), use psychotherapeutic behaviors to convey a sense of partnership and positive regard, and actively facilitate patients' involvement in decision making about their care. (For a review of effective medical communication strategies applied to headache treatment, see Buse & Lipton, 2008; Hahn, 2008.)

In applying the biopsychosocial model to assessment of the headache patient, the core tenets of the humanistic approach to counseling (i.e., genuineness/congruence, unconditional positive regard, and empathetic understanding) (Rogers, 1967) should be applied to the assessment process. Suspending one's own frame of reference and suspending judgment are important in order to attend fully to the speaker and to make the correct diagnosis and treatment plan. Empathetic understanding can be established through active listening strategies, such as reflection and clarification. *Reflection* is the act of repeating what the patient has said, conveying a nonjudgmental understanding of his or her statements (e.g., "I understand that your headaches have caused you to miss many days of work, as well as important family activities, and this makes you unhappy"). *Clarification* is the act of abstracting the core or essence of the information a patient gives, summarizing and repeating it back to the patient (e.g., "It sounds like you are telling me that your headaches are having a significant negative effect on the quality of your life").

Active listening is a structured way of listening and responding that incorporates the strategies reviewed (Robertson, 2005). Active listening involves utilizing the following four strategies: (1) listening to and understanding verbal messages; (2) listening to and interpreting nonverbal messages (e.g., posture, affect, tone of voice); (3) considering the patient within his or her relative context (which may include socioeconomic factors, cultural beliefs and practices, family and support group [or the lack thereof], among other factors); and (4) listening with empathy. The "Ask–Tell–Ask" strategy is another effective approach to medical communication and assessment (Back, Arnold, Baile, Tulsky, & Fryer-Edwards, 2005; Hahn, 2008). The underlying tenet is that effective education requires assessing what the patient already knows and believes, then building on (or correcting, when necessary) that knowledge. It demonstrates care and respect toward the patient in that the HCP is willing to take the time to discuss medical diagnoses, assessment, and treatment plans, and engage in a partnership with the patient in making medical decisions and planning treatment. The "Ask–Tell–Ask" strategy includes three basic steps (see Table 18.1). Back and colleagues (2005) advise following the "Ask–Tell–Ask" strategy with the "Tell me more" statement. This request provides an open forum for the patient to express his or her understanding, concerns, feelings, questions, and emotions. Some examples of useful invitations to "Tell me more" include the following:

TABLE 18.1. The "Ask–Tell–Ask" Strategy

- Step 1: *"Ask"* the patient to describe his or her current understanding of the issue. The information gained from the patient will assist you in tailoring an appropriate explanation for the patient taking into account his or her current level of understanding, emotional state, and degree of education.

- Step 2: Following the patient's description, *"Tell"* the patient the relevant facts in language and at a level that he or she will understand. Use this opportunity to clarify any misperceptions or incorrect information on the patient's part. Reinforce and validate the correct information that the patient shared. Do not overwhelm the patient. A good heuristic is to offer three key pieces of information.

- Step 3: *"Ask"* the patient if he or she understood the information that you just gave. Ask him or her to rephrase, explain, or tell you what you just told him or her. Use this opportunity to assess the patient's attitudes and motivation, and problem-solve around potential barriers. This will give you the opportunity to confirm that he or she understands and also offer the patient an opportunity to ask any remaining questions or express any remaining concerns. Ask the patient how he or she feels about the diagnosis or treatment plan: whether he or she plans to comply, and if not, what the barriers, challenges, or concerns are.

- Step 4: Repeat the "Ask–Tell–Ask" strategy as long as appropriate.

Note. Based on Hahn (2008).

"How are you feeling about what we have discussed/your diagnosis/the treatment plan?"
"What does this mean for you?"
"Do you have any additional concerns/questions/needs today?"

EVALUATION OF HEADACHE

Neurological Evaluation

Assessment and treatment should start with a complete medical evaluation by the HCP with experience in headache to rule out headache due to an acute medical condition, disease state, or structural abnormality, and to evaluate the patient for appropriate medical and pharmacological treatment of headache. It is imperative that patients be evaluated for the presence of underlying structural defects or diagnosable physical conditions other than a primary headache disorder. Once an acute problem is ruled out, a primary headache disorder can be diagnosed using ICHD-II criteria. (See Lipton et al., 2004, for a clinical algorithm to assist with diagnosis.) Understanding the impact of headache on the patient's occupational and social functioning, psychological status, medical and psychiatric comorbidities, HRQoL, attitudes, beliefs, and preferences is also a necessary element of evaluation.

Initial evaluation of the patient with headache requires a thorough neurological and general physical examination, and a complete medical and social history. The goal in obtaining the history and physical evaluation is to rule out findings suggestive of secondary headache pathology. The basic elements of the exam should include vital signs; palpation of the cranium for abnormalities or tenderness; ophthalmoscopic examination (including fundi); examination of the ears, nose, and throat; and a complete neurological examination. Other physical examination elements should be performed as indicated by the history and clinical presentation of the patient. Abnormal findings warrant neuroimaging to rule out intracranial pathology. If suspected, the preferred imaging modality to evaluate for subarachnoid hemorrhage is noncontrast computed tomographic (CT) scanning of the head, followed by lumbar puncture if the CT scan is normal. Magnetic resonance imaging (MRI) is more expensive than CT scanning and less widely available; however, MRI reveals more detail and is necessary for imaging the posterior fossa. Cerebrospinal fluid (CSF) analysis can help to confirm or rule out hemorrhage, infection, and disorders related to CSF hypertension or hypotension. Laboratory evaluation may be considered to rule out thyroid disease, anemia, or other conditions.

Important elements of the history include onset and progression; intensity, location, and duration of pain; exacerbating factors; relieving factors; associated features; and current and previous treatments and provider information. Triggers, prodromal symptoms, and medical and psychological comorbidities should be assessed. Lifestyle habits, sleep patterns, nicotine use, substance use (e.g., illicit drugs, alcohol, and caffeine),

and psychosocial stressors should also be addressed. In addition, the initial evaluation should include assessment of headache-related disability, including both ictal and interictal burden; impact of headache on occupational, academic, social, family, and personal functioning; and assessment of quality of life. Research has demonstrated that gathering information about headache-related disability leads to a more accurate recognition of the severity of the effect of migraine on the patient's life and tends to result in more aggressive and comprehensive treatment plans (Holmes et al., 2001).

Even after the neurological evaluation is complete and findings indicate an ICHD-II diagnosis of primary headache and not one suggesting acute pathology, we recommend that all HCPs maintain an ongoing relationship and open communication with the patient. Although medical factors may have been ruled out prior to beginning treatment, they may surface as significant factors during the course of treatment. An aid to remembering a list of "red flags" for the presence of serious underlying disorders as a cause of acute or subacute headache is the mnemonic SNOOP (Systemic symptoms, Neurological signs, Onset, Other associated conditions, and Prior headache history) (Dodick, 2003), presented in Table 18.2. When these "red flags" are present, neuroimaging is indicated

TABLE 18.2. "SNOOP" Mnemonic for "Red Flags"

Systemic symptoms or illness (including fever, persistent or progressive vomiting, stiff neck, pregnancy, cancer, immunocompromised state, anticoagulated).

Neurological signs or symptoms (including altered mental status, focal neurological symptoms or signs, seizures, or papilledema).

Onset is new (especially in those age 40 years or older) or sudden.

Other associated conditions (e.g., headache is subsequent to head trauma, awakens patient from sleep, or is worsened by Valsalva maneuvers).

Prior headache history that is different (e.g., headaches now are of a different pattern or are rapidly progressive in severity or frequency).

Note. From Dodick (2003). Reprinted with permission from *Advanced Studies in Medicine.* Available at *www. jhasim.com.*

to make an appropriate diagnosis and treatment plan.

Headache Pain Rating and Description

Headache and pain are private events, and no method yet exists that can reliably quantify headache parameters. Headache pain can be assessed using any of the pain scales reviewed in Jensen and Karoly, Chapter 2, and Katz and Melzack, Chapter 3, this volume. Simply asking the patient to rate his or her head pain on a scale of 0 ("no pain") to 10 ("worst pain imaginable") can be extremely useful. The question and rating scale should be kept uniform, so that ratings can be compared across time and across attacks. Patients should also be asked to describe the quality of their pain. Many patients use metaphors that may provide valuable clues to headache subtype and etiology (e.g., "It feels like my head is being squeezed in a vise" or "It feels like an ice pick in my eye"). Some patients (especially children and adolescents) best express their pain experience through drawing, in which case the simple instruction "Please draw your headache/pain," without any other parameters, may yield useful information. Patients should be asked about common prodromal symptoms, triggers, and qualities of pain, which are the criteria for diagnosing the various subtypes of headache.

Headache Diary

One simple and very useful way to gather data and monitor treatment is to have patients keep a "headache diary." Headache diaries can be maintained for 1–2 months to gain a more complete and accurate picture of a patient's health, functioning, and quality of life (Andrasik, Lipchik, McCrory, & Wittrock, 2005). These diaries may initially include virtually any data of interest to aid understanding, such as headache frequency, severity (rated on a scale of 0–10), duration, medications taken, presence of aura or focal neurological symptoms, associated features, hormonal factors and menstrual cycle, mood ratings, information about sleep, diet including meals, caffeine use, and alcohol, nicotine, weather (with a focus on barometric change), life events, and other potential triggers and exacerbators of interest.

Throughout the treatment process, diaries may be used to record medication use and habits, sleep, mood, practice of techniques taught, analysis of dysfunctional cognitions, and other relevant data. Diaries may be kept on paper, in a computer, or on a handheld electronic device (e.g., an application on a cellular phone), and may be completed by other interested parties, such as parents of children with headaches (Andrasik, Burke, Attanasio, & Rosenblum, 1985). Ratings obtained from the headache diary correlate moderately with ratings of improvement provided by significant others (Blanchard, Andrasik, Neff, Jurish, & O'Keefe, 1981). They may vary in level of detail according to patient and HCP preference, and may be customized or modified as appropriate. In early investigations, researchers required patients to monitor headache parameters on an hourly basis. More recently, recording demands have been reduced such that patients are asked to make recordings at just a few highly discriminable times (e.g., wake-up/breakfast, lunch, dinner, and bedtime) or even a single reading to represent the entire day. These reduced-demand approaches come at the price of reduced precision, because it is no longer possible to track actual frequency, duration, and so forth. Maintaining a headache diary can provide a wealth of information to both the HCP and the patient, and help to map out targets for behavioral intervention and predict (and avoid) future attacks.

Medication Consumption

Medication consumption can be monitored as another way to assess behavior motivated by pain. It is important to monitor medication consumption for several reasons. First is to be on guard for excessive use that may be triggering rebound headache. Second, many patients specifically request nonpharmacological treatment because of a desire to reduce or eliminate their need for medication. Systematic measures are necessary to evaluate progress toward this goal. Finally, concurrent tracking of pain parameters and medication allows the HCP to determine whether observed improvements in pain level are due in part to increased use of medications or enhanced compliance to a prescribed prophylactic medication regimen.

Special attention should be paid to narcotic or opioid medication use to monitor for signs of overuse, misuse, dependence, or abuse (Silberstein et al., 2005). Several instruments have been developed for monitoring opioid use with chronic pain and headache patients. The Screener and Opioid Assessment for Patients with Pain (SOAPP) helps clinicians assess the suitability of long-term opioid therapy for chronic pain patients (Akbik et al., 2006). The Current Opioid Misuse Measure (COMM) is a self-assessment that assists clinicians in identifying current pain patients who misuse their opioid medications (Butler et al., 2007). Finally, the Medication Dependence Questionnaire, based on DSM-IV criteria for dependence, was developed specifically for headache patients. Originally developed in French, it has since been translated into English (Radat et al., 2006).

The most direct way to assess this aspect is to ask patients to record or count the number of pills consumed. However, simple pill counts become problematic when patients take more than one medication, switch medications during treatment, or when comparison across patients is desired. Timing is also important. Some classes of acute mediations for headache are most effective when taken early (Holroyd et al., 1988); however, patients may wait to take their medication until they are sure about the type and severity of headache they are experiencing. A patient's individual headache diary may be customized to facilitate this documentation.

Headache Symptoms/Screening/Diagnosis

A number of measures have been developed to facilitate initial screening and diagnosis. Some of the most commonly used and well-validated measures are discussed here.

ID-Migraine

The ID-Migraine, a migraine screening instrument, was designed and validated for use in the outpatient primary care setting, but it is applicable to other settings as well (Lipton, Dodick, et al., 2003). There are nine diagnostic questions total, with a three-item subset addressing the migraine-defining symptoms of disability, nausea, and photophobia. The three-item subset can stand alone as a screen, with a sensitivity of .81 and specific-

ity of .75, or be used in the longer form for additional diagnostic criteria. There is, however, no improvement in sensitivity or specificity using the nine-item screen in addition to the three-item subset. This instrument has demonstrated good test–retest reliability (kappa = .68) and a positive predictive value of 93.3%.

Brief Headache Screen

The Brief Headache Screen (BHS) is a seven-item, self-administered headache screening tool. The BHS discriminates between EM syndromes, daily headache syndromes, and MOH, and has demonstrated 82.6% agreement with migraine diagnoses made with the ID-Migraine (Maizels & Houle, 2008).

Computerized Headache Assessment Tool

The Computerized Headache Assessment Tool (CHAT) is a computer-administered, branching screen developed to diagnose primary headache disorders (Maizels & Wolfe, 2008). It can also distinguish between episodic, chronic, and daily disorders, and recognize medication overuse. The CHAT was developed with an expert systems approach to headache diagnosis, with initial branch points determined by headache frequency and duration. When compared to results of a clinician diagnostic interview (the "gold standard"), the CHAT correctly identified patients with EM, CM, episodic TTH (ETTH), and chronic TTH (CTTH) with 100% accuracy. The most commonly misdiagnosed headache syndromes were transformed migraine (85.7%, $n = 49$), MOH (82.7%, $n = 52$), and new daily persistent headache (42.9%, $n = 7$).

Migraine Severity Scale

The Migraine Severity Scale (MIGSEV) is a seven-item scale designed for measuring migraine severity (El Hasnaoui et al., 2003). Questions include items on pain, tolerability, disability in daily activities, presence of nausea or vomiting, resistance to treatment, duration of attacks, and frequency of attacks, and can be categorized into three dimensions: intensity of attacks, resistance to treatment, and frequency of attacks. A prospective study of 287 migraineurs demonstrated high levels of external validity (between MIGSEV scores and "gold standard" clinician diagnoses) and strong test–retest reliability.

Headache-Related Functional Impairment, Burden, and Disability

Outcome measures for specific chronic diseases are largely based on mortality as the major endpoint. Because headache is not associated with premature death, traditional measures of burden (e.g., incidence/prevalence and mortality) are not applicable. To measure the burden of headache disorders accurately, headache disease-specific outcome measures must assess important dimensions of functioning and headache-related disability, including physical, emotional, social, and economic considerations. Measuring headache-related disability is challenging due to the episodic nature of the disease, and variation in severity and features of attacks both within and among individuals. Many validated headache instruments use a 1- or 3-month recall period to capture a representative period of time, while others use a single day. Measures may focus on the ictal or interictal burden or migraine, or both. The choice of instrument should be guided by the purposes of the assessment (e.g., research vs. clinical use) and headache type or subtype (e.g., EM vs. CM or chronic daily headache [CDH]).

Migraine Disability Assessment Scale

The Migraine Disability Assessment Scale (MIDAS), used to assess headache-related disability, is the most frequently used disability instrument in migraine research and clinical practice (Stewart, Lipton, Dowson, Sawyer, & Sawyer, 2001). It is a self-administered questionnaire that comprises five items that assess days of missed activity or substantially reduced activity due to headache in three domains: schoolwork/paid employment, household work or chores, and nonwork (family, social, and leisure) activities, plus two optional items: headache frequency in number of days over the preceding 3 months, and an average pain rating on a scale of 0 (*no pain*) to 10 (*worst pain ever*) for the same time period. Responses to the first five items are summed, with these scores falling into one of four grades of headache-related disability: *none, mild, moderate,* and *severe.*

The MIDAS questionnaire has been shown to be internally consistent, highly reliable, valid, and to correlate with physicians' clinical judgment. Test–retest reliability coefficients ranging from .59 to .80 have been reported and internal consistency, as measured by Cronbach's alpha, was .83. Convergent validity with diary-based measures was .66. The MIDAS has been validated for adults age 18 and older, and has been translated and validated in multiple languages. The MIDAS is available for use free of charge and may be accessed on the American Headache Society website at *www.achenet.org/tools/migraine/index. asp.* There is also a version developed for use with pediatric and adolescent patients: the PedMIDAS (Hershey et al., 2001).

Headache Needs Assessment Survey

The Headache Needs Assessment Survey (HANA) is a brief, self-administered questionnaire that assesses two dimensions of the impact of migraine: frequency and bothersomeness (Cramer, Silberstein, & Winner, 2001). This instrument has seven questions (with the corresponding subscales of Anxiety/Worry, Depression/Discouragement, Self-Control, Energy, Function/Work, Family/Social Activities, and Overall Impact). For each item, the respondent provides data on both frequency and "bothersomeness." The HANA has demonstrated good test–retest reliability (.77) and internal consistency (.92). There is a statistically significant correlation between HANA and Headache Disability Inventory total scores (.73, $p < .0001$), and high correlations with disease and treatment characteristics.

Headache Impact Test

The Headache Impact Test (HIT) is a brief, self administered questionnaire, developed to assess impact of headache on functional health and well-being. It is available in paper-and-pencil (HIT-6) and computerized (Dynamic Health Assessment [DYNHA] HIT) formats. The HIT-6 is a six-item questionnaire that measures lost time in three domains and other areas of impact (e.g., pain severity, fatigue, and mood) (Kosinski et al., 2003). It is valid for adults age 18 and older, and has been translated and validated in multiple languages. (It is available in 28 languages at *www.headachetest.com/ hit6translations.html*.) It has a 4-week recall period and response options ranging from *never* (6 points) to *always* (13 points), with a range of 36–78. Responses are summed and fall into the following categories: 49 or less, *no impact*; 50–55, *some impact*; 56–59, *substantial impact*; 60 or greater, *severe impact*. The HIT-6 has demonstrated good discriminatory validity (migraine vs. nonmigraine headache and mild vs. moderate vs. severe headache) and external validity. Cronbach's alpha for this instrument is .79. Test–retest reliability was also evaluated at approximately 21 days, with moderate reliability for EM and strong reliability for CM.

Headache Impact Questionnaire

The Headache Impact Questionnaire (HImQ) is a 16-item, self-administered instrument that combines measures of pain and disability into a single scaled measure of severity (Stewart, Lipton, Simon, Von Korff, & Liberman, 1998). The HImQ measures the cumulative impact of headache on an individual over a 3-month period. Questions include total number of headaches, headache duration, last headache, pain intensity, need for bed rest, disability in specific domains of activity, and symptoms. The HImQ score is derived from eight items and is the sum of average pain intensity (on a scale of 0 to 10) and total lost days in all three defined domains of activity (work for pay, housework, and nonwork activities). Reduced effectiveness day equivalents are also considered. Score calculation involves both addition and multiplication. This instrument has an internal consistency of .83 (Cronbach's alpha), and test–retest correlation at an average of 6 weeks for all eligible subjects was .77. There is moderate convergent validity (.49), with a 90-day daily headache diary and moderate to high convergent validity with the physician's judgment of disability. The highest convergent validity was for frequency-based items.

Functional Assessment in Migraine Questionnaire

The Functional Assessment in Migraine (FAIM) questionnaire is a migraine-specific, self-administered instrument derived from the WHO International Classification of Impairments, Disabilities, and Handicaps, Version 2 (ICIDH-2; Pathak, Chisolm, & Weis, 2005). The ICIDH-2 model includes three dimensions: (1) Body Structure and Function, including Mental Functioning, (2) Activity, and (3) Participation. Items include nine Mental Functioning items measuring the dimensions of Attention/Thought (five items) and Perception (four items), and a list of 28 Activity and Participation items from which respondents chose the five items most relevant to their lifestyle. Cronbach's alpha values were greater than .70 for all Mental Functioning items. Construct validity analysis of FAIM dimensions found significant positive correlations with self-reported symptom severity and significant negative correlations with functional status. There were moderately significant positive correlations with dimensions of the Migraine-Specific Quality of Life (MSQoL) questionnaire. The lowest correlations were seen between FAIM and the Emotional dimension of the MSQoL questionnaire and the Short Form Health Survey (SF-12) component scores.

Migraine Interictal Burden Scale

The Migraine Interictal Burden Scale (MIBS) is unique in that it measures *interictal burden* (i.e., burden related to headache in the time between attacks). The MIBS-4 is a four-item, self-administered questionnaire for clinical use or screening purposes (Buse et al., 2007). The MIBS-4 measures between-attack migraine burden across four domains: Disruption at Work and School, Diminished Family and Social Life, Difficulty Planning, and Emotional Difficulty. This instrument was developed and validated in a large survey-based study with 30 candidate items identified from existing outcome measures and focus groups. Test–retest reliability was high across all retest intervals (rho = .69). Moderate positive correlations were seen between the MIBS-4, MIDAS, and nine-item Patient Health Questionnaire (PHQ-9), and moderate negative correlations were seen between the MIBS-4 and MSQOL (total score and subscales), which would be expected; as interictal burden increases, quality of life decreases. The correlation between ictal burden as measured by MIDAS and the MIBS-4 was .35, which demonstrated that the burden of migraine during attacks only partially predicts the burden between attacks.

Henry Ford Hospital Disability Inventory

While the preceding instruments assess either ictal or interictal burden, the Henry Ford Disability Inventory (HDI) assesses both the ictal and interictal burden of headache (Jacobson, Ramadan, Aggarwal, & Newman, 1994). The HDI is a self-administered, 25-item inventory designed as a treatment outcome measure to quantify the impact of recurrent headache on activities of daily living. The instrument has two subscales addressing both Functional (12 items) and Emotional (13 items) Impairment. Patients are instructed to respond *yes* (4 points), *sometimes* (2 points), or *no* (0 points) to each of the 25 statements. The total score is the summation of the responses, with a maximum score of 100, which correlates with the highest level of disability. The HDI has proven to have good internal consistency (.94), 6-week test–retest reliability (.83), and 1-week test–retest reliability (.76). There is high convergent validity with both migraine severity and spouse's perceptions, but low convergent validity with HANA (Jacobson, Ramadan, Norris, & Newman, 1995).

Quality of Life

There is a trend toward looking at HRQoL in diseases that do not negatively influence life expectancy including primary headache. Quality of life (QoL) is a quantification of global well-being. HRQoL relates to health state, as well as physical and mental functional status (Fayers & Machin, 2000; Guyatt, Feeny, & Patrick, 1993). Migraineurs have demonstrated significantly lower SF-36 scores than nonmigraineurs, and migraine adversely affects functioning at least as much as depression, diabetes, and recent myocardial infarction (Solomon, Skobieranda, & Gragg, 1993). Also, migraineurs have significantly lower HRQoL than people in the general population without any chronic condition (Bussone et al., 2004). HRQoL can be measured by general instruments (e.g., Medical Outcomes Study 36-Item Short Form Health Survey–36 [MOS SF-36; Ware & Sherbourne, 1992] and 12-item Short Form Health Survey [SF-12; Ware, Kosinski, & Keller, 1996]) or disease-specific instruments. Several disease-specific instruments have been developed to assess HRQoL in those affected by migraine and other types of headache, which we describe briefly below (Andrasik, 2001; Solomon, 1997).

Migraine-Specific Quality of Life Questionnaire

The MSQoL is a 20-item self-administered questionnaire designed to assess the long-term effects of migraine on HRQoL (Wagner, Patrick, Galer, & Berzon, 1996). It consists of three domains: Avoidance, Social Relationships, and Feelings. Each of the 20 items is rated from 1 (*very much*) to 4 (*not at all*). Total scores range from 20 to 80; a transformed scale is achieved by subtraction, division, and multiplication, with a transformed score of 100 indicating maximum (best) QoL. Internal consistency as measured by Cronbach's alpha was .90 for total MSQoL scale, and test–retest validity at 24 days was .90. There was a high convergent validity with migraine symptom severity and moderate convergent validity with the MOS SF-36. There was a negative correlation with QoL and more migraine symptoms, medical appointments per year to treat migraine, and annual migraine frequency (Patrick, Hurst, & Hughes, 2000).

Migraine-Specific Quality of Life Questionnaire, Version 2.1

The Migraine-Specific Quality of Life Questionnaire, Version 2.1 (MSQoL-2.1) is a 14-item questionnaire that measures functional limitations and restrictions related to migraine through three dimensions: Role Function–Restriction, Role Function–Preventive, and Emotional Function over a 4-week period (Martin et al., 2000). Scores are reported on a 0- to 100-point scale, with higher scores correlating with better QoL. Internal consistency (Cronbach's alpha) of this instrument ranged from .86 to .96

across dimensions. The ICC of the dimensions ranged from .57 to .63, as measured by the test–retest reliability at 4 weeks. The Pearson correlation coefficients between baseline and 4 weeks ranged from .62 to .65. There was a low-to-moderate correlation with SF-36 scores.

24-Hour Migraine Quality-of-Life Questionnaire

The 24-Hour Migraine Quality-of-Life Questionnaire (24-hr-MQoLQ) was developed for use in clinical trials of acute migraine treatment (Santanello, Hartmaier, Epstein, & Silberstein, 1995). This 15-item self-administered questionnaire, requiring less than 10 minutes to complete, can be used clinically to measure the impact of migraine treatment on HR-QoL in the first 24 hours postadministration. The questionnaire has five domains: Work Functioning, Social Functioning, Energy/Vitality, Feelings/Concerns, and Migraine Symptoms, each with three items. Respondents are asked to rate each item on a 7-point scale, with 1 indicating *maximum impairment* and 7 indicating *no impairment*. The 24-hr-MQoLQ instrument has an internal consistency between .74 and .91 (Cronbach's alpha). There is a low-to-moderate convergent validity with a migraine diary. Longer duration of migraine negatively correlated with 24-hr-MQoLQ scores, as did the presence of nausea and/or vomiting. There is an overall negative correlation between an acute migraine attack and QoL. The 24-hr-MQoLQ showed good internal consistency, construct and discriminant validity, and responsiveness to acute migraine attacks.

Treatment Advice, Satisfaction, and Optimization

A number of scales have been developed to help HCPs assess clinical treatment needs, monitor therapeutic efficacy and patient satisfaction once initiated, and provide clinical suggestions for ways to optimize treatment outcomes.

Migraine Assessment of Current Therapy Questionnaire

The Migraine Assessment of Current Therapy (Migraine-ACT) is a four-item, yes–no questionnaire designed for use in the pri-

mary care setting to assess the efficacy of acute migraine treatment and evaluate the need for a change in current acute treatment (Dowson et al., 2004). It contains questions regarding consistency of response, global assessment of relief, headache impact, and emotional response. Test–retest reliability at 1 week, as measured by Pearson correlation coefficient, was high ($r = .82$). There is good correlation with items from the SF-36 and MIDAS.

Patient Perception of Migraine Questionnaire—Revised Version

The Patient Perception of Migraine Questionnaire—Revised (PPMQ-R) is a 29-item, migraine-specific, self-administered questionnaire designed to evaluate patient satisfaction with acute migraine treatment (Revicki et al., 2006). The questionnaire has five domains measuring satisfaction with Efficacy, Functionality, Ease of Use, Medication Cost, and Bothersomeness of Medication Side Effects. The total score is the average of Efficacy, Functionality, and Ease of Use scores and is reported on a 0- to 100-point scale, with higher scores indicating higher satisfaction. The PPMQ-R scale scores and total score demonstrated internal consistency reliability (Cronbach's alpha = .80 to .98) at baseline and following the first migraine attack. Test–retest reliability, as determined by ICC at an average of 8 weeks was .79 to .91. The PPMQ-R has demonstrated statistically significant negative correlations between migraine pain severity levels and levels of impairment in ability to work and perform usual activities.

Migraine Treatment Optimization Questionnaire

The five-item Migraine Treatment Optimization Questionnaire (MTOQ-5) is a questionnaire for assessing efficacy and patient satisfaction with current treatment based on five domains: Functioning, Consistency of Relief, Rapid Relief, Recurrence, and Side Effects (Lipton et al., 2009). The MTOQ-5 is intended to help HCPs assess the adequacy of acute headache treatment and to identify areas where improvements can be made. If all five questions are answered "yes," treatment is considered satisfactory; an answer of "no" to an item suggests a deficiency, and that a change in treatment should be considered. Strategies are suggested based on the area(s) of deficiency and include both pharmacological and nonpharmacological treatment strategies. Cronbach's alpha is .66 for the MTOQ-5. Test–retest reliability based on ICCs was over .80. Convergent validity with scales including the MIDAS, HIT-6, and MSQoL ranged from .35 to .44.

Migraine Therapy Assessment Questionnaire

The Migraine Therapy Assessment Questionnaire (MTAQ) is a self-administered, nine-item questionnaire developed to identify migraine patients in a primary care setting whose migraine management may be suboptimal (Chatterton et al., 2002). Individual questions fall into one of three identified domains: Migraine Control, Knowledge/Behavior/Treatment Satisfaction, and Economic Burden. Responses are scored based on a dichotomous scale (yes = 1, no = 0). A higher total score indicates deficiencies in current treatment. Test–retest reliability at 2 weeks for all MTAQ questions had a Cohen's kappa of at least .5 and an average Pearson's r of .72. There were significant negative correlations between MTAQ items and SF-36 scores and satisfaction. There were significant positive correlations between MTAQ items and work loss, disability, and health care resource use.

Migraine Prevention Questionnaire

The Migraine Prevention Questionnaire (MPQ-5) was developed to facilitate the clinical implementation of the Consensus Guidelines for Preventive Pharmacotherapy for Migraine Treatment in Clinical Practice and to highlight suboptimal clinical treatment of migraine (Lipton, Serrano, et al., 2007). The MPQ-5 assesses headache frequency, acute medication use, headache-related impairment in several domains, and headache-related anxiety. Responses are summed into a total score, which falls into one of three categories: preventive treatment not indicated, consider preventive treatment, and offer preventive treatment. Recommendations include both pharmacological and nonpharmacological therapies. In addition to a total score, each of the five questions has

individual cutoff scores, which may raise a "yellow flag" or "red flag" in one or more of the specific areas. This information should be used as an indicator that the HCP should gather additional information and consider appropriate treatment and/or referral in that specific area. Psychometric testing has demonstrated good reliability and validity.

Cognitive Status and Psychiatric Evaluation

The neuropsychological status of the patient deserves special attention to identify conditions (e.g., formal thought disorder, certain personality disorders) that might interfere with successful treatment. When significant cognitive deficits or diminished cognitive capacities are observed or suspected (e.g., in the case of posttraumatic headache), it may be helpful to obtain a thorough neuropsychological assessment. Penzien, Rains, and Holroyd (1993) recommend use of the Cognitive Capacities Screening Examination (Jacobs, Bernhard, Delgado, & Strain, 1977) or the Mini-Mental State Examination (MMSE; Folstein, Folstein, & McHugh, 1975) to screen for this purpose. However, there seems to be little point in using these measures on a routine basis in a headache practice. When tested in such a setting, only two of 88 patients scored in the range suggesting significant organic involvement (Lawson et al., 1988).

It is also important to assess and monitor psychiatric status and symptomology. Several forms of headache have demonstrated increased rates of comorbidity with many psychiatric disorders, including depression, anxiety, panic disorder, bipolar disorder, obsessive–compulsive disorder, and suicide attempts (Hamelsky & Lipton, 2006; Jette et al., 2008). Anxiety and depression are correlated with greater impairment in functional ability and HRQoL in migraineurs (Lanteri-Minet et al., 2005) as well as worse outcome to behavioral treatment (Blanchard et al., 1985; Jacob, Turner, Szekely, & Eidelman, 1983; Werder, Sargent, & Coyne, 1981) and pharmacological treatment (Holroyd et al., 1988).

Screening, assessment, referral, and education about common psychiatric comorbidities should be included in headache assessment and care. Psychiatric screening instruments can be used to assess and monitor psychological functioning and comorbid conditions. The Primary Care Evaluation of Mental Disorders (PRIME-MD) is a brief, self-administered questionnaire that provides screening for several of the primary Axis I psychological disorders based directly on DSM-IV criteria (Spitzer, Kroenke, Williams, & the Patient Health Care Primary Study Group, 1999). The Patient Health Questionnaire–2 (PHQ-2) of the PRIME-MD is a two-item screening instrument that has been empirically shown to detect the presence of depression (Kroenke, Spitzer, & Williams, 2003). The PHQ-9 can be used to conduct a more detailed yet still time-efficient evaluation for depression (Kroenke, Spitzer, & Williams, 2001). Clinically significant anxiety can be evaluated using the Generalized Anxiety Disorder–7 (GAD-7), a seven-item, self-administered questionnaire (Spitzer, Kroenke, Williams, & Lowe, 2006). Once these questionnaires are completed, the HCP can review them with the patient during the visit. Having this information may facilitate discussion about other areas of concern and further inform treatment decisions, which may include a multidisciplinary and multimodal approach. Questionnaires may also be used at every visit to track progress or changes over time.

Psychological Variables and Stress

The relationship between stress and headache has long been noted in the literature (Henryk-Gutt & Rees, 1973; Howarth, 1965). Stress-induced migraine may occur either at the peak of stress or during a period of relaxation immediately following stress (e.g., April 16 for tax accountants, at the end of the term for teachers). Stress likely interacts with other precipitants to increase vulnerability to migraine, without necessarily precipitating any particular migraine episode. It is important to realize that a patient's stress experience is idiosyncratic; stress rests within the individual's cognitive interpretive framework; that is, what determines whether any given event is stressful is more a function of how the patient appraises the event. Lazarus and Folkman (1984) distinguish two types of appraisal: primary—whether a given event is judged to be significant to the patient's well-being, and secondary—whether the patient possesses the available resources or options to respond successfully to the event. What is appraised as significant by one individual may not be by another.

For any given person with headaches, stress most likely operates in multiple ways and in concert with other, various biological influences. Take, for example, the person with headaches who is able to drink a glass or two of red wine and escape a headache when feeling "on top of the world" but is not able to do so when overworked, eating on the run, and so on. HCPs need to recognize that major stressful life events are not always the main culprit. Rather, more recent evidence indicates that everyday "ups and downs" or "hassles" are sufficient to engage biological headache mechanisms (Andrasik, Wittrock, & Passchier, 2006; De Benedittis & Lorenzetti, 1992; Holm, Holroyd, Hursey, & Penzien, 1986; Levor, Cohen, Naliboff, MacArthur, & Heuser, 1986).

The prolonged presence of headache or chronic pain exerts a psychological toll on the patient over time, such that the patient becomes "sick and tired of feeling sick and tired." The negative thoughts and emotions arising from the repeated experience of headache can become further stressors or trigger factors in and of themselves (referred to as *headache-related distress*), serving at that point both to help maintain the disorder and to increase the severity and likelihood of future attacks.

In the biopsychosocial model of headache management, cognitive processes, including thoughts, beliefs, attributions, and attitudes, play a key role in the conceptualization and treatment for each patient with headache. Although numerous cognitive processes can influence headache and disability, three areas that have been empirically demonstrated to be especially important include locus of control, self-efficacy, and catastrophizing (Martin, Holroyd, Rokicki, 1993; Nicholson, Houle, Rhudy, & Norton, 2007). These constructs have been demonstrated to be related to headache-related disability, QoL, adherence, and response to treatment. Specific cognitive goals of cognitive-behavioral therapy (CBT) for headache management include enhancing self-efficacy (i.e., the patient's belief in his or her ability to succeed or accomplish a certain task), helping the patient gain an *internal locus of control* (i.e., a belief that the mechanism for change lies within oneself) as opposed to an *external locus of control* (i.e., the belief that only the physician, medication, or medical procedures have the power to create change), and replacing catastrophizing with more realistic and positive ways of thinking (Andrasik, 2003; Buse & Andrasik, 2009).

Locus of Control

Locus of control (LoC) refers to the degree to which an individual perceives that an event is under his or her personal control. These beliefs range from a completely internal LoC (the individual perceives the event as totally under his or her control), to a completely external LoC (the event is perceived as totally outside the individual's realm of influence). In most cases an individual's perception falls in between these two extremes. Research has demonstrated that an external LoC (e.g., "The doctor is the only one that can take manage my headaches," "Only medication can cure my headaches. Nothing that I do matters") is related to poor outcome, passive coping, less active participation in treatment, and physiological responses including depletion of norepinephrine and increased serotonin sensitization (Heath, Saliba, Mahmassani, Major, & Khoury, 2008; Scharff, Turk, & Marcus, 1995; Weiss et al., 1981).

To facilitate measuring and monitoring perceived LoC among headache sufferers, Martin, Holroyd, and Penzien (1990) developed the Headache-Specific Locus of Control (HSLC), a 33-item questionnaire designed for use with recurrent headache sufferers. Response options range from 1 (*strongly disagree*) to 5 (*strongly agree*). The HSLC consists of three subscales with 11 items each: Health Care Professionals' Locus of Control, Internal Locus of Control, and Chance Locus of Control. A total score is derived, as well as scores on the three subscales. The instrument has good internal consistency (with alpha coefficients ranging from .84 to .88 among the three subscales), and test–retest reliability over a 3-week interval (from $r = .72$ to $r = .78$) among the three subscales.

Self-Efficacy

Self-efficacy (SE) refers to an individual's belief that he or she can successfully accomplish an action or behavior to produce a desired outcome (Bandura, 1986). Poor SE has been demonstrated to be related to poor treatment outcome and decreased QoL in headache management (French et al., 2000; Marlowe, 1986; Nicholson, Hursey, & Nash, 2005). SE has been demonstrated to predict differential response to combined pharmacological and behavioral treatment (Smith & Nicholson, 2006), and changes in SE correlate with changes in headache frequency (Bond, Dirge, Rubingh, Durrant, & Baggaley, 2004; Nicholson, Nash, & Andrasik, 2005).

French and colleagues (2000) developed the Headache Management Self-Efficacy Scale (HMSE), a 25-item questionnaire used to assess patients' levels of SE in regard to headache prevention and management. In the HMSE, 25 headache management statements are rated by respondents on a Likert-type scale, from 1, *strongly disagree,* to 7, *strongly agree.* Responses are summed to produce a total score, with higher scores reflecting greater perceived SE. The HMSE has demonstrated good internal consistency (Cronbach's alpha = .90) and construct validity (i.e., scores were positively associated with the use of psychological coping strategies both to prevent and to manage headache episodes, and negatively associated with anxiety).

Catastrophizing

Catastrophizing refers to a hopeless and overwhelming thinking pattern, characterized by rumination, magnification, and helplessness. Catastrophizing has been demonstrated to be associated with poor outcomes, increased impairment, and reduced QoL across many chronic pain conditions, including headache (Burns, Kubilus, Bruehl, Harden, & Lofland, 2003; Holroyd, Drew, Cottrell, Romanek, & Heh, 2007; Sullivan et al., 2001). Holroyd and colleagues (2007) examined catastrophizing, comorbid anxiety, depression, QoL, and headache characteristics among 232 migraine sufferers. They found that catastrophizing and severity of associated symptoms (photophobia, phonophobia, nausea) independently predicted QoL, demonstrating that not just headache severity and frequency predict QoL, but that patient perception also is directly related to QoL.

The Pain Catastrophizing Scale (PCS; (Sullivan, Bishop, & Pivik, 1995) is a 13-item questionnaire designed to assess chronic pain patients' tendency toward catastrophizing as a cognitive style. More specifically, it assesses rumination, magnification, and helplessness. Holroyd and colleagues (2007) modified the PCS for use with a headache population (substituting "headache" for "pain"). Maintaining the original PCS scoring system, items are rated on a 5-point scale from 0 ("not at all") to 4 ("all the time") and summed for a total score ranging from 0 to 52, with higher scores reflecting a greater likelihood of engaging in catastrophizing. The PCS demonstrated good reliability (alpha = .87) and construct validity.

Many pain-specific measures are useful in headache assessment and management (see Chapter 4 by DeGood & Cook, this volume). Two measures that are especially useful in headache assessment and management include the Chronic Pain Coping Inventory (CPCI; Hadjistavropoulos, MacLeod, & Asmundson, 1999; Jensen, Turner, Romano, & Strom, 1995) and the Survey of Pain Attitudes (SOPA; Jensen, Karoly, & Huger, 1987). The CPCI measures strategies used by patients to cope with chronic pain. The CPCI is a 70-item self-report instrument on which the individual is asked to indicate the number of days during the past week he or she employed specific coping strategies to deal with pain. It is validated for use with adults ages 21–80 and takes approximately 10–15 minutes to complete. The CPCI consists of nine scales divided into two domains—the Illness-Focused Coping Domain and the Wellness-Focused Coping Domain. The SOPA, a 57-item self-response instrument, assesses patient attitudes in seven areas: Pain Control, Solicitude (solicitous responses from others in response to one's pain), Medication (as appropriate treatment for pain), Pain-Related Disability, Pain and Emotions (the interaction between emotions and pain), Medical Cures for Pain, and Pain-Related Harm (pain as an indicator of physical damage or harm). The SOPA has been validated in several languages. The Survey of Pain Attitudes—Brief Version (SOPA-B; Tait & Chibnall, 1997) is a 30-item version of the original SOPA.

Pediatric and Adolescent Headache Instruments

Children and adolescents with headache should be treated by HCPs with training and experience with this specific population. Children and adolescents are not simply "small adults"; rather, they may have qualitatively different medical, psychological, family, and educational presentations and needs (Andrasik & Schwartz, 2006; Powers & Andrasik, 2005; White & Farrell, 2006; Winner, Hershey, & Li, 2008). Several disease-specific outcome measures exist for patients or study participants under the age of 18. The PedMIDAS can be used to assess functional impairment and burden caused by migraine (Hershey et al., 2001). Quality of Life Headache in Youth (QoL-Y) is a self-administered questionnaire developed by Langeveld, Koot, Loonen, Hazebroek-Kampschreur, and Passchier (1996) to assess psychological, physical, and social functioning, and functional status in patients ages 12–18. Hartmaier, DeMuro-Mercon, Linder, Winner, and Santanello (2001) also developed a brief migraine-specific outcome measure to determine QoL and functioning in adolescent patients with headache.

SUMMARY

In this chapter we have reviewed the classification, diagnosis, and assessment of primary headache disorders and related comorbidities. Our chapter is guided by the biopsychosocial model, which posits that biological, psychological, and social or environmental factors all play significant roles in medical disorders. This model provides an ideal framework to conceptualize management of patients with primary headache disorders, in which factors of biology, environment, behaviors, and beliefs are interwoven with the development, maintenance, progression, and remission of headache disorders (Andrasik, Flor, & Turk, 2005).

Headache is multidetermined, requiring a comprehensive, multifactorial assessment approach. The headache assessor needs to be mindful of a patient's need for information, understanding, and reassurance. Thus, early on, patient education and information exchange become an important part of the assessment process. Assessment begins with a thorough physical and neurological evaluation to rule out permanent structural defects or diagnosable physical conditions other than a primary headache disorder. HCPs need to remain on alert status for a developing physical problem and to maintain close medical collaboration throughout treatment to monitor such problems and to obtain assistance with medication management and modification as needed. A primary headache diagnosis is necessary to determine the proper treatment, to identify patients whose headaches may in part be due to medication abuse; to identify headache types found to be resilient to nonpharmacological approaches alone (e.g., CH and chronic daily headache); and to decide when a comprehensive, multidisciplinary approach (e.g., posttraumatic headache) or even hospitalization is needed. In addition to completing a thorough medical and headache history, the HCP also needs to obtain a thorough qualitative understanding of the patient's experience and beliefs, headache-related disability and impairment in all areas of life, QoL, level of SE, and information about related comorbidities. This information leads to a more accurate recognition of the severity of the effect of headache on the patient's life, which in turn tends to result in more effective and comprehensive treatment plans.

Assessment of the psychological status of the patient deserves special attention in order to identify conditions that might preclude direct treatment of headache at the moment (e.g., a significant psychiatric problem or traumatic brain injury) or complicate current treatment and compromise progress (e.g., depression, anxiety, or personality disorder). Assessment of psychiatric comorbidities should be included in routine headache care and treatment, and referral to a specialist should be initiated whenever appropriate. Identification of stress factors, both major and minor, are often helpful in suggesting targets for intervention. A minority of patients may require specialized neuropsychological assessment.

Finally, we have briefly reviewed assessment instruments developed for use with children and adolescents with headache.

These patients should be treated by HCPs with specialty training and experience, because children and adolescents may have qualitatively different medical, psychological, family, and educational needs and issues.

REFERENCES

Aamodt, A. H., Stovner, L. J., Langhammer, A., Hagen, K., & Zwart, J. A. (2007). Is headache related to asthma, hay fever, and chronic bronchitis?: The Head-HUNT Study. *Headache*, *47*, 204–212.

Akbik, H., Butler, S. F., Budman, S. H., Fernandez, K., Katz, N. P., & Jamison, R. N. (2006). Validation and clinical application of the Screener and Opioid Assessment for Patients with Pain (SOAPP). *Journal of Pain and Symptom Management*, *32*, 287–293.

American Academy on Communication in Healthcare. (2009). Relationship-centered quality healthcare: Moving patients' experiences from "good" to "very good." Retrieved May 25, 2009, from *www.aachonline.org*.

Andrasik, F. (2001). Migraine and quality of life: Psychological considerations. *Journal of Headache and Pain*, *2*, S1–S9.

Andrasik, F. (2003). Behavioral treatment approaches to chronic headache. *Neurological Sciences*, *24*(Suppl. 2), S80–S85.

Andrasik, F. (2006). Psychophysiological disorders: Headache as a case in point. In F. Andrasik (Ed.), *Comprehensive handbook of personality and psychopathology: Vol. 2. Adult psychopathology* (pp. 409–422). Hoboken, NJ: Wiley.

Andrasik, F., Burke, E. J., Attanasio, V., & Rosenblum, E. L. (1985). Child, parent, and physician reports of a child's headache pain: Relationships prior to and following treatment. *Headache*, *25*, 421–425.

Andrasik, F., Flor, H., & Turk, D. C. (2005). An expanded view of psychological aspects in head pain: The biopsychosocial model. *Neurological Sciences*, *26*, S87–S91.

Andrasik, F., Grazzi, L., Usai, S., Buse, D. C., & Bussone, G. (2009). Non-pharmacological approaches to treating chronic migraine with medication overuse. *Neurological Sciences*, *30*(Suppl. 1), S89–S93.

Andrasik, F., Lipchik, G. L., McCrory, D. C., & Wittrock, D. A. (2005). Outcome measurement in behavioral headache research: Headache parameters and psychosocial outcomes. *Headache*, *45*, 429–437.

Andrasik, F., & Schwartz, M. S. (2006). Behavioral assessment and treatment of pediatric headache. *Behavior Modification, 30,* 93–113.

Andrasik, F., Wittrock, D. A., & Passchier, J. (2006). Psychological mechanisms of tension-type headache. In J. Olesen, P. J. Goadsby, N. M. Ramadan, P. Tfelt-Hansen, & K. M. A. Welch (Eds.), *The headaches* (3rd ed., pp. 663–667). Philadelphia: Lippincott Williams & Wilkins.

Back, A. L., Arnold, R. M., Baile, W. F., Tulsky, J. A., & Fryer-Edwards, K. (2005). Approaching difficult communication tasks in oncology. *CA: A Cancer Journal for Clinicians, 55,* 164–177.

Bandura, A. (1986). *Social foundations of thought and action: A social cognitive theory.* Englewood Cliffs, NJ: Prentice-Hall.

Bigal, M. E., Rapoport, A. M., Lipton, R. B., Tepper, S. J., & Sheftell, F. D. (2003). Assessment of migraine disability using the Migraine Disability Assessment (MIDAS) questionnaire: A comparison of chronic migraine with episodic migraine. *Headache, 3,* 336–342.

Bigal, M. E., Serrano, D., Reed, M., & Lipton, R. B. (2008). Chronic migraine in the population: Burden, diagnosis, and satisfaction with treatment. *Neurology, 71,* 559–566.

Blanchard, E. B., Andrasik, F., Evans, D. D., Neff, D. F., Appelbaum, K. A., & Rodichok, L. D. (1985). Behavioral treatment of 250 chronic headache patients: A clinical replication series. *Behavior Therapy, 16,* 308–327.

Blanchard, E. B., Andrasik, F., Neff, D. F., Jurish, S. E., & O'Keefe, D. M. (1981). Social validation of the headache diary. *Behavior Therapy, 12,* 711–715.

Bond, D., Dirge, K., Rubingh, C., Durrant, L., & Baggaley, S. (2004). Impact of a self-help intervention on performance of headache management behaviors: A self-efficacy approach. *Internet Journal of Allied Health Sciences and Practice, 2*(1), 1–12.

Breslau, N., & Davis, G. C. (1993). Migraine, physical health and psychiatric disorder: A prospective epidemiologic study in young adults. *Journal of Psychiatric Research, 27,* 211–221.

Burns, J. W., Kubilus, A., Bruehl, S., Harden, R. N., & Lofland, K. (2003). Do changes in cognitive factors influence outcome following multidisciplinary treatment for chronic pain?: A cross-lagged panel analysis. *Journal of Consulting and Clinical Psychology, 71,* 81–91.

Buse, D. C., & Andrasik, F. (2009). Behavioral medicine for migraine. *Neurologic Clinics, 27,* 321–582.

Buse, D. C., Bigal, M. E., Rupnow, M. F. T., Reed, M. L., Serrano, D., Biondi, D. M., et al. (2007). The Migraine Interictal Burden Scale (MIBS): Results of a population-based validation study. *Headache, 47,* 778.

Buse, D. C., & Lipton, R. B. (2008). Facilitating communication with patients for improved migraine outcomes. *Current Pain and Headache Reports, 12,* 230–236.

Buse, D. C., Manack, A., Serrano, D., Turkel, C., & Lipton, R. B. (2010). Sociodemographic and comorbidity profiles of chronic migraine and episodic migraine sufferers. *Journal of Neurology, Neurosurgery, and Psychiatry, 81,* 428–432.

Buse, D. C., Rupnow, M. F., & Lipton, R. B. (2009). Assessing and managing all aspects of migraine: Migraine attacks, migraine-related functional impairment, common comorbidities, and quality of life. *Mayo Clinic Proceedings, 84,* 422–435.

Bussone, G., Usai, S., Grazzi, L., Rigamonti, A., Solari, A., & D'Amico, D. (2004). Disability and quality of life in different primary headaches: Results from Italian studies. *Neurological Science, 25*(Suppl. 3), S105–S107.

Butler, S. F., Budman, S. H., Fernandez, K. C., Houle, B., Benoit, C., Katz, N., et al. (2007). Development and validation of the Current Opioid Misuse Measure. *Pain, 130,* 144–156.

Chatterton, M. L., Lofland, J. H., Shechter, A., Curtice, W. S., Hu, X. H., Lenow, J., et al. (2002). Reliability and validity of the migraine therapy assessment questionnaire. *Headache, 42,* 1006–1015.

Cook, N. R., Bensenor, I. M., Lotufo, P. A., Lee, I. M., Skerrett, P. J., Chown, M. J., et al. (2002). Migraine and coronary heart disease in women and men. *Headache, 42,* 715–727.

Cramer, J. A., Silberstein, S. D., & Winner, P. (2001). Development and validation of the Headache Needs Assessment (HANA) survey. *Headache, 41,* 402–409.

Dahlof, C. G. H., & Dimenäs, E. (1995). Migraine patients experience poorer subjective well-being/quality of life even between attacks. *Cephalalgia, 15,* 31–36.

Dayno, J. M., Silberstein, S. D., & Lipton, R. B. (1996). Migraine comorbidity: Epilepsy and stroke. *Advances in Clinical Neurosciences, 6,* 365–385.

De Benedittis, G., & Lorenzetti, A. (1992). Minor stressful life events (daily hassles) in chronic primary headache: Relationship with MMPI personality patterns. *Headache, 32,* 330–332.

Dodick, D. W. (2003). Clinical clues and clinical rules: Primary versus secondary headache. *Advanced Studies in Medicine, 3,* S550–S555.

Dowson, A. J., Tepper, S. J., Baos, V., Baudet, F., D'Amico, D., & Kilminster, S. (2004). Identifying patients who require a change in their current acute migraine treatment: The Migraine Assessment of Current Therapy (Migraine-ACT) questionnaire. *Current Medical Research and Opinion*, *20*, 1125–1135.

El Hasnaoui, A., Vray, M., Richard, A., Nachit-Ouinekh, F., & Boureau, F., and the MIG-SEV Group. (2003). Assessing the severity of migraine: Development of the MIGSEV scale. *Headache*, *43*(6), 628–635.

Fayers, P. M., & Machin, D. (2000). *Quality of life: Assessment, analysis and interpretation.* New York: Wiley.

Finkel, A. G. (2003). Epidemiology of cluster headache. *Current Pain and Headache Reports*, *7*, 144–149.

Folstein, M. F., Folstein, S. E., & McHugh, P. R. (1975). "Mini-Mental State": A practical method for grading the cognitive state of patients for the clinician. *Journal of Psychiatric Research*, *12*, 189–198.

French, D. J., Holroyd, K. A., Pinell, C., Malinoski, P. T., O'Donnel, F., & Hill, K. R. (2000). Perceived self-efficacy and headache-related disability. *Headache*, *40*, 647–656.

Grazzi, L., Andrasik, F., Usai, S., & Bussone, G. (2009). Treatment of chronic migraine with medication overuse: Is drug withdrawal crucial? *Neurological Sciences*, *30*(Suppl. 1), S85–S88.

Guyatt, G. H., Feeny, D. H., & & Patrick, D. L. (1993). Measuring health-related quality of life. *Annals of Internal Medicine*, *118*, 622–629.

Hadjistavropoulos, H. D., MacLeod, F. K., & Asmundson, G. J. (1999). Validation of the Chronic Pain Coping Inventory. *Pain*, *80*, 471–481.

Hahn, S. R. (2008). Communication in the care of the headache patient. In S. D. Silberstein, R. B. Lipton, & D. W. Dodick (Eds.), *Wolff's headache and other head pain* (8th ed., pp. 805–824). New York: Oxford University Press.

Hamelsky, S. W., & Lipton, R. B. (2006). Psychiatric comorbidity of migraine. *Headache*, *46*, 1327–1333.

Hartmaier, S. L., DeMuro-Mercon, C., Linder, S., Winner, P., & Santanello, S. C. (2001). Development of a brief 24-hour adolescent migraine functioning questionnaire. *Headache*, *41*, 150–60.

Headache Classification Committee of the International Headache Society. (1988). Classification and diagnostic criteria for headache disorders, cranial neuralgias, and facial pain. *Cephalalgia*, *8*(Suppl. 7), 1–96.

Headache Classification Committee of the International Headache Society, Olesen, J., Bousser, M. G., Diener, H. C., Dodick, D., First, M., et al. (2006). New appendix criteria open for a broader concept of chronic migraine. *Cephalalgia*, *26*, 742–746.

Heath, R. L., Saliba, M., Mahmassani, O., Major, S. C., & Khoury, B. A. (2008). Locus of control moderates the relationship between headache pain and depression. *Journal of Headache and Pain*, *9*, 301–308.

Henryk-Gutt, R., & Rees, W. C. (1973). Psychological aspects of migraine. *Journal of Psychosomatic Research*, *17*, 141–153.

Hershey, A. D., Powers, S. W., Vockell, A. L., LeCates, S., Kabbouche, M. A., & Maynard, M. K. (2001). PedMIDAS: Development of a questionnaire to assess disability of migraines in children. *Neurology*, *57*, 2034–2039.

Holm, J. E., Holroyd, K. A., Hursey, K. G., & Penzien, D. (1986). The role of stress in recurrent tension headaches. *Headache*, *26*, 160–167.

Holmes, W. F., MacGregor, E. A., Sawyer, J. P., & Lipton, R. B. (2001). Information about migraine disability influences physicians' perceptions of illness severity and treatment needs, *Headache*, *41*, 343–350.

Holroyd, K. A., Drew, J. B., Cottrell, C. K., Romanek, K. M., & Heh, V. (2007). Impaired functioning and quality of life in severe migraine: The role of catastrophizing and associated symptoms. *Cephalalgia*, *27*, 1156–1165.

Holroyd, K. A., Holm, J. E., Hursey, K. G., Penzien, D. B., Cordingley, G. E., Theofanous, A. G., et al. (1988). Recurrent vascular headache: Home-based behavioral treatment vs. abortive pharmacological treatment. *Journal of Consulting and Clinical Psychology*, *56*, 218–223.

Howarth, E. (1965). Headache, personality, and stress. *British Journal of Psychiatry*, *111*, 1193–1197.

Jacob, R. G., Turner, S. M., Szekely, B. C., & Eidelman, B. H. (1983). Predicting outcome of relaxation therapy in headaches: The role of "depression." *Behavior Therapy*, *14*, 457–465.

Jacobs, J. W., Bernhard, M. R., Delgado, A., & Strain, J. J. (1977). Screening for organic mental syndromes in the medically ill. *Annals of Internal Medicine*, *86*, 40–46.

Jacobson, G. P., Ramadan, N. M., Aggarwal, S. K., & Newman, C. K. (1994). The Henry Ford Hospital Disability Inventory (HDI). *Neurology*, *44*(5), 837–842.

Jacobson, G. P., Ramadan, N. M., Norris, L., & Newman, C. W. (1995). Headache Disability Inventory (HDI): Short-term test–retest reliability and spouse perceptions. *Headache*, *35*, 534–539.

Jensen, M. P., Karoly, P., & Huger, R. (1987). The development and preliminary validation of an instrument to assess patients' attitudes toward pain. *Journal of Psychosomatic Research*, *31*, 393–400.

Jensen, M. P., Turner, J. A., Romano, J. M., & Strom, S. E. (1995). The Chronic Pain Coping Inventory: Development and preliminary validation. *Pain, 60*, 203–216.

Jette, N., Patten, S., Williams, J., Becker, W., & Wiebe, S. (2008). Comorbidity of Migraine and Psychiatric Disorders—a national population-based study. *Headache, 48*, 501–516.

Juang, K. D., Wang, S. J., Fuh, J. L., Lu, S. R., & Su, T. P. (2000). Comorbidity of depressive and anxiety disorders in chronic daily headache and its subtypes. *Headache, 40*, 818–823.

Kosinski, M., Bayliss, M. S., Bjorner, J. B., Ware, J. E., Jr., Garber, W. H., Batenhorst, A., et al. (2003). A six-item short-form survey for measuring headache impact: The HIT-6. *Quality of Life Research, 12*, 963–974.

Kroenke, K., Spitzer, R. L., & Williams, J. B. (2001). The PHQ-9: Validity of a brief depression severity measure. *Journal of General Internal Medicine, 16*, 606–613.

Kroenke, K., Spitzer, R. L., & Williams, J. B. (2003). The Patient Health Questionnaire–2: Validity of a two-item depression screener. *Medical Care, 41*, 1284–1292.

Langeveld, J. H., Koot, H. M., Loonen, M. C., Hazebroek-Kampschreur, A. A., & Passchier, J. (1996). A quality of life instrument for adolescents with chronic headache. *Cephalalgia, 16*, 183–196.

Lanteri-Minet, M., Radat, F., Chautard, M. H., & Lucas, C. (2005). Anxiety and depression associated with migraine: Influence on migraine subjects' disability and quality of life, and acute migraine management. *Pain, 118*, 319–326.

Lawson, P., Kerr, K., Penzien, D. B., Hursey, K. G., Ray, S. E., Arora, R., et al. (1988, November). *Caveats in using mental status examinations: Factors that influence performance.* Paper presented at the annual meeting of the Association for Advancement of Behavior Therapy, New York.

Lazarus, R. S., & Folkman, S. (1984). Coping and adaption. In W. D. Gentry (Ed.), *The handbook of behavioral medicine* (pp. 282–325). New York: Guilford Press.

Lemstra, M., Stewart, B., & Olszynski, W. (2002). Effectiveness of multidisciplinary intervention in the treatment of migraine: A randomized clinical trial. *Headache, 42*, 845–854.

Leonardi, M., Steiner, T. J., Scher, A. T., & Lipton, R. B. (2005). The global burden of migraine: Measuring disability in headache disorders with WHO's Classification of Functioning, Disability, and Health (ICF). *Journal of Headache and Pain, 6*, 429–440.

Levor, R. M., Cohen, M. J., Naliboff, B. D., MacArthur, D., & Heuser, G. (1986). Psycho-social precursors and correlates of migraine headache. *Journal of Consulting and Clinical Psychology, 54*, 347–353.

Lipton, R. B., Bigal, M. E., Diamond, M., Freitag, F., Reed, M. L., & Stewart, W. F. (2007). American Migraine Prevalence and Prevention (AMPP) Advisory Group: Migraine prevalence, disease burden, and the need for preventive therapy. *Neurology, 68*, 343–349.

Lipton, R. B., Bigal, M. E., Kolodner, K., Stewart, W. F., Liberman, J. N., & Steiner, T. J. (2003). The family impact of migraine: Population-based studies in the USA and UK. *Cephalalgia, 23*(6), 429–440.

Lipton, R. B., Bigal, M. E., Steiner, T. J., Silberstein, S. D., & Olesen, J. (2004). Classification of primary headaches. *Neurology, 63*, 427–435.

Lipton, R. B., Dodick, D., Sadovsky, R., Kolodner, K., Endicott, J., Hettiarachi, J., et al. (2003). A self-administered screener for migraine in primary care: The ID Migraine™ validation study. *Neurology, 61*, 375–382.

Lipton, R. B., Kolodner, K., Bigal, M. E., Valade, D., Láinez, M. J., Pascual, J., et al. (2009). Validity and reliability of the Migraine-Treatment Optimization Questionnaire. *Cephalalgia, 29*, 751–759.

Lipton, R. B., Serrano, D., Buse, D. C., Rupnow, M. F. T., Reed, M. L., & Bigal, M. E. (2007). The Migraine Prevention Questionnaire (MPQ): Development and validation. *Headache, 47*, 770–771.

Lipton, R. B., Stewart, W. F., Diamond, S., Diamond, M. L., & Reed, M. (2001). Prevalence and burden of migraine in the United States: Data from the American Migraine Study II. *Headache, 41*, 646–657.

Maizels, M., & Houle, T. (2008). Results of screening with the brief headache screen compared with a modified ID-Migraine. *Headache, 48*, 385–394.

Maizels, M., & Wolfe, W. J. (2008). An expert system for headache diagnosis: The Computerized Headache Assessment tool (CHAT). *Headache, 48*, 72–78.

Marlowe, N. (1986). Stressful events, appraisal, coping, and recurrent headache. *Journal of Clinical Psychology, 54*, 247–256.

Martin, B. C., Pathak, D. S., Sharfman, M. I., Adelman, J. U., Taylor, F., Kwong, W. J., et al. (2000). Validity and reliability of the Migraine-Specific Quality of Life Questionnaire (MSQ Version 2.1). *Headache, 40*, 204–215.

Martin, N. J., Holroyd, K. A., & Penzien, D. B. (1990). The Headache-Specific Locus of Control Scale: Adaptation to recurrent headaches. *Headache, 30*, 729–734.

Martin, N. J., Holroyd, K. A., & Rokicki, L. A. (1993). The Headache Self-Efficacy Scale: Adaptation to recurrent headaches. *Headache*, *33*, 244–248.

Nicholson, R. A., Houle, T. T., Rhudy, J. L., & Norton, P. J. (2007). Psychological risk factors in headache. *Headache*, *47*, 413–426.

Nicholson, R. A., Hursey, K. G., & Nash, J. (2005). Moderators and mediators of behavioral treatment for headache. *Headache*, *45*, 513–519.

Nicholson, R. A., Nash, J., & Andrasik, F. (2005). A self-administered behavioral intervention using tailored messages for migraine. *Headache*, *45*, 1124–1139.

Ottman, R., & Lipton, R. B. (1994). Comorbidity of migraine and epilepsy. *Neurology*, *44*, 2105–2110.

Pathak, D. S., Chisolm, D. J., & Weis, K. A. (2005). Functional Assessment in Migraine (FAIM) questionnaire: Development of an instrument based upon the WHO's International Classification of Functioning, Disability, and Health. *Value Health*, *8*, 591–600.

Patrick, D. L., Hurst, B. C., & Hughes, J. (2000). Further development and testing of the Migraine-Specific Quality of Life (MSQOL) measure. *Headache*, *40*, 550–560.

Penzien, D. B., Rains, J. C., & Holroyd, K. A. (1993). Psychological assessment of the recurrent headache sufferer. In C. D. Tollison & R. S. Kunkel (Eds.), *Headache: Diagnosis and interdisciplinary treatment* (pp. 39–49). Baltimore: Williams & Wilkins.

Platt, F. W., Gaspar, D. L., Coulehan, J. L., Fox, L., Adler, A. J., Weston, W. W., et al. (2001). "Tell me about yourself": The patient-centered interview. *Annals of Internal Medicine*, *134*, 1079–1085.

Powers, S. W., & Andrasik, F. (2005). Biobehavioral treatment, disability, and psychological effects of pediatric headache. *Pediatric Annals*, *34*, 461–465.

Radat, F., Irachabal, S., Lafittau, M., Creac'h, C., Dousset, V., & Henry, P. (2006). Construction of a medication dependence questionnaire in headache patients (MDQ-H) validation of the French version. *Headache*, *46*, 233–239.

Rasmussen, B. K. (1995). Epidemiology of headache. *Cephalalgia*, *15*, 45–68.

Revicki, D. A., Kimel, M., Beusterien, K., Kwong, J. W., Varner, J. A., Ames, M. H., et al. (2006). Validation of the revised Patient Perception of Migraine Questionnaire: Measuring satisfaction with acute migraine treatment. *Headache*, *46*, 240–252.

Robertson, K. (2005). Active listening. More than just paying attention. *Australian Family Physician*, *34*, 1053–1055.

Rogers, C. R. (1967). *On becoming a person: A psychotherapist's view of psychotherapy*. London: Constable.

Santanello, N. C., Hartmaier, S. L., Epstein, R. S., & Silberstein, S. D. (1995). Validation of a new quality of life questionnaire for acute migraine headache. *Headache*, *35*, 330–337.

Scharff, L., Turk, D. C., & Marcus, D. A. (1995). The relationship of locus of control and psychosocial–behavioral response in chronic headache. *Headache*, *35*, 527–533.

Scher, A. I., Bigal, M. E., & Lipton, R. B. (2005). Comorbidity of migraine. *Current Opinions in Neurology*, *18*, 305–310.

Scher, A. I., Stewart, W. F., & Lipton, R. B. (2006). The comorbidity of headache with other pain syndromes. *Headache*, *46*, 1416–1423.

Schwartz, B. S., Stewart, W. F., Simon, D., & Lipton, R. B. (1998). Epidemiology of tension-type headache. *Journal of the American Medical Association*, *279*, 381–383.

Silberstein, S. D., & Lipton, R. B. (1993). Epidemiology of migraine. *Neuroepidemiology*, *12*, 179–194.

Silberstein, S. D., Olesen, J., Bousser, M.-G., Diener, H.-C., Dodick, D., First, M., et al. (2004). The international classification of headache disorders, 2nd edition. *Cephalalgia*, *24*(Suppl. 1), 1–160.

Silberstein, S. D., Olesen, J., Bousser, M.-G., Diener, H.-C., Dodick, D., First, M., et al. (2005). The international classification of headache disorders, 2nd edition (ICHD-II)— Revision of criteria for 8.2 medication-overuse headache. *Cephalalgia*, *25*, 460–465.

Smith, T., & Nicholson, R. (2006). Are changes in cognitive and emotional factors important in improving headache impact and quality of life? *Headache*, *46*, 878.

Solomon, G. D. (1997). Evolution of the measurement of quality of life in migraine. *Neurology*, *48*, S10–S15.

Solomon, G. D., Skobieranda, F. G., & Gragg, L. A. (1993). Quality of life and well-being of headache patients: Measurement by the medical outcomes study instrument. *Headache*, *33*, 351–358.

Spitzer, R. L., Kroenke, K., Williams, J. B., & Lowe, B. (2006). A brief measure for assessing generalized anxiety disorder: The GAD-7. *Archives of Internal Medicine*, *166*, 1092–1097.

Spitzer, R. L., Kroenke, K., Williams, J. B. W., & the Patient Health Questionnaire Primary Care Study Group. (1999). Validation and utility of a self-report version of PRIME-MD: The PHQ Primary Care Study. *Journal of the American Medical Association*, *282*, 1737–1744.

Stewart, W. F., Lipton, R. B., Dowson, A. J., Sawyer, J., & Sawyer, M. B. (2001). Development and testing of the Migraine Disability

Assessment (MIDAS) questionnaire to assess headache-related disability. *Neurology, 56,* S20–S28.

Stewart, W. F., Lipton, R. B., Simon, D., Von Korff, M., & Liberman, J. (1998). Reliability of an illness severity measure for headache in a population sample of migraine sufferers. *Cephalalgia, 18,* 44–51.

Sullivan, M. J., Thorn, B., Haythornthwaite, J. A., Keefe, F., Martin, M., Bradley, L. A., et al. (2001). Theoretical perspectives on the relation between catastrophizing and pain. *Clinical Journal of Pain, 17,* 52–64.

Sullivan, M. J. L., Bishop, S. C., & Pivik, J. (1995). The Pain Catastrophizing Scale: Development and validation. *Psychological Assessment, 7,* 524–532.

Tait, R. C., & Chibnall, J. T. (1997). Development of a brief version of the Survey of Pain Attitudes. *Pain, 70,* 229–235.

Torelli, P., Castellini, P., Cucurachi, L., Devetak, M., Lambru, G., & Manzoni, G. (2006). Cluster headache prevalence: methodological considerations: A review of the literature. *Acta Biomedico Ateneo Parmense, 77,* 4–9.

Waggoner, C. D., & Andrasik, F. (1990). Behavioral assessment and treatment of recurrent headache. In T. W. Miller (Ed.), *Chronic pain* (pp. 319–361). Madison, CT: International Universities Press.

Wagner, T. H., Patrick, D. L., Galer, B. S., & Berzon, R. A. (1996). A new instrument to assess the long-term quality of life effects from migraine: Development and psychometric testing of the MSQOL. *Headache, 36,* 484–492.

Ware, J., Jr., Kosinski, M., & Keller, S. D.

(1996). A 12-item Short-Form Health Survey: Construction of scales and preliminary tests of reliability and validity. *Medical Care, 34,* 220–233.

Ware, J. E., Jr., & Sherbourne, C. D. (1992). The MOS 36-item Short-Form Survey (SF-36): I. Conceptual framework and item selection. *Medical Care, 30,* 473–483.

Weiss, J., Goodman, P., Losito, B., Corrigan, S., Charry, J., & Bailery, W. (1981). Behavioral depression produced by an uncontrollable stressor: Relationship to norepinephrine, dopamine, and serotonin levels in various regions of the rat brain. *Brain Research Reviews, 3,* 167–205.

Werder, D. S., Sargent, J. D., & Coyne, L. (1981). MMPI profiles of headache patients using self-regulation to control headache activity. *Headache, 21,* 164–169.

White, K., & Farrell, A. (2006). Anxiety and psychosocial stress as predictors of headache and abdominal pain in urban early adolescents. *Journal of Pediatric Psychology, 31,* 582–596.

Winner, P., Hershey, A. D., & Li, Z. (2008). Headaches in children. In S. D. Silberstein, R. B. Lipton, & D. W. Dodick (Eds.), *Wolff's headache and other head pain* (8th ed., pp. 665–690). New York: Oxford University Press.

Zwart, J. A., Dyb, G., Hagen, K., Odegard, K. J., Dahl, A. A., Bovim, G., et al. (2003). Depression and anxiety disorders associated with headache frequency: The Nord-Trondelag Health Study. *European Journal of Neurology, 10,* 147–152.

CHAPTER 19

Assessment of Patients with Cancer-Related Pain

KAREN O. ANDERSON

Poorly controlled pain has such deleterious effects on the patient with cancer and the patient's family that its proper management should have the highest priority in the routine care of anyone with cancer. Not only do mood and quality of life deteriorate in the presence of pain, but pain has adverse effects on measures of disease status such as appetite and daily function. A review of studies evaluating the prevalence of pain in patients with cancer concluded that the prevalence of pain across all cancer types is greater than 50% (van den Beuken-van Everdingen et al., 2007). Among the patients with pain, more than one-third rated their pain intensity as moderate or severe.

There is strong evidence that the majority of patients with cancer can get pain relief if adequate treatment is provided. Studies of the World Health Organization's (1986, 1996) guidelines for cancer pain relief indicate that 70 to 90% of patients are relieved if this simple protocol for oral analgesic medications is followed (Grond et al., 1993, 1999; Schug, Zech, & Dorr, 1990; Ventafridda, Tamburini, Caraceni, De, & Naldi, 1987; Zech, Grond, Lynch, Hertel, & Lehmann, 1995). When oral analgesics are not effective, a variety of supplemental pain management techniques can provide pain control.

It is estimated that approximately 95% of cancer patients could be free of significant pain (Foley, 2005). Unfortunately, multiple studies document undertreatment of cancer-related pain (Anderson et al., 2000; Cleeland et al., 1994; Cleeland, Gonin, Baez, Loehrer, & Pandya, 1996; Vainio & Auvinen, 1996; Zenz, Zenz, Tryba, & Strumpf, 1995; Zhukovsky, Gorowski, Hausdorff, Napolitano, & Lesser, 1995). A review of studies on the undertreatment of cancer pain found that from 8 to 82% of patients were receiving inadequate analgesics to control the intensity of their pain (Deandrea, Montanari, Moja, & Apolone, 2008). The authors found substantial variability in undertreatment of pain. For example, patients treated in developing countries in Asia or Europe were more likely to be undertreated than patients treated in wealthier nations. Also, patients who were rated less ill or in an early disease stage were more likely to receive inadequate pain treatment.

Although there are multiple barriers to good pain control for the patient with cancer, inadequate assessment is the most obvious. Unrecognized pain will not be treated, and pain whose severity is underestimated will not be treated aggressively enough. Over 800 Eastern Cooperative Oncology

Group (ECOG)-affiliated physicians responded to a survey designed to determine their knowledge and practice of cancer pain management (von Roenn, Cleeland, Gonin, Hatfield, & Pandya, 1993). Survey respondents ranked a list of potential barriers to optimal cancer pain management in their own practice settings. By far the most frequently identified barrier was lack of pain assessment; 76% of respondents rated inadequate assessment as one of the top barriers to good pain management. Patient reluctance to report pain, intimately related to inadequate assessment, was the next most frequently cited barrier. Similarly, surveys of physicians in public hospitals and in the Radiation Therapy Oncology Group found that poor pain assessment and patient reluctance to report pain were identified as top barriers to optimal pain management (Anderson et al., 2000; Cleeland, Janjan, Scott, Seiferheld, & Curran, 2000).

Despite the recognition that it is important, formal pain assessment is rarely practiced in most cancer care settings. The primary reason is that health care providers do not have the time to assess pain and its impact fully. Moreover, many health care providers do not have the necessary skills to assess pain and pain treatment effects adequately. Pain assessment is not a standard part of most patient appointments, and other priorities supplant symptom evaluation. When providers do ask about pain, they rarely attempt to quantify the severity of the pain or to document its characteristics and determinants. Even rarer is any attempt to assess the impact that pain is making on the emotional, social, or functional status of the patient.

In this chapter I examine some of the methodological and practical issues in the assessment of cancer pain and its impact, and describe a "minimal dataset" of information needed for treatment planning, and suggest how pain questionnaires might be used to improve assessment. While the focus is on the clinical assessment of pain, I describe how similar pain assessment procedures can be used in areas such as clinical trials and quality assurance, and deal only with information that can be obtained by questionnaires, interview, and observation of the patient. However, pain assessment should include a medical evaluation and the possible addition of appropriate diagnostic procedures. A retrospective survey of cancer patients found that two-thirds of patients referred for pain assessment had new (and often treatable) pathology diagnosed as a result of the medical evaluation and follow-up (Gonzales, Elliott, Portenoy, & Foley, 1991).

PREVALENCE OF CANCER PAIN

Cancer is a generic term applied to a variety of different diseases that have in common mutation of cell development leading to unregulated proliferation of cell growth that in turn results in invasion and metastases. The primary site and cell type of a cancer dictates many of its features, including rate of development; response to anticancer therapies; common sites of metastatic spread of disease; and the location, course, and quality of pain.

Early studies of the prevalence of pain in patients with cancer reported rates that ranged from 52 to 77% (Lempinen, 1971; Ross, Braasch, & Warren, 1973; Twycross, 1973). An international study of patients with advanced cancer found that one-half of patients with lung and breast cancer had at least moderate pain. Prevalence of moderate or severe pain was highest in the gynecological cancers, head and neck cancers, and prostate cancer (Vainio & Auvinen, 1996). A recent meta-analysis of studies evaluating the prevalence of pain in patients with cancer concluded that the pooled prevalence rate of pain for patients in active treatment was 59%. For patients with advanced disease, the pooled prevalence rate was 64%, and the rate was 33% for patients after curative treatment (van den Beuken-van Everdingen et al., 2007).

Clinicians have long been aware that near the end of life the majority of cancer patients will need pain management, but less attention has been paid to the problem of pain for patients during and after cancer treatments. Of the patients who achieve a cure, a substantial percentage will have indefinite periods of treatment-related pain (Andrykowski et al., 1999). For example, surveys of women who undergo breast cancer surgery reveal a high incidence of postmastectomy and postlumpectomy pain (Smith, Bourne, Squair,

Phillips, & Chambers, 1999; Wallace, Wallace, Lee, & Dobke, 1996). Because more than 60% of patients now survive cancer, while many live longer with more aggressive treatments, greater numbers of patients have to face extended periods of coping with pain from their cancer or its treatments (Burton, Fanciullo, Beasley, & Fisch, 2007).

PHYSICAL BASIS OF CANCER PAIN

Pain in cancer patients can be due to diverse causes (Chang, Janjan, Jain, & Chau, 2006a; Portenoy & Lesage, 1999). Since treatment is determined by the etiology of the pain, establishing the physical cause of the pain is an important goal of assessment. In a prospective study of over 2,000 patients with cancer referred to a pain service, 70% of the patients had pain due to multiple sources (Grond, Zech, Diefenbach, Radbruch, & Lehmann, 1996). In this study, the source of pain was classified (in decreasing frequency) as soft tissue invasion, bone pain, nerve damage or infiltration, and visceral pain. Other studies have found that bone pain and visceral pain are the most frequent etiologies of cancer pain (Banning, Sjogren, & Henriksen, 1991; Caraceni & Portenoy, 1999).

An important distinction needs to be made between primary *nociceptive pain* (pain caused by stimulation of pain receptors) and *neuropathic pain* (painful sensations caused by an injury or dysfunction of peripheral or central nervous system structures). Many cancer pain syndromes involve both neuropathic and nociceptive pain (Chang et al., 2006a; Urch & Dickenson, 2008). Since pain syndromes that include neuropathic pain may respond to different pharmacological interventions than do syndromes involving only nociceptive pain, it is crucial to specify the types of pain involved in each case.

Many patients have pain caused by cancer treatments (Caraceni & Portenoy, 1999; Chang, Janjan, Jain, & Chau, 2006b; Grond et al., 1996). By necessity, many cancer treatments are destructive, whether in the form of surgery, chemotherapy, or radiation therapy. Pain is often the product of these destructive procedures. In some cases treatment-related pain is time-limited, while in other cases a more permanent treatment-related pain syndrome, such as peripheral neuropathy, may develop. Although pain generally becomes worse with progression of the disease, pain can also improve if the disease is responsive to anticancer therapies.

THE CONTEXT OF CANCER PAIN ASSESSMENT

Historically, most pain assessment procedures were developed for patients with pain due to noncancer causes. Pain assessment evolved along with the development of multidisciplinary pain clinics that, for the most part, treated patients with noncancer pain who commonly reported pain as their primary health problem. The assessment of pain due to cancer requires some reorientation, dictated by the nature of the disease, the types of pain that cancer causes, and the medical and psychosocial context of having cancer. The dynamic and progressive nature of both the disease and its treatment must be integrated concurrently with treatment of the pain. In this context of multiple symptoms, potential organ system and metabolic instabilities, as well as intense focus on disease treatment, management of pain can be a moving target, with treatment needs changing rapidly and dramatically.

Because most pain assessment procedures have evolved from the needs of patients with chronic noncancer pain, it is important to point out some major differences between the majority of patients seen in traditional pain clinics and those seen in cancer treatment settings. Patients seen in multidisciplinary pain clinics most often freely complain of pain, and some treatment programs are designed to reduce the frequency and tenacity of pain complaints because of the negative social consequences of persistent pain reporting. In contrast, patients with cancer frequently underreport pain and pain severity. A number of patient-related barriers to the assessment of cancer pain have been identified (Reid, Gooberman-Hill, & Hanks, 2008; Thomason et al., 1998; Ward et al., 1993; Ward & Hernandez, 1994). Patients with cancer often do not want to be labeled as complainers, do not want to distract their health care provider from attending to the cancer, or are afraid that their pain means that the cancer is getting worse. Some patients are fatalistic and believe that pain is an inevitable part of having cancer (Anderson et al., 2002). Patients are often concerned about having to take potent opioids and may fear they will become addicts or develop tolerance to the effects of analgesics (Ersek, Kraybill, & Pen, 1999; Ward et al., 1993).

TARGETS OF PAIN ASSESSMENT

For the patient with cancer, what do we need to know about pain to plan treatment? In assessing the pain itself, we depend in large measure on patient self-report. In this realm, we first need to know the *location* of each pain and how *severe* it is. Guidelines for cancer pain treatment from the Agency for Healthcare Research and Quality, the American Pain Society, the National Comprehensive Cancer Network, and the World Health Organization all use a determination of pain severity as the primary item of information in specifying treatment (American Pain Society, 1999; Benedetti et al., 2000; Gordon et al., 2005; Jacox, Carr, & Payne, 1994; World Health Organization, 1986, 1996). The recommended analgesics change in type and increase in potency as pain increases in severity.

In addition to location and severity, patients need to be able to report the *quality* of their pain. They do this by using various descriptors, words such as "aching," "cramping," or "burning." The temporal *pattern* (onset, duration, predictability, aggravating factors) of the pain also is important. Is it constant, constant with intermittent exacerbations, or only episodically severe? Information on pain quality, pattern, and location are helpful in determining the physical bases or mechanisms of the pain.

An adequate pain assessment goes beyond information on pain characteristics and physical mechanisms. Information about the *impact* of pain on activities essential to living can be as valuable as severity ratings by indicating the extent to which pain causes disruptions in daily life. Some patients are reluctant to report their pain as severe. A patient who reports pain severity of 3 on a scale of 0 to 10 but is unable to sleep or walk may need treatment as urgently as another patient who reports pain at a level of 8.

Comprehensive treatment plans also need to be based on information about the patient's and family's *beliefs* about cancer pain treatment. These beliefs can determine whether patients will take medications prescribed or whether family members will inhibit or discourage pain treatments. Finally, a *pain history* is needed. Most patients have already been treated for pain. We need information about how long the pain has existed, what aggravates or alleviates the pain, what treatments did not work or did work, and for how long. A *physical exam* is required, along with relevant laboratory and imaging tests that are essential to determining etiology, mechanisms and, therefore, treatment. *Other symptoms* need to be evaluated. Pain treatment frequently causes side effects, and many symptoms that are common in patients with cancer can confound pain treatment.

PAIN ASSESSMENT MATERIALS

Using standardized, reliable, and validated pain assessment instruments minimizes many patient reporting biases and assists clinicians and researchers in obtaining complete and reliable information. Using pain scales that assign a metric to pain intensity and interference makes pain more of an "objective" symptom, similar to other signs and symptoms, such as blood pressure and heart rate. By "measuring" pain, patients feel freer (and more obligated) to report pain presence and severity. Standard measurement also readily allows patients to indicate when treatment is not working. "How is your medication working?" provokes a response of "Fine" or "OK" from a patient who wants to please, whereas "Rate your pain from 0 to 10" does not require the patient to judge the success or failure of the health care provider's treatment.

Using pain questionnaires or pain measurement scales also can minimize staff biases related to language, cultural variables, or the unfamiliar style of an individual patient. Multiple studies have found that minority patients with cancer are at risk for inadequate assessment and undertreatment of their pain (Anderson et al., 2000; Cleeland et al., 1994, 1997; Green, Anderson, et al., 2003; Green, Baker, Sato, Washington, & Smith, 2003). For example, a longitudinal study of over 1,000 women with metastatic breast cancer and bone metastases found that pain severity worsened more rapidly among nonwhite compared to white women (Castel et al., 2008). Documenting regular pain assessments is a crucial step in improving pain management for vulnerable and underserved minority populations (Green, Anderson, et al., 2003). The use of pain questionnaires also greatly reduces the amount of staff time required for the assessment process. The medical staff can use the extra time to pursue the specific needs of an individual patient, based on the patient's responses to the questionnaire.

Pain Scales

Several ways of scaling the severity or intensity of pain and associated symptoms have been advocated. Numerical rating scales (NRSs) are the most widely used in clinical settings and are easily adaptable to research needs. They typically measure pain severity by asking the patient to select a number from 0 to 10 (an 11-point scale) to represent how severe the pain is. The numbers can be arrayed along a horizontal line, with 0 on the left and labeled "no pain" and 10 on the right, labeled with a phrase such as "pain as bad as can be." Since pain due to cancer can be quite variable over a day, patients can be asked to rate their pain at the time of responding to the questionnaire, and at its "worst," and "usual" or "average" pain over the last 24 hours. The NRS has demonstrated good test–retest reliability for ratings of average and worst pain, strong concurrent and criterion validity, and sensitivity to changes in cancer-related pain (Jensen, 2003).

Verbal descriptor scales (VDSs) have a long history in pain research, and have demonstrated good concurrent and criterion validity in studies of patients with cancer (Jensen, 2003). The patient is asked to pick a category, such as "none," "mild," "moderate," "severe," and "excruciating," that best describes severity. Pain relief can be categorized in a similar way, such as "none," "slight," "moderate," "lots," and "complete." A number is associated with each descriptor (e.g., "none" = 0, "complete" = 4), and the patient's score is the number associated with the word. As a research tool, VDSs are limited by unequal distances between descriptors and dependence on language comprehension.

Visual analogue scales (VASs) often are used in clinical research comparing the effectiveness of analgesic drugs and other pain treatments (Cleeland, 1990a; Jensen, 2003; Wallenstein, 1984). Using the VAS, the patient makes a judgment as to how much of the length of a 10-cm line is equivalent to the severity of the pain. One end of the line represents "no pain" and the other end some concept such as "pain as bad as you can imagine." The advantages of the VAS are the ability to repeat measurement with less influence of past measures than with recall of a number or word, and the potentially infinite number of points on the line. The VAS has demonstrated good test–retest reliability, concurrent and criterion validity, and sensitivity to changes in cancer-related pain (Cleeland, 1990b). The disadvantages of the VAS include the need to have someone measure the line and the greater number of patients who have difficulty completing this type of pain assessment (Bruera, Kuehn, Miller, Selmser, & Macmillan, 1991; Ferraz et al., 1990).

In clinical settings, these three scales of severity approach equivalency, so that ease of use becomes the primary factor in scale selection (De Conno et al., 1994; Jensen, Karoly, & Braver, 1986). In clinical trials, the NRS has been found to be more reliable than the VAS, especially with less educated patients (Ferraz et al., 1990). With very sick patients and patients with limited literacy skills, oral versions of the NRS are easily administered. Guidelines for pain assessment increasingly recommend the NRS given its ease of use with the largest proportion of patients.

Pain Questionnaires

Several pain measurement instruments incorporate most of the relevant questions and can help to standardize pain assessment. These instruments are short enough to be considered for routine clinical use with cancer patients but have established reliability and validity for research purposes as well. The Brief Pain Inventory (BPI; Cleeland, 1989) was designed to assess pain in patients with cancer (see Appendix 19.1). Using the 0- to 10-point NRS, the BPI asks patients to rate the severity of their pain at its "worst," "least," "average," and "now." Using an

NRS, with 0 being "no interference" and 10 being "interferes completely," the BPI asks patients to rate how much pain interferes with mood, walking, general activity, work, relations with others, sleep, and enjoyment of life. It also asks patients to indicate the location of their pain on a pain drawing, and asks about treatments for pain and the extent of pain relief. In a somewhat longer form, the BPI provides a list of descriptors to help the patient describe pain quality. The short form of the BPI is widely used for frequent pain monitoring in clinical settings and in clinical trials.

The Short-Form McGill Pain Questionnaire (SF-MPQ; Melzack, 1987) has been developed for assessments using verbal descriptors. The main component of the SF-MPQ consists of 15 descriptors (11 sensory, 4 affective) rated on an intensity scale as 0 = "none," 1 = "mild," 2 = "moderate," or 3 = "severe." Three pain scores are derived from the sum of the intensity ratings of the Sensory, Affective, and Total descriptors. The SF-MPQ also includes the Present Pain Intensity (PPI) index of the standard MPQ and a VAS. An innovative touch screen, electronic version of the SF-MPQ also is available (Cook et al., 2004). VASs have been adapted for repeated clinical use in the Memorial Pain Assessment Card (MPAC; Fishman et al., 1987). The MPAC consists of three VASs for Pain Intensity, Pain Relief, and Mood, and one VDS. The MPAC and SF-MPQ are valuable scales, but they do not include all of the core information we have defined as necessary for a brief but complete assessment. Missing components are the location of pain, impact, pattern, and pain history.

Patient and Family Education

Patient and family education is usually not thought of as part of the assessment process, but it is a natural corollary and consequence of adequate assessment. For patients with cancer pain, it is critical to recognize some patients' reluctance to report pain and to contact their health care providers if they do not get pain relief. Patients must be active partners in their pain assessment and treatment. They need to be made aware that many myths about addiction, rapid development of tolerance, and unmanageable side effects associated with opioid analgesics do not apply to the majority of patients with cancer. They have to be assured that, in most instances, pain relief can be obtained, and that it is part of the health care professional's role to provide that relief.

Assessment is the first step in education. Patients learn how to report pain, and how their information is essential to determining proper treatment. They see that the outcome of assessment is improved treatment, and this facilitates ongoing communication with their health care providers. Assessment, along with educating patients about cancer pain, improves the outcome of pain treatment. Several randomized clinical trials with cancer patients experiencing pain have found that brief education on pain management produces significant reductions in pain intensity ratings (Allard, Maunsell, Labbe, & Dorval, 2001; de Wit et al., 1997; Syrjala et al., 2008).

PAIN ASSESSMENT METHODS

Working within the typical limitations of a cancer treatment setting, pain assessment needs to be focused on those aspects of pain that lead to differential treatment decisions. Rarely will there be the professional time or patient acceptance, or endurance to complete the type of assessment typically done in multidisciplinary pain clinics. It may be helpful to think of cancer pain assessment in a decision analysis model. Some branches of the decision tree need not be followed if appropriate screening does not indicate a treatment need. I have broken the assessment procedure down into three steps. Although I consider a comprehensive assessment to include screening at all steps, I have assigned Step 1 the highest priority.

Step 1: Assessing Pain Severity

Standard assessment of the multidimensional aspects of cancer pain makes it clear that pain severity is the primary factor determining the impact of pain on the patient and the urgency of the treatment process. Many adults, both with and without cancer, function quite effectively with a background level of pain that does not seriously impair them. As pain severity increases, however, it passes a threshold beyond which it cannot be ignored and becomes disruptive to many aspects of the patient's life (Serlin, Mendoza, Nakamura, Edwards, & Cleeland, 1995). Figure 19.1 presents the method for assessment of pain severity.

Simple pain scales make it possible to assess pain on each outpatient contact and at least once in every 24-hour period a patient is in the hospital (or more frequently, if pain is severe). The model presented should be thought of as being repeated until optimal pain control is achieved. The Step 1 diagram defines "mild," "moderate," and "severe" pain as ranges of patient response to a numerical rating of pain at its "worst" or "usual." These categories of pain severity are based on the degree of interference with function associated with each category (Serlin et al., 1995).

Mild pain (1–4, "worst" pain; 1–3, "usual" pain) that previously has been untreated may call for a "mild" analgesic (acetaminophen or a nonsteroidal anti-inflammatory), or "moderate" analgesic such as hydrocodone (Benedetti et al., 2000). This is the optimal time for education about the need to report pain when it occurs, when it gets worse, or if it is not relieved by current treatment. A mild pain level requires the least assessment, since it causes the least interference with function. However, the clinician must evaluate the nature of the pain problem. In clinical practice, it is valuable also to assess the impact of pain when the level is 3 or 4, since a small proportion of patients underrepresent their pain levels. Also, if the pain etiology and syndrome are understood, the clinician can determine whether the pain is likely to be progressive or subject to frequent exacerbations.

Moderate pain (5–6, "worst" pain; 4–6, "usual" pain) mandates Steps 2 and 3 of the assessment process and calls for a more aggressive analgesic program. Since pain at this level impairs multiple areas of function, a follow-up contact should be made within 72 hours to assess the efficacy of the pain treatment provided. For patients at home, this requires a phone call.

When pain is *severe* (7–10, "worst" or "usual" pain) the steps are similar to those for moderate pain, except that the analgesic selection and titration need to be aggressive, and follow-up contact (reassessment) needs to occur more quickly, within 24 hours after the initial assessment is made. In some cases, pain at this level constitutes a pain emergency and mandates hospital admission for more rapid medical workup and intravenous (IV) analgesic titration.

Step 2: Assessing Pain Characteristics

Information about aspects of cancer pain other than its severity helps to refine treatment plans. Much of this information can also be gathered through standard questionnaires that guide the patient's subjective

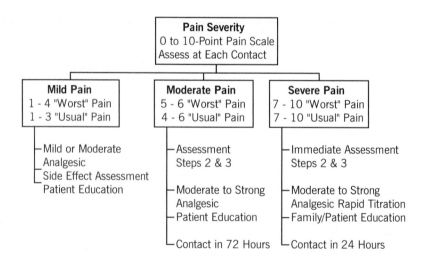

FIGURE 19.1. Step 1: Assessment of cancer pain severity.

reports of these additional characteristics. Further information needs to be obtained by clinical interview. The essential elements of Step 2 are presented in Figure 19.2.

Pain Location

Aiding patients in describing the location(s) of the pain they are experiencing is an essential part of pain assessment. This is most easily accomplished by asking the patient to mark on a body drawing the location of pain. The patient is given a front and back view of a human figure and asked to shade in areas of pain. This can provide a wealth of information about possible physical mechanisms contributing to the pain. It may also help to determine why pain is more of a problem with particular movements or positions. For example, patients may draw the pain in the distribution of a particular nerve, suggesting that the mechanism of pain is tumor impingement on that nerve.

Temporal Pattern of the Pain

Not all cancer pain remains at a constant level over a 24-hour period. While most pain is felt constantly, with periodic increases, some pain occurs only episodically. Some patients have significant *incident pain*, exacerbation of their pain with movement, which is common when the pathological process responsible for the pain is influenced by movement or position. Some types of pain (especially neuropathic pain) may have periods when pain spontaneously becomes more intense. These periodic increases in pain are often referred to as *breakthrough*

pain, defined as a transitory increase in pain occurring in the context of stable baseline pain (Portenoy, Payne, & Jacobsen, 1999). It is standard practice to include additional analgesia for the patient to take during breakthrough or incident episodes, or even before episodes, if it is possible to anticipate when they will occur. For some patients, however, the presence of breakthrough pain consistently prior to the next around-the-clock dose of medication may indicate only that the dose or potency of the analgesic is inadequate (Petzke, Radbruch, Zech, Loick, & Grond, 1999; Portenoy et al., 1999).

The temporal pattern of pain often is clearly described by the patient in an interview. If patients are unsure of the pattern or timing of increased pain, it may be necessary to have them rate their pain, along with medication use, in a log book or diary for a 1- to 7-day period to determine its pattern.

Pain Quality

Pain of different etiologies produces differences in the patient's subjective experience of the pain. For example, pain caused by destruction of nerve pathways may be described as "numb," "pins and needles," "burning," or "shooting." Pain from tumor destruction of soft tissue or bone is often described as "aching." Some pain problems can be mixed and include multiple characteristics (Dy et al., 2008; Urch & Dickenson, 2008). Establishing the qualities of a pain is an essential part of determining the physical basis of the pain, which will, in turn, determine the types of therapies to be used (Laird, Colvin, & Fallon, 2008). People often find it difficult

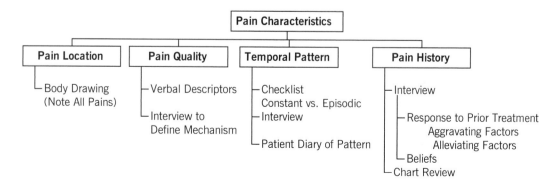

FIGURE 19.2. Step 2: Assessment of cancer pain characteristics.

to describe their pain spontaneously. Word lists of potential descriptors help the patient portray pain quality. Some questionnaires, such as the long forms of the BPI and the SF-MPQ, include lists of words for the patient to select.

Pain History

The patient's response to prior pain treatment is an additional variable that needs to be considered. When assessing response to prior analgesic treatments, patients' adherence to their prescribed analgesic medications must be determined, along with beliefs that might dictate future adherence. A recent study of outpatients with cancer-related pain found that patients adhered to their opioid therapy only 62–72% of the time (Du Pen et al., 1999). Nonadherence was significantly correlated with higher levels of symptom distress and lower quality-of-life scores. In interviews examining why patients did not take analgesics prescribed, side effects were the most common reasons, but other beliefs, such as addiction fear, also influenced patient choices (Ersek et al., 1999). Thus, it is important to determine whether a patient has taken or plans to take analgesic medications as prescribed, and if not, why. Careful assessment of the reasons for nonadherence can identify targets for patient education.

Treatments tried and other factors that alleviate or aggravate pain can help to determine both pain etiology and the next treatment steps. Pain that is severe and changing rapidly may require immediate laboratory and imaging studies to diagnose fracture, infection, obstruction, epidural metastases, or other medical emergencies. Patients whose pain does not respond to oral medications or those with unacceptable side effects may require alternative routes of analgesic administration (epidural, intrathecal, subcutaneous). Such patients obviously require greater clinical assessment. Prognosis, concurrent symptoms, ongoing disease treatment, and organ system complications may influence pain treatment choices. For example, if pain has a predictable course as a result of cancer therapy, then treatment methods may anticipate that course (e.g., use of IV patient-controlled analgesia with an opioid at the start of mucositis pain).

Step 3: Assessing Pain Impact

Step 3 of pain assessment (see Figure 19.3) measures the degree to which pain interferes with areas of the patient's life, and the degree to which other symptoms or problems interact with pain to disrupt the patient's pain relief or functioning. The suggested assessment steps are again tailored to elicit information that will lead to specific treatment recommendations. Whenever pain is moderate to severe, or concurrent with other symptoms, an effective intervention for pain control should be based on evaluation of more than pain severity and pain mechanism. As examples, if a patient suffers from uncontrolled nausea, an oral opioid may exacerbate nausea. The patient, therefore, may require an antiemetic a half-hour before the opioid or, alternatively, the patient may need a nonoral route of administration. If a patient has relatively good pain control but only if lying down, then treatment may

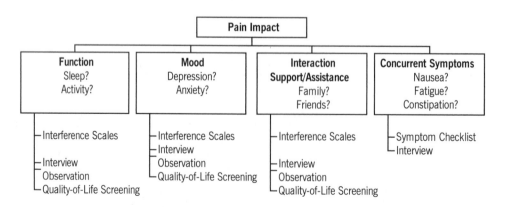

FIGURE 19.3. Step 3: Assessment of cancer pain impact.

be inadequate. A review of only pain severity and mechanism might inappropriately indicate that adequate treatment has been prescribed. As these examples demonstrate, Step 3 assessments for chronic cancer pain can provide valuable information even when pain, on initial screening, appears mild.

Assessing Quality of Life

The measurement of quality of life (QoL) for patients with cancer has received much research attention during the past two decades and is part of the context in which cancer pain must be understood. *Health-related QoL* has been defined as the perceived value of life as modified by impairments, functional states, perceptions, and social opportunities influenced by disease, injury, treatment, or policy (Patrick, 1992). Extensive work has been done to define and test measures of QoL related to cancer (Cella & Tulsky, 1993; Moinpour, Donaldson, & Redman, 2007). Although it is beyond the scope of this chapter to review the entire field of instruments available to measure QoL, several measures have been selected for review. The measures described below include evaluation of physical functioning, psychological status, social relationships, and in most cases, symptoms. These domains coincide with those listed under Step 3 of the pain assessment model: functioning, mood, social interaction, and concurrent symptoms.

The European Organization for Research and Treatment of Cancer–Quality of Life Questionnaire (EORTC-QLQ) has 28 items plus two global QoL items (Aaronson et al., 1993). Disease or problem-specific modules (e.g., lung cancer supplement) can be added to the scale (Bergman, Aaronson, Ahmedzai, Kaasa, & Sullivan, 1994). The core questionnaire includes Functional and Symptom subscales, an overall QoL assessment, and a question about financial concerns. The EORTC-QLQ has good psychometric properties and has been used successfully in clinical trials with cancer patients (Aaronson et al., 1993).

The Functional Assessment of Cancer Therapy (FACT) measurement system is a comprehensive group of scales that measure health-related QoL in patients with cancer or other chronic illnesses (Cella et al., 1993). The 34-item General Version (FACT-G) contains five subscales that assess Physical Well-Being, Functional Well-Being, Social/Family Well-Being, Emotional Well-Being, and the Patient's Relationship with the Physician. Additional subscales are added to the FACT-G to address issues specific to a disease site, treatment, or symptom. The FACT-G instrument and the multiple available subscales demonstrate good reliability and validity (Cella et al., 1993).

Several psychometrically sound QoL instruments were developed from the Medical Outcomes Study (MOS). Two broad QoL tools are the Short Form–36 (SF-36) Health Survey and the Short Form–12 (SF-12) Health Survey (Ware, Kosinski, & Keller, 1996; Ware & Sherbourne, 1992). These instruments include sections assessing Physical Functioning, Role Functioning, Social Functioning, Mental Health, Health Perceptions, and Pain. The SF-36 is reliable, valid and has been tested in widely diverse populations (Stewart, Hays, & Ware, 1988). Similarly, the SF-12 demonstrates sound psychometric properties, although the subscale scores may be less reliable due to the limited number of items.

Any of these QoL measures will provide a good screening tool and indicate any further need to assess mood, concurrent symptoms, social support, or function. A QoL scale can be combined with the BPI and a symptom assessment instrument to evaluate patients with moderate to severe pain. In the areas of psychological functioning and concurrent symptoms, one of the QoL scales alone is unlikely to sufficiently determine treatment needs, but it should be adequate to identify the need for further follow-up.

Function

The self-report measures described here—BPI, FACT, EORTC-QLQ, and SF-36 or SF-12—are designed to assess function. The BPI measures function related to pain, while the other measures do not assign a source for interference with function, measuring instead the level of activity a patient is able to perform. Both aspects of function may be relevant if a patient is ambulatory and likely to be living with pain for some time.

Observation measures within the field of cancer have historically focused on global measures of functioning. The most well-known of these is the Karnofsky Performance Status (Karnofsky, 1950), but other, similar 5- or 10-point global assessments are available, such as the ECOG Performance Status Scale (Oken et al., 1982). These scales have good interrater reliabilities but are not useful for specifying difficulties or determining treatment needs. Their primary value seems to be as outcome measures for clinical trials. Observer ratings are also available for more specific activities of daily living, behaviors related to coping with pain, and well-behaviors (Chapko, Syrjala, Bush, Jedlow, & Yanke, 1991; Wilkie, Keefe, Dodd, & Copp, 1992). I suggest observer ratings only in cases where patients are unable to provide their own self-report, or in combination with self-report.

Mood

The majority of cancer patients adjust to the stresses of the disease and its symptoms without diagnosable anxiety, depression, or other psychiatric disorders (Derogatis et al., 1983; Raison & Miller, 2003). However, patients with pain report significantly more depression, anxiety, and emotional distress than those without pain (Glover, Dibble, Dodd, & Miaskowski, 1995; Heim & Oei, 1993; Zaza & Baine, 2002). Among the many symptoms possible during the course of cancer, mood disorders can be among the most difficult to identify. Difficulty in recognizing mood disruptions results from the similarity of presentation of some mood symptoms and common disease-related somatic complaints, such as fatigue and weight loss. In my experience, assessment of mood in patients with cancer-related pain requires a focus on the affective components of mood disturbance, with somewhat more cautious evaluation of cognitive, behavioral, and somatic components. An assessment of mood is cursorily accomplished with the QoL measures or the BPI. If these measures suggest that mood disturbance exists, I recommend further assessment of mood, using either one of the many available standardized tools or a clinical interview.

Social Interaction

Social relationships are acknowledged to be very important to the functioning and well-being of patients with cancer (Moinpour et al., 2007; Syrjala, Stover, Yi, Artherholt, & Abrams, 2010). Nonetheless, social support

has been one of the most difficult areas for investigators to measure. In my experience, cancer patients tend to rate their supports very positively, resulting in a ceiling effect for measurement. QoL instruments or the BPI provides an initial screen of social support or pain interference with social interaction. A clinician assessing a patient with moderate to severe pain will also want to consider the availability of a family caregiver to assist the patient with prescribed treatments and to provide help if needed. Knowing the availability of assistance and support, as well as family members' beliefs related to pain treatment, can be as important as the assessment of the patient.

Concurrent Symptoms

Patients with cancer-related pain are liable to have other symptoms that need management and complicate the treatment picture. The negative side effects of analgesic drugs are numerous, especially if aggressive side effect prophylaxis and management are not included in treatment plans. The most common negative side effects of analgesic treatment include constipation, nausea, fatigue, and sedation. Cancer, especially if it advances, produces fatigue, weakness, cachexia, and, often, cognitive deficits. Disease treatment may produce fatigue, along with nausea and sleep disturbance. Many symptoms can be treated either pharmacologically or behaviorally. At a minimum, a checklist of potential concurrent symptoms, such as the M. D. Anderson Symptom Inventory (Cleeland, Mendoza, et al., 2000; see Appendix 19.2), the Edmonton Symptom Assessment Scale (Bruera et al., 1991), or the Memorial Symptom Assessment Scale (Portenoy et al., 1994), needs to be included at this step of assessment. As with pain, it is important to evaluate these symptoms over time to monitor changes in severity and response to treatment.

Interview Assessment of Pain Impact

The physical examination is a cornerstone of pain assessment. As part of this examination, a clinician can gather information on physical, emotional, and social functioning from an interview format. The advantage of an interview is that some patients will feel more understood or perceive fewer burdens with this format. Suicidal ideation is a risk for patients with severe uncontrolled pain and can best be assessed in an interview. The interview also can be used to screen for beliefs that disrupt treatment and a history of drug or alcohol abuse. Individuals with active or past substance abuse should not be denied appropriate treatment for their pain, and experience indicates that their pain can be managed successfully using appropriate medications and methods (Passik & Webster, 2008). The purpose of screening is to identify patients who may need additional psychosocial assessment and treatment, as well as monitoring of their medication use.

PAIN ASSESSMENT IN CHILDREN WITH CANCER

In most clinical settings, pain assessment in children with cancer is even more neglected than that in adults with cancer (Linton & Feudtner, 2008; Ljungman et al., 1996). Assessment is often more difficult, because it has to be tailored to the developmental stage of the child. The World Health Organization (1998) has developed guidelines for the assessment and treatment of cancer-related pain in children. These guidelines recommend regular assessment and documentation of the child's pain level as an essential vital sign. As with adults, treatment recommendations are based on the child's pain level.

The assessment of pain in infants often relies on physiological measures and observer reports of behaviors that indicate probable pain (Duhn & Medves, 2004; Stevens, 2007). Developmentally appropriate pain intensity measures also can be used with toddlers and preschool children. A variety of pain intensity measures are available for young children, including the Faces Pain Scale (Hicks, von Baeyer, Spafford, van Korlaar, & Goodenough, 2001) and a novel Poker Chip Tool (Hester, Foster, & Kristensen, 1990). Children over the age of 8 also can be given standard NRSs and VASs, although NRSs have not been validated for children (McGrath et al., 2008).

The child's self-report of pain should be considered the "gold standard" of pediatric pain assessment and be used whenever possible. However, behavioral observations are critical in pain assessment of very young children and children who do not have the ability to report their pain due to disability or disease. A number of reliable, valid behavioral observation methods have been developed for the assessment of pediatric behaviors related to pain, such as crying, clinging, and reduction in normal activity (Merkel, Voepel-Lewis, Shayevitz, & Malviya, 1997; Tarbell, Cohen, & Marsh, 1992; Voepel-Lewis et al., 2008; von Baeyer & Spagrud, 2007).

The three steps of assessment outlined in this chapter should work equally well for children, with the provisions recommended by the World Health Organization (1998) guidelines. In addition, a special panel of the American Academy of Pediatrics has suggested that a Pain Problem List be formulated for every child with cancer (McGrath et al., 1990). The goal of this list is to identify problems amenable to treatment, and to be sure that the multiple sources and dimensions of pain are addressed.

PAIN ASSESSMENT IN OLDER ADULT PATIENTS WITH CANCER

Sixty percent of all cancers occur in persons age 65 years and older (Yancik & Ries, 2000). Because the prevalence of cancer increases with age, many older adult individuals have to deal with this life-threatening illness and its related symptoms. Several recent studies have found that older adult patients are at risk for undertreatment of cancer-related pain. In a survey of outpatients with metastatic cancer who were experiencing pain, Cleeland and colleagues (1996) found that patients 70 years of age and older were more likely than younger patients to receive inadequate analgesics. Similarly, a survey of over 13,000 nursing home residents with cancer found that 26% of patients experiencing daily pain received no analgesics (Bernabei et al., 1998).

The undertreatment of cancer pain in older adults is often due to inadequate assessment (Balducci, 2003). In the nursing home study by Bernabei and colleagues (1998), regular pain assessments were not included in most patient charts. However, 86% of the patients, including cognitively impaired individuals, were able verbally to report pain to the research staff. Similarly, Ferrell, Ferrell, and Rivera (1995) found that 83% of older adult patients in a nursing home setting could complete at least one pain intensity scale.

The three steps of assessment outlined in this chapter apply to older adults, as well as to younger patients. However, many older patients require careful instruction and practice in the use of pain assessment instruments (Horgas & Elliott, 2004). Prior to assessing pain, all older adult patients should be screened to identify any sensory, motor, and/or cognitive deficits that affect their ability to report pain and related symptoms (Herr & Mobily, 1991). The Faces Pain Scale can be used for individuals who have difficulty understanding NRS or VAS formats (Herr, Mobily, Kohout, & Wagenaar, 1998). Pain assessment instruments also can be administered in an oral format for patients who have visual or motor impairments that prevent completion of paper-and-pencil measures. When cognitive deficits are severe and prevent self-report of pain, observation of pain-related behaviors is an alternative strategy. Several observation systems to assess pain behaviors in older adult patients have been developed (Fuchs-Lacelle, Hadjistavropoulos, & Lix, 2008; Horgas, Elliott, & Marsiske, 2009; Husebo et al., 2007; Kaasalainen, 2007).

In summary, the measurement of pain in older cancer patients involves special considerations and challenges that researchers and clinicians are beginning to address. The substantial growth of the older adult population mandates continued work in this area.

OTHER APPLICATIONS OF PAIN MEASUREMENT

Cancer pain measurement forms the basis of several applications in addition to clinical assessment, including efforts to ensure the quality of pain management and clinical trials to examine the effectiveness of cancer pain treatments. A brief review of these areas illustrates the application of pain assessment techniques.

Pain Measurement for Quality Assurance

Patients with cancer should be guaranteed the best possible pain management; therefore, poorly treated pain is a quality assurance issue. The development of specific practice guidelines for pain management has led to quality assurance standards for pain treatment (American Pain Society, 1999; Benedetti et al., 2000; Gordon et al., 2005; Jacox et al., 1994). In addition, the Joint Committee on Accreditation of Healthcare Organizations has developed standards for the assessment and management of pain. Hospitals and other health care facilities are expected to demonstrate compliance with these standards when they are reviewed for accreditation. The standards include the regular assessment and recording of patients' pain levels. Pain assessment tools provide a method for routine monitoring and charting of pain in the hospital or clinic setting.

Clinical Trials Applications

A major barrier to treatment of cancer pain has been a lack of rigorous clinical trials in cancer pain management. Controlled clinical trials are necessary to evaluate the effectiveness of analgesics, nonpharmacological interventions for pain control, and treatments involving multiple methods. In addition, variability in outcome measures across clinical trials has impeded the evaluation of treatment efficacy. The Initiative on Methods, Measurement, and Pain Assessment in Clinical Trials (IMMPACT) has recommended that six core outcome domains be considered when designing clinical trials for treatment of cancer or noncancer pain (Turk et al., 2003). These core outcome domains are pain, physical functioning, emotional functioning, participant ratings of improvement and satisfaction with treatment, symptoms and adverse events, and participant disposition. With regard to pain assessment, a review of cancer pain assessment in clinical trials concluded that detailed information on pain assessment procedures is often lacking (Caraceni, Brunelli, Martini, Zecca, & De, 2005). Recommendations for clinical trial reports included precise descriptions of the pain measurement instrument and assessment procedures, including the time frame for assessment, frequency, and mode of administration.

CONCLUSION

Although most patients with cancer-related pain should be able to get pain relief, many are poorly managed. Inadequate pain assessment is most often the reason. In the typical cancer care setting, health care professionals rarely have training in pain assessment, nor do they have time for the assessment that is typical in multidisciplinary pain clinics. Patients may be too ill to endure lengthy assessment procedures, or they may not complain about their pain. Recognizing these constraints, I have presented three steps of assessment. Components at each step are designed to lead to treatment decisions. Where possible, the assessment is structured around questionnaires designed for the patient with cancer. These questionnaires minimize patient and health professional biases and time, while standardizing the assessment process. Steps 2 and 3 of the assessment only need to be followed if pain intensity is 4 or above on a 0- to 10-point scale, or if screening suggests a potential treatment need.

In clinical practice, an assessment based on questionnaires needs to be supplemented by interview of the patient with, if possible, the primary family caregiver, as well as observation and medical examination. Proper assessment based on subjective report needs the full cooperation of the patient, yet cancer patients may be reluctant to complain of pain or other symptoms. To be full partners in their pain assessment and treatment, patients need education about their rights to symptom relief and the availability of effective treatment, and exploration of barriers that may inhibit assessment or treatment.

Cancer pain is dynamic and ever changing. Although pain sometimes improves with tumor regression, cancer remission, or conclusion of treatment, pain may become progressively worse, requiring more aggressive use of pain therapy. Once a patient develops pain, assessment needs to be repeated regularly. The steps presented in the model have additional applications outside of clinical assessment and can be used effectively in quality assurance and in clinical trials examining the effectiveness of pain treatments.

ACKNOWLEDGMENT

This work was supported by American Cancer Society Grant No. RSGT-05-219-01-CPPB.

REFERENCE

Aaronson, N. K., Ahmedzai, S., Bergman, B., Bullinger, M., Cull, A., Duez, N. J., et al. (1993). The European Organization for Research and Treatment of Cancer QLQ-C30: A quality-of-life instrument for use in international clinical trials in oncology. *Journal of the National Cancer Institute*, 85, 365–376.

Allard, P., Maunsell, E., Labbe, J., & Dorval, M. (2001). Educational interventions to improve cancer pain control: A systematic review. *Journal of Palliative Medicine*, 4, 191–203.

American Pain Society. (1999). *Principles of analgesic use in the treatment of acute pain and cancer pain*. Glenview, IL: Author.

Anderson, K. O., Mendoza, T. R., Valero, V., Richman, S. P., Russell, C., Hurley, J., et al. (2000). Minority cancer patients and their providers: Pain management attitudes and practice. *Cancer*, 88, 1929–1938.

Anderson, K. O., Richman, S. P., Hurley, J., Palos, G., Valero, V., Mendoza, T. R., et al. (2002). Cancer pain management among underserved minority outpatients: Perceived needs and barriers to optimal control. *Cancer*, 94, 2295–2304.

Andrykowski, M. A., Curran, S. L., Carpenter, J. S., Studts, J. L., Cunningham, L., & McGrath, P. C., et al. (1999). Rheumatoid symptoms following breast cancer treatment: A controlled comparison. *Journal of Pain and Symptom Management*, 18, 85–94.

Balducci, L. (2003). Management of cancer pain in geriatric patients. *Journal of Supportive Oncology*, 1, 175–191.

Banning, A., Sjogren, P., & Henriksen, H. (1991). Pain causes in 200 patients referred to a multidisciplinary cancer pain clinic. *Pain*, 45, 45–48.

Benedetti, C., Brock, C., Cleeland, C., Coyle, N., Dube, J. E., Ferrell, B., et al. (2000). NCCN Practice Guidelines for Cancer Pain. *Oncology (Williston Park)*, 14, 135–150.

Bergman, B., Aaronson, N. K., Ahmedzai, S., Kaasa, S., & Sullivan, M. (1994). The EORTC QLQ-LC13: A modular supplement to the EORTC Core Quality of Life Questionnaire (QLQ-C30) for use in lung cancer clinical trials: EORTC Study Group on Quality of Life. *European Journal of Cancer*, 30A, 635–642.

Bernabei, R., Gambassi, G., Lapane, K., Landi, F., Gatsonis, C., Dunlop, R., et al. (1998). Management of pain in elderly patients with cancer: SAGE Study Group: Systematic Assessment of Geriatric Drug Use via Epidemiology. *Journal of the American Medical Association*, 279, 1877–1882.

Bruera, E., Kuehn, N., Miller, M. J., Selmser, P., & Macmillan, K. (1991). The Edmonton

Symptom Assessment System (ESAS): A simple method for the assessment of palliative care patients. *Journal of Palliative Care, 7,* 6–9.

Burton, A. W., Fanciullo, G. J., Beasley, R. D., & Fisch, M. J. (2007). Chronic pain in the cancer survivor: A new frontier. *Pain Medicine, 8,* 189–198.

Caraceni, A., Brunelli, C., Martini, C., Zecca, E., & De, C. F. (2005). Cancer pain assessment in clinical trials: A review of the literature (1999–2002). *Journal of Pain and Symptom Management, 29,* 507–519.

Caraceni, A., & Portenoy, R. K. (1999). An international survey of cancer pain characteristics and syndromes: IASP Task Force on Cancer Pain: International Association for the Study of Pain. *Pain, 82,* 263–274.

Castel, L. D., Saville, B. R., Depuy, V., Godley, P. A., Hartmann, K. E., & Abernethy, A. P. (2008). Racial differences in pain during 1 year among women with metastatic breast cancer: A hazards analysis of interval-censored data. *Cancer, 112,* 162–170.

Cella, D. F., & Tulsky, D. S. (1993). Quality of life in cancer: Definition, purpose, and method of measurement. *Cancer Investigations, 11,* 327–336.

Cella, D. F., Tulsky, D. S., Gray, G., Sarafian, B., Linn, E., Bonomi, A., et al. (1993). The Functional Assessment of Cancer Therapy Scale: Development and validation of the general measure. *Journal of Clinical Oncology, 11,* 570–579.

Chang, V. T., Janjan, N., Jain, S., & Chau, C. (2006a). Regional cancer pain syndromes. *Journal of Palliative Medicine, 9,* 1435–1453.

Chang, V. T., Janjan, N., Jain, S., & Chau, C. (2006b). Update in cancer pain syndromes. *Journal of Palliative Medicine, 9,* 1414–1434.

Chapko, M. K., Syrjala, K. L., Bush, N., Jedlow, C., & Yanke, M. R. (1991). Development of a behavioral measure of mouth pain, nausea, and wellness for patients receiving radiation and chemotherapy. *Journal of Pain and Symptom Management, 6,* 15–23.

Cleeland, C. S. (1989). Measurement of pain by subjective report. In C. R. Chapman & J. D. Loeser (Eds.), *Issues in pain measurement* (pp. 391–403). New York: Raven Press.

Cleeland, C. S. (1990a). Assessment of pain in cancer: Measurement issues. In K. M. Foley (Ed.), *Advances in pain research and therapy* (pp. 47–55). New York: Raven Press.

Cleeland, C. S. (1990b). Pain assessment. In S. Lipton (Ed.), *Issues in pain management* (pp. 287–291). New York: Raven Press.

Cleeland, C. S., Gonin, R., Baez, L., Loehrer, P., & Pandya, K. J. (1997). Pain and treatment of pain in minority patients with cancer: The Eastern Cooperative Oncology Group Minor-

ity Outpatient Pain Study. *Annals of Internal Medicine, 127,* 813–816.

Cleeland, C. S., Gonin, R., Hatfield, A. K., Edmonson, J. H., Blum, R. H., Stewart, J. A., et al. (1994). Pain and its treatment in outpatients with metastatic cancer. *New England Journal of Medicine, 330,* 592–596.

Cleeland, C. S., Janjan, N. A., Scott, C. B., Seiferheld, W. F., & Curran, W. J. (2000). Cancer pain management by radiotherapists: A survey of radiation therapy oncology group physicians. *International Journal of Radiation Oncology–Biology–Physics, 47,* 203–208.

Cleeland, C. S., Mendoza, T. R., Wang, X. S., Chou, C., Harle, M. T., Morrissey, M., et al. (2000). Assessing symptom distress in cancer patients: The M. D. Anderson Symptom Inventory. *Cancer, 89,* 1634–1646.

Cook, A. J., Roberts, D. A., Henderson, M. D., Van Winkle, L. C., Chastain, D. C., & Hamill-Ruth, R. J. (2004). Electronic pain questionnaires: A randomized, crossover comparison with paper questionnaires for chronic pain assessment. *Pain, 110,* 310–317.

Deandrea, S., Montanari, M., Moja, L., & Apolone, G. (2008). Prevalence of undertreatment in cancer pain: A review of published literature. *Annals of Oncology, 19,* 1985–1991.

De Conno, F., Caraceni, A., Gamba, A., Mariani, L., Abbattista, A., Brunelli, C., et al. (1994). Pain measurement in cancer patients: A comparison of six methods. *Pain, 57,* 161–166.

Derogatis, L. R., Morrow, G. R., Fetting, J., Penman, D., Piasetsky, S., Schmale, A. M., et al. (1983). The prevalence of psychiatric disorders among cancer patients. *Journal of the American Medical Association, 249,* 751–757.

de Wit, R., van Dam, F., Zandbelt, L., van Burren, A., van der Heijden, K., Leenhouts, G., et al. (1997). A pain education program for chronic cancer pain patients: Follow-up results from a randomized controlled trial. *Pain, 73,* 55–69.

Duhn, L. J., & Medves, J. M. (2004). A systematic integrative review of infant pain assessment tools. *Advances in Neonatal Care, 4,* 126–140.

Du Pen, S. L., Du Pen, A. R., Polissar, N., Hansberry, J., Kraybill, B. M., Stillman, M., et al. (1999). Implementing guidelines for cancer pain management: Results of a randomized controlled clinical trial. *Journal of Clinical Oncology, 17,* 361–370.

Dy, S. M., Asch, S. M., Naeim, A., Sanati, H., Walling, A., & Lorenz, K. A. (2008). Evidence-based standards for cancer pain management. *Journal of Clinical Oncology, 26,* 3879–3885.

Ersek, M., Kraybill, B. M., & Pen, A. D. (1999). Factors hindering patients' use of medications for cancer pain. *Cancer Practice, 7,* 226–232.

Ferraz, M. B., Quaresma, M. R., Aquino, L. R., Atra, E., Tugwell, P., & Goldsmith, C. H. (1990). Reliability of pain scales in the assessment of literate and illiterate patients with rheumatoid arthritis. *Journal of Rheumatology, 17*, 1022–1024.

Ferrell, B. A., Ferrell, B. R., & Rivera, L. (1995). Pain in cognitively impaired nursing home patients. *Journal of Pain and Symptom Management, 10*, 591–598.

Fishman, B., Pasternak, S., Wallenstein, S. L., Houde, R. W., Holland, J. C., & Foley, K. M. (1987). The Memorial Pain Assessment Card: A valid instrument for the evaluation of cancer pain. *Cancer, 60*, 1151–1158.

Foley, K. M. (2005). Advances in cancer pain management in 2005. *Gynecological Oncology, 99*, S126.

Fuchs-Lacelle, S., Hadjistavropoulos, T., & Lix, L. (2008). Pain assessment as intervention: A study of older adults with severe dementia. *Clinical Journal of Pain, 24*, 697–707.

Glover, J., Dibble, S. L., Dodd, M. J., & Miaskowski, C. (1995). Mood states of oncology outpatients: Does pain make a difference? *Journal of Pain and Symptom Management, 10*, 120–128.

Gonzales, G. R., Elliott, K. J., Portenoy, R. K., & Foley, K. M. (1991). The impact of a comprehensive evaluation in the management of cancer pain. *Pain, 47*, 141–144.

Gordon, D. B., Dahl, J. L., Miaskowski, C., McCarberg, B., Todd, K. H., Paice, J. A., et al. (2005). American Pain Society recommendations for improving the quality of acute and cancer pain management: American Pain Society Quality of Care Task Force. *Archives of Internal Medicine, 165*, 1574–1580.

Green, C. R., Anderson, K. O., Baker, T. A., Campbell, L. C., Decker, S., Fillingim, R. B., et al. (2003). The unequal burden of pain: Confronting racial and ethnic disparities in pain. *Pain Medicine, 4*, 277–294.

Green, C. R., Baker, T. A., Sato, Y., Washington, T. L., & Smith, E. M. (2003). Race and chronic pain: A comparative study of young black and white Americans presenting for management. *Journal of Pain, 4*, 176–183.

Grond, S., Radbruch, L., Meuser, T., Sabatowski, R., Loick, G., & Lehmann, K. A. (1999). Assessment and treatment of neuropathic cancer pain following WHO guidelines. *Pain, 79*, 15–20.

Grond, S., Zech, D., Diefenbach, C., Radbruch, L., & Lehmann, K. A. (1996). Assessment of cancer pain: A prospective evaluation in 2266 cancer patients referred to a pain service. *Pain, 64*, 107–114.

Grond, S., Zech, D., Lynch, J., Diefenbach, C., Schug, S. A., & Lehmann, K. A. (1993). Validation of World Health Organization guidelines for pain relief in head and neck cancer: A prospective study. *Annals of Otology, Rhinology and Laryngology, 102*, 342–348.

Heim, H. M., & Oei, T. P. (1993). Comparison of prostate cancer patients with and without pain. *Pain, 53*, 159–162.

Herr, K. A., & Mobily, P. R. (1991). Complexities of pain assessment in the elderly: Clinical considerations. *Journal of Gerontological Nursing, 17*, 12–19.

Herr, K. A., Mobily, P. R., Kohout, F. J., & Wagenaar, D. (1998). Evaluation of the Faces Pain Scale for use with the elderly. *Clinical Journal of Pain, 14*, 29–38.

Hester, N., Foster, R., & Kristensen, K. (1990). Measurement of pain in children: Generalizability and validity of the pain ladder and poker chip tool. *Advance in Pain Research and Therapy, 15*, 79–84.

Hicks, C. L., von Baeyer, C. L., Spafford, P. A., van Korlaar, I., & Goodenough, B. (2001). The Faces Pain Scale—Revised: Toward a common metric in pediatric pain measurement. *Pain, 93*, 173–183.

Horgas, A. L., & Elliott, A. F. (2004). Pain assessment and management in persons with dementia. *Nursing Clinics of North America, 39*, 593–606.

Horgas, A. L., Elliott, A. F., & Marsiske, M. (2009). Pain assessment in persons with dementia: Relationship between self-report and behavioral observation. *Journal of the American Geriatrics Society, 57*, 126–132.

Husebo, B. S., Strand, L. I., Moe-Nilssen, R., Husebo, S. B., Snow, A. L., & Ljunggren, A. E. (2007). Mobilization–Observation–Behavior–Intensity–Dementia Pain Scale (MOBID): Development and validation of a nurse-administered pain assessment tool for use in dementia. *Journal of Pain and Symptom Management, 34*, 67–80.

Jacox, A., Carr, D. B., & Payne, R. (1994). New clinical practice guidelines for the management of pain in patients with cancer. *New England Journal of Medicine, 330*, 651–655.

Jensen, M. P. (2003). The validity and reliability of pain measures in adults with cancer. *Journal of Pain, 4*, 2–21.

Jensen, M. P., Karoly, P., & Braver, S. (1986). The measurement of clinical pain intensity: A comparison of six methods. *Pain, 27*, 117–126.

Kaasalainen, S. (2007). Pain assessment in older adults with dementia: Using behavioral observation methods in clinical practice. *Journal of Gerontological Nursing, 33*, 6–10.

Karnofsky, D. A. (1950). Nitrogen mustards in the treatment of neoplastic disease. *Advances in Internal Medicine, 4*, 1–75.

Laird, B., Colvin, L., & Fallon, M. (2008). Management of cancer pain: Basic principles and neuropathic cancer pain. *European Journal of Cancer, 44,* 1078–1082.

Lempinen, M. (1971). Carcinoma of the stomach: I. Diagnostic considerations. *Annales Chirurgiae et Gynaecologiae Fenniae, 60,* 135–140.

Linton, J. M., & Feudtner, C. (2008). What accounts for differences or disparities in pediatric palliative and end-of-life care?: A systematic review focusing on possible multilevel mechanisms. *Pediatrics, 122,* 574–582.

Ljungman, G., Kreuger, A., Gordh, T., Berg, T., Sorensen, S., & Rawal, N. (1996). Treatment of pain in pediatric oncology: A Swedish nationwide survey. *Pain, 68,* 385–394.

McGrath, P. J., Beyer, J., Cleeland, C., Eland, J., McGrath, P. A., & Portenoy, R. (1990). American Academy of Pediatrics Report of the Subcommittee on Assessment and Methodologic Issues in the Management of Pain in Childhood Cancer. *Pediatrics, 86,* 814–817.

McGrath, P. J., Walco, G. A., Turk, D. C., Dworkin, R. H., Brown, M. T., Davidson, K., et al. (2008). Core outcome domains and measures for pediatric acute and chronic/recurrent pain clinical trials: PedIMMPACT recommendations. *Journal of Pain, 9,* 771–783.

Melzack, R. (1987). The Short-Form McGill Pain Questionnaire. *Pain, 30,* 191–197.

Merkel, S. I., Voepel-Lewis, T., Shayevitz, J. R., & Malviya, S. (1997). The FLACC: A behavioral scale for scoring postoperative pain in young children. *Pediatric Nursing, 23,* 293–297.

Moinpour, C. M., Donaldson, G. W., & Redman, M. W. (2007). Do general dimensions of quality of life add clinical value to symptom data? *Journal of the National Cancer Institute Monograph, 37,* 31–38.

Oken, M. M., Creech, R. H., Tormey, D. C., Horton, J., Davis, T. E., McFadden, E. T., et al. (1982). Toxicity and response criteria of the Eastern Cooperative Oncology Group. *American Journal of Clinical Oncology, 5,* 649–655.

Passik, S. D., & Webster, L. R. (2008). Pain and addiction interface. *Pain Medicine, 9,* 631–633.

Patrick, D. L. (1992). Health-related quality of life in pharmaceutical evaluation: Forging progress and avoiding pitfalls. *Pharmacoeconomics, 1,* 76–78.

Petzke, F., Radbruch, L., Zech, D., Loick, G., & Grond, S. (1999). Temporal presentation of chronic cancer pain: Transitory pains on admission to a multidisciplinary pain clinic. *Journal of Pain and Symptom Management, 17,* 391–401.

Portenoy, R. K., & Lesage, P. (1999). Management of cancer pain. *Lancet, 353,* 1695–1700.

Portenoy, R. K., Payne, D., & Jacobsen, P. (1999). Breakthrough pain: Characteristics and impact in patients with cancer pain. *Pain, 81,* 129–134.

Portenoy, R. K., Thaler, H. T., Kornblith, A. B., Lepore, J. M., Friedlander-Klar, H., Kiyasu, E., et al. (1994). The Memorial Symptom Assessment Scale: An instrument for the evaluation of symptom prevalence, characteristics and distress. *European Journal of Cancer, 30A,* 1326–1336.

Raison, C. L., & Miller, A. H. (2003). Depression in cancer: New developments regarding diagnosis and treatment. *Biological Psychiatry, 54,* 283–294.

Reid, C. M., Gooberman-Hill, R., & Hanks, G. W. (2008). Opioid analgesics for cancer pain: Symptom control for the living or comfort for the dying?: A qualitative study to investigate the factors influencing the decision to accept morphine for pain caused by cancer. *Annals of Oncology, 19,* 44–48.

Ross, A. P., Braasch, J. W., & Warren, K. W. (1973). Carcinoma of the proximal bile ducts. *Surgical Gynecology and Obstetrics, 136,* 923–928.

Schug, S. A., Zech, D., & Dorr, U. (1990). Cancer pain management according to WHO analgesic guidelines. *Journal of Pain and Symptom Management, 5,* 27–32.

Serlin, R. C., Mendoza, T. R., Nakamura, Y., Edwards, K. R., & Cleeland, C. S. (1995). When is cancer pain mild, moderate or severe?: Grading pain severity by its interference with function. *Pain, 61,* 277–284.

Smith, W. C., Bourne, D., Squair, J., Phillips, D. O., & Chambers, W. A. (1999). A retrospective cohort study of postmastectomy pain syndrome. *Pain, 83,* 91–95.

Stevens, B. (2007). Pain assessment and management in infants with cancer. *Pediatric Blood Cancer, 49,* 1097–1101.

Stewart, A. L., Hays, R. D., & Ware, J. E., Jr. (1988). The MOS Short-Form General Health Survey: Reliability and validity in a patient population. *Medical Care, 26,* 724–735.

Syrjala, K. L., Abrams, J. R., Polissar, N. L., Hansberry, J., Robison, J., DuPen, S., et al. (2008). Patient training in cancer pain management using integrated print and video materials: A multisite randomized controlled trial. *Pain, 135,* 175–186.

Syrjala, K. L., Stover, A. C., Yi, J. C., Artherholt, S. B., & Abrams, J. R. (2010). Measuring social activities and social function in long-term cancer survivors who received hematopoietic stem cell transplantation. *Psycho-oncology, 19,* 462–471.

Tarbell, S. E., Cohen, I. T., & Marsh, J. L. (1992). The Toddler–Preschooler Postoperative Pain

Scale: An observational scale for measuring postoperative pain in children aged 1–5: Preliminary report. *Pain, 50,* 273–280.

Thomason, T. E., McCune, J. S., Bernard, S. A., Winer, E. P., Tremont, S., & Lindley, C. M. (1998). Cancer Pain Survey: Patient-centered issues in control. *Journal of Pain and Symptom Management, 15,* 275–284.

Turk, D. C., Dworkin, R. H., Allen, R. R., Bellamy, N., Brandenburg, N., Carr, D. B., et al. (2003). Core outcome domains for chronic pain clinical trials: IMMPACT recommendations. *Pain, 106,* 337–345.

Twycross, R. G. (1973). The terminal care of patients with lung cancer. *Postgraduate Medicine Journal, 49,* 732–737.

Urch, C. E., & Dickenson, A. H. (2008). Neuropathic pain in cancer. *European Journal of Cancer, 44,* 1091–1096.

Vainio, A., & Auvinen, A. (1996). Prevalence of symptoms among patients with advanced cancer: An international collaborative study: Symptom Prevalence Group. *Journal of Pain and Symptom Management, 12,* 3–10.

van den Beuken-van Everdingen, M. H., de Rijke, J. M., Kessels, A. G., Schouten, H. C., van Kleef, M., & Patijn, J. (2007). Prevalence of pain in patients with cancer: A systematic review of the past 40 years. *Annals of Oncology, 18,* 1437–1449.

Ventafridda, V., Tamburini, M., Caraceni, A., De, C. F., & Naldi, F. (1987). A validation study of the WHO method for cancer pain relief. *Cancer, 59,* 850–856.

Voepel-Lewis, T., Malviya, S., Tait, A. R., Merkel, S., Foster, R., Krane, E. J., et al. (2008). A comparison of the clinical utility of pain assessment tools for children with cognitive impairment. *Anesthesia and Analgesia, 106,* 72–78.

von Baeyer, C. L., & Spagrud, L. J. (2007). Systematic review of observational (behavioral) measures of pain for children and adolescents aged 3 to 18 years. *Pain, 127,* 140–150.

von Roenn, J. H., Cleeland, C. S., Gonin, R., Hatfield, A. K., & Pandya, K. J. (1993). Physician attitudes and practice in cancer pain management: A survey from the Eastern Cooperative Oncology Group. *Annals of Internal Medicine, 119,* 121–126.

Wallace, M. S., Wallace, A. M., Lee, J., & Dobke, M. K. (1996). Pain after breast surgery: A survey of 282 women. *Pain, 66,* 195–205.

Wallenstein, S. L. (1984). Measurement of pain and analgesia in cancer patients. *Cancer, 53,* 2260–2266.

Ward, S. E., Goldberg, N., Miller-McCauley, V., Mueller, C., Nolan, A., Pawlik-Plank, D., et al. (1993). Patient-related barriers to management of cancer pain. *Pain, 52,* 319–324.

Ward, S. E., & Hernandez, L. (1994). Patient-related barriers to management of cancer pain in Puerto Rico. *Pain, 58,* 233–238.

Ware, J., Jr., Kosinski, M., & Keller, S. D. (1996). A 12-Item Short-Form Health Survey: Construction of scales and preliminary tests of reliability and validity. *Medical Care, 34,* 220–233.

Ware, J. E., Jr., & Sherbourne, C. D. (1992). The MOS 36-Item Short-Form Health Survey (SF-36): I. Conceptual framework and item selection. *Medical Care, 30,* 473–483.

Wilkie, D. J., Keefe, F. J., Dodd, M. J., & Copp, L. A. (1992). Behavior of patients with lung cancer: Description and associations with oncologic and pain variables. *Pain, 51,* 231–240.

World Health Organization. (1986). *Cancer pain relief.* Geneva: Author.

World Health Organization. (1996). *Cancer pain relief and palliative care.* Geneva: Author.

World Health Organization. (1998). *Cancer pain relief and palliative care in children.* Geneva: Author.

Yancik, R., & Ries, L. A. (2000). Aging and cancer in America: Demographic and epidemiologic perspectives. *Hematolology and Oncology Clinics of North America, 14,* 17–23.

Zaza, C., & Baine, N. (2002). Cancer pain and psychosocial factors: A critical review of the literature. *Journal of Pain and Symptom Management, 24,* 526–542.

Zech, D. F., Grond, S., Lynch, J., Hertel, D., & Lehmann, K. A. (1995). Validation of World Health Organization Guidelines for cancer pain relief: A 10-year prospective study. *Pain, 63,* 65–76.

Zenz, M., Zenz, T., Tryba, M., & Strumpf, M. (1995). Severe undertreatment of cancer pain: A 3-year survey of the German situation. *Journal of Pain and Symptom Management, 10,* 187–191.

Zhukovsky, D. S., Gorowski, E., Hausdorff, J., Napolitano, B., & Lesser, M. (1995). Unmet analgesic needs in cancer patients. *Journal of Pain and Symptom Management, 10,* 113–119.

APPENDIX 19.1. Brief Pain Inventory (Short Form)

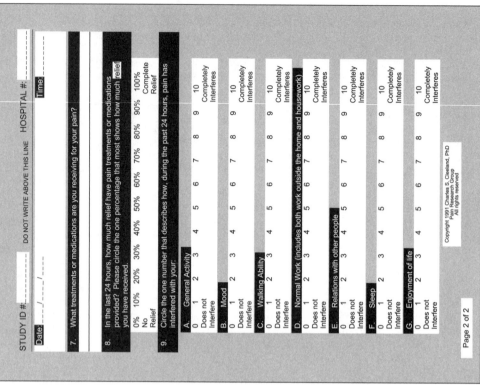

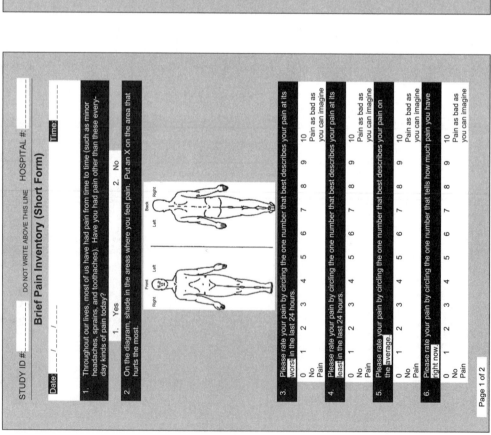

APPENDIX 19.2. M. D. Anderson Symptom Inventory (MDASI)

Date: _____

Participant Initials: _____

Participant Number: _____

Institution: _____

Hospital Chart #: _____

M. D. Anderson Symptom Inventory (MDASI) Core Items

Part I. How **severe** are your symptoms?

People with cancer frequently have symptoms that are caused by their disease or by their treatment. We ask you to rate how severe the following symptoms have been *in the last 24 hours.* Please fill in the circle below from 0 (symptom has not been present) to 10 (the symptom was as bad as you can imagine it could be) for each item.

Scale: Not Present (0) 1 2 3 4 5 6 7 8 9 10 As Bad As You Can Imagine

1. Your **pain** at its WORST?
2. Your **fatigue (tiredness)** at its WORST?
3. Your **nausea** at its WORST?
4. Your **disturbed sleep** at its WORST?
5. Your **feelings of being distressed (upset)** at its WORST?
6. Your **shortness of breath** at its WORST?
7. Your **problem with remembering things** at its WORST?
8. Your **problem with lack of appetite** at its WORST?
9. Your **feeling drowsy (sleepy)** at its WORST?
10. Your having a **dry mouth** at its WORST?

Scale: Not Present (0) 1 2 3 4 5 6 7 8 9 10 As Bad As You Can Imagine

11. Your **feeling sad** at its WORST?
12. Your **vomiting** at its WORST?
13. Your **numbness or tingling** at its WORST?

Part II. How have your symptoms interfered with your life?

Symptoms frequently interfere with how we feel and function. How much have your symptoms interfered with the following items in the last 24 hours:

Scale: Did Not Interfere (0) 1 2 3 4 5 6 7 8 9 10 Interfered Completely

14. **General activity?**
15. **Mood?**
16. **Work (including work around the house)?**
17. **Relations with other people?**
18. **Walking?**
19. **Enjoyment of life?**

PART V

SPECIAL ISSUES AND APPLICATIONS

CHAPTER 20

Assessment of Psychiatric Disorders

MARK D. SULLIVAN
JENNIFER BRENNAN BRADEN

Psychiatric disorders are common but still poorly understood in patients with chronic, nonmalignant pain. Epidemiologic evidence of high rates of psychiatric disorders in all kinds of chronic pain conditions supports the use of inclusive ("both–and") rather than exclusive ("either–or") models of psychiatric diagnosis in medical settings. But often psychiatric disorders are not considered in the differential diagnosis of physical symptoms such as pain until medical disorders have been "ruled-out." This stigma-driven policy can lead to unnecessary testing, iatrogenic injury, and poor clinical management of patients. Whenever a pain problem has become chronic and disabling, psychiatric disorders should be considered.

Any discussion of psychiatric disorders in patients with chronic pain is haunted by the concept of psychogenic pain. We are drawn to the concept of psychogenic pain because it fills the gaps left when our attempts to explain clinical pain exclusively in terms of tissue pathology fail. Psychogenic pain, however, is an empty concept. Positive criteria for the identification of psychogenic pain, mechanisms for the production of psychogenic pain, and specific therapies for psychogenic pain are lacking. Psychiatric diagnosis of many disorders, such as depression, can be very helpful to clinician and patient by pointing toward specific effective therapies. But the diagnosis of psychogenic pain too often only serves to stigmatize further the patient who experiences chronic pain.

In the discussion that follows, psychiatric disorders as defined in the fourth edition of the *Diagnostic and Statistical Manual of Mental Disorders* (DSM-IV) of the American Psychiatric Association (1994) are used as an organizing strategy. It is important to note, however, that the categorical model of mental disorder favored by psychiatrists and used in DSM-IV can imply more discontinuity between those with and without mental disorder than is actually the case. For example, it is common for patients with chronic pain partially to meet criteria for a number of mental disorders. It is therefore sometimes useful to think of these disorders as dimensions rather than as categories. DSM-IV nevertheless provides a well-recognized and systematic template for the discussion of psychiatric disorders in those with chronic pain.

When asked to evaluate patients at our Center for Pain Relief, we typically consider the following issues: depression, anxiety (panic, posttraumatic stress disorder [PTSD], and abuse history), substance abuse, somatization disorder, and personality disorders. Other issues are addressed as indicated, such as: obsessive–compulsive disorder, attention-deficit/hyperactivity disorder, dementia, psychosis, and antisocial behavior. We do not usually use a structured interview for psychiatric diagnosis. But for those who prefer some guidance and structure, the most useful interviews in the general medical setting are the PRIME-MD (Spitzer et al., 1994), and its self-administered version, the Patient Health Questionnaire (Spitzer, Kroenke, & Williams, 1999) or the Mini-International Neuropsychiatric Interview (MINI), a short, structured diagnostic interview developed jointly by psychiatrists and clinicians in the United States and Europe for DSM-IV and ICD-10 psychiatric disorders (Sheehan et al., 1998). These both have an administration time of approximately 15 minutes and are designed to meet the need for a short but accurate structured psychiatric interview for multicenter clinical trials and epidemiology studies, and as a first step in outcome tracking in nonresearch clinical settings These instruments screen for depression (major and minor), anxiety (panic disorder, generalized anxiety disorder), somatoform disorders, alcohol abuse, and eating disorders (bulimia, binge-eating disorder). There are several instruments available for screening for PTSD. The PTSD Checklist (PCL), a 17-item instrument, has been used in military and civilian populations (Blanchard, Jones-Alexander, Buckley, & Forneris, 1996). Recently, abbreviated versions of this instrument (Gerrity, Corson, & Dobscha, 2007; Lang & Stein, 2005) have been developed, and there is also a four-item Primary Care PTSD Screen (Ouimette, Wade, Prins, & Schon, 2008).

DEPRESSION

One must begin by distinguishing between depressed mood and the clinical syndrome of major depression. It is important to note, especially when working with patients with chronic pain, that depressed mood or dysphoria is not necessary for the diagnosis of major depression. *Anhedonia*, the inability to enjoy activities or experience pleasure, is an adequate substitute. It is common for patients with chronic pain to deny dysphoria but to acknowledge that enjoyment of

all activities has ceased, even those without obvious relation to their pain problem (e.g., watching TV for a patient with low back pain).

The DSM-IV criteria for major depressive episode include both psychological symptoms (worthlessness or guilt, thoughts of death or dying) and somatic symptoms (insomnia or hypersomnia, change in appetite, fatigue, trouble concentrating, psychomotor agitation or retardation). The presence of five or more symptoms is required for diagnosis of a major depressive episode. It is important to note that somatic symptoms count toward a diagnosis of major depression unless they are due to "the direct physiological effects of a general medical condition" or medication (American Psychiatric Association, 1994, p. 327). The poor sleep, poor concentration, and lack of enjoyment often experienced by patients with chronic pain are frequently attributed to pain rather than to depression. However, since they are not a direct physiological effect of pain, these symptoms should count toward a diagnosis of depression. In fact, studies of depression in medically ill populations have generally found greater sensitivity and reliability with "inclusive models" of depression diagnosis that accept all symptoms as relevant to the diagnosis than with models that try to identify the cause of each symptom (Koenig, George, Peterson, & Pieper, 1997).

Patients with chronic pain often dismiss a depression diagnosis, stating that their depression is a "direct reaction" to their pain problem. Psychiatry has long debated the value of distinguishing a "reactive" form of depression caused by adverse life events and an endogenous form of depression caused by biological and genetic factors (Frank, Anderson, Reynolds, Ritenour, & Kupfer, 1994). Life events are important in many depressive episodes, though they play a less important role in recurrent and very severe or melancholic or psychotic depressions (Brown, Harris, & Hepworth, 1994). Currently, the only life event that excludes someone who otherwise qualifies for a depression diagnosis is bereavement. Determining whether a depression is a "reasonable response" to life's stress may be very important to patients seeking to decrease the stigma of a depression diagnosis, and it has been of interest to pain investigators. It is not, however, important in deciding whether treatment is necessary and appropriate. Indeed, in assessment there is no clarity to be gained from debating whether the depression caused the pain or the pain caused the depression. If patients meet the criteria outlined earlier, they can likely benefit from appropriate treatment.

When considering the diagnosis of depression in the patient with chronic pain, important alternatives include bipolar disorder, substance-induced mood disorder, and dysthymic disorder. Patients with bipolar disorder have extended periods of abnormally elevated or irritable, as well as abnormally depressed, mood. These periods of elevated mood need to last several, continuous days (4 days for a hypomanic episode, 1 week for a manic episode) and include features such as inflated self-esteem, decreased need for sleep, and racing thoughts. A history of manic or hypomanic episodes predicts an atypical response to antidepressant medication and increases the risk of antidepressant-induced mania. Bipolar disorder is less common (12-month prevalence in the general population 2.6 vs. 6.7%; Kessler, Berglund, et al., 2005) than unipolar depression, but it is important to recognize because it requires a different treatment approach. Individuals with bipolar disorder have been reported to have higher rates of migraine headaches compared to those without bipolar disorder.

Substance-induced mood disorders can also occur in those with pain. Patients with chronic pain may be taking medications such as steroids, dopamine-blocking agents (including antiemetics), or sedatives (including "muscle relaxants") that produce a depressive syndrome. Patients' current medication lists should be scrutinized before additional medications are prescribed. For patients with a pure substance-induced mood disorder, symptoms can persist for up to a month after discontinuation of the substance but will eventually resolve. It should be noted that some patients with an underlying mood disorder "self-medicate" with other substances (drugs, alcohol), hence establishing the temporal relationship (as much as possible) between the onset of mood symptoms and substance abuse is important for treatment planning.

Dysthymic disorder is a chronic form of depression lasting 2 years or longer. Individuals with dysthymia are at high risk to develop major depression as well. This combined syndrome has often been called "double depression" (Keller, Hirschfeld, & Hanks, 1997). It is important to note that dysthymia is frequently invisible in medical settings, often dismissed as "just the way that patient is." Dysthymia has been shown to respond to many antidepressants, including the selective serotonin reuptake inhibitors (SSRIs; Thase et al., 1996). Treatment of double depression can be particularly challenging due to treatment resistance and concurrent personality disorders (Rush & Thase, 1997). Psychiatric consultation may be useful when any of these disorders is suspected.

Twelve-month prevalence rates for major depression and dysthymia in the general population are 6.7 and 1.5%, respectively (Kessler, Chiu, Demler, Merikangas, & Walters, 2005). Among individuals endorsing one or more chronic pain conditions in the general population (back/neck, arthritis, migraine/chronic headaches), 12-month rates are generally higher, 10–30% (Braden et al., 2008; McWilliams, Cox, & Enns, 2003; Stang et al., 2006; Von Korff et al., 2005). Prevalence rates of depression among patients in pain clinics have varied widely depending on the method of assessment and the population assessed. Rates as low as 10% and as high as 100% have been reported (Romano & Turner, 1985). The reason for the wide variability may be attributable to a number of factors, including the methods used to diagnose depression (e.g., interview, self-report instruments), the criteria used (e.g., DSM-IV, cutoff scores on self-report instruments), the set of disorders included in the diagnosis of depression (e.g., presence of depressive symptoms, major depression), and referral bias (e.g., higher reported prevalence of depression in studies in psychiatry clinics compared to rehabilitation clinics). The majority of studies report depression in over 50% of sampled patients with chronic pain (Fishbain, Goldberg, Meagher, Steele, & Rosomoff, 1986).

Studies of primary care populations (where generalization is less problematic) have revealed a number of factors that appear to increase the likelihood of depression in patients with chronic pain. Dworkin, Von Korff, and LeResche (1990) reported that patients with two or more pain complaints were much more likely to be depressed that those with a single pain complaint. Number of pain conditions reported was a better predictor of major depression than pain severity or pain persistence. Von Korff, Ormel, Keefe, and Dworkin (1992) developed a four-level scale for grading chronic pain severity based on pain disability and pain intensity: (1) low disability and low intensity, (2) low disability and high intensity, (3) high disability–moderately limiting, and (4) high disability–severely limiting. Depression, use of opioid analgesics, and doctor visits all increased as chronic pain grade increased. When dysfunctional primary care patients with back pain were followed for a year, those whose back pain improved also showed improvement of depressive symptoms to normal levels (Von Korff, Deyo, Cherkin, & Barlow, 1993).

These epidemiological studies provide solid evidence for a strong association between chronic pain and depression, but they do not address whether chronic pain causes depression or depression causes chronic pain. As indicated earlier, this question has more importance in medicolegal contexts than in clinical contexts. But since it is a perennial question, some attempt should be made to answer it. Prospective studies of patients with chronic musculoskeletal pain have suggested that chronic pain can cause depression (Atkinson, Slater, Patterson, Grant, & Garfin, 1991), that depression can cause chronic pain (Magni, Moreschi, Rigatti-Luchini, & Merskey, 1994), and that they exist in a mutually reinforcing relationship (Rudy, Kerns, & Turk, 1988).

One fact often raised to support the idea that pain causes depression is that the current depressive episode often begins after the onset of the pain problem. The majority of studies appear to support this contention (Brown, 1990). However, many patients with documented chronic pain (especially disabled patients seen in pain clinics) often have had episodes of depression that predated their pain problem by years (Katon, Egan, & Miller, 1985). This has led to some investigators to propose that there may exist a common trait of susceptibility to dysphoric physical symptoms (including pain) and to negative psychological symptoms (anxiety, as well as depression). Von Korff and Simon (1996, p. 106) concluded that "pain and psychological illness should be viewed as having

reciprocal psychological and behavioral effects involving both processes of illness expression and adaptation."

Patients with chronic pain often feel they are battling to have their suffering recognized as real. They resist a depression diagnosis if they see it as a way to dismiss their suffering. Even if clinicians are sensitive to these issues, they must recognize that legal proceedings, insurance companies, and workers' compensation boards can look on a depression diagnosis with prejudice. Traditional and industrial societies appear to hold individuals less responsible for somatic symptoms than for psychological symptoms. This difference may be especially prominent in modern Western biomedicine, where symptom complexes are validated or invalidated through their correspondence with objective disease criteria (Fabrega, 1990). A somatic "idiom of distress" therefore becomes the favored means for communicating distress of any origin that is overwhelming or disabling (Good, 1992). Pain is a more acceptable reason for disability than depression in many cultures. Therefore, cultural incentives exist for translation of depression into pain. Since depressed patients have many physical symptoms, these can become the focus of clinical communication and concern. Giving patients with chronic pain permission to talk of distress in the clinical setting using nonsomatic terms can facilitate treatment as long as they do not feel that somatic elements of their problem are being neglected or discounted. We try to validate depression as an understandable response to a chronic pain problem.

ANXIETY DISORDERS

It is not unusual for patients with symptoms of pain to be anxious and worried. This, however, is not synonymous with a psychiatric diagnosis of an anxiety disorder. When patients with chronic pain do suffer from an anxiety disorder, it is rare that this is their sole psychiatric diagnosis. Most patients with pain and chronic anxiety also meet criteria for either major depression or dysthymia. In these cases, treatment should be directed toward the mood disorder. With successful treatment of the mood disorder, the anxiety should be relieved as well. Benzodiazepines should almost always be avoided because of their association with tolerance, dependence, and withdrawal. Prolonged use may promote inactivity and cognitive impairment.

Panic Disorder

Panic disorder is a common, disabling psychiatric illness associated with high medical service utilization and multiple medically unexplained symptoms. In the pain clinic setting, panic disorder should be considered especially in patients with chest pain, abdominal pain, or headaches. The diagnosis of panic disorder requires that recurrent, unexpected panic attacks be followed by at least a month of worry about having another panic attack, about the implications or consequences of the panic attacks, or behavioral changes related to the attacks. A *panic attack* is defined as a discrete period of intense fear or discomfort in which four or more symptoms are present. As with major depression, DSM-IV criteria include symptoms that are somatic (increased heart rate, palpitations, sweating, shortness of breath, chest pain, trembling, dizziness, chills or hot flushes, nausea, feeling of choking, paresthesias) and psychological (fear of dying, fear of losing control or going crazy). These attacks should not be the direct physiological consequence of a substance or other medical condition. The panic attacks should not be better accounted for by another mental disorder, such as PTSD (described below) or obsessive–compulsive disorder. At least two unexpected attacks are required for the diagnosis, though most patients have more.

One of the most common problems with panic disorder is fear of undiagnosed, life-threatening illness. Patients with panic disorder can receive extensive medical testing and treatment for their somatic symptoms before the diagnosis of panic disorder is made and appropriate treatment is initiated.

Lifetime prevalence of panic disorder throughout the world is estimated to be 1.5 to 4.7% (Kessler, Berglund, et al., 2005). One year prevalence rates are from 1 to 2.7% (Kessler, Berglund, et al., 2005). Panic disorder is two to three times more common in women than in men. Age of onset is variable, but most cases typically occur between late adolescence and the mid-30s. Of all common mental disorders in the primary care setting, panic disorder is most likely to produce moderate to severe occupational dysfunction and physical disability (Ormel et al., 1994). It is also associated with the greatest number of disability days in the past month.

The most common complication of panic disorder is *agoraphobia*, or fear of public places. Patients with panic disorder learn to fear places where escape might be difficult or help may not be available in case they have an attack. One-half to two-thirds of patients with panic disorder also suffer from major depression. These are the most disabled patients with panic disorder. The differential diagnosis of patients presenting with panic symptoms in the medical setting includes thyroid, parathyroid, adrenal, and vestibular dysfunction, seizure disorders, cardiac arrhythmias, and drug intoxication or withdrawal. Patients with panic disorder typically present in the medical setting with cardiological, gastrointestinal, or neurological complaints (Zaubler & Katon, 1996).

Chest pain is one of the most common complaints presented to primary care physicians, but a specific medical etiology is identified in only 10–20% of cases. From 43 to 61% of patients with normal coronary arteries at angiography and 16 to 25% of patients presenting to emergency rooms with chest pain have panic disorder. A number of these patients eventually receive the diagnoses of vasospastic angina, costochondritis, esophageal dysmotility, or mitral valve prolapse. High rates of psychiatric disorders have been found in some of these groups as well (Carney, Freedland, Ludbrook, Saunders, & Jaffe, 1990). Many of these patients remain symptomatic and disabled 1 year later despite reassurance concerning coronary artery disease (Beitman et al., 1991).

Approximately 11% of primary care patients present with the complaint of abdominal pain to their physician each year. Less than one-fourth of these symptoms is associated with a definite physical diagnosis in the following year. Among the most common reasons for abdominal pain is irritable bowel syndrome. It is estimated that irritable bowel syndrome accounts for 20–52% of all referrals to gastroenterologists. Various studies have found that 54–74% of these patients with irritable bowel syndrome have associated psychiatric disorders. Walker, Gelfand,

Gelfand, and Katon (1995) determined that patients with irritable bowel syndrome have much higher current (28 vs. 3%) and lifetime (41 vs. 25%) rates of panic disorder than a comparison group with inflammatory bowel disease. This suggests that the psychiatric disorder was not simply a reaction to the abdominal distress.

Among 10,000 persons assessed in a community survey who consulted their physicians for headache, 15% of females and 13% of males had a history of panic disorder. Further studies have suggested that migraine headache is most strongly associated with panic attacks (Stewart, Breslau, & Keck, 1994). Often anxiety symptoms precede the onset of the headaches, whereas depressive symptoms often have their onset after the headaches. Some authors have suggested that people with panic attacks have a common predisposition to headaches (especially migraines and chronic daily headache), anxiety disorders, and major depression.

Posttraumatic Stress Disorder

Following direct personal exposure to an extreme traumatic event, some individuals develop a syndrome that includes reexperiencing the event, avoidance of stimuli associated with the event, and persistent heightened arousal. PTSD was originally described following exposure to military combat, but it is now recognized that it occurs following sexual or physical assault, natural disasters, accidents, life-threatening illnesses, and other events that induce feelings of intense fear, hopelessness, or horror. Persons may develop the disorder after experiencing or just witnessing these events. DSM-IV diagnostic criteria require that the person either experienced or witnessed an event that involved actual or threatened death, serious injury, or threat to the physical integrity of the self or others, and responded with intense fear, helplessness or horror. Posttraumatic symptoms must last more than 1 month. The event can be reexperienced in the form of recurrent nightmares, flashbacks, or intense psychological distress or physical reactivity in response to internal or external cues resembling the event. Three or more avoidance symptoms (e.g., avoiding thoughts or conversations about the event, avoiding people or places associated with

the event, a sense of foreshortened future, inability to recall important aspects of the trauma, restricted range of affect, diminished interest in people or activities, a feeling of detachment) and two or more symptoms of increased arousal (e.g., disturbed sleep, irritability, hypervigilance, increased startle response, difficulty concentrating) should also be present.

Up to 80% of Vietnam veterans with PTSD report chronic pain in limbs, back, torso, or head (Beckham et al., 1997). Increased physical symptoms, including muscle aches and back pain, are also more common in Gulf War Veterans with PTSD than in those without PTSD (Baker, Mendenhall, Simbartl, Magan, & Steinberg, 1997). The 12-month prevalence of PTSD in the general population is 3.5% (Kessler, Berglund, et al., 2005). The prevalence of PTSD in medical populations has been shown to be quite high. Averaging the prevalence rates of PTSD across a number of studies reveals that following motor vehicle accidents sufficiently severe to require medical attention, 29.5% of patients met the criteria for PTSD (Blanchard & Hickling, 2003). For over one-half of these patients, the symptoms resolved within 6 months. In one study, 15% of patients seeking treatment for idiopathic facial pain were found to have PTSD (Aghabeigi, Feinmann, & Harris, 1992). In another study 21% of patients with fibromyalgia were found to have PTSD (Amir et al., 1997). Case reports have associated reflex sympathetic dystrophy (complex regional pain syndrome) with PTSD. Other studies suggest that 50–100% of patients presenting at pain treatment centers meet the diagnostic criteria for PTSD (Sharp & Harvey, 2001). Pain patients with PTSD have been shown to have more pain and affective distress than those without PTSD (Geisser, Roth, Bachman, & Eckert, 1996), so it is not surprising that PTSD rates among patients with pain increase in more specialized treatment settings.

The relationship between pain and PTSD is multifaceted. Pain and PTSD may both result from a traumatic event. Sometimes acute pain can constitute the traumatic event, as described in a case of traumatic eye enucleation (Schreiber & Galai-Gat, 1993). PTSD also appears to permit induction of an opioid-mediated, stress-induced analgesia. PTSD-related stimuli can result in a naloxone-reversible decreased sensitivity to noxious stimuli in affected individuals (Pitman, van der Kolk, Orr, & Greenberg, 1990).

The relation between childhood abuse and chronic pain has received a lot of attention in recent years. Multiple studies have demonstrated higher rates of childhood maltreatment in patients with chronic pain than in comparison groups. They have also shown poorer coping among abused patients with pain (Spertus, Burns, Glenn, Lofland, & McCracken, 1999). However, the relationship between childhood psychological trauma and adult somatic symptoms is complex and multifaceted (Walker, Unutzer, & Katon, 1998). PTSD, dissociation, somatization, and affect dysregulation represent a spectrum of adaptations to trauma. They may occur together or separately (van der Kolk et al., 1996). The best way to incorporate information about childhood maltreatment into the treatment of the adult patient with chronic pain is as yet unclear. At minimum, it signals caregivers that establishing a therapeutic alliance may be difficult. It may also signal that the "here-and-now" focus of the cognitive-behavioral therapy frequently used for patients with pain will not be adequate. But chronic pain treatment trials have not yet grouped patients by trauma history or attempted treatment matching.

SUBSTANCE ABUSE

Diagnosis of substance abuse and substance dependence in patients with chronic pain is controversial, because it is difficult to achieve consensus on what constitutes a *maladaptive* pattern of substance use. DSM-IV distinguishes between substance dependence and substance abuse. The essential feature of *substance dependence* is continued use of a substance despite a cluster of cognitive, behavioral, and physiological problems. It is characterized by tolerance, withdrawal, and compulsive drug-taking behavior. DSM-IV diagnostic criteria for substance dependence require three or more symptoms or behaviors (e.g., withdrawal, tolerance, continued use despite having a physical or psychological problem caused or exacerbated by the substance, spending a significant amount of time obtaining, using or recovering from

the substance effects) occurring within a 12-month period.

Traditionally, opioids have been considered appropriate for terminal cancer pain, with tolerance, dependence, and dose escalation limited in their importance by the impending death of the patient. But they have been considered problematic for the chronic noncancer patient with pain whose long-term function is an essential issue. A large percentage of patients referred to multidisciplinary pain centers report taking opioids at the time of assessment. Following treatment, the majority of these patients report significantly reduced pain concurrent with elimination of opioid medication (Flor, Fydrich, & Turk, 1992; Hooten, Townsend, Sletten, Bruce, & Rome, 2007; Rome et al., 2004).

Portenoy (1990) and others have argued forcefully that chronic opioid therapy can be appropriate and beneficial in *some* patients with chronic noncancer pain. One of the current, unanswered questions is what factors characterize those patients who are likely to benefit from long-term opioids without problems of addiction, tolerance, or increased disability? To date there have been no long-term, double-blind studies that help to select the group for whom long-term opioids are beneficial. Nevertheless, in recent years, there has been a marked increase in the use of opioids for chronic noncancer pain. Several recent studies have found that individuals with underlying depressive, anxiety, or substance use disorders are more likely than those without these disorders to receive opioids for noncancer pain (Sullivan, Edlund, Zhang, Unutzer, & Wells, 2006). Hence, screening for and treating these disorders in individuals on, or being considered for, opioid therapy is important.

The essential feature of substance abuse is a maladaptive pattern of substance use characterized by recurrent and significant adverse consequences. These include impaired role function, substance use in physically hazardous situations, and legal problems.

The lifetime and 12-month prevalences of substance use disorders in the general population are 14.6% (Kessler, Berglund, et al., 2005) and 3.8% (Kessler, Chiu, et al., 2005), respectively. Prevalence rates for substance abuse in patients with chronic pain are variable due to differences in definitions used and populations assessed. Studies completed to date suggest that substance abuse and dependence occur in a minority of chronic pain patients on opioids. They do not answer the more difficult question of whether opioids are, on balance, beneficial treatment for these patients. Future studies involving random assignment of patients with chronic pain to opioid treatment will be necessary to determine which patients are able to obtain benefits (pain reduction and improvement of function) from long-term opioids without developing deleterious effects.

Since small amounts of alcohol use can retard response to antidepressant medication, it is important to inquire about alcohol use that may not otherwise meet criteria for abuse in patients who are candidates for antidepressant medication. We encourage patients we place on antidepressant medication to limit alcohol use to one or two drinks per week. Significant others and other third parties are an indispensable source of information about substance abuse. We routinely include a significant other in the initial evaluation of new patients disabled by chronic pain. We are also quite liberal in our use of urine toxicology screens in any patients with histories of substance abuse or possible current substance abuse. Often this is the only way to be sure about the cause of a patient's altered mental status, such as affective lability, cognitive impairment, and treatment nonresponse. Unfortunately, toxicology screens detect highly lipid-soluble compounds such as tetrahydrocannabinol (THC) from marijuana for a much longer time than other compounds, such as cocaine, more critical to treatment planning.

PERSONALITY DISORDERS

DSM-IV (American Psychiatric Association, 1994) defines a *personality disorder* as "an enduring pattern of inner experience and behavior that deviates markedly from the expectations of the individual's culture" (p. 633), that is manifested in two or more of the following areas: cognition, affectivity, interpersonal functioning, and impulse control. The pattern is inflexible and pervasive across a broad range of personal and social situations, is stable and of long duration, has an onset in adolescence or early adulthood,

and leads to clinically significant distress or impairment in functioning. Personality disorders are further divided into three clusters and 11 specific disorders (see Table 20.1 for a summary of the disorders; specific criteria can be found in DSM-IV).

The prevalence of any personality disorder in the general population ranges from 9.0 to 15.7% (Lenzenweger, Lane, Loranger, & Kessler, 2007). The prevalence in clinical settings is higher, reported to be around 25% in primary care (Moran, Jenkins, Tylee, Blizard, & Mann, 2000) and as high as 45% in psychiatric settings (Zimmerman, Rothschild, & Chelminski, 2005). In general, borderline personality disorder is the most commonly seen disorder in clinical settings; DSM-IV criteria for this disorder are listed in Table 20.1. In studies of patients with chronic pain seen in specialty settings, 40–70% met criteria for a DSM-IV personality disorder, most commonly paranoid and borderline disorders (Conrad et al., 2007; Dersh, Gatchel, Mayer, Polatin, & Temple, 2006). Genetic factors and adverse child-

TABLE 20.1. DSM-IV Personality Disorders

Cluster A personality disorders

Paranoid—pattern of distrust and suspiciousness
Schizoid—pattern of social detachment and restricted emotional expression
Schizotypal—pattern of social discomfort, cognitive/perceptual distortions, eccentricities

Cluster B personality disorders

Borderline—pattern of unstable relationships, self-image, and affect, and impulsivity
Antisocial—pattern of disregard for and violation of the rights of others occurring since age 15 years
Histrionic—pattern of excessive emotionality and attention-seeking
Narcissistic—pattern of grandiosity, need for admiration, and lack of empathy

Cluster C personality disorders

Avoidant—pattern of social inhibition, feelings of inadequacy, and hypersensitivity to negative evaluation
Dependent—pattern of excessive need to be taken care of
Obsessive–Compulsive—pattern of preoccupation with orderliness, perfection, and control

Personality disorder not otherwise specified

hood experiences (e.g., abuse, neglect) likely interact to bring about the development of personality disorder characteristics. In particular, a history of sexual abuse in childhood is more common among individuals with borderline personality disorder, as it is among individuals with chronic pain.

When assessing for the presence of a personality disorder, it is important to keep in mind the distinction between trait and state. In the midst of an acute depressive episode, individuals can present with behaviors or characteristics that are consistent with a personality disorder but that resolve once the depression has been treated. To diagnose a personality disorder in the context of an untreated or undertreated Axis I disorder, there must be a clear history of a pattern in thoughts, emotions, and behavior that predated the onset of a depressive or other Axis I disorder. On the other hand, comorbid Axis I disorders are very common among individuals with personality disorders (particularly mood, anxiety, and substance use disorders), and the presence of an underlying personality disorder may explain what appears to be inadequate response to treatment of the Axis I disorder. Effective treatment of an Axis II disorder typically requires psychotherapeutic interventions aimed at improving coping skills, interpersonal communication, and impulse control. For the patient with chronic pain, these areas of intervention may have relevance for not only mood but also pain management. For example, patients with borderline personality disorder have difficulty regulating emotions and controlling behaviors linked to emotions. Physical pain that may be a more acceptable expression of emotional pain may at the same time become overwhelming and lead to self-destructive behaviors (e.g., suicidal gestures, substance abuse). Thus, strategies to regulate and cope with strong emotions can also be directed toward the management of pain symptoms. In general, when assessing personality in patients with chronic pain, it is probably most useful to focus on identifying the particular patterns of thought and behavior that contribute to functional impairment. Many patients who may not meet criteria for a specific DSM personality disorder diagnosis may have personality traits that serve to reinforce pain and/or limit their ability to cope with pain.

SOMATOFORM DISORDERS

Current psychiatric theory dictates diagnoses of somatoform disorders rather than "abnormal illness behavior" or "misuse of the sick role." The essential feature of the somatoform disorders is the presence of physical symptoms that suggest a general medical condition but are not fully explained by a general medical condition. These symptoms must cause impairment in social and occupational functioning. The somatoform disorders are distinguished from factitious disorders and malingering in that the symptoms are not intentionally produced or feigned. The most valuable diagnosis among the somatoform disorders in our experience is somatization disorder.

Somatization disorder is a chronic condition characterized by a pattern of multiple and recurrent somatic complaints resulting in medical treatment and impairment in role functioning but not explained by a general medical condition. For this particular somatoform diagnosis, the somatic symptoms must be persistent and pervasive. These complaints must begin before 30 years of age and last for a period of years. Criteria include four pain symptoms, two gastrointestinal symptoms, one sexual symptom, and one pseudoneurological symptom (e.g., pseudoseizures, blindness).

Somatization disorder must be distinguished from medical disorders producing multiple and scattered symptoms, such as multiple sclerosis or systemic lupus erythematosus. It must also be distinguished from panic disorder. This also produces multiple somatic symptoms but is a more acute and treatable psychiatric disorder.

The prevalence of somatization disorder in the community has been reported to be between 0.13 and 0.4%, with the vast majority of cases being women (Smith, 1991). Prevalence estimates in the primary care setting have ranged from 0.2 to 5.0%. Studies of patients referred to pain clinics have produced estimates from 8 to 12%. Although prevalence rates clearly increase when moving from community to primary care to tertiary care settings, patients with somatization disorder remain in the clear minority in all settings, including pain clinics.

Unexplained somatic symptoms are a common problems in medical settings that extend far beyond the bounds of somatization disorder. Various attempts have been made to assess the prevalence of an abridged version of somatization disorder in primary care, requiring four to six unexplained symptoms (4.4% of patients) or three symptoms persistent over a 2-year period (8.2% of patients) (Jackson & Kroenke, 2008; Kroenke et al., 1997; Liu, Clark, & Eaton, 1997). Even these abridged forms of somatization disorder are associated with increased rates of disability, health care utilization, and mood and anxiety disorders.

Although the initial emphasis in somatization disorder was on a discrete, familial, even genetic disorder, recent evidence suggests that somatization is a process that exists along a spectrum of severity (Liu et al., 1997). A large international study confirms that whereas medically unexplained somatic symptoms are very common, full somatization disorder is quite rare (Gureje, Simon, Ustun, & Goldberg, 1997). A great deal of confusion exits between somatization as a process and somatization as a disorder. Somatization as a process, meaning the somatic experience of distress, is ubiquitous (Sullivan & Katon, 1993). It accounts for the majority of symptoms presented to primary care physicians. It is most frequently associated with transient stressors (and is therefore time-limited) or acute psychiatric disorders (which are very treatable). Somatization disorder is a rare, chronic, treatment resistant condition that characterizes the most severely and chronically distressed individuals. When clinicians use the term "somatizer" to refer to a patient with unexplained symptoms, it is unclear whether they are implying the process or the disorder. The primary value in diagnosing somatization disorder in the pain clinic setting is that it identifies a treatment-resistant group. This is the only group in which we have seen "symptom substitution" in response to cognitive-behavioral pain treatment that has been predicted by psychodynamic theorists. Full rehabilitation of patients with somatization disorder is extremely difficult. Often treatment must focus on preventing iatrogenic injury.

Although somatization disorder frequently occurs within families and may have a genetic component, it also appears to have a strong association with childhood physical and sexual abuse (Pribor, Yutzy, Dean, & Wetzel, 1993). A significant percentage of patients who meet criteria for somatization disorder also meet criteria for borderline personality disorder (Hudziak et al., 1996). This has led some investigators to question the independence of these diagnoses and others to stress their common origin in severe childhood abuse.

PAIN DISORDER

In many common pain syndromes (e.g., low back pain, headache, fibromyalgia), it is difficult to identify the tissue pathology giving rise to symptoms. When a somatic cause for pain cannot be identified, many clinicians begin to seek psychological causes. The identification of "psychogenic pain" is a difficult, and perhaps impossible, task. "Pain disorder" is the current psychiatric diagnosis that most closely corresponds to the concept of psychogenic pain.

Since "pain disorder" is an important but problematic concept at the interface of pain medicine and psychiatry, it is important to understand some of the history of the concept. In DSM-II (American Psychiatric Association, 1968), there was no specific diagnosis pertaining to pain. Painful conditions caused by emotional factors were considered part of the "psychophysiological disorders." DSM-III (American Psychiatric Association, 1980) introduced a new diagnostic category for pain problems, "psychogenic pain disorder." To qualify, a patient needed to have severe and prolonged pain inconsistent with neuroanatomical distribution of pain receptors, or without detectable organic etiology or pathophysiologic mechanism. Related organic pathology was allowed but the pain had to be "grossly in excess" of what was expected on the basis of physical examination. Accepted evidence that psychological factors were involved in the production of the pain were (1) a temporal relationship between pain onset and an environmental event producing psychological conflict, (2) pain appears to allow avoidance of some noxious event or responsibility, and (3) pain promotes emotional support or attention the individual would not have otherwise received. It is important to note that this kind of evidence never *proves* that psychological factors have caused a pain complaint.

Difficulties in establishing that pain was psychogenic led to changes in the diagnosis for DSM-IIIR (American Psychiatric Association, 1987). In DSM-III-R, the diagnosis was renamed "somatoform pain disorder," and three major changes were made in the diagnostic criteria. The requirements for etiological psychological factors and lack of other contributing mental disorders were eliminated, and a requirement for "preoccupation with pain for at least six months" was added. The diagnostic criteria (American Psychiatric Association, 1987, p. 266) were thus reduced to:

A. Preoccupation with pain for at least six months.
B. Either (1) or (2):
(1) appropriate evaluation uncovers no organic pathology or pathophysiologic mechanism . . . to account for the pain.
(2) when there is related organic pathology, the complaint of pain or resulting social or occupational impairment is grossly in excess of what would be expected from the physical findings

In DSM-III-R, therefore, somatoform pain disorder becomes purely a diagnosis of exclusion. The diagnosis is made when medical disorders are excluded in a patient "preoccupied" with pain.

The DSM-IV subcommittee on pain disorders found that despite these changes, "somatoform pain disorder" was rarely used in research projects or clinical practice. They identified a number of reasons for this: (1) the meaning of "preoccupation with pain" is unclear, (2) whether pain exceeds that expected is difficult to determine, (3) the diagnosis does not apply to many patients disabled by pain in which a medical condition is contributory, (4) the term "somatoform pain disorder" implies that this pain is somehow different from organic pain, and (5) acute pain of less than 6 months' duration was excluded (King & Strain, 1992). They therefore proposed the DSM-IV category of "pain disorder," which states that: pain is the predominant focus of the clinical presentation, that psychological factors are judged to have an important role in the onset, severity exacerbation or maintenance of the pain, and that the pain causes clinically significant distress or impairment in important areas of functioning. The disorder can be further coded as pain disorder associated with psychological factors, or pain disorder associated with psychological factors and a general medical condition.

The DSM-IV subcommittee tried to devise a broader diagnostic grouping to encompass both acute and chronic pain problems. They wanted to have all the factors relevant to the onset or maintenance of the pain delineated *and* also to have a diagnostic category that would not require more training than the majority of DSM-IV users would be expected to have. These two requirements may not be compatible. Furthermore, no guidance is given in determining when psychological factors have a major role in pain or are considered important enough in the presence of a painful medical disorder to be coded as a separate mental disorder. Given the high rates of mood and anxiety disorders among disabled patients with chronic pain, many for whom the diagnosis is most appropriate would be excluded. Although depression and anxiety diagnoses point toward specific proven therapies, this is not true for pain disorder. Thus, the diagnosis continues covertly as a diagnosis of exclusion, with neither clear inclusion criteria nor implications for therapy. Multiple studies have also demonstrated the association between medically unexplained symptoms (pain and nonpain) and psychiatric disorders. A linear relationship has been demonstrated between the lifetime number of medically unexplained physical symptoms and the lifetime number of depressive and anxiety disorders, or the degree of neuroticism or harm avoidance the patient demonstrates on psychological testing (Russo, Katon, Sullivan, Clark, & Buchwald, 1994).

Increased psychiatric morbidity has been repeatedly demonstrated for levels of unexplained medical symptoms far below the number required for a DSM diagnosis of somatization disorder (Escobar, Burnam, Karno, Forsyth, & Golding, 1987). This suggests that the somatoform disorders may be less distinct than implied by their separate DSM categories, and that they have a strong kinship with the depressive and anxiety disorders. It may be more accurate and productive to think of somatization as a process present in varying degrees throughout the population rather than as a set of disorders affecting a small subset of the population (Sullivan & Katon, 1993).

CONVERSION DISORDER

The essential feature of *conversion disorder* is an alteration in voluntary motor or sensory function that suggests a neurological or general medical disorder. Classical examples include hysterical paralysis, blindness, or mutism. Psychological factors must be associated with the initiation or exacerbation of this deficit. Great caution must be exercised in making the diagnosis of conversion disorder, because the presence of relevant psychological factors does not exclude the possibility of a concurrent organically caused condition.

In "Psychogenic Pain and the Pain-Prone Patient," George Engel (1959) proposed that psychogenic pain arises from guilt and an intolerance of success. He indicated that it functions as a substitute for loss or a replacement for aggression. He furthermore stated that "patients with conversion hysteria constitute the largest percentage of the pain-prone population" (p. 911). Others have also contended that pain is probably the most common conversion symptom encountered clinically (Ziegler, Imboden, & Meyer, 1960). However, only case reports support this contention. Pain is not a classic conversion disorder symptom, because it is not a neurological deficit or incapacity. It is controversial whether chronic pain can ever qualify as a conversion disorder by itself. Some, for example, have contended that reflex sympathetic dystrophy (RSD)/complex regional pain syndrome (CRPS) can be understood as a conversion reaction; however, this is highly controversial (Ochoa & Verdugo, 1995). Some elements of conversion disorders appear to be present in patients with RSD/CRPS (e.g., indifference or neglect toward the affected body part), though it is highly unlikely that the condition is entirely psychogenic.

Rather than labeling some and not other chronic pain problems as conversion reactions, it may be more useful to understand what components of conversion reaction may be present in chronic pain problems. Being ill surely creates problems in living for those affected. Being ill, however, can also solve problems in living. For example, being ill provides an excuse for not being at school or not meeting a deadline at work. These interpersonal advantages of illness were originally recognized by Freud and termed *secondary gain*. The term has been distorted and misunderstood in the care of chronic pain, probably due to medicolegal pressures. A number of corrections are in order. First, all illnesses are characterized by some secondary gain, not just illnesses considered to be psychogenic. Being sick *always* has advantages as well as disadvantages. Second, secondary gain includes all potential interpersonal benefits of illness, not just monetary advantages. Many of the advantages of illness are quite subtle and individualized. Third, secondary gain must be understood in the context of *primary gain*, the intrapersonal advantages of illness. For example, focusing on pain rather than depression may allow patients to avoid self-blame and thereby achieve primary gain. This is a common phenomenon in chronic pain. Indeed, blame avoidance has been hypothesized by some to be one of the main functions of somatization (Fackler, Anfinson, & Rand, 1997). Thus, some traditional elements of conversion disorder may be present in many chronic pain problems, without many pain problems qualifying as conversion disorders per se.

Purely psychogenic or conversion models of chronic pain have some questionable implications for diagnosis and therapy of chronic pain disorders. Interview of the patient with a suspected conversion disorder with the aid of an amytal (sodium amobarbital) infusion has been a standard tool in psychiatric diagnosis (Fackler et al., 1997). It is more common that motor and sensory deficits rather than pain will resolve under amytal sedation. Furthermore, some patients have had violent or suicidal reactions to abrupt resolution of their somatic symptoms under amytal, possibly due to loss of face-saving "primary gain" aspects of the illness. Psychodynamic theories of the origin of conversion symptoms imply that psychological treatments alone will be effective. Psychodynamic treatments for chronic pain, however, have little documented success. The most effective psychological treatments, such as cognitive-behavioral therapy, include a reactivation component that addresses the profound disuse and deconditioning found in many patients with chronic pain.

CONCLUSION

Psychiatric diagnosis and treatment can add an essential and often neglected component to the conceptualization and treatment of chronic pain problems. However, it is absolutely critical to avoid a dualistic model postulating that pain is *either physical or mental* in origin. This model alienates patients who feel blamed for their pain. It also is inconsistent with modern models of pain causation. Since the gate control theory of pain, multiple lines of evidence suggest that pain is a product of efferent, as well as afferent, activity in the nervous system. Tissue damage and nociception are neither necessary nor sufficient for pain. Indeed, it is now widely recognized that the relationship between pain and nociception is highly complex and must be understood in terms of the situation of the organism as a whole.

We are only beginning to understand the complexities of the relationship between pain and suffering. Pain usually, but not always, produces suffering. Suffering can, through somatization, produce pain. We have traditionally understood this suffering, as we have understood nociception, as arising from a form of pathology intrinsic to the sufferer; hence, the traditional view that pain is due either to tissue pathology (nociception) or to psychopathology (suffering). An alternative model that allows us to escape this dualism is to think of pain as a *transdermal process*, with causes outside as well as inside the body. For humans, social pathology can be as painful as tissue pathology. We can investigate the physiology and the psychology of this "sociogenic" pain without losing sight of its origins in relations *between* people.

Psychiatric and psychological care for patients with chronic pain should occur within the medical treatment setting whenever possible. This is the most effective way to reassure patients that the somatic elements of their problems are not neglected. It also allows integration of somatic and psychological treatments in the most effective manner. Effective treatment of the psychiatric disorders that often accompany chronic pain can be the difference between living well despite chronic pain and being overwhelmed by chronic pain.

REFERENCES

American Psychiatric Association. (1968). *Diagnostic and statistical manual of mental disorders* (2nd ed.). Washington, DC: Author.

American Psychiatric Association. (1980). *Diagnostic and statistical manual of mental disorders* (3rd ed.). Washington, DC: Author.

American Psychiatric Association. (1987). *Diagnostic and statistical manual of mental disorders* (3rd ed., rev.). Washington, DC: Author.

American Psychiatric Association. (1994). *Diagnostic and statistical manual of mental disorders* (4th ed.). Washington, DC: Author.

Aghabeigi, B., Feinmann, C., & Harris, M. (1992). Prevalence of post-traumatic stress disorder in patients with chronic idiopathic facial pain. *British Journal of Oral and Maxillofacial Surgery, 30*, 360–364.

Amir, M., Kaplan, Z., Neumann, L., et al. (1997). Posttraumatic stress disorder, tenderness and fibromyalgia. *Journal of Psychosomatic Research, 42*, 607–613.

Atkinson, J. H., Slater, M. A., Patterson, T. L., Grant, I., & Garfin, S. R. (1991). Prevalence, onset, and risk of psychiatric disorders in men with chronic low back pain: A controlled study. *Pain, 45*, 111–121.

Baker, D. G., Mendenhall, C. L., Simbartl, L. A., Magan, L. K., & Steinberg, J. L. (1997). Relationship between posttraumatic stress disorder and self-reported physical symptoms in Persian Gulf War veterans. *Archives of Internal Medicine, 157*, 2076–2078.

Beckham, J. C., Crawford, A. L., Feldman, M. E., et al. (1997). Chronic posttraumatic stress disorder and chronic pain in Vietnam combat veterans. *Journal of Psychosomatic Research, 43*, 379–389.

Beitman, B. D., Kushner, M. G., Basha, I., et al. (1991). Follow-up status of patients with angiographically normal coronary arteries and panic disorder. *Journal of the American Medical Association, 265*, 1545–1549.

Blanchard, E. B., & Hickling, E. J. (2003). *After the crash: psychological assessment and treatment of survivors of motor vehicle accidents* (2nd ed.). Washington, DC: American Psychological Association.

Blanchard, E. B., Jones-Alexander, J., Buckley, T. C., & Forneris, C. A. (1996). Psychometric properties of the PTSD Checklist (PCL). *Behaviour Research and Therapy, 34*, 669–673.

Braden, J. B., Zhang, L., Fan, M. Y., et al. (2008).

Mental health service use by older adults: The role of chronic pain. *American Journal of Geriatric Psychiatry, 16*, 156–167.

Brown, G. K. (1990). A causal analysis of chronic pain and depression. *Journal of Abnormal Psychology, 99*, 127–137.

Brown, G. W., Harris, T. O., & Hepworth, C. (1994). Life events and endogenous depression: A puzzle reexamined. *Archives of General Psychiatry, 51*, 525–534.

Carney, R. M., Freedland, K. E., Ludbrook, P. A., Saunders, R. D., & Jaffe, A. S. (1990). Major depression, panic disorder, and mitral valve prolapse in patients who complain of chest pain. *American Journal of Medicine, 89*, 757–760.

Conrad, R., Schilling, G., Bausch, C., et al. (2007). Temperament and character personality profiles and personality disorders in chronic pain patients. *Pain, 133*, 197–209.

Dersh, J., Gatchel, R. J., Mayer, T., Polatin, P., & Temple, O. R. (2006). Prevalence of psychiatric disorders in patients with chronic disabling occupational spinal disorders. *Spine, 31*, 1156–1162.

Dworkin, S. F., Von Korff, M., & LeResche, L. (1990). Multiple pains and psychiatric disturbance: An epidemiologic investigation. *Archives of General Psychiatry, 47*, 239–244.

Engel, G. L. (1959). Psychogenic pain and painprone patient. *American Journal of Medicine, 26*, 899–918.

Escobar, J. I., Burnam, M. A., Karno, M., Forsythe, A., & Golding, J. M. (1987). Somatization in the community. *Archives of General Psychiatry, 44*, 713–718.

Fabrega, H., Jr. (1990). The concept of somatization as a cultural and historical product of Western medicine. *Psychosomatic Medicine, 52*, 653–672.

Fackler, S. M., Anfinson, T. J., & Rand, J. A. (1997). Serial sodium amytal interviews in the clinical setting. *Psychosomatics, 38*, 558–564.

Fishbain, D. A., Goldberg, M., Meagher, B. R., Steele, R., & Rosomoff, H. (1986). Male and female chronic pain patients categorized by DSM-III psychiatric diagnostic criteria. *Pain, 26*, 181–197.

Flor, H., Fydrich, T., & Turk, D. C. (1992). Efficacy of multidisciplinary pain treatment centers: A meta-analytic review. *Pain, 49*, 221–230.

Frank, E., Anderson, B., Reynolds, C. F., III, Ritenour, A., & Kupfer, D. J. (1994). Life events and the research diagnostic criteria endogenous subtype: A confirmation of the distinction using the Bedford College methods. *Archives of General Psychiatry, 51*, 519–524.

Geisser, M. E., Roth, R. S., Bachman, J. E., & Eckert, T. A. (1996). The relationship between symptoms of post-traumatic stress disorder and pain, affective disturbance and disability among patients with accident and non-accident related pain. *Pain, 66*, 207–214.

Gerrity, M. S., Corson, K., & Dobscha, S. K. (2007). Screening for posttraumatic stress disorder in VA primary care patients with depression symptoms. *Journal of General Internal Medicine, 22*, 1321–1324.

Good, M. D. (1992). *Pain as human experience: An anthropological perspective*. Berkeley: University of California Press.

Gureje, O., Simon, G. E., Ustun, T. B., & Goldberg, D. P. (1997). Somatization in crosscultural perspective: A World Health Organization study in primary care. *American Journal of Psychiatry, 154*, 989–995.

Hooten, W. M., Townsend, C. O., Sletten, C. D., Bruce, B. K., & Rome, J. D. (2007). Treatment outcomes after multidisciplinary pain rehabilitation with analgesic medication withdrawal for patients with fibromyalgia. *Pain Medicine, 8*, 8–16.

Hudziak, J. J., Boffeli, T. J., Kreisman, J. J., et al. (1996). Clinical study of the relation of borderline personality disorder to Briquet's syndrome (hysteria), somatization disorder, antisocial personality disorder, and substance abuse disorders. *American Journal of Psychiatry, 153*, 1598–1606.

Jackson, J. L., & Kroenke, K. (2008). Prevalence, impact, and prognosis of multisomatoform disorder in primary care: A 5-year follow-up study. *Psychosomatic Medicine, 70*, 430–434.

Katon, W., Egan, K., & Miller, D. (1985). Chronic pain: Lifetime psychiatric diagnoses and family history. *American Journal of Psychiatry, 142*, 1156–1160.

Keller, M. B., Hirschfeld, R. M., & Hanks, D. (1997). Double depression: A distinctive subtype of unipolar depression. *Journal of Affective Disorders, 45*, 65–73.

Kessler, R. C., Berglund, P., Demler, O., et al. (2005). Lifetime prevalence and age-of-onset distributions of DSM-IV disorders in the National Comorbidity Survey Replication. *Archives of General Psychiatry, 62*, 593–602.

Kessler, R. C., Chiu, W. T., Demler, O., Merikangas, K. R., & Walters, E. E. (2005). Prevalence, severity, and comorbidity of 12-month DSM-IV disorders in the National Comorbidity Survey Replication. *Archives of General Psychiatry, 62*, 617–627.

King, S. A., & Strain, J. J. (1992). Revising the category of somatoform pain disorder. *Hospital and Community Psychiatry, 43*, 217–219.

Koenig, H. G., George, L. K., Peterson, B. L., &

Pieper, C. F. (1997). Depression in medically ill hospitalized older adults: Prevalence, characteristics, and course of symptoms according to six diagnostic schemes. *American Journal of Psychiatry, 154,* 1376–1383.

Kroenke, K., Spitzer, R. L., deGruy, F. V., III, et al. (1997). Multisomatoform disorder: An alternative to undifferentiated somatoform disorder for the somatizing patient in primary care. *Archives of General Psychiatry, 54,* 352–358.

Lang, A. J., & Stein, M. B. (2005). An abbreviated PTSD Checklist for use as a screening instrument in primary care. *Behaviour Research and Therapy, 43,* 585–594.

Lenzenweger, M. F., Lane, M. C., Loranger, A. W., & Kessler, R. C. (2007). DSM-IV personality disorders in the National Comorbidity Survey Replication. *Biological Psychiatry, 62,* 553–564.

Liu, G., Clark, M. R., & Eaton, W. W. (1997). Structural factor analyses for medically unexplained somatic symptoms of somatization disorder in the Epidemiologic Catchment Area study. *Psychological Medicine, 27,* 617–626.

Magni, G., Moreschi, C., Rigatti-Luchini, S., & Merskey, H. (1994). Prospective study on the relationship between depressive symptoms and chronic musculoskeletal pain. *Pain, 56,* 289–297.

McWilliams, L. A., Cox, B. J., & Enns, M. W. (2003). Mood and anxiety disorders associated with chronic pain: An examination in a nationally representative sample. *Pain, 106,* 127–133.

Moran, P., Jenkins, R., Tylee, A., Blizard, R., & Mann, A. (2000). The prevalence of personality disorder among UK primary care attenders. *Acta Psychiatrica Scandinavica, 102,* 52–57.

Ormel, J., Von Korff, M., Ustun, T. B., et al. (1994). Common mental disorders and disability across cultures: Results from the WHO Collaborative Study on Psychological Problems in General Health Care. *Journal of the American Medical Association, 272,* 1741–1748.

Ouimette, P., Wade, M., Prins, A., & Schohn, M. (2008). Identifying PTSD in primary care: Comparison of the Primary Care–PTSD screen (PC-PTSD) and the General Health Questionnaire-12 (GHQ). *Journal of Anxiety Disorders, 22,* 337–343.

Pitman, R. K., van der Kolk, B. A., Orr, S. P., & Greenberg, M. S. (1990). Naloxone-reversible analgesic response to combat-related stimuli in posttraumatic stress disorder: A pilot study. *Archives of General Psychiatry, 47,* 541–544.

Portenoy, R. K. (1990). Chronic opioid therapy in nonmalignant pain. *Journal of Pain and Symptom Management, 5,* S46–S62.

Pribor, E. F., Yutzy, S. H., Dean, J. T., & Wetzel, R. D. (1993). Briquet's syndrome, dissociation, and abuse. *American Journal of Psychiatry, 150,* 1507–1511.

Romano, J. M., & Turner, J. A. (1985). Chronic pain and depression: Does the evidence support a relationship? *Psychological Bulletin, 97,* 18–34.

Rome, J. D., Townsend, C. O., Bruce, B. K., et al. (2004). Chronic noncancer pain rehabilitation with opioid withdrawal: Comparison of treatment outcomes based on opioid use status at admission. *Mayo Clinic Proceedings, 79,* 759–768.

Rudy, T. E., Kerns, R. D., & Turk, D. C. (1988). Chronic pain and depression: Toward a cognitive-behavioral mediation model. *Pain, 35,* 129–140.

Rush, A. J., & Thase, M. E. (1997). Strategies and tactics in the treatment of chronic depression. *Journal of Clinical Psychiatry, 58*(Suppl. 13), 14–22.

Russo, J., Katon, W., Sullivan, M., Clark, M., & Buchwald, D. (1994). Severity of somatization and its relationship to psychiatric disorders and personality. *Psychosomatics, 35,* 546–556.

Schreiber, S., & Galai-Gat, T. (1993). Uncontrolled pain following physical injury as the core-trauma in post-traumatic stress disorder. *Pain, 54,* 107–110.

Sharp, T. J., & Harvey, A. G. (2001). Chronic pain and posttraumatic stress disorder: Mutual maintenance? *Clinical Psychology Review, 21,* 857–877.

Sheehan, D. V., Lecrubier, Y., Sheehan, K. H., et al. (1998). The Mini-International Neuropsychiatric Interview (M.I.N.I.): The development and validation of a structured diagnostic psychiatric interview for DSM-IV and ICD-10. *Journal of Clinical Psychiatry, 59*(Suppl. 20), 22–33; quiz 4–57.

Spertus, I. L., Burns, J., Glenn, B., Lofland, K., & McCracken, L. (1999). Gender differences in associations between trauma history and adjustment among chronic pain patients. *Pain, 82,* 97–102.

Spitzer, R. L., Kroenke, K., & Williams, J. B. (1999). Validation and utility of a self-report version of PRIME-MD: The PHQ Primary Care Study: Primary Care Evaluation of Mental Disorders. Patient Health Questionnaire. *Journal of the American Medical Association, 282,* 1737–1744.

Spitzer, R. L., Williams, J. B., Kroenke, K., et al. (1994). Utility of a new procedure for diagnosing mental disorders in primary care: The PRIME-MD 1000 Study. *Journal of the American Medical Association, 272,* 1749–1756.

Stang, P. E., Brandenburg, N. A., Lane, M. C., et al. (2006). Mental and physical comorbid conditions and days in role among persons with arthritis. *Psychosomatic Medicine, 68,* 152–158.

Stewart, W., Breslau, N., & Keck, P. E., Jr. (1944). Comorbidity of migraine and panic disorder. *Neurology, 44,* S23–S27.

Sullivan, M. D., Edlund, M. J., Zhang, L., Unutzer, J., & Wells, K. B. (2006). Association between mental health disorders, problem drug use, and regular prescription opioid use. *Archives of Internal Medicine, 166,* 2087–2093.

Sullivan, M. D., & Katon, W. J. (1993). Somatization: The path from distress to somatic symptoms. *American Pain Society Journal, 2,* 141–149.

Thase, M. E., Fava, M., Halbreich, U., et al. (1996). A placebo-controlled, randomized clinical trial comparing sertraline and imipramine for the treatment of dysthymia. *Archives of General Psychiatry, 53,* 777–784.

van der Kolk, B. A., Pelcovitz, D., Roth, S., et al. (1996). Dissociation, somatization, and affect dysregulation: The complexity of adaptation of trauma. *American Journal of Psychiatry, 153,* 83–93.

Von Korff, M., Crane, P., Lane, M., et al. (2005). Chronic spinal pain and physical–mental comorbidity in the United States: Results from the National Comorbidity Survey Replication. *Pain, 113,* 331–339.

Von Korff, M., Deyo, R. A., Cherkin, D., & Barlow, W. (1993). Back pain in primary care: Outcomes at 1 year. *Spine, 18,* 855–862.

Von Korff, M., Ormel, J., Keefe, F. J., & Dworkin, S. F. (1992). Grading the severity of chronic pain. *Pain, 50,* 133–149.

Von Korff, M., & Simon, G. (1996). The relationship between pain and depression. *British Journal of Psychiatry Supplement, 30,* 101–108.

Walker, E. A., Gelfand, A. N., Gelfand, M. D., & Katon, W. J. (1995). Psychiatric diagnoses, sexual and physical victimization, and disability in patients with irritable bowel syndrome or inflammatory bowel disease. *Psychological Medicine, 25,* 1259–1267.

Walker, E. A., Unutzer, J., & Katon, W. J. (1998). Understanding and caring for the distressed patient with multiple medically unexplained symptoms. *Journal of the American Board Family Practice, 11,* 347–356.

Zaubler, T. S., & Katon, W. (1996). Panic disorder and medical comorbidity: A review of the medical and psychiatric literature. *Bulletin of the Menninger Clinic, 60,* A12–A38.

Ziegler, F. J., Imboden, J. B., & Meyer, E. (1960). Contemporary conversion reactions: A clinical study. *American Journal of Psychiatry, 116,* 901–910.

Zimmerman, M., Rothschild, L., & Chelminski, I. (2005). The prevalence of DSM-IV personality disorders in psychiatric outpatients. *American Journal of Psychiatry, 162,* 1911–1918.

CHAPTER 21

Disability Evaluation in Painful Conditions

JAMES P. ROBINSON

Patients with painful conditions often receive work disability benefits as well as medical or surgical care for their problems. Typically, a physician must assert that such patients are disabled from work in order for them to receive disability benefits. The information and opinions provided by physicians are used by adjudicators in disability agencies to determine whether the patients are eligible for benefits under various work disability programs.

Physicians perform disability evaluations on patients in two different contexts. Sometimes they interact with patients solely for the purpose of performing disability evaluations. For example, insurance companies and disability agencies often retain independent medical examiners to do the evaluations. However, most disability evaluations are performed by treating physicians; that is, a physician who is treating a patient also evaluates the patient's ability to work and communicates this information to a disability agency or insurance company.

The judgments a physician must make during a disability evaluation are the same, regardless of whether he or she is a treating physician or an independent medical examiner. However, there are significant differences between challenges faced by treating physicians and those faced by independent medical examiners. First, independent medical examiners have no ongoing contact with the patients they evaluate, and no responsibility to provide treatment. In contrast, treating physicians have the challenge of blending the *adjudicative role* they play when they perform disability evaluations with the *clinical role* they play in other interactions with patients (Robinson, 2002). Second, physicians who choose to become independent medical examiners do so only because they are willing to perform disability evaluations. They often make disability evaluation an important part of their professional activities, and take courses to enhance their ability to perform the evaluations. In contrast, treating physicians often have a distaste for performing disability evaluations, and have only minimal knowledge about how the evaluations should be performed.

This chapter focuses on practical strategies treating physicians use when they perform disability evaluations. It is important to note at the outset that it is impossible to write a step-by-step "guidebook" for conducting disability evaluations. The question "How do you evaluate disability in a patient with chronic pain?" is just as complex as the question "How do you provide medical or surgical care for a patient with chronic pain?" In both instances, a chapter can describe general principles, but the application of these principles to specific patients requires a good deal of clinical judgment.

One factor that contributes greatly to the complexity of disability evaluation is the diversity of the insurance companies and governmental agencies that administer disability programs. For example, in the United States, there are 50 state workers' compensation systems, three federal workers' compensation systems, two disability programs operated by the Social Security Administration (SSA), a Veterans Administration disability program, and several disability programs offered by private insurance companies. Also, many public assistance (welfare) programs provide disability benefits, and miscellaneous other programs (e.g., Medicare and Medicaid) deal to some extent with disability (Demeter, Andersson, & Smith, 1996; Rondinelli & Katz, 2000; Williams, 1991; Wolfe & Potter, 1996). Because of the multitude of disability programs, virtually any statement about disability is likely to have exceptions, and it is difficult even to define concepts unambiguously.

PROGRESS SINCE THE SECOND EDITION

Since the publication of this chapter in the second edition of *Handbook of Pain Assessment* in 2001, a few publications relevant to the assessment of pain-related impairment and disability have appeared. In particular, the American Medical Association (AMA) *Guides to the Evaluation of Permanent Impairment*, fifth edition (Cocchiarella & Andersson, 2001), and the AMA *Guides* sixth edition (Rondinelli, 2008), provide detailed discussions of problems in assessing impairment associated with pain. Also, the primary authors of the chapter on pain-related impairment in the fifth edition subsequently published a paper addressing conceptual issues regarding the evaluation of pain-related impairment (Robinson, Turk, & Loeser, 2004). The World Health Organization (2001) published an important conceptual model that addresses relations among impairment, activity restrictions, and disability. This has been adopted by other organizations, such as the AMA. Two law professors have published a detailed discussion of SSA regulations related to pain, along with crucial legal judgments regarding these regulations (Schneider & Simeone, 2001). Waddell (2004) has published a fascinating historical review of efforts by various jurisdictions in Canada to address pain-related disability. Finally, Robinson and Tait (2009) have written a chapter that describes the kinds of research that determine the validity of systems for rating pain-related impairment/disability, and summarizes the meager research to date.

Overall, though, a striking fact about impairment/disability evaluation in the context of chronic pain is that the scientific literature on the subject is so sparse. It is difficult to find empirical studies that address the reliability and validity of systems to assess impairment or disability among patients with chronic pain, or theoretical discussions of the issues involved in such assessments. The paucity of the scientific literature in this area is particularly striking when we consider the high prevalence of disability secondary to pain. For example, data from the Bureau of Labor Statistics (*www.bls.gov/iif/oshcdnew. htm*; retrieved January, 21, 2008) indicate that in 2003, 1,315,920 work injuries and occupational illnesses in the United States required a worker to take time off work. Of these, 43% were coded as sprains/strains, and 18% as back injuries. (These two categories overlap, since most back injuries are coded as back strains/sprains.) Bureau of Labor Statistics data on claims that require prolonged time away from work (more than 30 days) indicate similar trends: 43% of such claims were for sprains/strains, and 21.4% were for back injuries. These data on low back pain disorders and sprains/strains estimate the magnitude of the problem of pain-related disability, since there are typically few or no objective findings to corroborate patients' complaints of incapacitating pain in both kinds of disorders.

As a result of the lack of progress in either scientific research or conceptual analysis of pain-related impairment/disability, the concepts outlined in my chapter in the second edition of this handbook continue to be relevant, and the dilemmas faced by treating physicians who navigate the difficult waters of impairment/disability determination are the same as when the original chapter was published.

BASIC CONCEPTS

Disability

The two fundamental concepts in the area of disability are "impairment" and "disability." These terms do not have unique definitions, because different disability agencies define them in slightly different ways.

In its broadest meaning, *disability* refers to an inability to carry out necessary tasks in any important domain of life because of a medical condition. For example, a person with C5 quadriplegia is disabled in the sense of being unable to carry out many basic activities of daily living. This chapter focuses on the more restricted concept of *work disability*, which can be informally defined as the inability to work because of a medical condition.

Work disability can be subcategorized in several ways. The most important distinctions are between total and partial disability, and between temporary and permanent (or long-term) disability. Various disability agencies have programs tailored to these different categories of work disability. For example, the SSA programs are designed for people who are permanently and totally disabled; workers' compensation time loss benefits are paid to individuals who are totally, temporarily disabled; many private disability insurance policies provide benefits when an individual is disabled from performing his or her usual work, even if he or she is not totally disabled.

Impairment

In the United States, the most widely used system for assessing impairment is the one developed by the AMA and described in *Guides to the Evaluation of Permanent Impairment* (Rondinelli, 2008). The discussion of impairment in this chapter is based on concepts described in the *Guides*.

The *Guides* defines *impairment* as "A significant deviation, loss, or loss of use of any body structure or body function in an individual with a health condition, disorder, or disease" (p. 5). Impairment is important,

because it permits disability agencies to distinguish between medical and nonmedical causes of workplace failure. Disability programs provide benefits to people who fail in the workplace because of a medical condition (i.e., who have an impairment), but not to ones who fail in the workplace because of poor job skills or other nonmedical factors. If an applicant is judged to have no impairment, his or her application for disability is likely to be rejected.

The AMA *Guides* system permits a physician to make a qualitative judgment about whether a claimant has any impairment. Also, among claimants judged to have impairment, the system permits physicians to indicate *how much* impairment they have. To do this, an examining physicians starts by determining the severity of dysfunction in the organ or body part that is affected by a claimant's medical condition. He or she then consults a table that indicates the amount of *whole-person impairment* the claimant has. Whole-person impairment is measured on a scale from 0% (when there is no impairment) to 100% (when a person is completely incapacitated). In principle, this system permits physicians to quantify the burden of illness imposed by different types of disorders within an organ system (e.g., to compare impairment secondary to a fracture of the lumbar spine to impairment secondary to a persistent lumbar radiculopathy). It also permits comparisons between individuals with completely different kinds of medical disorders.

It should be noted that the AMA's quantitative system is difficult to interpret, because it is extremely abstract and embodies assumptions that have not been empirically validated. Consider, for example, one individual with significant cardiovascular disease and another with significant visual impairment. An examiner following the *Guides'* procedures might conclude that both individuals have whole-person impairment of 50%. But it is obvious that the functional limitations imposed by cardiovascular disease are entirely different from those imposed by visual impairment. There is no validated method for comparing the burden of illness borne by these two individuals.

The assessment of impairment is best construed as an intervening step in the determination of the issue that is most important to society—whether an individual is disabled from work. The linkages between severity of impairment and severity of work incapacitation (or probability of work incapacitation) have not been subjected to systematic research. Although disability agencies routinely assume that linkages exist, the *Guides* is much more cautious regarding this issue. It states:

> The Guides is not intended to be used for direct estimates of work participation restrictions. Impairment percentages derived according to the Guides' criteria do not directly measure work participation restrictions. ... In disability evaluation, the impairment rating is one of several determinants of disablement. (p. 6)

A few practical points need to be made about impairment and disability. First, despite rhetoric that can be found in various monographs (e.g., Rondinelli, 2008), the distinction between impairment and disability is often unclear (Robinson, 2002). Second, when a person seeking disability benefits is evaluated, the "bottom line" of the evaluation is the decision about whether he or she is actually disabled. The assessment of impairment is important, because it is an intervening step in the broader task of assessing disability. Finally, physicians are typically asked questions about both impairment and disability when they perform evaluations on patients. The discussion below focuses on disability evaluations; it assumes that when a physician performs a disability evaluation, the evaluation includes an impairment assessment.

Issues Addressed in Disability Evaluations

Physicians are typically asked to address the following when they conduct disability evaluations:

1. Diagnosis
2. Causation
3. Need for further treatment
4. Impairment
5. Physical capacities
6. Ability to work

Examples of the questions posed by disability agencies are listed in Table 21.1. The second column presents questions addressed to an independent medical examiner by a workers' compensation board. The patient was a woman who had sustained a non-catastrophic neck injury in the course of her work. The third column lists questions addressed to a physician treating a man for a non-work-related median neuropathy. The patient had a disability policy through a private insurance company, and the questions were written by the company. Table 21.1 is organized to show how questions were worded by the two agencies, and which key issues the questions addressed. Note that the questions from the workers' compensation board addressed all five of the issues listed earlier, whereas the questions from the private insurance company addressed only three of them. This reflects the different mandates of the two agencies: For example, workers' compensation programs are responsible only for injuries that occur at work, whereas many private disability programs provide benefits regardless of how a policyholder became disabled.

A fundamental goal of the disability evaluation process is to determine whether a patient can work. From this perspective, items 1–4 presented earlier can be viewed as preliminary items that set the stage for addressing the fifth and crucial question. For example, Figure 21.1 displays the type of algorithm that many disability agencies follow, at least when a patient is being evaluated for long-term or permanent disability.

Problems Associated with Disability Evaluation in Painful Conditions

Disability evaluation is a complex area for many reasons that have been discussed in other publications (Robinson, 2001, 2002, 2005, 2007b; Robinson & Seroussi, 2007; Robinson & Tait, 2009; Robinson & Turk, 2007), and are mentioned only briefly here.

1. Disability agencies have to a large extent defined the concepts and procedures to be used in disability evaluations. However sensible these concepts may be from a bureaucratic standpoint, they are often difficult for physicians to apply.

2. One central tenet of disability agencies is that impairment should be public and objectively measurable; that is, a skilled physi-

TABLE 21.1. Typical Issues Addressed and Specific Questions Asked in Disability Evaluations

Issue addressed	Specific questions asked	
	Workers' compensation system: Questions to independent medical examiner	Private insurance company: Questions to treating physician
Diagnosis	What are the diagnoses based on objective findings?	Diagnoses_____ Subjective Symptoms_____ Objective findings _____
Causation	Please state which, if any, of the diagnosed conditions are work related?	
Maximal medical improvement	Is Ms. X medically stable or has she reached preinjury status? What treatment would you recommend?	Has patient reached maximal medical improvement? Would any further therapy be reasonably expected to result in full or partial recovery?
Impairment rating	If Ms. X is medically stable, does she have a ratable permanent partial impairment according to the AMA *Guides*, fourth edition?	
Ability to work	Can Ms. X return to her job of injury? (Her job description is attached.)	1. Rate patient's physical impairment • Class 1—No limitation • Class 2—Capable of medium work • Class 3—Capable of light work • Class 4—Capable of sedentary work • Class 5—Incapable of minimal activity or sedentary work 2. Please describe fully how patient's symptoms/limitations affect ability to work. 3. Would job modification enable patient to work with impairment? 4. Would vocational counseling and/or retraining be recommended?

cian should be able to determine the nature and severity of a patient's impairment.

3. As a corollary of item 2 presented earlier, disability agencies focus on what might be called a "mechanical failure" model of impairment (Osterweis, Kleinman, & Mechanic, 1987). The assumption is that activity limitations of people are (or should be) closely linked to measurable evidence of failure or dysfunction in certain organs or body parts rather than to self-reported subjective barriers, such as anxiety or pain.

4. Disability is particularly difficult to evaluate in painful conditions precisely because they violate the assumption that impairment is objectively measurable and closely linked to mechanical failure of an organ or body part. Patients with chronic pain routinely complain of activity restrictions that cannot be fully understood in terms

of mechanical failure of some body part or organ. The mismatch between the subjective reports of patients with chronic pain and the objective evidence of mechanical failure of their organs creates a fundamental dilemma for a disability evaluator. At one extreme, the disability evaluator might ignore a patient's subjective appraisals and rely strictly on objective evidence of organ dysfunction. At the opposite extreme, the evaluator might rely strictly on the subjective appraisals and apparent activity restrictions of the patient, regardless of whether they can be objectified in terms of measurable failure or dysfunction of an organ. Finally, the evaluator might rate impairment on the basis of some composite of objective and subjective factors. No disability agency or disability evaluation system has offered an acceptable resolution to this dilemma.

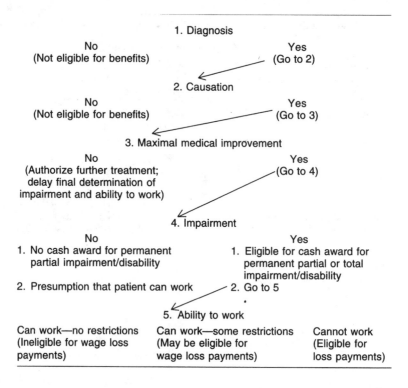

FIGURE 21.1. An algorithm for the evaluation of long-term disability.

PRACTICAL STRATEGIES FOR DISABILITY EVALUATION

Preliminaries: A Word of Caution

The discussion below is largely based on my experiences as a private practitioner, an attending physician at a university-based pain center, an independent medical examiner, and a consultant to the Washington State Department of Labor and Industries. It is *not* based on scientific data, because such data do not exist. For example, data on the reliability of disability evaluations are scanty (Clark et al., 1988; Clark & Haldeman, 1993). Research on concurrent or predictive validity of disability evaluations is also scanty, and suggests that they are fraught with error and bias. For example, studies have found that disability ratings at the time of closure of workers' compensation claims correlate poorly with functional and work status 2 years later (Tait, Chibnall, Andresen, & Hadler, 2006), and fail to compensate adequately for future earnings losses the workers experience (Reville, Seabury, Neuhauser, Burton, & Greenberg, 2005).

Also, there is evidence that physicians' judgments about disability are affected by the race of the claimants (Chibnall, Tait, Andresen, & Hadler, 2005). Given the paucity of scientific data, it is impossible to say what decision-making strategies are appropriate when one performs disability evaluations. In this ambiguous situation, it is easy for practitioners (and authors of chapters) to fall into the trap of believing they are making valid judgments, when in fact their judgments are based on a variety of biases (Gilovich, 1991; Robinson, 2001).

Conceptual Issues

• *What ethical issues do you encounter when you perform disability evaluations?* It is beyond the scope of this chapter to discuss ethical dilemmas in disability evaluation in any detail. Suffice it to say that such dilemmas abound, and that they are particularly acute when a physician evaluates a patient he or she is treating. Many of these dilemmas are discussed in a thoughtful paper by Sullivan and Loeser (1992).

Some of the most difficult dilemmas involve trust. Patients put their trust in treating physicians, because they expect their physicians to be advocates for them. Although physicians are often forced to balance the needs of patients against other factors, such as the cost of medical care, most of them perceive themselves as putting the needs of their patients first. Thus, a kind of symmetry exists: Patients place their trust in physicians, and physicians reciprocate by acting as agents for patients.

When physicians perform disability evaluations on patients they are treating, there is a potential for them to abuse the trust that patients have placed in them. Sullivan and Loeser (1992) describe the dilemma as follows:

> Encounters between physician and patient for the purposes of treating and rating disability create fundamentally different relationships. When the aim of medical diagnosis is the selection of effective treatment for the patient's pain, the physician acts as agent for the patient. When the aim of diagnosis is rating the patient's disability, the physician acts as agent for the state. The purpose of the former encounter is to reduce suffering; the purpose of the latter encounter is to assign compensation as mandated by law or regulation. If two different physicians perform these tasks, there is little chance for confusion about the nature of the relationship on the part of the patient. If one individual is performing both functions, the potential for confusion and exploitation of trust is higher. (p. 1830)

Sullivan and Loeser (1992) conclude that physicians should refuse to perform disability evaluations on patients they are treating. Unfortunately, this option is frequently not available to a treating physician. If a physician refuses to complete a disability form, several adverse consequences ensue. Sometimes, the patient's disability benefits are summarily halted. In other situations, the disability agency refuses to pay the physician for his or her clinical services. Some disability agencies have the legal right to impose fines on physicians who do not submit disability forms. In essence, physicians frequently have no choice other than to fill out a disability form on patients they are treating. When they do this, however, they need to be aware that they are treading on morally ambiguous terrain.

• *What are your attitudes toward disability?* Some physicians empathize with patients who are applying for disability. They believe that the patients are likely to experience severe emotional and physical stress if economic circumstances force them to remain in the workforce. At the opposite extreme, some physicians perceive disability applicants as con artists who are trying to manipulate "the system" and get benefits they do not deserve. The available evidence suggests that both of these perspectives are oversimplified.

First, for most workers, the workplace provides many benefits. In addition to financial rewards, work provides social contacts and binds people to the community. The psychosocial benefits of work can best be appreciated by the extensive research on unemployment among people who are not disabled. The general thrust of this research is that when people are separated from the workplace, for example, by being laid off during an economic recession, they and their families are at increased risk for a number of adverse outcomes, including depression, anxiety, substance abuse, social isolation, family dissolution, and suicide (Atkinson, Liem, & Liem, 1986; Hammarstrom & Janlert, 1997; Kaplan, Roberts, Camacho, & Coyne, 1987; Mrazek & Haggerty, 1994; Rahmqvist & Carstensen, 1998). The implication of this research is clear: The mental health of most people—even those with significant medical problems—is better served by remaining in the workforce than by leaving it.

Second, in addition to the psychological losses associated with separation from the work environment, injured workers suffer severe economic losses when they go on disability (Reno, Mashaw, & Gradison, 1997). Thus, the notion that disabled people are "milking the system" is almost certainly wrong (Robinson & Loeser, in press). In fact, one of the tragedies of disability is that everyone seems to lose—the injured workers, their families, the people who pay disability insurance premiums, and society at large.

Third, many observers of disability systems have speculated that the process of interacting with disability agencies has detrimental effects on patients (Robinson & Loeser, in press; Robinson, Rondinelli, & Scheer, 1997). For example, Hadler (1996) has argued that as patients try to prove their incapacitation to disability adjudicators, they become more and more convinced that they really are disabled. Some observers have suggested the term "disability syndrome" to describe the set of dysfunctional attitudes and beliefs that develops over time as a person adapts to the role of being a disabled person. Thus, patients who seem straightforward and highly motivated soon after injuries often become more resistant to rehabilitation later on (Krause & Ragland, 1994; Robinson et al., 1997).

"Disability syndrome" is an inferred construct that is difficult to validate. But it is at least consistent with studies demonstrating that a significant number of people seem to get "stuck" in disability systems. For example, research indicates that after a person has been awarded disability benefits by the SSA, the probability is only about 3% that he or she will ever return to the workforce (Muller, 1992). Also, numerous studies on disabled workers with industrial compensation claims have shown that the while vast majority of them return to work within a few weeks after injury, those who are still disabled 6 months after injury have a high probability of protracted disability (Cheadle et al., 1994; Robinson, 1998).

• *How much do you know about the disability agencies with which you interact?* When physicians perform disability evaluations on their patients, they act as intermediaries between the patients and various agencies that provide benefits for people who are disabled from work. To understand disability evaluation, one needs to have some understanding of these disability agencies, since they typically define the issues that must be addressed in a disability evaluation.

Unfortunately, this understanding is difficult to achieve, in part because of the enormous heterogeneity of disability agencies and the programs they administer. Also, the policies and practices a disability agency follows when it determines eligibility for benefits are generally not available to physicians. In this ambiguous situation, physicians can increase their understanding substantially by reviewing monographs that deal with disability agencies and disability evaluation (Demeter et al., 1996; Osterweis et al., 1987; Rondinelli & Katz, 2000). Also,

if physicians are observant as they perform disability evaluations on patients, they can learn a lot about the disability agencies with which they interact.

• *How do you integrate disability EVALUATION into an overall strategy of disability MANAGEMENT?* This chapter focuses on disability evaluation. In practical situations, however, treating physicians do not do disability evaluations in isolation. Broadly speaking, a treating physician needs to develop strategies for disability *management* for patients he or she is treating (Robinson, 2005). Disability management encompasses at least four areas: assessment of disability risk, establishment of a treatment contract with a patient, prevention of disability, and evaluation of disability. These areas are linked; thus, if a physician fails to assess disability risk adequately or to develop reasonable disability prevention strategies, he or she will probably find disability evaluation particularly difficult.

• *How much importance do you give to the subjective appraisals that patients make regarding their ability to work?* At one extreme, a physician might accept more or less at face value what patients say about their physical capacities. Such a physician would run the risk of being duped by patients with chronic pain and/or greatly underestimating capacities of the patients. At the opposite extreme, a physician might try to make decisions about the disability status of patients strictly on the basis of objective findings, and react skeptically to reports of incapacitation that are not closely linked to objective findings.

A position somewhere between these two extremes is probably most appropriate. The perceptions patients have about their abilities certainly should not be ignored or automatically discounted. As a practical matter, research demonstrates that these self-appraisals are important predictors of whether patients with pain problems perform well on physical tests and/or succeed in getting off disability (Fishbain, Cutler, Rosomoff, Khalil, & Steele-Rosomoff, 1997, 1999; Hazard, Bendix, & Fenwick, 1991; Hidding et al., 1994; Hildebrandt, Pfingsten, Saur, & Jansen, 1997; Kaplan, Wurtele, & Gillis, 1996). Thus, physicians who make disability decisions without considering patients' appraisals are discarding valuable data. As a result, their decisions can go awry in two ways. First, they can pressure patients to return to work in jobs that the patients are realistically not capable of performing. Second, they may be completely ineffective in resolving disability issues. Consider, for example, a patient who is released to work by his physician, even though he is convinced that he is unable to work. Such a patient (or his attorney) is likely to seek out a different physician who will provide a different opinion regarding his disability. In this setting, the physician who released the patient for work might believe that he or she has successfully gotten the patient off disability, but the belief is illusory.

But the fact that patients' perceptions are important does not mean that they are valid, or that they are immutable. In fact, research suggests just the opposite, that is, that chronic pain patients often have distorted views of their capabilities, and that these views are modifiable (Alaranta et al., 1994; Estlander, Mellin, Vanharanta, & Hupli, 1991; Jensen, Turner, & Romano, 1994; Lipchik, Milles, & Covington, 1993). These results have implications for both the evaluation and the management of disability by a treating physician. When performing a disability evaluation, the physician needs to consider the validity of a patient's stated activity limitations in light of the biomedical information available and his or her assessment of the patient's credibility. He or she should reserve the right to challenge the patient's self-assessments and to make decisions that are discordant with these assessments. In the course of treatment, the treating physician needs to promote change in perceptions that are unduly self-defeating and medically unsubstantiated.

It is worth noting that such challenges are likely to be met with resistance. Patients with chronic pain generally do not welcome suggestions by physicians that their perceptions are inaccurate. Their message is often something like "I am the only one who really knows about my pain. You outsiders can only guess." Thus, a treating physician needs to approach the issue of inaccurate perceptions with a good deal of tact.

In summary, the treating physician should carefully assess pain patients' perceptions regarding their ability to perform various tasks, and, whenever feasible, should render disability judgments that are consistent with these perceptions. But this does not mean that the physician should let pain patients control the terms of discussion about disability or the outcomes of disability evaluations. Instead, the physician should be ready to challenge the appraisals of patients when he or she believes that they are inaccurate.

Mechanics

Overview

Table 21.2 provides an algorithm that can help you approach disability evaluations systematically. The major sections are as follows:

1. Before the disability form arrives
2. Initial review of the disability form
3. Getting additional data
4. Addressing the main questions
5. Objective findings
6. Psychogenic pain
7. Filling out the disability form
8. Follow-up

TABLE 21.2. Overview of Steps During Disability Evaluation

1. Before the disability form arrives
   a. Initial assessment of risk for protracted disability
   b. Contracting
2. Initial review of the disability form
   a. Who should fill out the form?
   b. What disability agency is requesting the form?
   c. What issues are you asked to address?
   d. Overall assessment of the patient
   e. Assessment of patient credibility
   f. Discussion of the form with the patient
3. Getting additional data
4. Addressing the main questions
   a. Diagnosis
   b. Causation
   c. Need for further treatment
   d. Impairment
   e. Ability to work
5. Objective findings
6. Psychogenic pain
7. Filling out the disability form
8. Follow-up

Before the Disability Form Arrives

INITIAL ASSESSMENT OF RISK
FOR PROTRACTED DISABILITY

You will do a better job of responding to disability requests if you have thought about the disability issues that might arise for a particular patient, and have done some preliminary work to resolve or mitigate these (Robinson, 2005). You should at least do a preliminary analysis of several issues at the time of initial evaluation of patients. You may well revise your assessment of these issues as you learn more about a patient.

1. A key issue is that you should assess the current disability status of every pain patient when you first evaluate him or her. Is the patient currently working? If so, is he or she struggling on the job because of pain, or missing a lot of time from work? If the patient is not working, is this because of his or her health or for some other reason? If the patient is disabled from work, how long has he or she been disabled? Is there any history of disability or work instability prior to the index injury for which the patient is seeing you?

2. In addition to obtaining factual information about the disability status of patients, you should assess their perceptions regarding disability. What barriers to return to work do they identify? Are they optimistic or pessimistic about the probability of returning to work? Do they believe that their employers and the workers' compensation system have treated them fairly? Remember that patients' perceptions are important predictors of the actual outcomes of claims.

3. You should look for risk factors for protracted disability as you carry out the history and physical examination. There is no single list of such risk factors. Research has demonstrated a few factors (Stover, Wickizer, Zimmerman, Fulton-Kehoe, & Franklin, 2007; Turner et al., 2008), and expert panels have proposed much longer lists of risk factors (Frymoyer & Cats-Baril, 1987; Washington State Department of Labor and Industries, 1999). Table 21.3 lists a set of risk factors identified on the basis of input from physicians in the Washington State Medical Association and senior claims adjudicators at the Washington State Department

of Labor and Industries. Note that the list includes factors in the environment around the patient, rather than just personal attributes of the patient. This reflects the opinion of experts that factors external to an individual patient have a substantial bearing on the likelihood that the patient will become chronically disabled. Some of these "systems issues" are difficult for a clinician to assess, especially when parties to a claim have a hidden agenda of some kind.

4. Without being unduly cynical, you need to be aware of the possibility that any participant in a disability claim can have a hidden agenda. Opportunities for deception are particularly rich in workers' compensation claims.

a. An extensive medical literature on secondary gain, compensation neurosis, and malingering has dealt with hidden agendas of patients (Bellamy, 1997; Fishbain, Rosomoff, Cutler, & Rosomoff, 1995; Loeser, Henderlite, & Conrad, 1995; Mendelson, 1988; Robinson & Loeser, in press; Voiss, 1995). Most experts in disability believe that frank malingering or deception is uncommon among patients who seem to report excessive disability, but you should be alert to the following:
   • Is there any evidence that a patient who claims to be disabled is "double dipping" (i.e., working at the same time he or she is getting disability benefits)?
   • Is there evidence from surveillance tapes or other collateral sources that a patient's physical capabilities are far greater than he or she claims?

b. Other parties to a workers' compensation claim—including employers and adjudicators for disability agencies—can have hidden agendas. Their agendas have been ignored almost completely in research on disability (Dembe & Boden, 2000), so you need to use clinical judgment in deciding whether participants in a disability claim are behaving in a deceptive manner. You should consider the following:
   • Is there evidence that the disability system is "playing hardball" with the patient? For example, does it appear that the patient has had his or her claim closed arbitrarily? Has the compensa-

TABLE 21.3. Proposed List of Risk Factors for Prolonged Disability

Group 1: Catastrophic—*Cases with catastrophic injuries are very likely to benefit from medical case management*
- ☐ 1. Catastrophic

Group 2A: High Risk—*Cases with any of these factors are likely to benefit from medical case management, unless there is clear evidence the worker is about to return to work.*
- ☐ 1. Hospitalized within 28 days of injury, for reasons related to industrial injury
- ☐ 2. Worker who is 45 years old or older with carpal tunnel syndrome
- ☐ 3. 90 or more days of time loss

Group 2B: High Risk—*The presence of one or more of the following may indicate an increased likelihood of long-term disability and, therefore, some potential benefit from case management or other intensive services.*

A. Medical Factors
- ☐ 1. Presence of secondary medical condition
- ☐ 2. Injury to dominant hand
- ☐ 3. Hospitalized within 28 days of injury for reasons unrelated to industrial injury
- ☐ 4. Pre-existing psychiatric conditions

B. Injury Descriptions
- ☐ 1. Non-overt injury—injury occurring in course of usual work activities
- ☐ 2. No objective findings on examinations
- ☐ 3. Diagnosis not consistent with injury description
- ☐ 4. Time gap in report of injury
- ☐ 5. Unwitnessed accident

C. Provider/Patient Factors
- ☐ 1. No identifiable treatment plan or goals
- ☐ 2. Over-utilization of health care delivery systems and services by either patient or provider, or over-referral by physician. May include frequent changes of attending physician
- ☐ 3. Misuse of scheduled medications by patient
- ☐ 4. Physician fostering illness beliefs
- ☐ 5. Number of surgeries both related and unrelated to work-related problem. May include a number of unsuccessful surgeries in the same area.
- ☐ 6. Spread of diagnosis over time; newly contended diagnosis
- ☐ 7. No documented medical progress

D. Psychosocial Factors
- ☐ 1. Exaggerated illness behavior: Presence of non-organic signs (Waddell signs); no objective findings.
- ☐ 2. Evidence of abuse of alcohol, illicit drug or prescription medication
- ☐ 3. Presence of depression or avoidance anxiety, post-traumatic disorder or other dysphoric affects (for example, anger at employer or supervisor or L&I [Washington State Department of Labor and Industries])
- ☐ 4. History of childhood abuse, physical or sexual abuse, substance abuse in caretaker or family instability
- ☐ 5. Presence of personality traits or disorders. For example, presence of specific somatization traits or problematic interpersonal relationships; arrests

E. Demographic Factors
- ☐ 1. Low educational level, including illiteracy
- ☐ 2. English not primary language
- ☐ 3. Age greater than 50 and employed in heavy industry
- ☐ 4. Back or lower extremity injury with medium or heavy labor employment
- ☐ 5. Nearing retirement age

F. Job Factors
- ☐ 1. Anger at employer
- ☐ 2. Employer anger at worker
- ☐ 3. Miscellaneous employer factors: seasonal work, strike, plant closure, job becoming obsolete, etc.
- ☐ 4. Loss of job in which the injury occurred
- ☐ 5. Singular work history in heavy industry
- ☐ 6. Complaints of inability to function

(cont.)

TABLE 21.3. *(cont.)*

☐ 7. History of poor job performance, frequent job change, short duration of employment, job
      dissatisfaction or job termination prior to claims filing
•   8. Employer or worker not active in return-to-work efforts
☐ 9. Worker is not clearly headed back to work
☐ 10. Perception of the worker that he or she will be retrained "for a better job" or other misperceptions
      of L&I vocational entitlement

G. Administrative Factors
☐ 1. Third-party involvement
☐ 2. Recent claim closures; application for reopening
☐ 3. Employer protest
☐ 4. Current income, including time-loss, compares favorably to net income prior to injury.
☐ 5. Multiple L&I claims (may include a number of previous claims)
☐ 6. Loss of driver's license or other credentials
☐ 7. Loss of medical insurance
☐ 8. Originally non-time-loss claim that has become time-loss
☐ 9. Non-compliance with medical or vocational treatment
☐ 10. Worker or physician perception that L&I is unresponsive or adversarial

Note. From Washington State Department of Labor and Industries (1999). In the public domain.

tion carrier refused to authorize services requested by the attending physician? Does it appear that the patient's claims manager is requesting multiple evaluations in order to maneuver the patient out of the disability system on the basis of "preponderance of evidence"?

• Is there any indication that the patient's former employer has created misleading job descriptions, put pressure on the patient not to file a workers' compensation claim, or fired the patient in apparent response to the patient's report of injury (Scherzer, Rugulies, & Krause, 2005; Shannon & Lowe, 2002)?

5. Based on items 1–4 above, you should formulate some preliminary assessment of the patient's risk for protracted disability.

CONTRACTING

Your ability to respond to disability forms is also enhanced if you establish ground rules with patients at the beginning of treatment. At the very least, it is advisable to describe your approach to disability management and disability evaluation to the patient. Also, indicate what you expect from the patient in the area of disability. For example, some physicians treat disabled patients only if the patients express a commitment to return to work.

Initial Review of the Disability Form

1. You should first consider whether you are the most appropriate person to fill out the form. For example, suppose you are acting as a pain consultant for a general physician who has been treating a patient for an extended period of time. In such a scenario, it might well be most appropriate for the general physician to fill out disability forms.

2. You should review the form and identify the disability agency that has sent it. Do you know anything about that agency? (If not, you may end up filling out the form in a way that leads to problems for you or your patient later.) Also, you should determine which of the six key issues—diagnosis, causation, need for further treatment, impairment, physical capacities, and ability to work—you are being asked to assess and try to formulate tentative answers, identifying in the process important information gaps.

3. As you consider your answers, formulate an overall assessment of the patient with respect to disability issues. It is often best to think of a narrative that you might write to describe the patient. This (imaginary) narrative should address the five basic issues to the extent that they are relevant to the patient you are evaluating.

4. Your overall assessment should include a consideration of the credibility of the patient you have been asked to evaluate. The rationale for this is simple but compelling.

As noted earlier, disability assessment of patients with chronic pain is difficult primarily because patients' statements about their activity limitations often cannot be easily rationalized in terms of objectively measurable organ pathology. As a practical matter, if you consider a patient's statements about his or her incapacitation to be valid, you will be more likely to judge him or her as being disabled than if you make a judgment based strictly on organ pathology. The question then becomes: Should your patient's statements be accepted as valid? To answer this, you must decide whether the statements are credible.

The importance of patient credibility has been acknowledged by the SSA, the administrative body that administers the largest disability programs in the United States (Social Security Ruling, 1996). However, neither the SSA nor any other disability agency (as far as I am aware) gives any specific guidelines about how to assess patient credibility. Table 21.4 lists factors thought to be relevant to patient credibility. Be aware, though, that the list has not been validated, and that research on deception by medical patients suggests that physicians are not particularly good at assessing patient credibility (Faust, 1995; Hall & Pritchard, 1996).

It is important to note that treating physicians have an advantage over independent medical examiners in the assessment of patient credibility. A major reason for this is that treating physicians have the opportunity to observe their patients over extended periods of time. As they observe the consistency of physical findings over repeated examinations and patients' responses to various therapies, physicians gradually gain a sense about the credibility of their patients.

5. Discuss the form with the patient. At the very least, let the patient know that you received a request for information about his or her disability status. To the extent feasible, find out how your patient believes you should answer questions on the disability form. In particular, it is helpful to the get the patient's view of his or her physical limitations. Also, it is important to see whether the patient challenges any of the factual information provided along with the disability form. For example, it is not uncommon for patients to object strenuously to the information provided in job analyses.

Getting Additional Data

Physicians sometimes find that they need additional information to fill out a disability form responsibly. For example, additional past medical records are sometimes crucial. These might include a report of the initial injury or records from physicians who treated the patient soon after the injury. Sometimes, medical records covering the period prior to the index injury are extremely informative (Mustard & Hertzman, 2001).

Sometimes a disability form will prompt you to do an overall clinical reassessment of your patient. This could consist of a thorough re-examination in your office, or updated radiological or laboratory tests.

You may also need objective data regarding the physical capacities of a patient. Objective performance data can be obtained from a functional capacities evaluation, or from a work hardening program or a pain center (see below).

Finally, you may need input from a patient's employer. This is particularly important when the patient alleges that the employer has provided distorted information about the demands of his job. One way to clarify the demands of a job is to meet with both the patient and a representative of the company for which he or she has worked.

TABLE 21.4. Characteristics Associated with High Patient Credibility

1. No preexisting condition
2. No medical comorbidities
3. Definite stimulus (e.g., crushed by a tree)
4. Definite tissue damage (e.g., fracture)
5. Symptoms, signs, activity limitations fit expectations for the medical problem
6. Consistent findings over repeated examinations
7. No exaggerated pain behavior
8. No inconsistencies between symptoms/signs noted in physician's office and behavior outside the office
9. No chronic psychiatric disorders or long-term psychosocial risk factors
10. No reactive psychiatric problems (e.g., anxiety disorder, depression)
11. Patient motivated to return to productivity
12. Job opportunities exist
13. No incentives for disability

Note. Adapted from Robinson (1997).

Addressing the Main Questions

DIAGNOSIS

You will generally not have difficulty providing a diagnosis for a patient. You should be aware, though, that adjudicators sometimes make inferences about causation on the basis of a diagnosis. For example, if you diagnose a patient as having lumbar degenerative disc disease (ICD 722.52), an adjudicator might take the position that the patient's back pain is not caused by a specific accident.

CAUSATION

Concepts that are helpful in the assessment of causation are given in Table 21.5. Causation is important when a patient is seeking disability benefits from an agency that is responsible only for medical conditions that arise in certain circumstances. For example, workers' compensation carriers are responsible only for conditions that arise out of employment; automobile insurance carriers are responsible only for injuries that occur in motor vehicle accidents. The assessment of causation is difficult both conceptually (Kramer & Lane, 1992; Lakoff & John-

TABLE 21.5. Factors to Consider in Assessing Causation

1. Did the patient have similar problem prior to index event?
2. Was the nature of the accident consistent with the patient's present problem?
3. Is there any biological marker that clearly and specifically ties the patient's problems to the accident (e.g., complete quadriplegia)?
   a. Alternatives:
      • Biological marker with uncertain relation to exposure (e.g., carpal tunnel syndrome)
      • No biological marker (e.g., headaches)
4. Is the patient's problem mentioned in initial medical evaluation following injury?
5. Is there a paper trail (i.e., a record of ongoing treatment, and consistency of symptoms and findings)?
6. Did the patient have any other injuries after the index injury?
7. Are symptoms/signs on your initial exam interpretable? Credible?
8. Are findings consistent over time on repeated examination?
9. Are there any reinforcers that might give the patient an incentive to manipulate you?
10. Overall, how credible do you find the patient?

son, 1999) and practically. This is particularly true for patients who have cumulative trauma disorders and/or disorders without clear-cut biological markers. Another difficult situation arises when a patient sustains an injury to a body part that has previously been injured. For example, a patient who has undergone a lumbar discectomy in the remote past may report a return of radicular symptoms after falling down. In this kind of setting, a disability agency may ask you to apportion causation of the patient's impairment between the index injury and his or her preexisting lumbar disc condition.

It is worth noting that disability agencies differ significantly in the standard they set for establishing causation. Some agencies follow the principle that for an index injury to be accepted as the cause of a patient's impairment, the injury must be the major factor contributing to the impairment. Others adopt a much lower standard of causation described as "lighting up." When this standard applies, an index injury may be viewed as the cause of an impairment even when the injury is minor and impairment is severe. For example, consider an individual with multiple knee surgeries who falls at work, develops an effusion in the knee, and is told by an orthopedist that he needs a total knee replacement. If the individual's workers' compensation carrier operates under the "lighting up" standard of causation, this person's knee symptoms and need for a total knee replacement would be viewed as being caused by his slip and fall.

Also, it is important to note that the legislative and regulatory bodies that determine standards for causation of injuries typically provide no guidance about how to apply the standards in specific cases. As an example, in 2006, the Alaska legislature mandated that a new standard be used to determine whether a work exposure caused an injury. Prior to 2006, an exposure was judged to be the cause of a condition (and, therefore, the responsibility of the workers' compensation system) if the exposure was "a substantial factor" in the onset of the condition. In 2006, the standard was changed, so that the exposure had to be "the substantial factor" in onset of the condition. However, no specific information was given by the legislature about how to apply this new standard. Thus, when evaluating a patient who presents with axial lumbar spine pain that he attributes to his work, a physician would understandably be uncertain about how to apply the new standard. Does it require objective evidence of damage to the spine, such as fracture? Does it require the worker to have been exposed to a very severe injury stimulus, such as falling from a roof? Does it require the worker to have engaged in some unusual work activity when his symptoms developed? Does it preclude workers who were receiving care for a lumbar spine disorder just prior to the alleged injury? Since the legislature did not address any of these questions when it established the new standard, the stage was set for different physicians to interpret the standard differently and, therefore, to disagree about whether an alleged injury is in fact the substantial cause of a worker's symptoms.

Physicians should indicate the factors they consider when they make a causation assessment, and indicate when their statements about causation are based on their medical training as opposed to common sense that a nonphysician would use. For example, suppose a patient has alleged that she injured her lower back in an automobile accident, and that review of records reveals that she was already receiving treatment for low back pain when the accident occurred. The historical information would cast ambiguity on the causal role of the motor vehicle accident in her current back pain. However, the ambiguity would be equally apparent to a nonphysician and a physician.

NEED FOR FURTHER TREATMENT

Table 21.6 lists factors to consider in determining whether a patient needs further treatment. It is important to be aware, though, that the determination of whether a patient needs additional treatment is fraught with ambiguity.

Disability agencies generally adopt an idealized model of the course of recovery following an injury. The model, shown in Figure 21.2, embodies the assumption that people show rapid improvement following injury, then level off and reach a plateau. Before patients reach this hypothetical plateau, they presumably can benefit from further treatment. When they reach the plateau, they are considered to have achieved maximal medical improvement (MMI). When a patient has

TABLE 21.6. Issues to Consider in Determining Whether a Patient Needs Further Treatment

1. Is the patient's condition best construed as:
   a. A distinct injury
   b. A repetitive strain (overuse) syndrome
   c. A disease
2. How long does it usually take for people with this condition to recover, or to reach a stable plateau?
   a. Is there a predictable course?
   b. Is patient's condition likely to get worse in the future?
3. How much time has elapsed since the index condition began?
4. What has been the trend over time with respect to function of the affected organ or body part?
   a. Steady improvement
   b. Steady
   c. Deterioration
   d. Widely fluctuating
5. What has been the trend of time with respect to the patient's symptoms?
   a. Steady improvement
   b. Steady
   c. Deterioration
   d. Widely fluctuating
6. Does the patient have concurrent medical conditions that obscure recovery curve from the index condition?
7. Has the patient had access to treatment approaches that are appropriate for his condition?

reached MMI, insurance companies and/or disability agencies typically refuse to pay for additional medical care, and attempt to make a final determination regarding a patient's impairment and work capacity. From an administrative perspective, the model is convenient, because it provides guidelines for intervention and decision making. For example, when a patient has reached a plateau in treatment, as demonstrated by a failure to improve during a significant period of time, curative treatment should be abandoned, and a permanent partial impairment rating should be made.

Unfortunately, patients frequently present with clinical problems that are hard to conceptualize in terms of the idealized recovery shown in Figure 21.2. The difficulties in this area are myriad. For example, it is not at all clear that patients with repetitive strain injuries should be expected to follow the trajectory shown in Figure 21.2. Another problem is that patients may have comorbidities that complicate recovery and make it difficult to

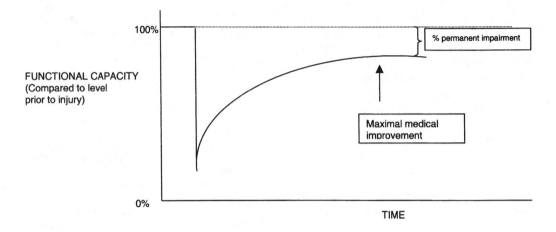

FIGURE 21.2. Hypothetical recovery curve following an injury.

determine when they have reached MMI. An example is a diabetic who has a work-related carpal tunnel syndrome in addition to a peripheral polyneuropathy.

A final complication of the MMI concept is that a patient who has reached maximal benefit from a particular kind of treatment may not have reached maximal benefit from treatment in general. For example, consider a patient who is examined 6 months after a low back injury. Assume that her treatment has consisted entirely of chiropractic care during the 6-month interval, and that she has not shown any measurable improvement during the past 2 months. This patient might be judged to have reached maximal medical benefit *from chiropractic care*, but an examining physician would understandably be uncertain about whether she could benefit from physical therapy, epidural steroids, lumbar surgery, aggressive use of various medications, or other therapies not provided by her chiropractor. This problem is not just a hypothetical one, since examiners routinely find that even patients with very chronic pain have not had exposure to all the plausible treatment approaches for their condition.

One other consideration that is extremely important for a treating physician does not bear on the process of determining MMI, but it does bear on the consequences that follow the determination that a patient has reached MMI. Disability and health insurance companies typically take the position that no more medical treatment should be authorized after a patient has reached MMI. This administrative perspective frequently does not match the clinical needs of the patient. For example, a patient may have reached MMI from a low back injury in the sense that a significant period of time has elapsed since injury, and no further curative treatment is available. But the individual might still need *maintenance* treatment for his condition—for example, ongoing medication. This issue is often ignored by agencies that administer benefits.

IMPAIRMENT

As described earlier, *impairments* are deficits in the functioning of organs or body parts. Disability agencies routinely insist that applicants for disability benefits have impairments. The logic of this requirement is straightforward. In order to carry out their mandate of providing benefits for people who are unable to work because of a medical condition, disability agencies must distinguish between people who are unemployed because of a medical condition and those who are unemployed for nonmedical reasons (e.g., lack of job skills or a depressed economy). Agencies rely on evidence of impairment when they make this distinction.

Disability systems typically indicate the procedures that physicians must follow in determining the presence and severity of patients' impairments. The most elaborate and widely used system to determine impairment is the one described in the American

Medical Association's *Guides to the Evaluation of Permanent Impairment* (Rondinelli, 2008). It is beyond the scope of this chapter to discuss this system in detail. However, it should be noted that the system in the *Guides* is extremely ambitious. It describes methods for rating impairments in a wide range of medical disorders. Also, it allows examiners not only to determine whether an impairment exists but also how severe (on a scale of 0–100%) the impairment is.

Although many disability agencies require physicians to rate impairment on the basis of the AMA's *Guides*, this is not always the case. An important exception is the SSA, which has a very different system for determining impairment in the evaluation of applicants for Social Security Disability Insurance (SSDI) or Supplemental Security Income (SSI; *Disability Evaluation under Social Security*, 2006). The SSA requires that an applicant have some impairment but eschews the quantification of impairment that is fundamental to the AMA *Guides*. Among applicants with evidence of some kind of impairment, the SSA has a two-tier system. It has created a set of "listings" that describe impairments severe enough to provide prima facie evidence that an applicant warrants SSDI or SSI benefits. If an applicant has an impairment that does not match one of the listings, he or she might still be awarded SSDI or SSI benefits, but the disability determination process becomes more complex.

PHYSICAL CAPACITIES

The assessment of physical capacities is a precursor to the determination of a patient's ability to work. Disability agencies typically request detailed physical capacities data and usually provide supplementary forms for this purpose. Figure 21.3 provides an example of a typical physical capacities form.

Table 21.7 outlines issues to consider in assessing the physical capacities of your patient. In general, a clinical evaluation in your office will not provide the detailed physical capacities information you will need to fill out a physical capacities form. You can supplement information gleaned from your clinical evaluation in a variety of ways.

The simplest way is to ask the patient to estimate his or her capacities. Consider filling out a physical capacities form on the basis of a patient's reports if you judge the patient to be highly credible, or if you do not have access to objective data regarding the patient's capacities. (If you follow this approach, you should indicate this on the form.)

Another way to obtain physical capacities data is to refer a patient for a functional capacity evaluation (FCE) (King, Tuckwell, & Barrett, 1998; Lechner, 1998; Rondinelli & Katz, 2000). An FCE is a formal, standardized assessment, typically performed by a physical therapist. It typically lasts from 2 to 5 hours. The therapist gathers information about a patient's strength, mobility, and endurance in tasks related to the work the patient is expected to do. As noted by King and colleagues (1998), FCEs are popular with insurance carriers and attorneys, because they provide objective performance data. However, in a comprehensive review, King and colleagues noted that virtually no data validate FCEs against actual job performance. In the past few years, some validity studies have been done on FCEs. They suggest that the ability of FCE results to predict recovery from work disability is modest at best (Gross & Battié, 2005, 2006).

Finally, a physician can get physical capacities data on a patient by referring him or her to a functional restoration program, a pain center, or a work-hardening program (Hildebrandt et al., 1997; Mayer, 1988; Niemeyer, Jacobs, Reynolds-Lynch, Bettencourt, & Lang, 1994). A common feature of both programs is that they assess physical capacities and provide treatment designed to improve those capacities. The performance data from one of these programs have more face validity than performance data from an FCE, because functional restoration programs, work-hardening programs, and pain centers typically observe performance over a few weeks, and indicate what patients can do after they have completed rehabilitative treatment.

ABILITY TO WORK

As noted earlier, the ability of a patient to work is in many respects the key issue in a disability evaluation. In essence, disability agencies are required to make wage compensation payments to patients if, and only if, the patients are judged not to be employ-

1. In an 8-hour workday, this patient can:

	TOTAL AT ONE TIME (hours)	TOTAL DURING 8-HR DAY (hours)
A. Sit	0 ½ 1 2 3 4 5 6 7 8	0 ½ 1 2 3 4 5 6 7 8
B. Stand	0 ½ 1 2 3 4 5 6 7 8	0 ½ 1 2 3 4 5 6 7 8
C. Walk	0 ½ 1 2 3 4 5 6 7 8	0 ½ 1 2 3 4 5 6 7 8

2. Patient can lift:

	Never	Occasionally	Frequently	Continuously
Up to 5 lbs				
5–10 lbs				
11–20 lbs				
21–25 lbs				
26–50 lbs				
51–100 lbs				

3. Patient can carry:

	Never	Occasionally	Frequently	Continuously
Up to 5 lbs				
5–10 lbs				
11–20 lbs				
21–25 lbs				
26–50 lbs				
51–100 lbs				

4. Patient is able to:

	Never	Occasionally	Frequently	Continuously
Bend				
Squat				
Crawl				
Climb				
Crouch				
Kneel				
Stoop				
Reach overhead				

5. Patient can use hands for repetitive actions such as:

	Simple Grasp	Push/Pull	Fine Manipulation
Right:	__Yes __No	__Yes __No	__Yes __No
Left:	__Yes __No	__Yes __No	__Yes __No

6. Patient can use feet for repetitive movements, as in operating foot controls:

Right	Left	Both
__Yes __No	__Yes __No	__Yes __No

KEY: "Occasionally" = 1%–33% of an 8-hour workday
     "Frequently" = 34%–66% of an 8-hour workday
     "Continuously" = 67%–100% of an 8-hour workday

FIGURE 21.3. A physical capacities form.

TABLE 21.7. Issues to Consider in Determining Physical Capacities

1. What physical capacities issues need to be addressed in order to determine the patient's eligibility for disability benefits? (Example: Most jobs do not require employees to run. Therefore, the ability of a patient to run is usually irrelevant to an evaluation of his or her disability.)
2. Does the patient have a clear diagnosis?
3. Does this diagnosis provide clear information about the nature and severity of the activity restrictions the patient is likely to have?
4. Are the patient's symptoms and physical findings consistent over time, and consistent with his or her diagnosis?
5. Does the patient describe activity limitations that are plausible, given the medical information you have on him or her?
6. Do you have reports or behavioral data on the patient's activities outside your medical office?
   a. Data from day-to-day life (e.g., reports from spouse or employer; surveillance tapes)?
   b. Data from a functional capacity evaluation?
   c. Data from a rehabilitation program, such as a work-hardening program or a pain center?
7. What is your overall assessment of the patient's credibility?

TABLE 21.8. Issues to Consider in Determining Employability

1. What specific questions about employability are you being asked to address?
   a. Can the patient work at a specified job?
   b. What general category of work can the patient perform (sedentary, light, medium, heavy, very heavy)?
   c. Is the patient employable in any capacity?
2. For work in a specific job:
   a. Is there a job analysis?
   b. Does the patient agree with the demands stated on the job analysis?
   c. Are there any collateral sources of information about the job (e.g., information from the employer)?
   d. Do you believe the patient can perform the job with modifications?
   e. Do you believe the patient needs assistance in transitioning to the job (e.g., a graduated reentry or a work-hardening program)?
3. Do you have reliable physical capacities data that permit you to determine the appropriateness of a specific job, or the appropriateness of a general work category?
4. Are there any "trick questions"?
   a. Description of a job with minimal physical requirements? (e.g., phone solicitor)?
   b. Description of a job that seems inappropriate for the patient from an economic and career standpoint (e.g., description of a cashiering job for a person who has spent the last 20 years working as an electrician)?
5. Based on the questions addressed to you, does it seem that the disability agency is making a sincere attempt to find a place in the workforce for the patient, as opposed to trying to "set the patient up" (i.e., contrive vocational options that will maneuver him or her out of the disability system)?
6. Does it appear that the patient is making a sincere effort to return to work, or is he or she exaggerating pain complaints and/or maneuvering in some way to get long-term disability?

able because of a medical condition. Unfortunately, assessing employability is difficult, and there is no simple set of techniques to apply when a decision about employability is requested. Table 21.8 outlines issues that you should consider when you judge a patient's employability.

As Figure 21.4 suggests, a physician makes a judgment about a patient's employability by balancing the patient's capacities (or limitations) against the demands of jobs for which the patient is being considered. Both sides of the balance involve difficult measurements. Issues related to assessing physical capacities were discussed earlier.

As far as the demands of jobs are concerned, the physician usually has to rely on information provided by vocational rehabilitation counselors (VRCs) or employers. In workers' compensation claims, VRCs often prepare formal job analyses. Figure 21.5 gives a sample job analysis. Note that the job analysis form includes a section in which the evaluating physician is asked to give his or her opinion about whether the worker can perform the job.

A detailed job analysis can be extremely helpful in the assessment of the work demands that a patient is likely to face. However, check with the patient to see whether he or she agrees with the physical requirements listed in a job analysis. If the patient vigorously disputes the job analysis, make an attempt to reconcile the discrepancy.

Several problems involving employability determinations occur frequently enough to warrant further discussion.

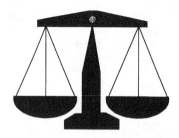

Capacities (Impairments)　　　　Work Demands

FIGURE 21.4. Balancing capacity against work demands.

1. Sometimes you will be asked whether your patient can do a specific job, and you will be provided with a job analysis. In other situations, you will be asked much broader questions. For example, you might be asked to rate the general "category" of work for which the patient is suited. Broad work categories defined in the *Dictionary of Occupational Titles* (U.S. Department of Labor Employment and Training Administration, 1977) and a supplementary publication by Field and Field (1992; Lechner, 1998) include sedentary, light, medium, heavy, and very heavy. The problem is that these work categories might not capture specific activity limitations of your patient. When you are asked to place your patient in a general work category, probably the best approach is to use physical capacities data to assign the patient.

2. Sometimes you will be presented with "trick questions" dealing with employability. As an example, imagine that you are treating a patient with chronic low back pain who has multiple spine surgery failures and continues to complain of relentless pain despite implantation of an intrathecal opiate delivery system. Imagine that you do not believe it is realistic for this patient to return to competitive employment. Suppose that a disability agency asks whether your patient can work as a telephone solicitor. This question poses a dilemma. If you indicate "yes," your patient will probably have his disability benefits terminated. If you say "no," you are implicitly saying that the patient's low back pain prevents him from doing a job that has essentially no physical demands. The "trick" in this type of situation is that disability ad-

judicators or VRCs sometimes concoct jobs specifically because they demand essentially nothing in the way of physical capacities. When you see a trick question like this one, you have good reason to be suspicious that the disability system is maneuvering to terminate the patient's benefits. In this situation, it is appropriate to be protective of your patient, and to demand details regarding the proposed job. For example, you should ask the adjudicator whether there is a market for the phone solicitor job, and whether the patient would have to commute to an office to perform the job.

3. Some patients drag their feet and emphasize the severity of their incapacitation. These behaviors should make you suspicious of their agendas. In such a situation, it is reasonable to stick closely to objective data regarding the patient's capacities rather than to be influenced strongly by the patient's subjective assessments.

It is important to make an employability determination that is acceptable to your patient whenever this is possible. As noted earlier, physicians sometimes feel that they have resolved a difficult disability claim when they say a patient is capable of employment. If the patient strongly disagrees with this conclusion, then he or she may simply go to another physician or retain an attorney. In many instances, the anticipated resolution of the claim turns out to be ephemeral. The recommendation here is *not* to let the patient dictate what you say on a disability form. But it is important to listen carefully to your patient's concerns about employment, and to look for an employment plan that is both medically sensible and acceptable to the patient and to the disability system.

It is worth noting that you can sometimes use disability evaluations as springboards to mobilize patients to take an active role in their vocational rehabilitation. Some chronically disabled patients passively wait for "the system" to solve their vocational dilemmas. When they see the jobs that are proposed during disability evaluations, they are often appalled. In this setting, a treating physician can encourage a patient to become more active in seeking vocational options on his or her own. Some patients take this advice and find jobs that fit their physical limitations

Job Title: Taxi Dispatcher
DOT: 913.367-010
GOE: 07.04.05
SVP: 3

Job Description: Dispatches taxicabs in response to telephone requests for service by entering client name and pick-up and drop-off locations into the computer. Directs calls to dispatch supervisor if needed.

Job Qualifications: Good customer service skills; ability to type and learn computer program.

Types of Machines, Tools, Special Equipment Used: Telephone with headset, computer.

Materials, Products, Subject Matter, Services: Local and suburban transit and interurban buses.

Work Schedule: Full time, 8-hour shifts.

Physical Demands:
1. Stand: Occasionally. Daily total 0.5 hours.
2. Walk: Occasionally. Daily total 0.5 hours.
3. Sit: Constantly with option to stand. Daily total 7 hours.
4. Lift/carry: Occasionally lift/carry ounces.
5. Push/pull: Occasionally with minimum force to open file drawers and keyboard trays.
6. Controls: Frequently use controls on telephone. Most calls are incoming.
7. Climb: Not required.
8. Balance: Not required.
9. Bend/stoop: Rarely to occasionally.
10. Crouch: Not required.
11. Twist: Occasionally at the neck while answering the phones.
12. Kneel: Not required.
13. Crawl: Not required.
14. Handle/grasp: Occasionally handle/grasp office supplies and handset.
15. Fine manipulation/fingering: Frequent to constant typing is involved during workday. Fingering to dial telephone.
16. Feeling: Not required.
17. Reach: Occasionally at mid-waist level, three-quarters to full arm extension.
18. Vision: Correctable vision is desirable.
19. Talk/hear: Speech and hearing are mandatory.
20. Taste/smell: Not required.
21. Environmental factors: Office environment. Floors are carpeted.
22. Work environment access: On-site parking available.

Physician's Judgment:
__ The injured worker can perform this job without restrictions and can return to work on _____.
__ The injured worker can perform this job without restrictions, but only on a part-time basis for __ hours per day, __ days per week. The worker can be expected to return to full-time work in __ days/weeks.
__ The injured worker can perform this job, but only with the following modifications: _____

   Modifications are needed on a __ permanent __ temporary basis.
__ The injured worker temporarily cannot perform this job, based on the following physical limitations: _____

   Anticipated release date: _____
__ The injured worker permanently cannot perform this job, based on the following physical limitations:

Comments:

_____   _____
Signature of Physician   Date

FIGURE 21.5. A job analysis.

and their economic needs. Thus, a disability evaluation can provide the stimulus for patients to become more actively involved in their own rehabilitation.

Objective Findings

It is routine for disability agencies to ask physicians to base their opinions on objective findings. This request may seem innocuous, but it has profound implications. As noted earlier, disability agencies attempt to make decisions based on objectively measurable evidence of incapacitation. But patients with painful conditions typically report incapacitation that goes beyond measurable damage to their organs. Even if you find a patient's pain complaints very credible, you invariably have difficulty stating objective findings that make his or her activity limitations inevitable. For example, consider a patient with low back pain who reports that he can sit for only 20 minutes at a time. There is no objective measure that would make this limitation inevitable.

The request for objective findings can create at least two kinds of problems for an examining physician. First, some patients (e.g., those with fibromyalgia or chronic headaches) may not have any unequivocally objective findings. Second, and far more important, even when patients have objective findings, the findings rarely explain the extent of the incapacitation the patients report.

As a step toward a strategy for dealing with requests for objective findings, it is important to note that the term *objective findings* is not precisely defined. In general it refers to laboratory or physical findings that are objectively measurable and are not subject to voluntary control or manipulation by a patient. Objective findings can be contrasted with *subjective findings*, such as patients' reports of pain intensity or activity restrictions caused by pain. However, as shown in Table 21.9, a lot of clinically important examination findings are "semiobjective." They are objective in the sense that they can be observed and measured. But they are not completely objective, since patients can to some extent voluntarily modify them. Most of the adjudicators who request objective findings are not aware of these subtleties.

TABLE 21.9. "Objective Findings" and "Subjective Findings" in Low Back Pain

Objective findings

1. X-ray abnormalities (e.g., fracture, scoliosis, spondylolisthesis, disc space narrowing, osteophytes)
2. MRI abnormalities (e.g., spinal stenosis, disc herniation)
3. Electromyographic abnormalities (e.g., positive waves and fibrillations, absent H-reflex)

Subjective findings

1. Patient-reported pain intensity
2. Activity restrictions reported by patient

Semiobjective findings

1. Posture (e.g., loss of lumbar lordosis, list)
2. Gait
3. Muscle spasms
4. Soft tissue hypersensitivity (myofascial pain)
5. Range of motion
6. Abnormal straight-leg raising
7. Some lower-extremity deep tendon reflex findings (e.g., reflexes difficult to elicit in patient who is tense)
8. Sensory function in lower extremities
9. Lower-extremity strength

There is a fairly simple way to finesse the objective findings issue. If you do not find your patient credible, it is perfectly reasonable to indicate that there are no objective findings to support his or her claimed incapacitation. But if your patient has consistent physical findings that you find credible, you can simply list them in the space where you are requested to give objective findings. In most instances, the findings you list will be accepted by the disability system, even if they are only semiobjective, or do not necessarily explain the activity restrictions your patient reports. If your findings are challenged, you can indicate that in your clinical judgment they represent valid indices of the patient's condition.

Psychogenic Pain

A physician who does disability evaluations of patients with chronic pain needs to have at least a rudimentary familiarity with psychogenic pain. Unfortunately, concepts surrounding psychogenic pain are generally ambiguous, and there is significant disagreement among experts regarding how to apply them (Fishbain, 1996; Hiller, Rief, & Fichter, 1997; Jackson, 1992; King, 1995; Sullivan & Katon, 1993).

A terminological issue needs to be addressed at the outset. *Psychogenic pain* can be used in a broad sense to refer to pain complaints that are best understood in psychological rather than biomedical terms (i.e., psychological factors appear to play a major role in the onset or maintenance of a patient's pain complaints). It can also be used in a more restricted sense to refer to two diagnoses given in the fourth edition of the American Psychiatric Association's *Diagnostic and Statistical Manual of Mental Disorders* (DSM-IV; 1994—pain disorder associated with psychological factors (307.80), and pain disorder associated with both psychological factors and a general medical disorder (307.89). DSM-IV indicates that these diagnoses should be considered when two conditions are met: (1) a patient's pain complaints can best be understood in psychological terms, and (2) the complaints *cannot* be "better accounted for by a Mood, Anxiety or Psychotic Disorder" (p. 458). Thus, pain disorder has the quality of a "wastebasket diagnosis": It is given only when a patient's pain complaints seem to be affected by psychological factors and no specific Axis I diagnosis can be made. For nonpsychiatrists, the broader concept of psychogenic pain is more useful.

It is appropriate for physicians to consider the possibility of psychogenic pain in patients with chronic pain for at least two reasons. First, as indicated earlier, patients with chronic pain routinely report symptoms and activity restrictions that cannot be rationalized in terms of objectively measurable biological deficits. There are multiple reasons for the mismatch between the restrictions a patient reports and the biomedical abnormalities a physician can observe, but one possibility is that psychological factors may be leading the patient to amplify his or her reports of incapacitation. Second, there is abundant research demonstrating high levels of psychopathology (Fishbain, Goldberg, Labbe, Steele, & Rosomoff, 1988; Robinson, Robinson, & Shelton, 1999) and psychological distress (Turk & Okifuji, 1997; Turk, Okifuji, Sinclair, &

Starz, 1996, 1998; Wells, 1994) in patients with chronic pain.

However, it is important to avoid the simplistic dichotomy of concluding something like "I'll find the source of my patient's pain either on the MRI [magnetic resonance imaging] or on the MMPI [Minnesota Multiphasic Personality Inventory]." Chronic pain is a dilemma for patients and physicians precisely because it often cannot be neatly compartmentalized into "biogenic" and "psychogenic" subgroups. In attempting to understand a patient's pain complaints, it is important for a physician to consider a variety of possible explanations, and to avoid premature closure. No one has developed a widely accepted framework in terms of which to conceptualize pain complaints that are not easily explained in terms of biological dysfunction (Robinson & Apkarian, 2009), but a prudent physician should consider the following general categories:

1. The patient's pain may be a manifestation of a pathophysiological process that is obscure enough to have eluded detection.
2. The patient's pain may reflect central nervous system sensitization.
3. The pain may best be construed in psychological terms—either as a manifestation of a pain disorder or as a manifestation of an anxiety, depressive, or psychotic disorder.
4. The pain may best be construed in terms of "systems issues" (Robinson, 2007a; Robinson et al., 1997) such as financial disincentives or poor employment opportunities.

If you are a nonpsychiatric physician, your best strategy is to ask for help with the assessment of patients who appear to have psychological or systems issues that may be influencing their pain complaints. To implement this strategy, you need to do at least a preliminary assessment of these factors. But if you maintain a high index of suspicion and a low threshold for seeking psychiatric or psychological consultation, you should be able to get the help you need. If you follow this strategy, do not be surprised if you get some puzzling reports back. As noted earlier, no one has been able to articulate a coherent, widely accepted perspective on psychogenic pain at a clinical level, and the forensic implications of psychogenic pain are even murkier.

Filling Out the Form

Once you have addressed the issues just described, your work in filling out a disability form is largely done. However, there are three other matters you should consider.

1. When you fill out a disability form, you are acting as an intermediary between the medical system and an administrative or legal system. The manner in which the disability agency responds to the form you submit will be governed by the administrative and legal mandate under which the agency functions. In many instances, the agency's response will depend on specific words you use in answering questions. For example, if you are writing a report on behalf of an applicant for SSDI benefits, your report will probably have a greater impact if you compare your patient's clinical findings to the appropriate "listing" the SSA uses when it determines whether an applicant is eligible for disability benefits. (Listings are described in the book *Disability Evaluation under Social Security* [2006].) In contrast, you may use language that is sensible from a medical standpoint when you fill out a disability form, then find that the disability agency to which it is submitted interprets it in a completely different way. There is no easy way to solve this problem. Ideally, you should be aware that it exists, and you should learn enough about the legal and administrative mandates of disability systems that you do not accidentally use wording that is misinterpreted or misused.

2. It is not unusual for disability forms to contain questions that physicians are simply unable to answer. For example, it is often impossible for a physician to determine causation in problems such as low back pain and cumulative trauma disorders of the upper extremities. When you encounter such an item, you should feel free to withhold judgment. However, it is often effective to indicate the difficulty of the item on the form, for example, to say "Neither I nor any other physician can answer this question on the basis of the information available."

3. Sometimes the questions in a disability form are so specific that they do not give you a chance to communicate an overall perspective on your patient. As a practical matter, you may find that the information you provided on the disability form does not convey the general assessment you constructed when you first reviewed the form. In this situation, you should write a cover letter to accompany the disability form. In it, you should communicate your overall perspective on the patient and any critical information not given when you answered the specific questions on the form.

Follow-Up

Sometimes your interaction with a disability system will end after you have sent in a single disability form. For example, the SSA generally asks a treating physician to fill out only a single form. Other agencies—such as the workers' compensation companies—ask you to participate in sequential disability determinations that may extend over months or even years.

In either case, your responses to a disability form may have ongoing consequences for your relationship with your patient. Some patients object if your statements on a disability form suggest that they are capable of working. They usually look for another physician if you give the "wrong" answers. In other situations, you and your patient may agree about the information you put on a disability form, but the disability agency to which the form is submitted may reach a decision that adversely affects to the patient's interests. The patient may then feel that you have sold him or her out. The best way to avoid such recriminations is to tell your patient at the outset that disability decisions are made by adjudicators rather by physicians, and that you cannot provide information that will guarantee a favorable outcome.

Another consequence of a disability evaluation is that the patient's medical and wage replacement payments may change dramatically. It is helpful to discuss this openly with a patient before a final decision has been made by the disability agency. For example, if you have been treating a patient under a workers' compensation claim, you should discuss whether the patient wants to continue treatment after the claim has been closed, and, if so, how he or she will pay for the treatment.

INTEGRATING DISABILITY EVALUATION INTO CLINICAL PRACTICE

The preceding discussion demonstrates that disability evaluations are difficult for treating physicians to perform. A physician who tries to incorporate disability evaluation into his or her practice must deal with several challenges:

1. Disability evaluations require information and skills that physicians typically do not acquire in their training. For example, they require a physician to know about the policies of various disability agencies.

2. Agencies that request disability evaluations typically challenge assumptions that are fundamental to clinical medicine. The clearest example of this is the demand for objective findings. This demand challenges the view that an essential task of a physician is to combine objective findings, semiobjective findings, and symptoms into a coherent picture of a patient. In essence, disability evaluation procedures embody skepticism about clinical judgments that are fundamental to the practice of medicine.

3. Even for physicians who have spent the time necessary to gain expertise in the area of disability evaluation, the evaluations are time-consuming and tedious. They frequently require extensive record reviews, efforts to reconcile conflicting opinions, and a lot of paperwork.

4. Disability evaluations can have significant effects on the doctor–patient relationship. In particular, patients frequently become hostile when they perceive that their treating physicians are understating the severity of their incapacitation.

5. Disability evaluations raise significant ethical challenges for a treating physician. Many physicians worry that in the course of performing the evaluations, they may misuse the trust that patients place in them. They may also be concerned about the outcomes of their disability evaluations. At one extreme, they are likely to feel angst if patients whom they perceive as severely incapacitated are denied disability benefits. At the opposite extreme, when patients with very minimal incapacitation receive disability benefits, treating physicians may feel that they have failed to represent the legitimate need of society to refuse disability benefits to individuals who do not have incapacitating medical problems.

6. These ethical concerns are aggravated by the lack of validation of disability evaluation procedures. Thoughtful physicians realize that their judgments about the ability of their patients to work have important consequences, but they have no way to determine whether their judgments are well founded.

Given these difficulties, some physicians are understandably tempted to avoid making judgments about whether their patients are disabled. Unfortunately, this is not a viable option. As noted earlier, society requires physicians to make disability determinations on patients whom they are treating. Physicians may do disability evaluations thoughtfully or thoughtlessly, but they do not have the option of simply not doing them.

Another option is for a physician to develop expertise in the area of disability evaluation. For example, a physician might gain familiarity with major disability agencies and attend courses on independent medical examinations (e.g., ones conducted by the American Board of Independent Medical Examiners).

Yet another option that is probably most appropriate for the majority of physicians is to get help from consultants. Clinicians are used to requesting consultation regarding medical care of their patients. Medical specialists have an important role to play, because they have more expertise than nonspecialists in certain areas of clinical medicine. In the same way, some physicians—especially ones trained in physical medicine and rehabilitation or occupational medicine—have enough expertise in disability evaluation to provide consultation to other physicians. If you decide that it is infeasible to acquire expertise in disability evaluation, you should identify physicians in your community who can assist you in making disability determinations on your patients.

REFERENCES

Alaranta, H., Rytokoski, U., Rissanen, A., Talo, S., Ronnemaa, T., Puukka, M. A., et al. (1994). Intensive physical and psychosocial training program for patients with chronic low back pain. *Spine, 19,* 1339–1349.

American Medical Association. (1993). *Guides to the evaluation of permanent impairment* (4th ed.). Chicago: American Medical Association.

American Psychiatric Association. (1994). *Diagnostic and statistical manual of mental disorders* (4th ed.). Washington, DC: Author.

Atkinson, T,, Liem, R., & Liem, J. (1986). The social cost of unemployment: Implications for social support. *Journal of Health and Social Behavior, 54,* 454–460.

Bellamy, R. (1997). Compensation neurosis. *Clinical Orthopedics & Related Research, 336,* 94–106.

Cheadle, A., Franklin, G., Wolfhagen, C., Savarino, J., Liu, P. Y., Salley, C., et al. (1994). Factors influencing the duration of work-related disability: A population-based study of Washington State workers' compensation. *American Journal of Public Health, 84,* 190–196.

Chibnall, J. T., Tait, R. C., Andresen, E. M., & Hadler, N. M. (2005). Race and socioeconomic differences in post-settlement outcomes for African American and Caucasian workers' compensation claimants with low back injuries. *Pain, 114,* 462–472.

Clark, W., & Haldeman, S. (1993). The development of guideline factors for the evaluation of disability in neck and back injuries. *Spine, 18,* 1736–1745.

Clark, W. L., Haldeman, S., Johnson, P., Morris, J., Schulenberger, C., Trauner, D., et al. (1988). Back impairment and disability determination: Another attempt at objective, reliable rating. *Spine, 13,* 332–341.

Cocchiarella, L. & Andersson, G. B. J. (Eds.). (2001). *Guides to the evaluation of permanent impairment* (5th ed.). Chicago: AMA Press.

Dembe, A. E., & Boden, L. I. (2000). Moral hazard: A question of morality? *New Solutions, 10,* 257–279.

Demeter, S. L., Andersson, G. B. J., & Smith, G. M. (1996). *Disability evaluation.* Chicago: AMA Press.

Disability evaluation under Social Security. (2006). SSA Publication No. 64-039. Washington, DC: U.S. Government Printing Office.

Estlander, A., Mellin, G., Vanharanta, H., & Hupli, M. (1991). Effects and follow-up of a multimodal treatment program including intensive physical training for low back pain patients. *Scandinavian Journal of Rehabilitation Medicine, 23,* 97–102.

Faust, D. (1995). The detection of deception. *Neurologic Clinics of North America, 13,* 255–265.

Field, J. E., & Field, T. F. (1992). *Classification of jobs.* Athens, GA: Elliott & Fitzpatrick.

Fishbain, D. A. (1996). Where have two DSM revisions taken us for the diagnosis of pain disorder in chronic pain patients? *American Journal of Psychiatry, 153,* 137–138.

Fishbain, D. A., Cutler, R. B., Rosomoff, H. L., Khalil, T., & Steele-Rosomoff, R. (1997). Impact of chronic pain patients' job perception variables on actual return to work. *Clinical Journal Pain, 13,* 197–206.

Fishbain, D. A., Cutler, R. B., Rosomoff, H. L., Khalil, T., & Steele-Rosomoff, R. (1999). Prediction of "intent," "discrepancy with intent," and "discrepancy with nonintent" for the patient with chronic pain to return to work after treatment at a pain facility. *Clinical Journal of Pain, 15,* 141–150.

Fishbain, D. A., Goldberg, M., Labbe, E., Steele, R., & Rosomoff, H. (1988). Compensation and non-compensation chronic pain patients compared for DSM-III operational diagnoses. *Pain, 32,* 197–206.

Fishbain, D. A., Rosomoff, H. L., Cutler, R. B., & Rosomoff, R. S. (1995). Secondary gain concept: A review of the scientific evidence. *Clinical Journal of Pain, 11,* 6–21.

Frymoyer, J. W., & Cats-Baril, W. (1987). Predictors of low back pain disability. *Clinical Orthopedics and Related Research, 221,* 89–98.

Gilovich, T. (1991). *How we know what isn't so.* New York: Free Press.

Gross, D. P., & Battié, M. C. (2005). Functional capacity evaluation performance does not predict sustained return to work in claimants with chronic back pain. *Journal of Occupational Rehabilitation, 15,* 285–294.

Gross, D. P., & Battié, M. C. (2006). Does functional capacity evaluation predict recovery in workers' compensation claimants with upper extremity disorders? *Occupational and Environmental Medicine, 63,* 404–410.

Hadler, N. M. (1996). If you have to prove you are ill, you can't get well: The object lesson of fibromyalgia. *Spine, 21,* 2397–2400.

Hall, H. V., & Pritchard, D. A. (1996). *Detecting malingering and deception.* Delray Beach, FL: St. Lucie Press.

Hammarstrom, A., & Janlert, U. (1997). Nervous and depressive symptoms in a longitudinal study of youth unemployment—selection or exposure? *Journal of Adolescence, 20,* 293–305.

Hazard, R. G., Bendix, A., & Fenwick, J. W.

(1991). Disability exaggeration as a predictor of functional restoration outcomes for patients with chronic low-back pain. *Spine*, *16*, 1062–1067.

Hidding, A., Van Santen, M., De Klerk, E., Gielen, X., Boers, M., Geenen, R., et al. (1994). Comparison between self-report measures and clinical observations of functional disability in ankylosing spondylitis, rheumatoid arthritis, and fibromyalgia. *Journal of Rheumatology*, *21*, 818–823.

Hildebrandt, J., Pfingsten, M., Saur, P., & Jansen, J. (1997). Prediction of success from a multidisciplinary treatment program for chronic low back pain. *Spine*, *22*, 990–1001.

Hiller, W., Rief, W., & Fichter, M. M. (1997). How disabled are patients with somatoform disorders? *General Hospital Psychiatry*, *19*, 432–438.

Jackson, J. E. (1992). After a while, no one believes you: Real and unreal pain. In M. E. Good, P. E. Brodwin, & B. J. Good (Eds.), (1992). *Pain as human experience: A anthropological perspective*. Los Angeles: University of California Press.

Jensen, M. P., Turner, J. A., & Romano, J. M. (1994). Correlates of improvement in multidisciplinary treatment of chronic pain. *Journal of Consulting and Clinical Psychology*, *62*, 172–179.

Kaplan, G. A., Roberts, R. E., Camacho, T. C., & Coyne, J. C. (1987). Psychosocial predictors of depression. *American Journal of Epidemiology*, *125*, 206–220.

Kaplan, G. M., Wurtele, S. K., & Gillis, D. (1996). Maximal effort during functional capacity evaluations: An examination of psychological factors. *Archives of Physical Medicine and Rehabilitation*, *77*, 161–164.

King, P. M., Tuckwell, N., & Barrett, T. E. (1998). A critical review of functional capacity evaluations. *Physical Therapy*, *78*, 852–866.

King, S. A. (1995). DSM-IV and pain. Clinical Journal of Pain, *11*, 171–176.

Kramer, M. S., & Lane, D. A. (1992). Causal propositions in clinical research and practice. *Journal of Clinical Epidemiology*, *45*, 639–649.

Krause, N., & Ragland, D. R. (1994). Occupational disability due to low back pain: A new interdisciplinary classification based on a phase model of disability. *Spine*, *19*, 1011–1020.

Lakoff, G., & Johnson, M. (1999). *Philosophy in the flesh*. New York: Basic Books.

Lechner, D. E. (1998). Functional capacity evaluation. In P. M. King (Ed.), *Sourcebook of occupational rehabilitation*. New York: Plenum Press.

Lipchik, G. L., Milles, K., & Covington, E. C.

(1993). The effects of multidisciplinary pain management treatment on locus of control and pain beliefs in chronic non-terminal pain. *Clinical Journal of Pain*, *9*, 49–57.

Loeser, J. D., Henderlite, S. E., & Conrad, D. E. (1995). Incentive effects of workers' compensation benefits: A literature synthesis. *Medical Care Research and Review*, *52*, 34–59.

Mayer, T. G. (1988). *Functional restoration for spinal disorders: The sports medicine approach*. Philadelphia: Lea & Febiger.

Mendelson, G. (1988). *Psychiatric aspects of personal injury claims*. Springfield, IL: Thomas.

Mrazek, P. J., & Haggerty, R. J. (Eds.). (1994). *Reducing risks for mental disorder*. Washington, DC: National Academy Press.

Muller, L. S. (1992). Disability beneficiaries who work and their experience under program work incentives. *Social Security Bulletin*, *55*, 2–19.

Mustard, C., & Hertzman, C. (2001). Relationship between health services outcomes and social and economic outcomes in workplace injury and disease: Data sources and methods. *American Journal of Industrial Medicine*, *40*, 335–343.

Niemeyer, L. O., Jacobs, K., Reynolds-Lynch, K., Bettencourt, C., & Lang, S. (1994). Work hardening: Past, present and future—the Work Programs Special Interest Section National Work-Hardening Outcome Study. *American Journal of Occupational Therapy*, *48*, 327–339.

Osterweis, M., Kleinman, A., & Mechanic, D. (1987). *Pain and disability*. Washington, DC: National Academy Press.

Rahmqvist, M., & Carstensen, J. (1998). Trend of psychological distress in a Swedish population from 1989 to 1995. *Scandinavian Journal of Social Medicine*, *3*, 214–222.

Reno, V. P., Mashaw, J. L., & Gradison, B. (Eds.). (1997). *Disability*. Washington, DC: National Academy of Social Insurance.

Reville, R. T., Seabury, S. A., Neuhauser, F. W., Burton, J. F., & Greenberg, M. D. (2005). *An evaluation of California's permanent disability rating system*. Santa Monica, CA: RAND Corporation.

Robinson, J. P. (1997, June). *Psychological aspects of disability*. Paper presented at the Employer Advisory Group, Valley Medical Center, Renton, WA.

Robinson, J. P. (1998). Disability in low back pain: What do the numbers mean? *American Pain Society Bulletin*, *8*, 9–13.

Robinson, J. P. (2001). Evaluation of function and disability. In J. D. Loeser, S. D. Butler, C. R. Chapman, & D. C. Turk (Eds.), *Bonica's management of pain* (3rd ed.). Philadelphia: Lippincott Williams & Wilkins.

Robinson, J. P. (2002). Pain and disability. In T. Jensen, P. Wilson, & A. Rice (Ed.), *Clinical pain management: Chronic pain.* London: Edward Arnold.

Robinson, J. P. (2005). Disability management in primary care. In B. McCarberg & S. D. Passik (Eds.), *Expert guide to pain management.* Philadelphia: American College of Physicians.

Robinson, J. P. (2007a). Chronic pain. *Physical Medicine and Rehabilitation Clinics of North America, 18,* 761–783.

Robinson, J. P. (2007b). Impairment, pain-related. In R. F. Schmidt & W. D. Willis (Eds.), *Encyclopedic reference of pain.* Berlin: Springer-Verlag.

Robinson, J. P., & Apkarian, A. V. (2009). Low back pain. In E. A. Mayer & M. C. Bushnell (Eds.), *Functional pain syndromes: Presentation and pathophysiology.* Seattle, WA: IASP Press.

Robinson, J. P., & Loeser, J. D. (in press). Effects of workers' compensation systems on recovery from disabling injuries. In M. Hasenbring, A. Rusu, & D. C. Turk (Eds.), *From acute to chronic back pain: Risk factors, mechanisms and clinical implications.* Oxford, UK: Oxford University Press.

Robinson, J. P., Robinson, K. A., & Shelton, J. L. (1999). *Psychiatric independent medical examinations on injured workers with back pain.* Poster presented at the Congress of the International Association for the Study of Pain, Vienna, Austria.

Robinson, J. P., Rondinelli, R. D., & Scheer, S. J. (1997). Industrial rehabilitation medicine: 1. Why is industrial rehabilitation medicine unique? *Archives of Physical Medicine and Rehabilitation, 78*(Suppl. 3), S3–S9.

Robinson, J. P., & Seroussi, R. E. (2007). Impairment rating and disability determination. In R. L. Braddom (Ed.), *Physical medicine and rehabilitation* (3rd ed.). Philadelphia: Elsevier.

Robinson, J. P., & Tait, R. C. (2009). Disability evaluation in painful conditions. In J. C. Ballantyne, J. P. Rathmell, & S. M. Fishman (Eds.), *Bonica's management of pain* (4th ed.). Philadelphia: Lippincott Williams & Wilkins.

Robinson, J. P., & Turk, D. C. (2007). Compensation, disability assessment, and pain in the workplace. In R. F. Schmidt & W. D. Willis (Eds.), *Encyclopedic reference of pain.* Berlin: Springer-Verlag.

Robinson, J. P., Turk, D. C., & Loeser, J. D. (2004). Pain, impairment, and disability in the AMA Guides. *Journal of Law, Medicine and Ethics, 32,* 315–326.

Rondinelli, R. D. (Ed.). (2008). *Guides to the evaluation of permanent impairment* (6th ed.). Chicago: AMA Press.

Rondinelli, R. D., & Katz, R. T. (Eds.). (2000). *Impairment rating and disability evaluation.* Philadelphia: Saunders.

Scherzer, T., Rugulies, R., & Krause, N. (2005). Work-related pain and injury and barriers to workers' compensation among Las Vegas hotel room cleaners. *American Journal of Public Health, 95,* 483–488.

Schneider, E. K., & Simeone, J. J. (2001). Pain and disability under Social Security: Time for a new standard. *Journal of Health Law, 34,* 459–485.

Shannon, H. S., & Lowe, G. S. (2002). How many injured workers do not file claims for workers' compensation benefits? *American Journal of Industrial Medicine, 42,* 467–473.

Social Security Ruling 96-7p. Federal Register, Vol. 61, No. 128 (2 July 1966) pp. 34483–34488.

Stover, B., Wickizer, T. M., Zimmerman, F., Fulton-Kehoe, D., & Franklin, G. (2007). Prognostic factors of long-term disability in a workers' compensation system. *Journal of Occupational and Environmental Medicine, 49,* 31–40.

Sullivan, M., & Katon, W. (1993). Somatization: The path between distress and somatic symptoms. *American Pain Society Journal, 2,* 141–149.

Sullivan, M. D. (2000). DSM-IV pain disorder: A case against the diagnosis. *International Review of Psychiatry, 12,* 91–98.

Sullivan, M. D., & Loeser, J. D. (1992). The diagnosis of disability. *Archives of Internal Medicine, 152,* 1829–1835.

Sullivan, M. D., & Turk, D. C. (2001). Psychiatric illness, depression, and psychogenic pain. In J. D. Loeser, S. D. Butler, C. R. Chapman, & D. C. Turk (Eds.), *Bonica's management of pain* (3rd ed.). Philadelphia: Lippincott Williams & Wilkins.

Tait, R. C., Chibnall, J. T., Andresen, E. M., & Hadler, N. M. (2006). Disability determination: Validity with occupational low back pain. *Journal of Pain, 7,* 951–957.

Turk, D. C., & Okifuji, A. (1997). Evaluating the role of physical, operant, cognitive, and affective factors in the pain behaviors of chronic pain patients. *Behavior Modification, 21,* 259–80.

Turk, D. C., Okifuji, A., Sinclair, J. D., & Starz, T. W. (1996). Pain, disability, and physical functioning in subgroups of patients with fibromyalgia. *Journal of Rheumatology, 23,* 1255–1262.

Turk, D. C., Okifuji, A., Sinclair, J. D., & Starz,

T. W. (1998). Differential responses by psychosocial subgroups of fibromyalgia syndrome patients to an interdisciplinary treatment. *Arthritis Care and Research, 11*, 397–404.

Turner, J. A., Franklin, G., Fulton-Kehoe, D., Sheppard, L., Stover, B., Wu, R., et al. (2008). Early predictors of chronic work disability: A prospective, population-based study of workers with back injuries. *Spine, 33*, 2809–2818.

U.S. Department of Labor Employment and Training Administration. (1977). *Dictionary of occupational titles* (4th ed.). Washington, DC: U.S. Government Printing Office.

Voiss, D. V. (1995). Occupational injury: Fact, fantasy, or fraud? *Neurologic Clinics of North America, 13*, 431–446.

Waddell, G. (2004). *Compensation for chronic pain*. London: Stationery Office.

Washington State Department of Labor and Industries. (1999). *Attending doctor's handbook* (rev. ed.). Olympia, WA: Author.

Wells, N. (1994). Perceived control over pain: Relation to distress and disability. *Research in Nursing and Health, 17*, 295–302.

Williams, C. A. (1991). *An international comparison of workers' compensation*. Boston: Kluwer Academic.

Wolfe, F., & Potter, J. (1996). Fibromyalgia and work disability. *Rheumatic Disease Clinics of North America, 22*, 369–391.

World Health Organization. (2001). *International classification of functioning, disability, and health: ICF*. Geneva: Author.

CHAPTER 22

The Importance of Biopsychosocial Screening before Surgical Intervention or Opioid Therapy for Patients with Chronic Pain

ROBERT J. GATCHEL

When pain becomes chronic in nature, many complex biopsychosocial interactions affect differences in how individuals report physical symptoms, how often they seek health care services, and their responses to the same treatments (Gatchel, 2004; Turk & Monarch, 2002). Indeed, quite frequently, the nature of a patient's response to treatment has little to do with his or her objective physical condition (Gatchel, Peng, Peters, Fuchs, & Turk, 2007). Even though interdisciplinary pain management programs (based on the biopsychosocial conceptualization of pain) have been demonstrated to be more therapeutic and cost-effective relative to monotherapies, such as surgery, injections, pharmacotherapy (Gatchel & Okifuji, 2006; Turk & Swanson, 2007), many patients often do not have access to, or knowledge about, such effective programs. Instead, when chronic pain becomes intractable in nature, referring physicians are in the habit of sending these patients for surgery or medication management, because these monotherapies have traditionally offered the prospect of dramatic improvement. However, as noted by Block, Gatchel, Deardorff, and Guyer (2003), in the context of spine surgery, such hopes are relatively brief because positive results:

are not easily, quickly, or uniformly achieved. Relief, even when it comes, does so slowly and with great effort. Although spine surgery is most often successful in ameliorating painful conditions, on average it leads to only about a 50% reduction in pain level and moderate increases in functional ability. . . . More significantly, about 25% of patients do not experience relief at all. (p. 3)

Unfortunately, those patients who have undergone unsuccessful surgery often continue along a path of more and increasingly invasive and unsuccessful interventions, leading ultimately to total functional disability and emotional distress, accompanied by significant financial, medical, and personal suffering costs.

FAILED BACK SURGERY SYNDROME

According to Hua and Levy (1999), over 300,000 Americans undergo spine surgery each year; of those, an estimated 20–40% result in unsuccessful outcomes. *Failed back surgery syndrome* (FBSS) is a somewhat vague term frequently applied to the condition in which a patient has undergone back surgery with a poor outcome. FBSS can arise from multiple etiologies:

- Misdiagnosis of the patient, resulting in an incorrect and possibly damaging surgery. A common example is arthritis misdiagnosed as a lumbar disc disease.
- Unnecessary surgery that may actually worsen a patient's condition. For example, an unnecessary excision of the nucleus pulposus from a normal disc may increase the risk for chronic pain by creating instability and malalignment problems. Nonoperative treatments may be more appropriate approaches with less risk.
- Improper or inadequate surgery (e.g., disc excision performed at the wrong level; improper removal of disc material fragments; inadvertent damage of nerve roots; excessive development of scar tissue)
- Finally, the most common cause is poor patient selection for surgery. Many patients have a poor biopsychosocial profile that contraindicates or is not appropriate for surgical intervention at this point in time.

Methods to avoid some of these causes of FBSS are further reviewed later in this chapter.

IMPLANTABLE DEVICES

During the past decade, we have witnessed an expanding role of two other surgical techniques for many patients with FBSS as an alternative to reoperations—implantable devices, such as spinal cord stimulators (SCSs), and intrathecal (IT) drug delivery systems. These have also been used to treat other chronic pain syndromes that are refractory to more conservative treatment techniques, such as reflex sympathetic dystrophy, postamputation pain, postherpetic neuralgia, spinal cord injury dysesthesias, and pain associated with multiple sclerosis (Gatchel, 2004). SCS and IT delivery systems are two semipermanent options for these patients. They are, though, rather invasive placement procedures that are also quite costly. Cost-effective analyses have shown SCSs and IT pumps are more costly at outset but, after 2.5 years, become less costly than conventional pain therapies (Kemler et al., 2000;

Kumar, Malik, & Demeria, 2002). However, their overall success rates have been questionable, hovering around only 50% (Kupers et al., 1994; North, Kidd, Zahurak, James, & Long, 1993). Again, these relatively low success rates are most likely due to a poor patient selection process, similar to that for spine surgery (Heckler et al., 2007; Schocket et al., 2008). A more successful selection process is discussed later in this chapter.

OPIOID THERAPY

A traditional stance taken by many pain specialists is that "when all else fails" chronic opioid therapy is the "fallback" alternative. However, Katz and Barkin (2008) have recently noted that although a variety of pharmacological treatments are currently available for patients suffering from chronic and persistent pain, such pain is often inadequately managed. Nicholson (2009) has further noted that in a recent American Pain Society survey of 800 patients with moderate to severe chronic pain, 47% reported that their pain was not under adequate control. As Gatchel (2008) has further elucidated, one of the many reasons for this inadequacy is the concern of many health care professionals of being perceived as complicit in increasing rates of abuse and addiction. Indeed, misuse/abuse of controlled substances, such as opiates, is escalating at a rate commensurate with the number of prescriptions in the United States (Reid et al., 2002; Soderstrom et al., 2001). In an effort to control this problem, prescribing physicians are now legally required to consider a number of issues prior to dispensing such prescriptions, as delineated below (from Gatchel, 2008):

- Justification for the medical use of this drug.
- Assessment of patients for possible current addictions prior to dispensing a prescription.
- The need for accurate records of prescribing practices in each patient's chart that are subject to a Drug Enforcement Agency (DEA) audit at any time.

Acting on these regulations, medical licenses of physicians have been revoked for failure to adhere to them. As a consequence, many physicians have developed *opiophobia*, a term coined by the pharamacologist John Morgan in 1986, which is defined as a fear of opiate prescribing, with an inherent prejudice against these types of drugs, regardless of their appropriate clinical utility (Bernstein et al., 2007; Gatchel, 2008). Clinicians, therefore, are faced with a major conundrum: Despite the known benefits of opioid therapy and the growing number of such drugs available for patients with chronic pain, many clinicians hesitate to prescribe them because they are either opiophobic or they do not have an adequate understanding of the risks of potential misuse and abuse. In order to address this conundrum, Gatchel (2008) and Turk, Swanson, and Gatchel (2008) have developed guidelines for evaluating potential opioid misuse/abuse. This also is reviewed later in this chapter.

BIOPSYCHOSOCIAL SCREENING

Not until recently, with the advent of the biopsychosocial model of chronic pain, has an important change in the *zeitgeist* of surgical and medication care of patients occurred. Regardless of the level of a surgeon's or clinician's diagnostic acumen and technical skill, psychosocial factors interact with biological factors in exerting very strong influences on the final treatment outcomes, and can either help to improve or to inhibit a patient's ultimate recovery (Block et al., 2003; Gatchel, 2004). For example, many manufacturers of implantable devices, as well as insurance companies, often require psychological clearance before a patient receives approval for implantation. Unfortunately, such "clearance" may not be based on an empirically derived and valid screening algorithm. However, compelling scientific evidence is now documenting how certain surgical results can be significantly augmented by the inclusion of certain predictive psychosocial components in both the assessment and preparation of patients for invasive procedures, such as spine surgery, and the postoperative care phase (Block et al., 2003; Gatchel, 2001). Similarly, such screening is of great importance when prescribing opioid therapy to monitor potential misuse of such medications.

At the outset, it should again be noted that the biopsychosocial model has been shown to be the most heuristic approach to the assessment and treatment of pain, especially chronic pain (e.g., Gatchel, 2004; Turk & Monarch, 2002). From a historical perspective, Gatchel and Okifuji (2006) noted that traditional interventions for chronic pain have predominantly involved monotherapies, such as surgery, injections, and a wide array of pharmacotherapeutic approaches. However, as highlighted by Turk and Gatchel (2002), a more comprehensive biopsychosocial approach was needed to address both the physical and psychosocial factors involved. George Engel (1977) is credited as being one of the first to call for a new approach to the traditional biomedical reductionistic philosophy that has dominated the field of medicine since the Renaissance. That older philosophy embraced a dualistic viewpoint that mind and body function separately and independently. However, there began a growing recognition that psychosocial factors, such as emotional stress, could impact medical disorders. This subsequently led to the growth of the field of behavioral medicine/health psychology (Gatchel & Baum, 1983). A major outgrowth, in turn, was the development of the biopsychosocial model. This model has been especially influential in the area of pain, and it focuses on both disease and illness, viewing illness as the complex interaction of biological, psychological, and social factors. Turk and Monarch (2002) define *disease* as "an objective biological event" involving the disruption of specific body structures or organ systems, caused by either anatomical, pathological or physiological changes. In contrast, *illness* refers to a "subjective experience or self-attribution" that a disease is present. Thus, illness refers to how a sick person and members of his or her family live with, and respond to, symptoms of disability. The distinction between disease and illness is analogous to the distinction between nociception and pain. *Nociception* involves the stimulation of nerves that convey information about possible tissue damage to the brain. On the other hand, *pain* is a more subjective perception that is the result of the transduction, transmission, and modulation of sensory input. This input may be filtered through an individual's genetic composition, prior learning history, current psychological status, and sociocultural influences. Thus, with this general perspective, a diversity of results of pain or illness can be expected (including its severity, duration, and psychosocial consequences). In order to fully understand a patient's perception and response to pain/illness, the interrelationships among these influences need to be considered.

Thus, by embracing this biopsychosocial model, one must approach the assessment process by conceptualizing pain as a complex and dynamic interaction among physiological, psychological, and social factors that often results in, or at least maintains, pain. It cannot be broken down into distinct, independent psychosocial or physical components. Also, each individual experiences pain uniquely. The complexity of pain is especially evident when it persists over time, as a range of psychological, social, and economic factors can interact with physical pathology to modulate a patient's report of pain and subsequent disability. As such, when assessing pain in a patient, one must consider physical, biological, cognitive, emotional, behavioral, and social factors, as well as their interplay, when explaining a patient's report of pain. Appropriate "tailored" interventions can then be prescribed. Although this may seem like a daunting task, major advances in recent years have delineated methods/instruments to use in the biopsychosocial assessment process (Gatchel, 2004; Gatchel et al., 2007).

How an appropriate biopsychosocial assessment can be used as a valuable screening tool for presurgical or opioid therapy interventions decision making is reviewed next. The resultant intervention plans can then be tailored more effectively to reduce pain, increase the longevity of pain relief and patients' expectations, as well as increase functioning. Moreover, as noted by Gatchel (2001), these preintervention evaluations can also "raise a flag" to the requirement of biopsychosocial interventions needed *before* the actual planned interventions in order to reduce patient stress levels, to improve motivation, and help to resolve unrealistic expectations, to solicit family support, and to provide effective coping skills required to maximize postintervention recovery. This additional use of such screening has been reiterated by Block and colleagues (2003).

BIOPSYCHOSOCIAL SCREENING BEFORE SURGICAL INTERVENTION

The number of back surgeries in the United States exceeds 250,000 per year (Epker & Block, 2001). In light of the traditional poor outcomes of traditional spine surgeries (such as fusions, laminectomies, discectomies, etc.), it became clear that long-overlooked psychosocial factors could potentially be used to identify patients who might not be suitable for such surgeries (Block et al., 2003). In fact, Block, Ohnmeiss, Guyer, Rashbaum, and Hochschuler (2001) were the first formally to use a presurgical psychological screening (PPS) method (using psychometric testing, clinical interviews, and medical history) to determine the spine surgical outcome of 204 surgical candidates. They were able to identify a number of risk factors for poor surgical outcomes, divided into "medical" and "psychosocial" risk factors. The medical risk factors included the following:

- The type of surgery now being contemplated
- History of previous surgeries
- Prior medical problems
- Presence of "non-organic signs" (Waddell, 1987)
- Duration of pain
- Abnormal pain drawings
- Smoking
- Obesity

The psychosocial risk factors included the following:

- Workers' compensation status or pending litigation
- Job dissatisfaction
- Spousal solicitousness and/or lack of support
- History of abuse and/or abandonment
- History of substance abuse
- History of psychological disturbance
- Chronic and/or reactive depression
- A pathological depression profile on the Minnesota Multiphasic Personality Inventory (MMPI)
- Anger
- Anxiety
- Pain sensitivity

Each of these risk factors was assigned an a priori weight of either "high" or "medium" risk based on past empirical research in the literature. The authors then constructed a "risk score card" to assign patients to "good," "fair," or "poor" outcome categories. Subsequent analysis of these data (Block et al., 2001) indicated that 82.3% of patients in the "poor" prognosis group actually achieved poor surgical outcome, while only 17% of patients with a "poor" prognosis achieved fair or good surgical outcomes. A follow-up analysis to the scorecard categorization involved using a hierarchical regression analysis to determine which variables significantly contributed to outcomes. The hierarchical regression analysis showed a success rate of 84.3%. This was only slightly more effective at predicting outcome when compared to their scorecard categorization method.

Block and colleagues (2003) later reported refining the scorecard approach into a more formal algorithm. In the algorithm, each risk factor was assigned a weight based on findings reported in the previous research literature. Strong risk factors were assigned a value of 2, and moderate risk factors were assigned a value of 1. The replacement of the categorical approach with the algorithm offered several additional features: (1) Psychosocial risk factors, most often found as strong predictors of surgical outcome, were placed above medical risk in the primary position; (2) the algorithm added adverse clinical features when considering surgical prognosis; and (3) the paths within the algorithm led to a set of general treatment conditions, as well as surgical prognosis. Thus, the algorithm comprised interview and testing data, medical risk factors, as well as adverse clinical features. According to this new algorithm, patients with a poor prognosis were recommended for either discharge or noninvasive treatment, and *not* surgery. On the other end of the spectrum, patients with a good prognosis were recommended for either *postoperative* biopsychosocial treatment or no treatment. Furthermore, patients with a fair prognosis were recommended for work with a psychologist on compliance and motivation issues *before* surgery was performed.

In summarizing the use of this presurgical psychological screening, Epker and Block (2001) have recommended two important uses of this approach. The first is that it allows the clinician to gather information regarding psychosocial and medical risk factors to help determine potential surgical outcome based on empirical data. The second is that the results of the screening provide information for the development of individualized treatment plans. Thus, outcomes for acceptable candidates are enhanced, motivation in marginal candidates can be improved, and those patients not recommended for a surgical procedure can begin more conservative, "less risky" treatment modalities for pain management.

BIOPSYCHOSOCIAL SCREENING BEFORE INSTALLATION OF SURGICALLY IMPLANTABLE DEVICES

As we know, many chronic pain patients are refractory to conservative medical care. After failing to improve with such care, such as opioids and other minimally invasive procedures, these patients are often then referred for more invasive procedures, including surgery and, ultimately, implantable devices, if the pain remains refractory. As noted earlier in this chapter, SCSs and IT drug delivery systems are the two semipermanent options for these refractory patients. However, as reviewed earlier, such options are quite costly, and their long-term success rates are still questionable. Therefore, just as spine surgery was a decade ago, there is now a realization of the need to develop preimplantation screening techniques to decide which patients have a better or worse prognosis for improvement with such intervention.

As a first step in this evaluation process, Schocket and colleagues (2008) conducted a preimplantation biopsychosocial screening assessment of patients being considered for IDT or SCS procedures. This screening method, derived from the algorithm developed by Block and colleagues (2003), was refined to place patients in one of four recommendation groups: Green, Yellow-I, Yellow-II, or Red. Based on this screening, patients in the Green group were cleared for implantation, with no accompanying biopsychosocial treatment being needed. Patients in the Yellow-I group were recommended for postoperative biopsychosocial treatment after implantation. Patients in the "Yellow-II" group were recommended for *preimplantation* biopsychosocial treatment, to work on compliance and motivation issues. Finally, patients in the "Red" group recommended for either noninvasive treatment exclusively or discharged. When subsequently examining the algorithm, Schocket and colleagues (2008) found the interview risk factors, psychological testing risk factors, adverse clinical features, and medical risk factors to be significantly different among the groups. Most interestingly, adverse clinical features were significant in predicting poor implantation outcome, thus suggesting a more significant role than previously thought by Block and colleagues (2003). This study was also able to collect 6-month follow-up data on a small cohort of patients (31 of the original 60) to determine some outcomes. Overall, it was found that 40% of patients the Green group were not taking medications at the 6-month follow-up, and this percentage decreased as prognosis worsened (Yellow-I, 27.3%; Yellow-II, 25%; and Red, 0%).

In a subsequent investigation by this same clinical research team, Heckler and colleagues (2007) further evaluated the utility of this prescreening algorithm for implantable devices, as well as conducting a 12-month follow-up of patients. Results again clearly showed significant biopsychosocial differences among the four groups. Results revealed significant linear trends across the four groups (Green, Yellow-I, Yellow-II, and Red), such that the best biopsychosocial functioning occurred in the Green group and the worst in the Red group for the following variables: visual analogue scores of pain; self-report measures of disability; depressive symptomology; catastrophizing; and scores on the Short Form–36 Health Survey (SF-36). Thus, these findings indicate clear biopsychosocial differences among the four groups based on the prescreening algorithm.

Overall, the results of both of the studies demonstrate that the algorithm, modified from the original one developed by Block and colleagues (2001, 2003), is generally applicable to patients undergoing examination for implantable devices to help manage their chronic pain. However, research is still needed to "tweak" the algorithm further to increase its predictive value, as well studies

using it further to assess long-term improvement rates. There can be no doubt, though, that patients with lower levels of biopsychosocial stress and dysfunction, specifically, with low levels of depression and more effective coping strategies, are the best candidates for such surgeries. They show the highest percentages of success in overall outcomes by increasing functional abilities and psychological functioning, decreasing pain levels, and decreasing medication intake. Patients exhibiting large amounts of biopsychosocial stress, specifically high levels of depression and the presence of adverse clinical features, are poor candidates for these procedures, because they are often unable to recover successfully and tend to have negative outcomes. Targeting those risk factors that appear most indicative of potential success or failure for implantable devices may allow patients to avoid undergoing procedures that are likely to be unsuccessful; help physicians avoid pitfalls with patients who may not be appropriate for these devices; and create an improved system on which third-party payers rely to compensate these costly procedures.

BIOPSYCHOSOCIAL SCREENING FOR, AND MONITORING OF, OPIOID THERAPY

It should again be kept in mind that the use of only opioid therapy, or some other pain-reducing medication (e.g., benzodiazepines, antidepressants, and neuroleptics), which simply amounts to monotherapy for patients with chronic pain, is not as effective as a more comprehensive interdisciplinary pain management program (Gatchel & Okifuji, 2006). Indeed, the consideration of such pharmacotherapy, if needed, should be only one aspect of a more comprehensive biopsychosocial evaluation in "tailoring" the interdisciplinary pain management for a particular patient. Such a program usually includes psychosocial treatment, physical therapy, occupational therapy, and pharmacotherapy, if needed—all coordinated by a physician–nurse team.

As Gatchel (2008) has recently highlighted, even though a variety of pharmacotherapies are currently available for use with patients suffering from chronic and persistent pain, such pain is often inadequately managed.

Nicholson (2009) has also noted this, even though there is evidence for the beneficial effects of extended-release opioid analgesic formulations for patients with chronic pain. Moreover, Katz and Barkin (2008) point out reasons for this inadequate treatment:

- The need for multiple doses for continuous pain relief, with the resultant inconvenience/time-compliance issues that may prevent patients from achieving adequate pain relief.
- Side effects, such as gastrointestinal, cardiovascular, and organ toxicity symptoms.
- The fear of abuse or addiction.

Of these three reasons, the one that is of special concern for many health care professionals is the fear of potential perceived complicity on their part in increasing abuse or addiction (Reid et al., 2002). Indeed, in an effort to control the potential misuse/abuse of controlled substances, such as opiates, in our society, which is escalating at a rate commensurate with the number of prescriptions (Joranson et al., 2002; Soderstrom et al., 2001), prescribing physicians are legally required to consider a number of issues prior to dispensing such prescriptions: The drug must be for justifiable medical use; patients must be assessed for possible current addiction prior to dispensing a prescription; and accurate records of prescribing practices for each patient must be kept in each patient's chart, which are subject to a DEA audit at any time (Gatchel, 2008). Medical licenses have actually been revoked for failure to adhere to these rules. As a consequence, many physicians have developed "opiophobia" (a term coined by the pharmacologist John Morgan in 1986), defined as a fear of opiate prescribing, with an inherent prejudice against these types of drugs, regardless of appropriate clinical utility.

Thus, today, we are faced with a major conundrum. That is to say, despite the benefits of opioid therapy for many patients, and the growing number of such medications available for patients with chronic pain, many physicians hesitate to prescribe them because they are either "opiophobic," or they do not have an adequate understanding of the risks for potential misuse or abuse. As

Turk and colleagues (2008) have noted, this has stimulated a search for strategies to identify patients who are at risk for the potential of misuse or abuse. Turk and colleagues also noted that a subset of patients (estimated to be anywhere from 2.8 to 62.2%), depending on the study and patient group evaluated, has such potential (e.g., Chabal, Erjavec, Jacobson, Marravo, & Chaney, 1997; Gilson, Ryan, Joranson, & Dahl, 2004; Joranson et al., 2002; Polatin & Gajraj, 2002). Of course, for these patients, *greater vigilance* is required. Thus, the following guidelines should be followed: (1) Have a single physician take the primary responsibility for the opioid medication; (2) do not refill prescriptions over the telephone; the patient needs to be evaluated in person when the prescription is to be refilled; and (3) a clear Medication Agreement is needed to delineate what "emergency" situations will allow an early refill of a prescription. These early refills need to be minimized and carefully monitored, using only one pharmacy.

With these issues in mind, an important goal for those advocating the use of opioid medication is the development of a reliable method to evaluate the patient risk associated with potential abuse/misuse. This is especially important for patients with chronic pain who use opioids, and whose urine toxicology screening results indicate that such abuse/misuse is a significant problem (with a range from 27.2 to 42%; Martell et al., 2007). Indeed, as noted by Ballantyne and Mao (2003), the optimally effective use of opioids must include an evaluation of the potential for abuse in all patients being considered for opioid therapy.

As a consequence of these issues, newer methods for helping to assess potentially at-risk patients for misuse/abuse of pain reduction medications are being developed. A number of recent reviews on this topic have been published by Bernstein and colleagues (2007), Schatman (2008), and Turk and colleagues (2008). Of course, the "gold standard" for detecting substance abuse is urine toxicology screens, which many suggest should be used routinely for all chronic patients who receive opioids. However, as noted by Turk and colleagues, even these results need to be interpreted with some caution because of the following:

- Lack of an initially positive urine screen cannot be mindlessly used as a predictor of all future drug abuse/misuse behavior in *all* patients.
- Katz and colleagues (2003) have shown that even patients with an initially negative screen may subsequently display behaviors indicative of substance abuse/misuse.
- Katz and colleagues have also shown that an initial positive urine toxicology screen may not predict future abuse/misuse problems.

One important "starting point" for avoiding the potential of medication abuse is to address the issue at the very beginning of the intervention. A Medication Agreement can help achieve this by clearly stating that it is the responsibility of the patient not to misuse any drugs, and having the patient sign an agreement to that effect. In passing, it should also be noted that the term "agreement" should be used rather than "contract," because the latter implies a legal document (which it is not; Gatchel, 2005). Moreover, if the patient has many medications prescribed over the years by many different physicians (e.g., benzodiazepine for anxiety/stress, a muscle relaxant, a medication for sleep, as well as multiple narcotic medications for pain), then a detoxification program (either inpatient or outpatient) may need to be prescribed so that the patient–physician team can start a new opioid intervention strategy with a "clean slate."

Of course, we are still left with the issue of what other measure(s) can be used to "flag" those patients who are potentially at risk for future medication abuse/misuse, so that physicians will be able to take special precautions in treating them. In response to this, a number of self-report instruments have been developed (see Turk et al., 2008). As a good example of one such instrument, the *Pain Medication Questionnaire* (PMQ) has been receiving a great deal of interest as a result of the initial studies by Adams and colleagues (2004) and Holmes and colleagues (2006). The PMQ was designed to assess the risk for medication misuse in chronic pain patients. Adams and colleagues initially found a positive relationship between higher PMQ scores and concurrent measures of substance abuse, psychopathology, and physical/life functioning. Holmes and colleagues subsequently replicated these results, and also found that patients with high PMQ scores

- Were 2.6 times more likely to have a known substance abuse problem, relative to patients with low PMQ scores.
- Were 3.2 times more likely to request early refills of prescription medications.
- Had diminished biopsychosocial functioning.
- Showed a significant decrease in PMQ scores 6 months following treatment discharge.

There are also a number of other important benefits of using the PMQ (Gatchel, 2008). For example, it has been shown to be psychometrically sound. The two core psychometric properties of any test are reliability and validity. *Reliability* refers to the reproducibility of a test from one administration to the next. One would expect that if a test is administered at two points in time, with no major intervening circumstances possibly affecting the test, then the test–retest reliability should be high. The PMQ has been shown to have good reliability. *Validity* refers to the appropriateness and usefulness of a particular test or measurement in making an inference about an individual's behavior (in this case, the potential for medication misuse by a patient). The PMQ has also been shown to have good validity.

The PMQ is also a brief, 26-item self-report instrument that can be easily filled out by patients (it also only requires a third-grade reading level). Finally, the other advantages of using the PMQ include the following (Gatchel, 2008):

- Demonstrates due diligence in monitoring substance use for any potential DEA audit.
- Increases quality assurance of the treatment program, as well as "tailoring" the program to specific needs of patients.
- Produces better overall program outcomes—good public relations to use with insurance carriers.
- Demonstrates high sensitivity (.90)

Of course, an instrument such as the PMQ should be only one part of a more comprehensive biopsychosocial evaluation of the patient with chronic pain. Besides the evaluation of both potential underlying pathophysiology and physical functioning, in order to truly understand and treat chronic pain, factors such as a patient's positive–negative coping skills, current level of stress, social support, negative cognitions (e.g., catastrophizing), and so forth, must be taken into account to get a "complete picture" of the patient's strengths and weaknesses. A treatment program can then be tailored to each patient to further minimize his or her strengths, and to help eliminate the weaknesses. Obviously, such assessment data are greatly needed by the health care professional to evaluate more effectively the potential benefits–risks of prescribing long-term opioid treatment.

CONCLUSIONS

As reviewed, many complex biopsychosocial interactions can significantly affect how individuals report physical symptoms and pain, their requirements for health care services, and their responses to the same treatments. Fortunately, there are now biopsychosocially based interdisciplinary pain management programs that have been demonstrated to be more therapeutic and cost-effective relative to monotherapies such as surgery, pharmotherapy, and so forth (Gatchel & Okifuji, 2006). Many patients, though, have neither knowledge of, nor access to, such effective programs. This leads, unfortunately, to the following scenario: When chronic pain becomes intractable in nature, referring physicians are in the habit to sending these patients for surgery or medication management, because these monotherapies are all they know, and they have offered in the past the prospect of dramatic improvement. However, in the case of one such widely used monotherapy, spinal surgery, postsurgical outcome results are not at all impressive (Block et al., 2003). Nevertheless, over 300,000 Americans undergo spine surgery each year at a great economic cost. In fact, in a recent survey report, Martin and colleagues (2008) reported that economic expenditures among adults with back and neck problems increased 65% (adjusted for inflation) from 1997 to 2005

(which was more rapid than overall health expenditures in the United States). More importantly, such expenditures were not associated with corresponding improvement in self-assessed health status of these patients.

What is a possible solution to this problem? One promising and major solution presented here is to conduct appropriate biopsychosocial screening before surgical intervention, or opioid therapy, in patients with chronic pain. Indeed, we are beginning to make promising inroads into this by developing such prescreening protocols. As discussed, Block and colleagues (2001, 2003) developed an impressive screening algorithm for patients being considered for spine surgery. As an extension of this, Gatchel and colleagues (Heckler et al., 2007; Schocket et al., 2008) developed a modified prescreening protocol for patients being considered for surgically installed implantable devices for pain reduction, specifically SCSs and IT devices. The results of this approach were found to be quite promising, but additional clinical research is needed both to refine it further and to examine long-term outcomes of its efficacy.

Finally, the "political hot potato" of opiophobia among physicians who hesitate to prescribe potentially therapeutically safe and effective pharmacotherapy was reviewed. However, this hesitancy can be addressed by educating health care physicians to demonstrate *due diligence* in documenting their patients' visits and prescriptions; to provide *greater vigilance* in monitoring the medications; and to "flag" patients who might potentially misuse these medications. A number of recently developed medication misuse screening approaches are now available. One such instrument, the PMQ, was reviewed. Of course, all of these recommendations are only one part of a more comprehensive biopsychosocial evaluation of the patient with chronic pain.

ACKNOWLEDGMENTS

The writing of this chapter was supported in part by grants to Robert J. Gatchel from the National Institutes of Health (Nos. 3R01 MH 046452, 1K05 MH 071892, 1U01 DE 010713-12A2) and from the Department of Defense (No. DAMD17-03-1-0055).

REFERENCES

Adams, L. L., Gatchel, R. J., Robinson, R. C., Polatin, P. P., Gajraj, N., Deschner, M., et al. (2004). Development of a self-report screening instrument for assessing potential opioid medication misuse in chronic pain patients. *Journal of Pain and Symptom Management, 27*, 440–459.

Ballantyne, J. C., & Mao, J. (2003). Opioid therapy for chronic pain. *New England Journal of Medicine, 349*, 1943–1953.

Bernstein, D., Stowell, A. W., Haggard, R., Worzer, W., Polatin, P. B., & Gatchel, R. J. (2007). Complex interplay of participants in opioid therapy. *Practical Pain Management, 7*, 10–36.

Block, A. R., Gatchel, R. J., Deardorff, W., & Guyer, R. D. (2003). *The psychology of spine surgery*. Washington, DC: American Psychological Association.

Block, A. R., Ohnmeiss, D. O., Guyer, R. D., Rashbaum, R. F., & Hochschuler, S. H. (2001). The use of presurgical psychological screening to predict the outcome of spine surgery. *Spine Journal, 1*, 274–282.

Chabal, C., Erjavec, M. K., Jacobson, L., Marravo, A., & Chaney, E. (1997). Prescription opiate abuse in chronic pain patients: Clinical criteria, incidence and predictors. *Clinical Journal of Pain, 13*, 150–155.

Engel, G. L. (1977). The need for a new medical model: A challenge for biomedicine. *Science, 196*, 129–136.

Epker, J., & Block, A. R. (2001). Presurgical psychological screening in back pain patients: A review. *Clinical Journal of Pain, 17*, 200–205.

Gatchel, R. J. (2001). A biopsychosocial overview of pre-treatment screening of patients with pain. *Clinical Journal of Pain, 17*, 192–199.

Gatchel, R. J. (2004). Comorbidity of chronic mental and physical health disorders: The biopsychosocial perspective. *American Psychologist, 59*, 792–805.

Gatchel, R. J. (2005). *Clinical essentials of pain management*. Washington, DC: American Psychological Association.

Gatchel, R. J. (2008). Methods for monitoring medication use in chronic pain patients. *Advances in Pain Management, 2*, 54–58.

Gatchel, R. J., & Baum, A. (1983). *An introduction to health psychology*. Reading, MA: Addison-Wesley.

Gatchel, R. J., & Okifuji, A. (2006). Evidence-based scientific data documenting the treatment- and cost-effectiveness of comprehensive pain programs for chronic nonmalignant pain. *Journal of Pain, 7*, 779–793.

Gatchel, R. J., Peng, Y., Peters, M. L., Fuchs, P. N., & Turk, D. C. (2007). The biopsychosocial approach to chronic pain: Scientific advances and future directions. *Psychological Bulletin, 133*, 581–624.

Gilson, A. M., Ryan, K. M., Joranson, D. E., & Dahl, J. L. (2004). A reassessment of trends in the medical use and abuse of opioid analgesics and implications for diversion control: 1997–2002. *Journal of Pain and Symptom Management, 28*, 176–188.

Heckler, D., Gatchel, R. J., Lou, L., Whitworth, T., Bernstein, D., & Stowell, A. W. (2007). Presurgical behavioral medicine evaluation (PBME) for implantable devices for pain management: A one-year prospective study. *Pain Practice, 7*(2), 110–122.

Holmes, C. P., Gatchel, R. J., Adams, L. L., Stowell, A. W., Hatten, A., Noe, C., et al. (2006). An opioid screening instrument: Long-term evaluation of the utility of the Pain Medication Questionnaire. *Pain Practice, 6*, 74–88.

Hua, S. E., & Levy, R. M. (1999). Spinal cord stimulation for failed back surgery syndrome. In H. T. Benyon, G. Srinivasa, D. Borsook, R. E. Malloy, & G. Strichartz (Eds.), *Essentials of pain medicine and regional anesthesia* (pp. 237–241). Philadelphia: Churchill Livingstone.

Joranson, D. E., Carrow, G. M., Ryan, K. M., Schaefer, L., Gilson, A. M., Good, P., et al. (2002). Pain management and prescription monitoring. *Journal of Pain and Symptom Management, 23*, 231–238.

Katz, N. P., Sherburne, S., Beach, M., Rose, R. J., Vielguth, J., Bradley, J., et al. (2003). Behavioral monitoring and urine toxicology testing in patients receiving long-term opioid therapy. *Anesthesia and Analgesia, 97*, 1097–1102.

Katz, W. A., & Barkin, R. L. (2008). Dilemmas in chronic/persistent pain management. *American Journal of Therapeutics, 15*, 256–264.

Kemler, M. A., Barendse, G. A. M., Van Kleef, M., De Vet, H. C. W., Rijks, C. P. M., Furnee, C. A., et al. (2000). Spinal cord stimulation in patients with chronic reflex sympathetic dystrophy. *New England Journal of Medicine, 343*, 618–624.

Kumar, K., Malik, S., & Demeria, D. (2002). Treatment of chronic pain with spinal cord stimulation versus alternative therapies: Cost-effectiveness analysis. *Neurosurgery, 51*(1), 106–116.

Kupers, R. C., Van den Oever, R., Van Houdenhove, B., Vanmechelen, W., Hepp, B., Nuttin, B., et al. (1994). Spinal cord stimulation in Belgium: A nation-wide survey on the incidence, indications, and therapeutic efficacy by the health insurer. *Pain, 56*(2), 211–216.

Martell, B. A., O'Ocoonr, P. G., Kerns, R. D.,

Becker, W. C., Morales, K H., Kosten, T. R., et al. (2007). Systematic review: Opioid treatment for chronic back pain: Prevalence, efficacy, and association with addiction. *Annals of Internal Medicine, 146*(2), 116–127.

Martin, B. I., Deyo, R. A., Mirza, S. K., Turner, J. A., Comstock, B. A., Hollingworth, W., et al. (2008). Expenditures and health status among adults with back and neck problems. *Journal of the American Medical Association, 299*, 656–664.

Nicholson, B. (2009). Benefits of extended-release opioid analgesic formulations in the treatment of chronic pain. *Pain Practice, 9*, 71–81.

North, R. B., Kidd, D. H., Zahurak, M., James, C. S., & Long, D. M. (1993). Spinal cord stimulation for chronic, intractable pain: Experience over two decades. *Neurosurgery, 32*, 384–395.

Polatin, P. B., & Gajraj, N. M. (2002). Integration of pharmacotherapy with psychological treatment of chronic pain. In D. C. Turk & R. J. Gatchel (Eds.), *Psychological approaches to pain management: A practitioner's handbook* (pp. 276–298). New York: Guilford Press.

Reid, M. C., Engles-Horton, L. L., Weber, M. B., Kerns, R. D., Rogers, E. L., & O'Conner, P. G. (2002). Use of opioid medications for chronic noncancer pain syndromes in primary care. *Journal of General Internal Medicine, 17*, 173–179.

Schatman, M. E. (2008). Identifying abusers prior to initiating chronic opioid therapy. *Practical Pain Management, 8*, 54–61.

Schocket, K. G., Gatchel, R. J., Stowell, A. W., Deschner, M., Robinson, R. C., Lou, L., et al. (2008). Presurgical behavioral medicine evaluation: Categorizing patients for potential treatment efficacy for spinal cord stimulation and intrathecal drug therapy. *Neuromodulation, 11*, 237–248.

Soderstrom, C. A., Dischinger, P. C., Kerns, T. J., Kufera, J. A., Mitchell, K. A., & Scalea, T. M. (2001). Epidemic increases in cocaine and opiate use by trauma center patients: Documentation with a large clinical toxicology database. *Journal of Trauma, 51*, 557–564.

Turk, D. C., & Gatchel, R. J. (Eds.). (2002). *Psychological approaches to pain management: A practitioner's handbook* (2nd ed.). New York: Guilford Press.

Turk, D. C., & Monarch, E. S. (2002). Biopsychosocial perspective on chronic pain. In D. C. Turk & R. J. Gatchel (Eds.), *Psychological approaches to pain management: A practitioner's handbook* (2nd ed., pp. 3–29). New York: Guilford Press.

Turk, D. C., & Swanson, K. (2007). Efficacy and cost-effectiveness treatment of chronic pain: An analysis and evidence-based synthesis. In M. E. Schatman & A. Campbell (Eds.), *Chronic pain management: Guidelines for multidisciplinary program development* (pp. 15–38). New York: Informa Healthcare.

Turk, D. C., Swanson, D. C., & Gatchel, R. J. (2008). Predicting opioid misuse by chronic pain patients: A systematic review and literature synthesis. *Clinical Journal of Pain, 24*, 487–508.

Waddell, G. (1987). Clinical assessment of lumbar impairment. *Clinical Orthopaedics and Related Research, 221*, 110–120.

CHAPTER 23

Assessment of Chronic Pain in Epidemiological and Health Services Research
Empirical Bases and New Directions

MICHAEL VON KORFF

This chapter reviews conceptual and empirical bases for assessment and classification of chronic pain in epidemiological and health services research, focusing on psychometric properties, scoring, and interpretation of Version 2.0 of the Graded Chronic Pain Scale (GCPS) and a three-item Graded Chronic Pain—Primary Care Scale (GCP-PCS). A new approach to classification of chronic pain is described, based on a Prognostic Risk Score and classification in terms of outcome probabilities. The methods discussed provide approaches to chronic pain assessment that are applicable across diverse anatomically defined pain conditions or chronic pain conditions in general. This chapter is organized in three parts:

- The first part describes a conceptual approach to defining chronic pain in terms of prognosis estimated from measures of pain severity, pain duration, and other variables.
- The second part reviews methodological underpinnings of standardized assessment of chronic pain severity and duration within the context of epidemiological and survey research. The psychometric bases of the GCPS are reviewed in depth. The GCPS can be used to obtain dimen-

sional measures of chronic pain intensity, interference with activities and pain duration, as well as an ordinal classification of chronic pain severity (Chronic Pain Grade).

- The third part describes Version 2.0 of the GCPS, and the three-item GCP-PCS for brief assessment of chronic pain in primary care settings. The revised, simplified scoring rules provided for Version 2.0 of the GCPS, and for the three-item GCP-PCS, facilitate hand scoring.

BACKGROUND

Over the past 20 years, epidemiology has made significant contributions to the field of chronic pain research (Crombie, Croft, Linton, Le Resche, & Von Korff, 1999). However, scientific progress in chronic pain epidemiology lags behind that achieved in other areas (e.g., cardiovascular, cancer, and mental disorder epidemiology). The lack of standardized classification criteria for chronic pain has been an impediment. Standardized diagnostic criteria have been developed for specific pain disorders, including migraine headache (International Headache Society, 2004), temporomandibular disorders (Truelove, Sommers, LeResche, Dworkin, & Von Korff, 1992), and fibromyalgia (Wolfe et al., 1990), but there are unique challenges in establishing standardized classification criteria for chronic pain as a general phenomenon.

Chronic pain subsumes diverse pain disorders that differ in causal mechanisms and distribution in populations by age, sex, and other risk factors. Cancer, cardiovascular disease, and mental disorder epidemiology employ standardized classification criteria for specific disorders but not for an entire class of disorders. While chronic pain epidemiology needs standardized diagnostic criteria for specific pain disorders, there is also a need for standardized classification criteria for chronic pain in general.

DEFINING CHRONIC PAIN BY PROGNOSIS

The traditional approach to defining chronic pain relies on pain duration alone (Merskey & Bogduk, 1994). Defining chronic pain solely by pain duration is based on the view that acute pain signals potential tissue damage, whereas chronic pain results from central and peripheral sensitization in which pain is sustained after nociceptive inputs have diminished (Bonica, 1990). While appealing, this approach has not led to reliable and valid methods for differentiating acute from chronic pain, nor has it led to standardized operational criteria for defining cases in epidemiological and health services research (Von Korff & Dunn, 2008). Defining chronic pain solely by duration is difficult to apply to recurrent pain. The duration-based approach is also contrary to the view that chronic pain is multidimensional (Turk & Rudy, 1988).

Duration-based definitions identify persons with chronic pain empirically as the passage of time sorts out patients with chronic pain from those with acute pain. There are four problems with duration-based definitions:

1. The elapsed time typically used to differentiate chronic from acute pain (3–6 months) does not correspond to the timescale of neurophysiological mechanisms hypothesized to result in chronic pain, which are thought to occur in millisec-

onds, minutes, hours, or days, rather than months.
2. Duration-based definitions of chronic pain do not provide a basis for targeting patients at risk of an unfavorable pain outcome early in its course, when prevention might be most effective.
3. Defining chronic pain by duration alone is insufficient to differentiate persons with clinically significant pain from those with long-lasting pain problems that have less substantial impact.
4. There is not compelling evidence that patients typically become progressively more dysfunctional simply as a function of increasing pain duration. Whereas key manifestations of chronic pain (e.g., severe pain, depression, activity limitations) are often present in the acute phase of pain, the transition to chronic pain is more often characterized by a failure of these manifestations to resolve, rather than by progressive worsening with the passage of time. For these reasons, the distinction between acute and chronic pain may not be adequately defined by pain duration alone.

An alternative approach to defining chronic pain combines information on pain severity *and* duration with information on other prognostic variables, defining chronic pain in terms of outcome probabilities. This approach was initially developed using data from a cohort of primary care patients with back pain (Von Korff & Miglioretti, 2006), and was subsequently replicated across multiple musculoskeletal pain conditions in independent studies (Dunn, Croft, Main, & Von Korff, 2008; Thomas et al., 2008; Von Korff & Dunn, 2008). Table 23.1 provides empirically derived and replicated scoring rules for a chronic pain Prognostic Risk Score based on items in the GCPS, along with the number of anatomically defined pain sites and depression severity. This Prognostic Risk Score permits the use of any of three depression severity scales: the Patient Health Questionnaire (PHQ-9 or PHQ-8; Kroenke et al., 2009), the Symptom Checklist 90—Revised (SCL-90-R; Derogatis, 1983), and the Hospital Anxiety and Depression Scale (HADS; Zigmond & Snaith, 1983). (Other depression scales could be

TABLE 23.1. Scoring Rules for a Chronic Pain Prognostic Risk Score and Classification Criteria for Possible and Probable Chronic Pain Based on Prognostic Risk Score and the GCPS (see Appendix 23.1)

Item			Item value	Risk Score value
Usual pain intensity (Q4)			0–3	0
			4–6	1
			7–10	2
Worst pain intensity (Q3)			0–4	0
			5–7	1
			8–10	2
Current pain intensity (Q2)			0–2	0
			3–4	1
			5–10	2
Interference with daily activities (Q6)			0–2	0
			3–4	1
			5–10	2
Interference with work/household activities (Q8)			0–2	0
			3–4	1
			5–10	2
Interference with family/social activities (Q7)			0–2	0
			3–4	1
			5–10	2
Days of activity limitation due to pain in the prior 3 months (Q5)			0–2	0
			3–6	1
			7–15	2
			16–24	3
			25–90	4
Number of (other) pain sites			0	0
			1	1
			2	2
			3	3
			4	4
Number of days with pain in the prior 6 months (Q1)			0–30	0
			31–89	1
			90–120	2
			121–160	3
			161–180	4

	PHQ-9 Depression	SCL-90-R Depression	Hospital Anxiety and Depression Scale	
Depression symptom severity scale	0–5	< 0.50	0–3	0
	6–9	0.50–< 1.00	4–7	1
	10–13	1.00–< 1.50	8–10	2
	14–18	1.50–< 2.00	11–12	3
	19+	2.00+	13+	4

(cont.)

TABLE 23.1. *(cont.)*

Cutoff points for classification of chronic pain based on Prognostic Risk Score
for primary care pain patients and for general population samples

General population samples	
Low risk	0–4 points
Intermediate risk	5–11 points
Possible chronic pain (50% + risk)	12–17 points
Probable chronic pain (80% + risk)	18+ points
Primary care samples	
Low risk	0–7 points
Intermediate risk	8–15 points
Possible chronic pain (50% + risk)	16–21 points
Probable chronic pain (80% + risk)	22+ points

Note. This algorithm for estimating a chronic pain Prognostic Risk Score has been placed in the Creative Commons and may be used without the author's permission with citation of this publication.

substituted by defining scoring rules comparable to those developed for the PHQ, the SCL-90-R, and the HADS.)

The ability of the Prognostic Risk Score to predict clinically significant pain at follow-up was assessed with use of a smoothed plot of the Baseline Risk Score against the probability of significant pain 1 year after an index pain consultation. *Probable chronic pain* was defined by an 80% or greater probability of future clinically significant pain. *Possible chronic pain* was defined by a 50% or greater probability. Cutoff points for low risk, intermediate risk, and for possible and probable chronic pain were then defined on the Prognostic Risk Score from the probability plot. For primary care patients with pain, *low risk* was defined by risk scores of 0–7; intermediate risk, by risk scores of 8–15; possible chronic pain by risk scores of 16–21; and probable chronic pain by risk scores of 22 or more (Von Korff & Dunn, 2008; Von Korff & Miglioretti, 2005). These categories strongly predicted long-term pain outcomes over a 5-year follow-up period.

Subsequent work suggested that different cutoff points should be employed in general population samples (Thomas, Dunn, Mallen, & Peat, 2008). Primary care patients are typically initially assessed in proximity to exacerbation of a pain problem (prompting treatment seeking), whereas persons in a general population sample are not. For this reason, lower cutoff points on the Prognostic Risk Score are appropriate when used in general population samples. Thomas and

colleagues (2008) suggested 0–4 for low risk; 5–11 for intermediate risk; 12–17 for possible chronic pain; and 18+ for probable chronic pain. These cutoff points were shown to achieve comparable positive predictive value for clinically significant pain at long-term follow-up as the cutoff points originally proposed for primary care patients with pain. Cutoff points for defining possible and probable chronic pain are summarized in Table 23.1.

The Prognostic Risk Score approach defines chronic pain in probabilistic terms (i.e., "possible" and "probable" chronic pain). Defining chronic pain in probabilistic terms is consistent with the observation from longitudinal studies that chronic pain outcomes are variable and uncertain. The fact that outcome probabilities are a function of multiple factors calls attention to the potential to improve chances of a favorable outcome in many different ways other than limiting the duration of pain. The likelihood of a favorable outcome may be increased by reducing pain intensity, by increasing activity levels, or by controlling depression.

A prognostic approach to defining chronic pain could be extended, based on empirical research, to include other factors that contribute to improved prediction of chronic pain outcomes. This might include additional self-report measures, psychophysical tests, genetic markers, or health history information from medical records. The probability of continuation of clinically significant pain provides a common metric for combining multiple prognostic variables. The criteria guiding selection of prognostic variables would be (1) improved accuracy of long-term prediction of pain outcomes and (2) generalizability across anatomically defined pain conditions.

EMPIRICAL RESEARCH ON ASSESSING CHRONIC PAIN SEVERITY AND PERSISTENCE

In assessing specific chronic pain conditions, signs and symptoms of the underlying disorder are typically included in a standardized case definition. For example, migraine headache diagnosis is based on specific symptoms, such as unilateral location and pulsating quality, as well as moderate to severe pain intensity (International Headache Society, 2004). In classifying and assessing chronic pain based on prognosis, key features that need to be assessed include anatomical location(s) and diffuseness; pain intensity, pain-related activity limitation, pain duration or persistence, and prognostic factors integral to chronic pain (e.g., depression). In this section, the methodological bases of assessing these chronic pain features in epidemiological and health services research are reviewed. The psychometric properties of the GCPS are discussed in depth. However, evaluation of measurement properties needs to be considered within the context of potential biases.

Case Ascertainment Biases

Sources of bias in epidemiological and health services research employing survey methods have been extensively studied (Bradburn, Rips, & Shevell, 1987; Cannel, 1977; Converse & Traugott, 1986). They include measurement bias in questionnaires, a variety of reporting biases, as well as sample biases, such as undercoverage (persons missed by the sampling method) and nonresponse (persons refusing the interview or not contacted).

Recall bias is a significant issue in epidemiological and health services research concerning pain, because it is often necessary to ask respondents whether they have experienced an anatomically defined pain condition over a defined period of time (e.g., 1 week, 1 month, 3 months, 6 months, 1 year). Means, Nigram, Zarrow, Loftus, and

Donaldson (1989), in a monograph on autobiographical memory for health-related events, drew a distinction between semantic memory and episodic memory. *Semantic memory* is conceptually structured information resistant to interference from other memory traces. *Episodic memory* is a temporally ordered set of autobiographical events that can be more difficult to retrieve. It is important to understand what features of a chronic pain condition (e.g., persistence, intensity, activity limitations) lead to encoding of the pain condition as a semantic or as an episodic memory. If the characteristic levels of pain intensity and of activity limitation related to pain are more likely to be encoded as semantic memories, then the accuracy of recall of these attributes of pain conditions may be adequate for a recall interval of 3, 6, or 12 months for clinically significant and long-lasting pain conditions. In contrast, mild episodic pain conditions that are less persistent or less severe may be more likely to be forgotten if semantic memories of these experiences are not formed.

In epidemiological and health services research, it is often necessary to ask respondents whether they have experienced pain at a given anatomical site. It is not possible to ask follow-up questions about intensity, persistence, and pain-related interference with activities until the respondent has reported the presence of a pain condition of interest. Based on research showing that memory for doctor visits decays rapidly with increasing time since the visit (Cannel, 1977), an important issue is how long a recall period should be employed in asking subjects about chronic pain conditions. There are tradeoffs for short versus long reporting intervals (Von Korff & Dworkin, 1989). A short reporting period, all else being equal, should minimize forgetting of pain conditions if the subject is not experiencing pain at the time of the interview. However, a short reporting period may not yield as reliable an estimate of a subject's characteristic chronic pain status because of large within-subject variability in pain status over time. For example, it may be more informative to know that a person experienced back pain on 90 days in the prior 6 months than to know that back pain was present on 4 days in the prior week, even though 1-week recall may be more accurate than 6-month recall. Similarly, it may be of greater research value to learn that a patient's average headache pain intensity was 5 over the past 3 months than to learn that average headache pain intensity was 4 over the past 24 hours, as assessed on several occasions with an electronic diary, even though the 24-hour measurement is more accurate than 3-month recall.

Other cognitive processes are relevant to the recall of pain in epidemiological and health services research. *Forward telescoping* is a tendency for respondents to report earlier events as having occurred during the reporting period. This may be particularly problematic in studies estimating first-onset rates of pain conditions. If subjects tend to report first onset as more recent than it actually was, incidence rate estimates could be substantially inflated. There is evidence that this phenomenon occurs for recall of mental disorder onset (Simon & Von Korff, 1995). Carey, Garrett, Jackman, Sanders, and Kalsbeek (1995) studied back pain recall among 235 patients with back pain who had made a back pain visit 4–16 months earlier. In this study, there was evidence that episodes of back pain occurring more than 8 months before the interview tended to be recalled as occurring more recently, suggesting forward telescoping.

In addition to the sources of bias encountered in survey interviews, investigators conducting longitudinal studies need to be aware of additional sources of bias, including loss to follow-up, missing data, and measurement biases introduced by repeated measurement. Missing data and loss to follow-up can substantially reduce sample size in a longitudinal survey, particularly if observations are made on more than two occasions. Such losses are generally not random; thus, they may introduce an important source of bias. Measures that may be biased by repeated measurement or that may "drift" over time also present problems in longitudinal studies, as do unreliable measures.

Assessment of Chronic Pain Status in a Defined Time Interval

Epidemiological and health services research on chronic pain often require assessment of the characteristic level and pattern of pain and associated interference with activities over a period of time (e.g., 1 month, 3 months) rather than measurement of an individual's pain status only at the time of assessment. Determining a person's characteristic chronic pain status is made difficult by the large across-time variability in individual pain status and the diverse sources of variation in pain measurement. Variation in pain measurement may be due to the measurement method, such as the scale or questions used (see Jensen & Karoly, Chapter 2, this volume), the scaling of responses, the length of the recall period, the method of prompting for condition or anatomical site, and/or the method of administration (e.g., personal interview, self-administered questionnaire, telephone interview). Additional variation may be due to timing of measurements: the number of different times pain status is measured; time of the day; day of the week; and timing of administration in relation to milestones in the natural history of the condition or treatment seeking. Context of pain measurement may also contribute to variation (e.g., work, home, health care or research settings).

In epidemiological and health services research, determining characteristic pain status by frequently repeated assessments (e.g., a 1-week or a 1-month daily diary) is rarely feasible in studies that require a large sample size. Rather, it is necessary to rely on retrospective report of key parameters of pain status over a defined time period, such as 1 week, 1 month, 3 months, 6 months, or 1 year. Key parameters of pain status evaluated by recall for a defined time period include the number of days a patient experiences pain, the average pain intensity level when in pain, the average level of interference with life activities, and the number of days of interference with daily activities (Von Korff, Ormel, Keefe, & Dworkin, 1992).

A possible approach to quantifying pain severity is by estimating the product of average pain intensity and the total duration of pain, as in "headache index"–type measures (Von Korff, Lipton, & Stewart, 1994). However, pain intensity and pain duration are not necessarily highly correlated (Von Korff et al., 1992). Their association with other measures of pain impact (e.g., disability, medicine use, depression) may be additive rather than multiplicative (Von Korff et al., 1994). For this reason, it is useful to view pain persistence and pain intensity as distinct, albeit moderately correlated, dimensions of chronic pain. In contrast, measures of pain intensity and pain-related interference with activities generally scale together, often forming an underlying unidimensional continuum of pain severity (Schmidt, Raspe, & Kohlmann, 2010).

Reliability and Validity of Retrospective Pain Report

Rigorous empirical studies have provided considerable information on the reliability and validity of retrospective report of pain intensity, persistence, and associated disability. While these studies suggest that retrospective pain report is not perfect, well-crafted questions about pain status for a 3-month recall period yield reliable and valid data. A National Center for Health Statistics monograph on pain assessment in health surveys evaluated recall bias (Salovey et al., 1992). This research consisted of experiments designed to investigate factors influencing accurate recall of pain and associated activity limitations. The investigators reached the following conclusions:

> Compared with the literature reviewed at the start of this paper, which reported, for the most part, considerable inaccuracy in recall of pain among small samples of patients undergoing treatment in pain clinics, recall among our subjects across most of the studies would be better characterized by its accuracy. Overall, we were impressed by how well subjects could report on their pain retrospectively. When biases in retrospective report were observed, they tended to be in the direction of overestimating rather than underestimating prior levels of pain.
>
> The severity of prior pain, its impact on daily activities and behaviors related to the pain problem are all recalled approximately equally well and seem to be equally stable over time among individuals with chronic pain problems. Survey researchers who seek more informative data than that provided by mere intensity ratings should feel comfortable querying respondents about these other pain related behaviors. ... One systematic source of bias in pain ratings is created by severity of pain at the time of recall. Controlling for original levels of pain and the amount that pain fluctuates during the applicable time period, greater pain at recall was associated with overestimating of prior pain experience. Survey researchers

who seek to include questions about prior experiences with pain may wish to include questions about current levels of pain as well. ... Mood may not be a major influence on pain recall, at least not under the specific circumstances investigated here. (Salovey et al., 1992, p. 26)

Similarly, Jamison, Raymond, Slawsby, McHugo, and Baird (2006, p. 192) reached the following conclusions from a comparison of pain recall to repeated pain assessment employing an electronic diary:

> Weekly recalled pain might be just as useful as momentary data collected through electronic data entry. Some believe that remembered pain is problematic because of recall bias and that data from frequent momentary pain ratings with electronic diaries are more valid. This study demonstrates that recalled pain is as valid as momentary data for many patients.

These results, and results from other studies reviewed below, provide strong empirical support for the validity of retrospective recall of key aspects of chronic pain status over time periods from 1 week to 6 months, depending on the nature of the recall task.

Validity of Recall of Anatomically Defined Pain

In an epidemiological survey, it is often necessary to ask subjects whether they have experienced pain at a particular anatomical site (e.g., back pain, headache) during a defined time period (e.g., 3 months, 1 year). It is not possible to ask follow-up questions about intensity, persistence, and disability until the subject has reported the presence of an anatomically defined pain condition.

Research by the National Center for Health Statistics provides estimates of the probability of recall of selected chronic conditions known to have been present in the prior year because they were treated (Madow, 1973). For example, diabetes, sinusitis, and hypertension were recalled by more than 80% of treated patients, while asthma, headache, and arthritis were recalled by more than 60% of treated patients. This research showed that the agreement of self-report and medical records data increased with the number of visits for a chronic condition and was higher if the subject had received medicines for the condition. This suggests that pain conditions with greater impact are more salient, and more likely to be remembered and reported. Experience with questioning patients about chronic conditions also suggests that they are much more likely to report them when asked about a list of specific conditions than when asked a general question about chronic illness. Higher yield in pain surveys is achieved if subjects are asked about each anatomically defined pain condition of interest than if they are asked a general question about the occurrence of pain (not anatomically defined).

In a study of high utilizers of health care who had made a health care visit for back pain in the prior year (Von Korff, 1991), recall of back pain was high (88%) if the visit occurred within the prior 6 months, but lower (73%) if the visit occurred more than 6 months before the interview. Persons with multiple visits were more likely to recall their back pain episode (92%) than were persons with a single visit (69%). Depressed persons (91%) were more likely to recall their back pain episode than were nondepressed individuals (74%), particularly among persons whose visit was more than 6 months before the interview (88 vs. 57%). In a survey of 235 patients with back pain who had made back pain visits, Carey and colleagues (1995) found that 79% reported having had back pain when asked 4 to 16 months after their visit. These results suggest that ability to recall prior episodes of pain is adequate, particularly if the episode occurred within the prior 6 months and had significant impact.

Validity of Retrospective Report of Average Pain Intensity

Salovey and colleagues (1992) reported correlations between different retrospective measures of pain intensity for the prior 2 weeks and 2 weeks of hourly pain ratings for persons undergoing assessment at a pain treatment center. They found the following correlations with the mean of the hourly pain ratings: current pain ($r = .74$); usual pain ($r = .83$); worst pain ($r = .68$); and least pain ($r = .87$). De Wit and colleagues (1999) conducted a diary study of 159 cancer patients and found correlations of .80 or higher between 1-week recall of average pain intensity and estimates of average pain intensity from a daily diary. Jensen, Turner, Turner, and Ro-

mano (1996) compared retrospective ratings of usual, least, worst, and current pain to hourly pain ratings made by 40 patients with chronic pain over a period of 6–14 days. They reported the following correlations between diary-estimated average pain and alternative measures based on patient recall: least pain ($r = .81$); usual pain ($r = .78$); current pain ($r = .64$); and worst pain ($r = .64$). They found that composite measures tended to produce modest increases in these correlations. In a subsequent study, Jensen, Turner, Romano, and Fisher (1999) found that single and composite pain measures were similar in their ability to detect change in pain status, but that composite pain measures showed greater across-time correlation (stability). Stewart, Lipton, Simon, Liberman, and Von Korff (1999) carried out a 3-month daily diary study in a population sample of 132 migraine sufferers. They found high correlations between diary-based estimates of pain intensity and retrospective report of average pain intensity ($r = .74$). Jamison and colleagues (2006) reported that the correlation of pain intensity recall over a 1-week period and pain ratings obtained at least once a day over a 1-week period were greater than .90. Broderick and colleagues (2008) found that the correlation of averaged momentary daily pain intensity ratings with 28-day recall of average pain intensity (rated on a 0- to 10-point scale) exceeded .80. Ratings of other symptoms (e.g., stabbing pain, aching pain, nagging pain, fatigue) were somewhat lower, suggesting that the specific rating task can influence recall accuracy. This study replicated prior research showing that recalled average pain intensity was higher than the average of daily momentary pain intensity assessments. However, studies comparing recalled average pain intensity to averaged daily momentary assessments have rarely taken into account that when subjects recall average pain intensity, they generally consider times when they are experiencing pain, not times when they are pain-free. There was less difference between recalled average pain intensity and averaged daily momentary pain ratings when pain-free observations were excluded from the daily momentary assessments (Stewart, Lipton, Simon, et al., 1999).

Across these studies, retrospective report of average pain intensity showed a high correlation with diary-based estimates of average pain intensity. Given the favorable results of several validity studies, there appears to be sufficient empirical support for using measures of average or usual pain intensity for up to a 3-month recall period. Research suggests that pain intensity measures on a 0- to 10-point scale provide adequate discrimination (Jensen, Karoly, O'Riordan, Bland, & Burns, 1989; Jensen, Turner, & Romano, 1994). However, there is evidence that increasing the number of occasions on which pain intensity is measured, up to three times per day for 4 days, can increase the reliability and validity of estimators of average pain (Jensen & McFarland, 1993). There is also evidence that composite measures of pain intensity (e.g., composites of average, least, worst, and current pain) can yield modest improvements in measurement properties relative to a single rating (Dworkin et al., 1990; Jensen et al., 1996, 1999).

Validity of Retrospective Report of Days with Pain

There has been less research evaluating the validity of retrospective report of days with pain over a fixed period of time than for average pain intensity. Salovey and colleagues (1992) reported a correlation of .70 between subject recall of the number of days in the prior 2 weeks with a pain rating greater than 5 and a diary-based estimate. In their 3-month daily diary study, Stewart, Lipton, Simon, and colleagues (1999) reported a correlation ($r = .67$) between diary data on days with headache and 3-month recall of days with headache.

These results support the validity of recall of days with pain over an extended period of time, but more research is needed. For purposes of differentiating persons with chronic versus recurrent or acute pain conditions, one can question whether a 3-month reporting period is sufficient. The International Headache Society (2004) defines *chronic headache* as headaches occurring on at least half the days in a 3-month period, or at least 180 days in a year. Similarly, *persistent back pain* has been defined as back pain present on at least half the days in a 6-month period (Von Korff & Saunders, 1996). This suggests the potential utility of asking about pain days over a 6-month or 1-year timeframe, even though daily diary studies to validate self-report over these lon-

ger time periods are not available and would be difficult to carry out.

Validity of Retrospective Report of Pain-Related Interference with Life Activities

There are three widely used types of questions to ask about pain-related interference with life activities. One form of question asks respondents to rate the degree of interference with daily activities due to pain during a definite or indefinite time period (Kerns, Turk, & Rudy, 1985). A variation on this form asks respondents to rate the percentage of reduction in their ability to perform a set of activities (Stewart, Lipton, Kolodner, Liberman, & Sawyer, 1999). A second form of question, typically with a yes–no response format, asks about limitations in activities due to pain (Roland & Morris, 1983). A third format asks about days of activity limitation during a 1-month, 3-month, or 6-month time period when the subject was unable to carry out usual activities due to pain (Von Korff et al., 1992).

There is considerable support for the internal consistency and convergent validity of these kinds of questions. However, relatively few studies have validated recall of pain-related disability in relation to daily diary measures. In a population-based study of persons with migraine, Stewart, Lipton, Simon, and colleagues (1999) found a correlation ($r = .62$) between diary and retrospective report of percentage of reduced effectiveness at work. They reported a correlation ($r = .48$) between recall of lost work days due to headache and the corresponding diary-based measure. They observed that questions about activity limitation days with lower yield had lower correlation between recall and diary-based measures than did questions with higher yield, likely reflecting the attenuation of correlation with highly skewed items. In a second validity study, they evaluated revised questions about activity limitation days (Stewart, Lipton, Whyte, et al., 1999). This study yielded the correlations between a 3-month daily diary and retrospective report (see Table 23.2).

Although there is a need for more research, these results from daily diary studies, in combination with prior research evaluating the internal consistency and convergent validity of pain disability measures, suggests

TABLE 23.2. Correlation of 3-Month Retrospective Report and Mean of 3-Month Daily Diary Estimate

	Pearson correlation
Number of days of missed work or school due to headache	.60
Work/school days productivity reduced by half due to headache	.67
Days of household work missed due to headache	.63
Days productivity in household work reduced by half due to headache	.61
Days missed in family, social, or leisure activities due to headache	.61

that retrospective report of interference with daily activities provides reliable and valid information. Information on internal consistency, test–retest reliability, and convergent validity is presented in the following section concerning the psychometric properties of the GCPS. Future research comparing retrospective report to employer records of absenteeism and work performance would be particularly useful.

Psychometric Evaluation of the GCPS

This section reviews evidence regarding the psychometric properties of a brief measure of pain status widely used in epidemiological and health services research—the GCPS (Von Korff et al., 1992).

The GCPS was developed to provide a brief and simple method of assessing the severity of chronic or recurrent pain in general population surveys and studies of patients with pain in primary care settings. The GCPS measures an underlying severity continuum defined by pain intensity and interference with daily activities (Chronic Pain Grade) that has a hierarchical structure in which lower levels of severity are differentiated by pain intensity, and higher levels of severity are differentiated by interference with activities. This structure suggests that patients at higher levels of severity, defined by moderate to severe interference with activities, can show improvement by reductions in disability even if pain intensity is not reduced.

Analyses carried out in developing the GCPS suggested a threshold effect for pain intensity. Respondents with moderate to severe interference with activities (Grades III and IV) almost always reported intensity ratings of 5 or greater on a 0- to 10-point Characteristic Pain Intensity scale (average pain + worst pain + current pain/3). In other words, high pain intensity levels were a necessary (but not sufficient) condition for the presence of moderate to severe interference with activities. This suggests that modest reductions in pain intensity might have substantial effects in reducing interference with functioning, if pain intensity were reduced below a threshold level necessary for disability. Although pain persistence per se is not used in determining Chronic Pain Grade, an item asking about pain days in the prior 6 months is included (Von Korff et al., 1992). The items included in Version 2.0 of the GCPS are provided in Appendix 23.1.

The GCPS can be used to assess pain intensity, pain-related interference with activities, and pain persistence at a defined anatomical location (e.g., back pain, headache) or to assess chronic pain status without reference to a particular anatomical location. The GCPS questions were initially developed with a 6-month reporting period. Subsequently, they have been administered with a 3-month reporting interval (Von Korff et al., 1998) or with a 1-month reporting interval (Underwood, Barnett, & Vickers, 1999). The shorter reporting intervals are useful in situations where respondents are being followed over time to assess change (e.g., in a study of clinical course or a clinical trial). This chapter focuses on the 3-month version of the GCPS.

The GCPS grades the severity of the pain condition into five ordered categories: Grade 0–Pain-Free; Grade I–Low Intensity, Low Interference; Grade II–High intensity; Grade III–Moderate Interference with Activities; Grade IV–Severe Interference with Activities. For patients with higher levels of disability (i.e., Grades III and IV), grading does not consider pain intensity scores. The ordered categories facilitate analysis of the spectrum of severity of chronic–recurrent pain in general population and primary care samples. Using the pain days question (Q1, Appendix 23.1), patients reporting pain on at least half the days in a 6-month time period are classified as having persistent pain, an additional descriptor of chronic pain status.

The GCPS can also be used to provide continuous measures of (1) pain intensity (Usual Pain Intensity or Characteristic Pain Intensity); (2) interference with activities (Disability Score); and (3) persistence (Pain Days). These continuous measures are more suitable for assessing the effectiveness of interventions (e.g., in clinical trials) than the ordered categories of Chronic Pain Grade, which are less responsive to change. The continuous measures of pain intensity, disability, and persistence may also be useful in situations where distinct measures of pain intensity, disability, and persistence are needed (e.g., as predictor variables in multivariate analyses, or in analyses of how different components of chronic pain status change with time).

The items used to grade chronic pain status have been evaluated in a large population survey with a 3-year follow-up and in large samples of primary care patients with pain (Von Korff et al., 1992). The grading criteria for GCPS may have limited utility in pain clinic populations, where most patients are likely to fall at Grade IV. Table 23.3 provides the distribution of Chronic Pain Grade for primary care patients with back pain, headache, and orofacial pain, and for a population sample of adult health plan en-

rollees, with patients were assigned to their highest pain grade across three pain conditions (back pain, headache, orofacial pain).

The GCPS has been used and evaluated in pain surveys carried out in diverse settings in the United States and Europe, and has been translated into numerous languages without difficulties. In its initial validation, Von Korff and colleagues (1992) showed that GCPS was associated with an independent measure of pain-related disability, with use of health care and medicines for pain, with severity of depressive symptoms, with frequent use of doctor visits and opioids for pain, and with unemployment in samples of primary care patients with back pain, headache, and temporomandibular pain. GCPS was also shown to be associated with increased likelihood of a poor functional outcome 1 year and 3 years later. In this initial work, it was shown that the pain intensity and disability items formed a unidimensional scale with good psychometric properties. Based on Pearson correlations of the seven items used in the GCPS, the internal consistency (Cronbach's alpha) was .84 for back pain, .79 for headache, and .84 for temporomandibular pain.

Smith and colleagues (1997) validated the GCPS in a postal survey of 293 persons drawn from a general practice roster (see also Purves et al., 1998). They confirmed that the

TABLE 23.3. Percentage at Chronic Pain Grade for Patients with Back Pain, Headache, and Orofacial Pain in Primary Care and for a Population Sample of Adult Health Maintenance Organization (HMO) Enrollees

Chronic Pain Grade	Back pain	Headache	Orofacial pain	Population sample
0: No pain (prior 6 months)	—	—	—	48.9
I: Low intensity, low interference	34.9	29.7	40.7	17.9
II: High intensity	27.9	40.1	43.5	20.3
III: Moderate interference	20.0	20.2	10.5	10.7
IV: Severe interference	17.2	10.0	5.4	2.3
(Sample size)	(1,213)	(779)	(397)	(803)

Note. The population prevalence rates are for back pain, headache, and/or orofacial pain based on a 6-month version of the GCPS. Persons are assigned to the highest pain grade across the three pain conditions. Persons classified as pain-free did not report back pain, headache, or orofacial pain in the prior 6 months. Primary care patients with pain were assessed 1–3 weeks after an initial visit.

GCPS was unidimensional, with an internal consistency coefficient (Cronbach's alpha) of .91. The eigenvalue of the first factor was 4.80, while remaining factors all had eigenvalues of less than .85. Chronic Pain Grade showed a correlation of −.84 with the Bodily Pain scale of the Short Form Health Survey (SF-36), and correlations of −.49 to −.65 with the Physical Function, Social Function, Physical Role, and Emotional Role scales of the SF-36 (these correlations are negative, because a lower score indicates greater disability on the SF-36, while a higher grade indicates greater disability on the GCPS). Chronic Pain Grade was also found to be significantly associated with use of health care and medicines for pain in this study.

A study of the GCPS was reported by Penny, Purves, Smith, Chambers, and Smith (1999) in a random sample of 3,605 persons drawn from general practice registers, supplemented by 3,335 persons drawn from a list of persons filling repeated prescriptions for analgesic medications. This study showed a strong relationship between Chronic Pain Grade and each of the subscales of the SF-36. This study also showed significant relationships between Chronic Pain Grade and each of the dimensions of the Glasgow Pain Questionnaire (including frequency, intensity, coping, emotional reactions, and restrictions).

Underwood and colleagues (1999) compared the GCPS and the Roland Disability Scale (Roland & Morris, 1983) in patients with back pain. They tested a version of the GCPS with a 1-month reporting period. They reported internal consistency coefficients of .91 for the Characteristic Pain scale and .89 for Disability Score. They assessed test–retest reliability with intraclass correlation coefficients (ICCs) based on a readministration at 1–2 weeks. They reported an ICC of .82 for Pain Intensity and .85 for Disability Score. They reported high correlations of these GCPS subscales with the SF-36 Pain scale (−.67 for Pain Intensity and −.76 for Disability Score) and with the SF-36 Physical Function subscale (−.64 for Pain Intensity and −.72 for Disability Score. The validity of the GCPS has also been established in persons with spinal cord injury (Raichle, Osborne, Jensen, & Cardenas, 2006).

The responsiveness to change of the GCPS has been evaluated in several studies (Elliott,

Smith, Smith, & Chambers, 2000; Elliott, Smith, Hannaford, Smith, & Chambers, 2002), and the GCPS has been used as an outcome measure in randomized controlled trials (Moore, Von Korff, Cherkin, Saunders, & Lorig, 2000; Von Korff et al., 1998, 2005), providing support for its responsiveness to change. As noted earlier, when used to assess outcomes in randomized controlled trials or in longitudinal studies, it is recommended to use the continuous pain intensity ratings and the disability score measures of the GCPS, rather than Chronic Pain Grade, as the continuous GCPS measures are likely to be more responsive to change than the ordinal Chronic Pain Grade.

Schmidt, Raspe, and Kohlmann (2010) evaluated psychometric properties of the GCPS in a survey of 8,756 persons with back pain in Germany, using latent-class analysis and confirmatory factor analysis. They found that average pain intensity ratings below 5 entailed no or only modest increases in pain-related disability, whereas pain intensity ratings of 5 or greater were more likely to be associated with significant disability. However, disability ratings increased gradually with pain intensity ratings across their range. They observed that high levels of pain intensity occurred infrequently in combination with low levels of pain-related disability (Grade II). This suggests that Grade II might be better characterized as reflecting high pain intensity levels, without characterizing the class as having low levels of interference with activities. They also found that pain intensity and pain-related interference with activities formed independent dimensions that shared substantial common variation, indicating that pain severity constitutes a second-order latent variable rather than regarding pain intensity and interference with activities as having a simple unidimensional factor structure.

The reliability and validity of the GCPS have now been established by numerous research groups in diverse populations. Normative data are available for general population samples (Elliot, Smith, Penny, Smith, & Chambers, 1999) and for primary care samples with back pain, headache, and orofacial pain (Von Korff et al., 1992). The GCPS is an efficient means of assessing and comparing the severity of different chronic–recurrent pain conditions. It can be used as an ordinal scale (Chronic Pain Grade) or as a set of continuous measures of pain intensity, interference with activities, and persistence.

THE GCPS

Version 2.0 of the GCPS assesses pain persistence (Q1), Characteristic Pain Intensity (Q2–Q4), and Pain-Related Interference with Life Activities (Q5–Q8). The use of a 6-month reporting period for pain days is advised to permit meaningful differentiation of persistent and recurrent pain conditions, even when the 3-month or 1-month version of the GCPS is being used. In research concerning chronic pain in general, the GCPS can assess pain severity and persistence in general by dropping the anatomical location modifier in the questions.

Scoring the GCPS Version 2.0

The scoring of the GCPS Version 2.0 has been simplified. Characteristic Pain Intensity is calculated by summing Pain Intensity Right Now (Q2), Worst Pain Intensity (Q3), and Usual Pain Intensity (Q4), resulting in a score with a range from 0 to 30. This change was made to facilitate hand scoring. When analyzing or reporting Characteristic Pain Intensity as a dimensional measure of pain intensity, the 0–30 score can be divided by 3 to yield a score with a conventional range of 0–10.

The Disability Score is calculated by summing the 0–10 score for Days Kept from Usual Activities (Q5), Interference with Daily Activities (Q6), Interference with Social Activities (Q7) and Interference with Work/Housework Activities (Q8), resulting in a score with a range from 0 to 40. It is important to observe that the score for Days Kept from Usual Activities (Q5) is the 0–10 score, not the reported number of activity limitation days. When analyzing or reporting Disability Score as a dimensional measure of pain-related interference with activities, the 0–40 score may be divided by 4 to yield a score with a conventional range of 0–10.

Using the GCPS Version 2.0, Chronic Pain Grade is determined using the Characteristic Pain Intensity and Disability Score according to the following rules (see Appendix 23.2).

The five GCPS Version 2.0 grades are Grade 0, pain-free; Grade I, Low pain intensity, low interference; Grade II, High pain intensity; Grade III, Moderate interference; and Grade IV, Severe interference. Persons with a Disability Score of 25 or greater are classified at Grade IV, regardless of their Characteristic Pain Intensity score. Persons with a Disability Score of 17–24 are classified at Grade III (regardless of their Characteristic Pain Intensity score). Persons with a Disability Score less than 17 are classified at Grade II if their Characteristic Pain Intensity score is between 15 and 30 (based on the 0–30 scoring of Characteristic Pain Intensity), and at Grade I if their Characteristic Pain Intensity score is less than 15. Persons who are pain-free are classified at Grade 0. The simplified scoring methods and classification algorithm employed for GCPS Version 2.0 yield a high level of agreement with Chronic Pain Grade based on the original scoring methods and classification algorithm. In primary care samples with back pain, headache, and orofacial pain, the weighted kappa coefficient for agreement of Chronic Pain Grade based on the original and the simplified scoring method was .88 for back pain, .76 for headache, and .88 for orofacial pain.

Three-Item GCP-PCS

For clinical applications in primary care settings, a very brief pain assessment is sometimes desired. For clinical applications, it is possible to employ a subset of three GCPS items, called the Graded Chronic Pain—Primary Care Scale (GCP-PCS). The three GCP-PCS items are denoted by the ♣ symbol in Appendix 23.1. The three-item GCP-PCS is scored as follows: The 0–10 Usual Pain Intensity item (Q4) is used in place of Characteristic Pain Intensity. Two interference ratings, Days Kept from Usual Activities (Q5) and Interference with Daily Activities (Q6), are summed to estimate a two-item Disability Score ranging from 0 to 20.

When the GCP-PCS is used, Chronic Pain Grade is determined from Usual Pain Intensity and the two-item Disability Score according to the following rules (see Appendix 23.2). Persons with a two-item Disability Score of 13–20 are classified at Grade IV, regardless of their Usual Pain Intensity score. Persons with a two-item Disability Score of

9–12 are classified at Grade III (regardless of their Usual Pain Intensity score). Persons with a two-item Disability Score less than 9 are classified at Grade II if their Usual Pain Intensity score is 5 or greater, and at Grade I if their Usual Pain Intensity score is less than 5. The classification algorithm employed for the GCP-PCS yields a high level of agreement with Chronic Pain Grade based on the original scoring methods applied to the full seven-item scale. In primary care samples with back pain, headache, and orofacial pain, the weighted kappa coefficient for agreement of the original scoring of the seven-item GCPS and simplified scoring of the three-item GCP-PCS was .84 for back pain, .77 for headache, and .82 for orofacial pain.

Use and Interpretation of GCPS Measures and Items

The 0- to 10-point numerical pain intensity and interference ratings in the GCPS are consistent with Initiative on Methods, Measurement, and Pain Assessment in Clinical Trials (IMMPACT) recommendations for pain assessment in randomized controlled trials (Dworkin et al., 2008). The GCPS and the three-item GCP-PCS are both appropriate for use in estimating the prevalence of clinically significant pain (i.e., Grades II–IV) and for describing the distribution of pain severity in primary care or general population samples. When using the GCPS or three-item GCP-PCS to assess change in randomized trials or longitudinal studies, the dimensional measures (e.g., Characteristic Pain Intensity, Usual Pain Intensity, Disability Score) should be employed. Consistent with IMMPACT recommendations, a 2-point change or 30% reduction in Usual Pain Intensity or in Characteristic Pain Intensity scored with a 0–10 range is regarded as moderate improvement in pain intensity (Dworkin et al., 2009). Based on recommendations from prior research using similar measures (Edelen & Saliba, 2010; Jones, Vojir, Hutt, & Fink, 2007), Usual Pain Intensity (Q4) is considered to be mild if rated 1–4, moderate if rated 5–6, and severe if rated 7–10. The Pain-Related Interference with Activities items (Q6, Q7, and Q8) are considered mild if rated 1–3, moderate if rated 4–6, and severe if rated 7–10.

SUMMARY

This review has considered how to assess and classify chronic pain in epidemiological and health services research. The approaches discussed are suitable for population surveys, longitudinal studies that assess the course of chronic pain over time, and for randomized controlled trials. The GCPS is not appropriate for assessing the onset (incidence) of anatomically defined pain conditions or of chronic pain in general, which involves complex measurement issues beyond the scope of this chapter.

Numerous methodological studies have now shown that recall of key parameters of chronic–recurrent pain (average intensity, interference with activities, activity limitation days, and days with pain) have acceptable levels of reliability and validity for at least a 3-month recall period. This suggests that self-report pain measures with up to a 3-month recall period can yield useful information on the distribution and burden of chronic pain. Available research provides strong support for the reliability and validity of brief self-report measures of pain severity based on assessment of pain intensity and interference with daily activities. There may be circumstances (e.g., epidemiological evaluation of genetic markers) in which achieving highly reliable differentiation of chronic pain phenotypes requires assessment of pain status on multiple occasions, for example, with electronic diary methods. However, electronic diaries have their own methodological difficulties and limitations, and use of daily diary methods typically requires a tradeoff between possible gains in the reliability of assessment of chronic pain status and sample size. For studies that require thousands of research subjects, such as genomewide association studies, the tradeoff between sample size and the number of occasions on which chronic pain status is assessed should be carefully considered.

In this chapter I have discussed a new direction in chronic pain assessment for epidemiological and health services research—the use of a Prognostic Risk Score to assess and classify chronic pain based on prospective outcome probabilities. Defining chronic pain based on risk of future clinically significant pain means using probabilistic terms (e.g., possible and probable chronic pain), indicating that change in pain status is expected over time. A prognostic approach to defining chronic pain suggests that the development of chronic pain is not a linear progression over time in which increasing pain duration defines a transition from acute to chronic pain. It has been found that the predictive value of a multifactorial Prognostic Risk Score for a range of pain-related outcomes exceeds that of pain duration alone. From this perspective, chronic pain is viewed as a continuum rather than as a distinct class. Because pain outcomes are highly variable across persons and over time, chronic pain should be viewed as having an inherently uncertain prognosis, not as a static trait that identifies patients whose pain is intractable.

In summary, there are now strong empirical and conceptual bases for assessment and classification of chronic pain in epidemiological and health services research. Further work will be needed to achieve consensus on standardized classification methods that can be used in epidemiological and health services research concerning chronic pain. Epidemiological research on chronic pain, in particular, would benefit if researchers achieved consensus on methods for assessing chronic pain in field research, and on criteria for classifying chronic pain based on standardized assessment methods.

REFERENCES

Bonica, J. J. (1990). General considerations of chronic pain. In *The management of pain* (2nd ed., pp. 180–196). Philadelphia: Lea & Febiger.

Bradburn, N. M., Rips, L. J., & Shevell, S. K. (1987). Answering autobiographical questions: The impact of memory and influence on surveys. *Science, 236*, 157–161.

Broderick J. E., Schwartz, J. E., Vikingstad, G., Pribbernow, M., Grossman, S., & Stone, A. A. (2008). The accuracy of pain and fatigue items across different reporting periods. *Pain, 139*, 146–157.

Cannel, C. F. (1977). A summary of research studies of interviewing methodology, 1959–1970. In Vital and health statistics: Series 2. Data evaluation and methods research (DHEW Publication No. 69, HRA 77-1343). Washington, DC: U.S. Government Printing Office.

Carey, T. S., Garrett, J., Jackman, A., Sanders, L., & Kalsbeek, W. (1995). Reporting of acute low back pain in a telephone interview: Identification of potential biases. *Spine, 20*, 787–790.

Converse, P. E., & Traugott, M. W. (1986). Assessing the accuracy of polls and surveys. *Science, 234*, 1094–1098.

Crombie, I. K., Croft, P. R., Linton, S. J., Le Resche L., & Von Korff, M. (Eds.). (1999). *Epidemiology of pain.* Seattle, WA: IASP Press.

Derogatis, L. R. (1983). SCL-90-R: Administration, scoring and procedures manual–II. Towson, MD: Clinical Psychometric Research.

De Wit, R., van Dam, F., Hanneman, M., Zabndbelt, L., van Buuren, A., van der Heijden, K., et al. (1999) Evaluation of the use of a pain diary in chronic cancer pain patients at home. *Pain, 79*, 89–99.

Dunn, K. M., Croft, P. R., Main, C. J., & Von Korff, M. (2008). A prognostic approach defining chronic pain: Replication in a UK primary care low back pain population. *Pain, 135*, 48–54.

Dworkin, R. H., Turk, D. C., McDermott, M. P., Peirce-Sandner, S., Burke, L. B., Cowan, P., et al. (2009). Interpreting the clinical importance of group differences in chronic pain clinical trials: IMMPACT recommendations. *Pain, 146*, 238–244.

Dworkin, R. H., Turk, D. C., Wyrwich, K. W., Beaton, D., Cleeland, C., Farrar, J. T., et al. (2008). Interpreting the clinical importance of treatment outcomes in chronic pain clinical trials: IMMPACT recommendations. *Journal of Pain, 9*, 105–121.

Dworkin, S. F., Von Korff, M., Whitney, C. W., Le Resche, L., Dicker, B. G., & Barlow, W. (1990). Measurement of characteristic pain intensity in field research. *Pain, 41*(Suppl. 5), S290.

Edelen, M. O., & Saliba, D. (2010). Correspondence of verbal descriptor and numeric rating scales for pain intensity: An item response theory calibration. *Journals of Gerontology A: Biological Sciences and Medical Sciences, 65*, 778–785.

Elliott, A. M., Smith, B. H., Hannaford, P. C., Smith, W. C., &Chambers, W. A. (2002). Assessing change in chronic pain severity: The chronic pain grade compared with retrospective perceptions. *British Journal of General Practice, 52*, 269–274.

Elliot, A. M., Smith, B. H., Penny, K. I., Smith, W. C., & Chambers, W. A. (1999). The epidemiology of chronic pain in the community. *Lancet, 354*, 1248–1252.

Elliott, A. M., Smith, B. H., Smith, W. C., & Chambers, W. A. (2000). Changes in chronic pain severity over time: The Chronic Pain Grade as a valid measure. *Pain, 88*, 303–308.

International Headache Society. (2004). The

international classification of headache disorders, 2nd edition. *Cephalalgia*, 24(Suppl. 1), 1–160.

Jamison, R. N., Raymond, S. A., Slawsby, E. A., McHugo, G. J., & Baird, J. C. (2006). Pain assessment in patients with low back pain: Comparison of weekly recall and momentary electronic data. *Journal of Pain*, 7, 192–199.

Jensen, M. P., Karoly, P., O'Riordan, E. F., Bland, F., Jr., & Burns, R. S. (1989). The subjective experience of acute pain: An assessment of the utility of 10 indices. *Clinical Journal of Pain*, 5, 153–159.

Jensen, M. P., & McFarland, C. A. (1993). Increasing the reliability and validity of pain intensity measurement in chronic pain patients. *Pain*, 55, 195–203.

Jensen, M. P., Turner, J. A., & Romano, J. M. (1994). What is the maximum number of levels needed in pain intensity measurement? *Pain*, 58, 387–392.

Jensen, M. P., Turner, J. A., Romano, J. M., & Fisher, L. D. (1999). Comparative reliability and validity of chronic pain intensity measures. *Pain*, 83, 157–162.

Jensen, M. P., Turner, L. R., Turner, J. A., & Romano, J. M. (1996). The use of multiple-item scales for pain intensity measurement in chronic pain patients. *Pain*, 67, 35–40.

Jones, K. R., Vojir, C. P., Hutt, E., & Fink, R. (2007). Determining mild, moderate and severe pain equivalency across pain-intensity tools in nursing home residents. *Journal of Rehabilitation Research and Development*, 44, 305–314.

Kerns, R. D., Turk, D. C., & Rudy, T. E. (1985). The West Haven–Yale Multidimensional Pain Inventory (WHYMPI). *Pain*, 23, 345–356.

Kroenke, K., Strine, T. W., Spitzer, R. L., Williams, J. B., Berry, J. T., & Mokdad, A. H. (2009). The PHQ-8 as a measure of current depression in the general population. *Journal of Affective Disorders*, 114, 163–173.

Madow, W. G. (1973). Net differences in interview data on chronic conditions and information derived from medical records. In *Vital and health statistics: Series 2. Data evaluation and methods research* (DHEW Publication No. 57, HSM 73-1331). Washington, DC: U.S. Government Printing Office.

Means, B., Nigam, A., Zarrow, M., Loftus, E. F., & Donaldson, M. S. (1989). Autobiographical memory for health-related events. In *Vital and health statistics: Series 6. Cognitive and survey measurement* (PHS 89-1077). Washington, DC: National Center for Health Statistics.

Merskey, H., & Bogduk, N. (1994). *Classification of chronic pain: Descriptions of chronic pain syndromes and definitions of pain terms*. Seattle, WA: IASP Press.

Moore, J. E., Von Korff, M., Cherkin, D., Saunders, K., & Lorig, K. (2000). A randomized trial of a cognitive-behavioral program for enhancing back pain self-care in a primary care setting. *Pain*, 88, 145–153.

Penny, K. I., Purves, A. M., Smith, B. H., Chambers, W. A., & Smith, W. C. (1999). Relationship between the chronic pain grade and measures of physical, social and psychological well-being. *Pain*, 79, 275–279.

Purves, A. M., Penny, K. I., Munro, C., Smith, B. H., Grimshaw, J., Wilson, B., et al. (1998). Defining chronic pain for epidemiologic research: Assessing a subjective definition. *Pain Clinic*, 10, 139–147.

Raichle, K. A., Osborne, T. L., Jensen, M. P., & Cardenas, D. (2006). The reliability and validity of pain interference measures in persons with spinal cord injury. *Journal of Pain*, 7, 179–186.

Roland, M., & Morris, R. (1983). A study of the natural history of back pain: I. Development of a reliable and sensitive measure of disability in low-back pain. *Spine*, 8, 141–144.

Salovey, P., Seiber, W. J., Smith, A. F., Turk, D. C., Jobe, J. B., & Willis, G. B. (1992). Reporting chronic pain episodes on health surveys (Vital Health Statistics No. 6). Washington, DC: National Center for Health Statistics.

Schmidt, C. O., Raspe, H., & Kohlmann, T. (2010). Graded back pain revisited-do latent variable models change our understanding of severe back pain in the general population? *Pain*, 149, 50–60.

Simon, G. E., & Von Korff, M. (1995). Recall of psychiatric history in cross-sectional surveys: Implications for epidemiologic research. *Epidemiologic Reviews*, 17, 221–227.

Smith, B. H., Penny, K. I., Purves, A. M., Munro, C., Wilson, B., Grimshaw, J., et al. (1997). The Chronic Pain Grade Questionnaire: Validation and reliability in postal research. *Pain*, 71, 141–147.

Stewart, W. F., Lipton, R. B., Kolodner, K., Liberman, J., & Sawyer, J. (1999). Reliability of the migraine disability assessment score in a population-based sample of headache sufferers. *Cephalagia*, 19, 107–114.

Stewart, W. F., Lipton, R. B., Simon, D., Liberman, J., & Von Korff, M. (1999). Validity of an illness severity measure for headache in a population sample of migraine sufferers. *Pain*, 79, 291–301.

Stewart, W. F., Lipton, R. B., Whyte, J., Kolodner, K., Liberman, J. N., & Sawyer, J. (1999). An international study to assess reliability of the Migraine Disability Assessment (MIDAS) score. *Neurology*, 53, 988–994.

Thomas, E., Dunn, K. M., Mallen, C., & Peat, G. (2008). A prognostic approach to defining chronic pain: Application to knee pain in older adults. *Pain, 139,* 389–397.

Truelove, E. L., Sommers, E. E., LeResche, L., Dworkin, S. F., & Von Korff, M. (1992). Clinical diagnostic criteria for TMD: New classification permits multiple diagnoses. *Journal of American Dental Association, 123*(4), 47–54.

Turk, D. C., & Rudy, T. E. (1988). Toward an empirically derived taxonomy of chronic pain patients: Integration of psychological assessment data. *Journal of Consulting and Clinical Psychology, 56,* 233–238.

Underwood, M. R., Barnett, A. G., & Vickers, M. R. (1999). Evaluation of two time-specific back pain outcome measures. *Spine, 24,* 1104–1112.

Von Korff, M. (1991). Memory for pain in epidemiologic research: Effects of depression on back pain recall. In *Proceedings of the 12th annual meeting of the Society of Behavioral Medicine* (Abstract C78, p. 142).

Von Korff, M., Balderson, B. H., Saunders, K., Miglioretti, D. L., Lin, E. H., Berry, S., et al. (2005). A trial of an activating intervention for chronic back pain patients in primary care and physical therapy settings. *Pain, 113,* 323–330.

Von Korff, M., & Dunn, K. (2008). Chronic pain reconsidered. *Pain, 138,* 267–276.

Von Korff, M., & Dworkin, S. (1989). Problems in measuring pain by survey: The classification of chronic pain in field research. In C. R. Chapman & J. D. Loeser (Eds.), *Advances in pain research and therapy: Vol. 12. Issues in pain management* (pp. 519–533). New York: Raven Press.

Von Korff, M., Lipton, R., & Stewart, W. E. (1994). Assessing headache severity: New directions. *Neurology, 44*(Suppl. 6), S40–S46.

Von Korff, M., & Miglioretti, D. L. (2005). A prognostic approach to defining chronic pain. *Pain, 117*(3), 304–313.

Von Korff, M., Moore, J. E., Lorig, K., Cherkin, D. C., Saunders, K., Gonzales, V. M., et al. (1998). A randomized trial of a lay-led self-management group intervention for back pain patients in primary care. *Spine, 23,* 2608–2615.

Von Korff, M., Ormel, J., Keefe, F., & Dworkin, S. F. (1992). Grading the severity of chronic pain. *Pain, 50,* 133–149.

Von Korff, M., & Saunders, K. (1996). The course of back pain in primary care. *Spine, 21,* 2833–2837.

Wolfe, F., Smythe, H. A., Yunus, M. B., Bennett, R. M., Bombardier, C., Goldenberg, D. L., et al. (1990). The American College of Rheumatology 1990 criteria for the classification of fibromyalgia (Report of the Multicenter Criteria Committee). *Arthritis and Rheumatism, 33,* 160–172.

Zigmond, A. S., & Snaith, R. P. (1983). The Hospital Anxiety and Depression Scale. *Acta Psychiatrica Scandinavica, 67,* 361–370.

APPENDIX 23.1. GCPS Version 2.0

The three-item GCP-PCS items are denoted by ♣.

Q1. On how many days in the **last 6 months** have you had *[ANATOMICAL SITE]* pain? _____ Days

Q2. How would you rate your *[ANATOMICAL SITE]* pain **RIGHT NOW**? Use a scale from 0 to 10, where 0 is "no pain" and 10 is "pain as bad as could be."

										PAIN AS BAD
NO PAIN										AS COULD BE
0	1	2	3	4	5	6	7	8	9	10

Q3. In the last 3 months, how would you rate your **WORST** *[ANATOMICAL SITE]* pain? Use the same scale, where 0 is "no pain" and 10 is "pain as bad as could be."

										PAIN AS BAD
NO PAIN										AS COULD BE
0	1	2	3	4	5	6	7	8	9	10

♣ Q4. In the last 3 months, **ON AVERAGE**, how would you rate your *[ANATOMICAL SITE]* pain? Use the same scale, where 0 is "no pain" and 10 is "pain as bad as could be." [*That is, your usual pain* at times you were in pain.]

										PAIN AS BAD
NO PAIN										AS COULD BE
0	1	2	3	4	5	6	7	8	9	10

♣ Q5. In the last 3 months, how many days did your *[ANATOMICAL SITE]* pain keep you from doing your **USUAL ACTIVITIES** like work, school or housework?

	☐	☐	☐	☐	☐	☐	☐	☐	☐	☐	☐
Days	None	1	2	3–4	5–6	7–10	11–15	16–24	25–60	61–75	76–90
(Score)	*(0)*	*(1)*	*(2)*	*(3)*	*(4)*	*(5)*	*(6)*	*(7)*	*(8)*	*(9)*	*(10)*

♣ Q6. In the last 3 months, how much has *[ANATOMICAL SITE]* pain interfered with your **DAILY ACTIVITIES**? Use a 0 to 10 scale, where 0 is "no interference" and 10 is "unable to carry on any activities."

										UNABLE TO CARRY ON
NO INTERFERENCE										ANY ACTIVITIES
0	1	2	3	4	5	6	7	8	9	10

Q7. In the last 3 months, how much has *[ANATOMICAL SITE]* pain interfered with your **RECREATIONAL, SOCIAL AND FAMILY ACTIVITIES**? Use the same scale, where 0 is "no interference" and 10 is "unable to carry on any activities."

										UNABLE TO CARRY ON
NO INTERFERENCE										ANY ACTIVITIES
0	1	2	3	4	5	6	7	8	9	10

Q8. In the last 3 months, how much has *[ANATOMICAL SITE]* pain interfered with your **ABILITY TO WORK**, including housework? Use the same scale, where 0 is "no interference" and 10 is "unable to carry on any activities."

										UNABLE TO CARRY ON
NO INTERFERENCE										ANY ACTIVITIES
0	1	2	3	4	5	6	7	8	9	10

APPENDIX 23.2. Scoring Rules and Classification Criteria for Version 2.0 of the GCPS (Appendix 23.1, Questions 1–8) and for the Three-Item GCP-PCS (Appendix 23.1, Questions 4–6)

Measures Used for GCPS Version 2.0

Characteristic Pain Intensity: Sum of Pain Right Now (Q2) + Worst Pain (Q3) + Usual Pain Intensity (Q4) [Range 0 to 30]

Four-Item Disability Score: Sum of Interference with Daily Activities (Q6) + Interference with Social Activities (Q7) + Interference with Work/Housework (Q8) + Score for Days Kept from Usual Activities (Q5) [Range 0 to 40]

Measures Used for GCP-PCS

Usual Pain Intensity (Q4) [Range 0 to 10]

Two-Item Disability Score: Sum of Interference with Daily Activities (Q6) + Score for Days Kept from Usual Activities (Q5) [Range 0 to 20]

CHRONIC PAIN GRADE based on GCPS Version 2.0	
PAIN FREE	
GRADE 0	No pain problem (prior 3 months)
GRADE I—Low intensity, Low interference	Characteristic Pain Intensity less than 15 *and* four-item Disability Score less than 17
GRADE II—High intensity	Characteristic Pain Intensity of 15 or greater *and* four-item Disability Score less than 17
GRADE III—Moderate interference	Four-item Disability Score of 17 to 24
GRADE IV—Severe interference	Four-item Disability Score of 25 to 40

CHRONIC PAIN GRADE based on three-item GCP-PCS	
PAIN FREE	
GRADE 0	No pain problem (prior 3 months)
GRADE I—Low intensity, Low interference	Usual Pain Intensity less than 5 *and* two-item Disability Score less than 9
GRADE II—High intensity	**Characteristic Pain Intensity of 5 or greater** *and* two-item Disability Score less than 9
GRADE III—Moderate interference	Two-item Disability Score of 9 to 12
GRADE IV—Severe interference	Two-item Disability Score of 13 to 20

PERSISTENCE CLASSIFICATION	
NONPERSISTENT PAIN	1–89 Pain Days (Question 1)
PERSISTENT PAIN	90–180 Pain Days (Question 1)

These scoring rules for the GCPS have been placed in the Creative Commons and may be used without the author's permission with citation of this publication.

473

CHAPTER 24

Assessment of Pain and Health-Related Quality of Life in Chronic Pain Clinical Trials

Alec B. O'Connor
Robert H. Dworkin

Clinical trials have been defined as "any research study that prospectively assigns human participants or groups of humans to one or more health-related interventions to evaluate the effects on health outcomes" (World Health Organization, 2009). This chapter focuses on how pain-related effects of interventions are measured within clinical trials.

The design, conduct, outcomes measurement, and reporting of clinical trials examining pain have evolved tremendously over the past three decades. In the recent past, clinical trials assessing the efficacy of analgesics in patients with chronic pain varied substantially in methods used (e.g., structure of the trial and the selection of patients), types of outcomes assessed (e.g., whether quality of life or mood were assessed), and outcome measures used for specific domains (e.g., how pain intensity was quantified, or how quality of life was measured). This variability created a number of problems in the interpretation of the results of the trials and, in many cases, prevented direct comparisons among them.

There has been significant attention to the methods of measuring outcomes in pain clinical trials over the last few years. For example, in 2002, a broad-based consensus group was created to establish consensus recommendations for types of outcomes to be measured in chronic pain trials, and how these outcomes should be assessed. The Initiative on Methods, Measurement, and Pain Assessment in Clinical Trials (IMMPACT) is sponsored by unrestricted educational grants from pharmaceutical companies and contains members from academia, governmental agencies (e.g., the U.S. Food and Drug Administration), pharmaceutical industry, and pain advocacy groups. To date, IMMPACT has published eight consensus recommendations about the design and interpretation of chronic pain clinical trials (*www.immpact.org*).

In this chapter, we discuss clinical trial design issues and summarize current recommendations for the assessment of pain and health-related quality of life (HRQoL) in chronic pain clinical trials. Readers may be struck by the large number of different types of recommended assessments, which creates an important problem: Investigators must balance the completeness of their data collection with subject burden resulting from a potentially large number of questionnaires and other measures that might adversely affect subject retention in trials and reliability of results. Clinical trial investigators will not be able to collect and report all of the outcomes suggested, but they should prioritize based on the specific aims of their trial.

CLINICAL TRIAL DESIGN AND ANALYSIS

The optimal design of a clinical trial depends heavily on the specific aims of the trial. Similarly, the types of patients enrolled and the methods of data analysis must be selected on the basis of the objectives of the trial.

Clinical Trial Design

Trial Aims

Several different factors affect the design of a chronic pain clinical trial. On a basic level, trials can typically be categorized as either explanatory or pragmatic. In general, *explanatory trials* seek to answer questions about disease etiology, the modes of action of treatment, or both. Explanatory trials often have numerous inclusion and exclusion criteria to try to obtain homogeneous samples of patients with the disease or to increase the likelihood of treatment response. Explanatory trials may assess interventions that are not practical in real-world settings and often use methods of assessment that are not used in clinical practice because they are invasive, time-consuming, expensive, or experimental. The range of options for assessment used in explanatory trials, such as quantitative sensory testing, functional magnetic resonance imaging (fMRI), and biopsy, can be quite broad.

In contrast, *pragmatic trials* seek to answer questions concerning how best to manage patients in real-world settings. Their enrollment criteria should be relatively liberal to promote generalizability; the interventions compared should be of practical use (e.g., oral medications administered in a titration scheme that promotes adherence to treatment); and their methods of assessment should include those that are the most clinically relevant. The remainder of this chapter focuses on assessments that are pertinent to pragmatic trials, but that also might be used in certain circumstances in explanatory trials.

Given the variability among patients in a well-designed pragmatic clinical trial, complete assessment of patient demographics, previous treatments, and comorbidities is essential. Differences in any of these variables between treatment groups can confound the results, and differences between different trials might explain the sometimes contradictory results of one trial compared with another.

Trial Phases

Clinical trials can be categorized according to their phase of research from a regulatory perspective. Phase I studies are the first to involve humans. They typically enroll small numbers of healthy volunteers and seek to provide preliminary information on drug safety, pharmacokinetics, and typical dose range, but do not typically assess efficacy.

If there are no significant safety concerns from the Phase I trials, then Phase II trials are conducted to assess the tolerability and pharmacokinetics of different dosages in relatively small numbers (e.g., 30–125) of patients with the disease of interest. Although Phase II trials may be uncontrolled, they often are designed to provide "proof of _____ concept" regarding treatment efficacy to obtain preliminary information that can be used in the design of subsequent, larger trials.

Phase III trials are conducted if Phase II trials do not raise significant tolerability concerns and suggest that the drug has efficacy. Phase III trials are much larger (often 200 or more patients from multiple centers) and are methodologically rigorous (e.g., randomized, double-blind, controlled) to provide the confirmatory evidence of efficacy and safety required for regulatory approval. Phase III trials of chronic pain treatments almost always have a placebo control group, although comparison with the existing standard of care would provide additional valuable information that a placebo group does not.

Phase IV trials are conducted after regulatory approval. They are often used to improve knowledge regarding the safety of a drug by expanding the numbers of patients enrolled in relatively controlled settings. However, they can also be conducted in patients with different diseases than those for which regulatory approval has been granted, sometimes as a prelude to seeking drug approval for another indication.

Trial Structure

There are two basic structures of randomized clinical trials, each of which has advantages and disadvantages. In general, parallel group trials are considered to be the most methodologically rigorous structure, and they are often required to obtain regulatory agency approval. They are performed by randomizing each eligible subject to only one of two or more treatment groups (also termed treatment *arms*), and differences between groups in treatment outcomes are evaluated after a prespecified duration of treatment. The primary disadvantage of parallel group design trials is the need for a large number of study subjects: A trial of sufficient size to ensure comparability between the randomized groups and sufficient power to detect treatment differences usually requires considerable resources; in addition, recruitment of large numbers of subjects can often be problematic.

In situations where the treatment effect has a relatively short and predictable duration (e.g., certain analgesics) and the condition being treated is relatively stable (e.g., chronic pain), researchers may use a crossover design in which each subject receives each intervention. In a crossover design, trial subjects are randomized to a treatment sequence (e.g., drug *A* first vs. drug *B* first), but each subject typically is administered each treatment being compared. The biggest advantage of crossover trials is that they require smaller study populations (e.g., as few as one-fourth of the patients required for a comparably powered parallel group trial) and are therefore substantially less expensive and more easily conducted than similarly powered parallel group trials.

However, a critical assumption of crossover trials is that treatment with the drug in the first treatment period will not affect treatment response in the second (and later) treatment period(s). This assumption can be violated if the treatment in the first period is not allowed sufficient time for its effects to "wash out" prior to initiating subsequent treatments. If there is "carryover" of effects from the first to the second period, the treatment effects in the second period may be ex-

aggerated, or interactions between lingering treatment effects from the first period may increase the perceived intolerance of the treatment in the second period.

Data Analysis and Interpretation

The analysis of clinical trials can be quite complicated, and the optimal analytic approach depends on the hypothesis being tested. However, several analytic principles are broadly applicable. First, the primary outcome variable and the method of data analysis should be specified prior to subject enrollment. For trials designed to demonstrate the superiority of one treatment over another (or over placebo), an *intention-to-treat* (ITT) analysis is best. ITT refers to an analysis in which all subjects are analyzed according to the treatment group to which they were randomized, regardless of the treatment they actually received. The other commonly used analytic plan, a "per protocol" analysis, only includes those subjects who completed the study taking the treatment they were assigned and typically also showed a prespecified level of adherence with study procedures. This type of analysis can introduce bias, because failure to take the assigned treatment may relate to the treatment itself (e.g., it causes excessive side effects relative to the comparator), and because the groups that remain after dropouts and non-protocol-adhering subjects are excluded are no longer truly randomized. In addition, attention must be paid to how endpoints are defined and how missing data will be handled, since certain approaches can lead to overestimations of treatment efficacy in chronic pain clinical trials (O'Connor, 2009a).

Whether a clinical trial finds a statistically significant difference between treatment arms depends on many factors that are both intrinsic and extrinsic to the trial. Some of the factors include the degree of efficacy of the intervention(s), the sample size, the placebo response rate in the trial, the dropout rate, the specific interventions compared (e.g., a too rapid titration scheme may lead to a greater number of dropouts), and the data analysis methods used, to name a few. In trials that fail to show a statistically significant treatment response, specific attention must be paid to the sample size and whether the trial was adequately powered. *Power* refers to the probability that a trial will be able to detect a difference in the treatments being compared when there is truly a difference; it is related to the number of subjects in each treatment group, the magnitude of the true difference between the treatment groups, and the variability in responses within a treatment group. Failure to demonstrate superiority of a treatment over placebo (or another comparison) should *not* be interpreted as evidence of equivalence between the treatments, unless the trial was specifically designed and powered to show equivalence (or noninferiority). Conversely, the presence of a statistically significant difference between interventions should not necessarily be interpreted as evidence of a clinically significant difference between the interventions (e.g., if a trial is overpowered, then it can show statistical differences without clear clinical meaning).

PAIN ASSESSMENT

Several different methods of measuring pain have been used in chronic pain clinical trials. IMMPACT recommendations have identified two critical types of pain measures that should be assessed in these clinical trials: pain intensity and use of rescue analgesics.

Pain Intensity

Patient report continues to be considered the best method for assessing pain intensity; other measures, such as clinician estimates and "objective" measures (e.g., the presence of verifiable pathology) have consistently been shown to be less accurate (Tait, Chibnall, & Kalauokalani, 2009).

Pain intensity is often measured with numerical rating scales (NRSs). Several different types of NRSs have been used in clinical trials. Most require patients to score pain intensity on a scale of either 0–10 or 0–100, with 0 indicating "no pain" and 10 or 100 indicating the "worst possible pain." NRSs can be obtained in different ways, including by verbal report or written questionnaire. Visual analogue scales (VASs), another common approach to the assessment of pain intensity, typically present to subjects a 100-mm line labeled "no pain" at

the left side and "worst possible pain" (or an equivalent phrase) at the right side. Subjects are then asked to mark their pain intensity on the line, and the responses are measured in millimeters and scored from 0–100 (see Jensen & Karoly, Chapter 2, this volume). Of the different methods, patients seem to prefer NRSs; there has been concern that the greater degree of abstraction required by VASs might compromise their validity in patients with cognitive impairments, so NRSs are often recommended for the assessment of pain intensity (Dworkin et al., 2005; see Katz & Melzack, Chapter 3, this volume).

The scale recommended by the IMMPACT authors for use in chronic pain trials, based on the frequency of its use and in order to standardize reporting (not because it is clearly better than all other methods), consists of a 0- to 10-point scale with the instructions "Please rate your pain by indicating the number that best describes your pain on average in the last 24 hours" with the numbers 0–10 and instructions that 0 means "no pain" and 10 means "pain as bad as you can imagine" (Dworkin et al., 2005). This basic scale can be adapted for use in other settings (e.g., for acute pain trials) by altering the instructions, such as "Please rate your pain by indicating the number that best describes your current pain level."

Pain intensity can also be measured with categorical scales (e.g., "none," "mild," "moderate," or "severe"). Categorical scales are a bit less abstract, and can sometimes be used by, for example, cognitively impaired patients who are unable to use an NRS (Dworkin et al., 2005). In addition, IMMPACT recommended reporting categorical scale ratings, if possible, to facilitate comparison with existing trials that have used categorical scales to assess pain intensity (Dworkin et al., 2005).

Alternative methods for measuring pain intensity may be needed for young children or cognitively impaired patients. Pain scales for children of different ages, cognitively impaired individuals, and sedated patients (e.g., in an intensive care unit) have been developed (Herr, Bjoro, & Decker, 2006; Li, Puntillo, & Miaskowski, 2008; McGrath et al., 2008; see Ruskin, Amaria, Warnock, & McGrath, Chapter 11, this volume).

IMMPACT recommends that changes in pain intensity be reported in specific ways to allow comparison of results between trials. The change in pain intensity from baseline to the endpoint of the trial should be reported, and this is often the primary endpoint in clinical trials, because it may offer the greatest power to detect between-group differences. In addition, the proportion of patients achieving ≥ 30% pain intensity reduction over the course of the trial should be reported, because this represents a clinically meaningful change in pain (Dworkin et al., 2005; Farrar, Young, LaMoreaux, Werth, & Poole, 2001). The proportion of patients reporting a ≥ 50% pain intensity reduction should also be reported, because this represents a substantial clinical response and has usually been reported in older trials and most meta-analyses (Dworkin et al., 2005; Farrar et al., 2001).

The frequency of pain assessment within a trial depends on a number of factors, including the acuity of the pain and the duration of the trial. Since no clear recommendations exist, the frequency of assessment should balance clinical relevance (e.g., how soon the treatment starts to work) with subject and researcher burden caused by frequent assessments. Many analgesic trials for chronic pain lasting from 8 to 12 weeks have documented pain intensity on a daily basis, which is a feasible approach, although substantially less burdensome weekly assessments have rarely been used.

Use of Rescue Analgesics

In chronic pain clinical trials, protocols often allow patients to use additional analgesics (e.g., acetaminophen) if needed. While this complicates trial interpretation, it is often necessary to retain subjects in a trial, and it does better reflect "real-life" usage of medications, which may promote the generalizability of trial results. Allowance of rescue medications also permits the use of a placebo group, which might otherwise be ethically problematic when studying patients who have moderate or severe chronic pain.

Quantification of the amount and timing of rescue analgesic use in pain clinical trials is recommended. Interpretation of trial results then requires consideration of both pain intensity changes and the amount of rescue medication consumed. Attempts to combine these two factors into a single measure have

been made, but these scales have not been validated and are not recommended (Dworkin et al., 2005).

Measurement of Pain Characteristics Other Than Intensity

Pain intensity can be thought of as one of the dimensions of pain. Additional dimensions of pain that may be appropriate to measure include its sensory, affective, and temporal characteristics, since treatments may differ in their effects on these aspects of a patient's pain. The sensory characteristics of different types of pain can vary; for example, pain can be described by different patients as "burning," "cold," "stabbing," or in a variety of other ways (see Katz & Melzack, Chapter 3, this volume). Pain affect can be thought of as the amount of distress or unpleasantness that pain causes, and it, too, can vary substantially between patients with the same pain intensity. The duration and time course of pain can also vary dramatically from patient to patient, present in some cases continuously at a constant level but episodic and transiently severe in other cases. For example, patients with significant *allodynia* (pain resulting from normally nonpainful stimuli, e.g., the light touch of clothes or wind) may not have much pain the majority of time but be very distressed by sudden and often unpredictable episodes of provoked pain.

The *Short-Form McGill Pain Questionnaire* (SF-MPQ) is an instrument that measures the sensory and affective characteristics of pain (Dworkin et al., 2005). It has been found to be responsive to treatment in chronic pain clinical trials and is recommended as a secondary outcome measure in clinical trials (Dworkin et al., 2005). The recently published SF-MPQ-2, a revised version of this measure, has been expanded to assess neuropathic pain characteristics (Dworkin et al., 2009; see Katz & Melzack, Chapter 3, this volume).

ASSESSMENT OF HRQoL

Pain can affect a number of different aspects of patients' lives, including their mood, ability to sleep, and ability to function physically. Pain can affect different patients very differently. In addition, different patients value certain activities or impairments differently. For example, severe chronic pain may reduce a patient's quality of life substantially, because it prevents him or her from being able to walk independently or have a good night's sleep. A given reduction in pain intensity in this patient may or may not substantially improve his or her ability to walk or sleep. In addition, chronic pain treatments have associated side effects and inconveniences (e.g., having to take pills three times per day), and may also produce different effects on different patients (e.g., sleep or mood changes), all of which may alter quality of life. Since chronic pain treatment is not known to affect mortality substantially, the primary goal of long-term treatment is overall symptom improvement, not just pain improvement. The most all-encompassing measure of overall symptom burden, including pain, associated limitations, side effects, mood, sleep, and inconvenience, is quality of life. Those

components of quality of life that relate to health are referred to as health-related quality of life (HRQoL).

Supporting the need to measure more than just pain in chronic pain clinical trials, IMMPACT has summarized literature that defines three "relatively independent" factors that seem to drive the overall experience of patients with pain: pain intensity, physical functioning, and emotional functioning (Turk et al., 2003). Physical and emotional functioning can be measured with validated overall HRQoL instruments or instruments specifically intended to measure physical or emotional function (Table 24.1).

Besides pain intensity, physical functioning, and emotional functioning, IMMPACT identified additional domains that should be considered for routine assessment in clinical trials for chronic pain: participant ratings of global improvement, symptoms and adverse events, and participant disposition (Turk et

TABLE 24.1. Provisional Benchmarks for Interpreting Changes in Chronic Pain Clinical Trial Outcome Measures

Outcome domain and measure	Type of improvement[a]	Method[b]	Change
Pain intensity			
0–10 numerical rating scale	Minimally important	Anchor	10–20% decrease
	Moderately important	Anchor	≥ 30% decrease
	Substantial	Anchor	≥ 50% decrease
Physical functioning			
Multidimensional Pain Inventory Interference scale	Clinically important	Distribution	≥ 0.6-point decrease
Brief Pain Inventory Interference scale	Minimally important	Distribution	1-point decrease
Emotional functioning			
Beck Depression Inventory	Clinically important	Distribution	≥ 5-point decrease
Profile of Mood States			
Total Mood Disturbance	Clinically important	Distribution	≥ 10- to 15-point decrease
Specific subscales	Clinically important	Distribution	≥ 2- to 12-point change[c]
Global rating of improvement			
Patient Global Impression of Change	Minimally important	Anchor	Minimally improved
	Moderately important	Anchor	Much improved
	Substantial	Anchor	Very much improved

Note. From Dworkin et al. (2008). Copyright 2008. Reprinted with permission from Elsevier.
[a]Because few studies have examined the importance of worsening on these measures, benchmarks are only provided for improvement in scores.
[b]Specific method used in determining benchmark is provided in final column; distribution-based methods were based on use of 0.5 standard deviation or 1.0 standard error of measurement, or both.
[c]The magnitude of a clinically important change depends on the specific subscale, as does the direction of change that reflects an improvement.

al., 2003). Another consensus group, the Outcome Measures in Rheumatoid Arthritis Clinical Trials (OMERACT), has recommended clinical trial outcome measures for specific rheumatological diseases with associated pain, including rheumatoid arthritis (Brooks et al., 2001), osteoarthritis (Brooks et al., 2001), psoriatic arthritis (Gladmann et al., 2007), and fibromyalgia syndrome (Mease et al., 2007). In general, OMERACT and IMMPACT recommendations have been similar, including measurement of pain, HRQoL, physical functioning, mood, sleep, and global measures, but OMERACT has also recommended the assessment of fatigue and domains specific to the disease in question, such as joint and skin activity in psoriatic arthritis (Gladmann et al., 2007).

HRQoL can be measured with either of two types of scales—generic HRQoL instruments, which can be used for any disease, or disease-specific HRQoL scales. Both approaches have advantages and disadvantages. Generic HRQoL scales are more versatile, because results on a scale can be compared across different diseases. In general, however, disease-specific HRQoL instruments are more sensitive to clinical changes in patients with the disease, and are therefore preferred over generic HRQoL scales when a choice between the two approaches must be made. IMMPACT has recommended the use of both generic and disease-specific measures whenever possible (Turk et al., 2003).

A strong argument can be made that improvements in HRQoL would be at least as clinically meaningful as improvements in pain intensity and in certain circumstances could therefore be the primary endpoint of chronic pain clinical trials. However, we have been unable to find evidence that any single measure of overall HRQoL is sufficiently responsive and reliable to serve as the primary endpoint in chronic pain clinical trials; in contrast, there is evidence suggesting limitations of current HRQoL measures in chronic osteoarthritis, rheumatoid arthritis, and fibromyalgia (Carville & Choy, 2008; Ruchlin & Insinga, 2008; Russel, 2008). For example, a recent systematic review of important outcome measures for patients with fibromyalgia concluded that there are sensitive instruments for measuring each of the critical domains for fibromyalgia patients except for HRQoL (Carville & Choy, 2008).

Generic Measures of HRQoL

In general, HRQoL instruments include multiple-choice questions about a number of different components of normal function and enjoyment of life. For clinical trials of chronic pain treatments, IMMPACT has emphasized the importance of measuring physical functioning (e.g., the ability to perform activities of daily living), as well as emotional functioning, including emotional distress or impaired mood but not necessarily psychiatric illness per se (Turk et al., 2003). IMMPACT considered other domains to be "supplemental," including role functioning and social functioning (Turk et al., 2003).

The Medical Outcomes Study 36-Item Short-Form Health Survey (SF-36) is the most commonly used generic measure of HRQoL in chronic pain clinical trials and clinical trials in general (Coons, Rao, Keininger, & Hays, 2000). The results of the SF-36 can be reported as eight subscale scores (Physical Functioning, Social Functioning, Role–Physical, Role–Emotional, Bodily Pain, General Health, Vitality, and Mental Health) or as two summary scores of Physical Health and Mental Health (Ware, 2009). The SF-36 has been shown to be fairly responsive in chronic neuropathic pain clinical trials, but there are examples of trials that found statistically significant improvements in pain intensity but not in the SF-36 Bodily Pain subscale score (O'Connor, 2009b). Of the eight subscales, the one that most commonly has improved in clinical trials of neuropathic pain has been Bodily Pain, followed by Mental Health and Vitality (O'Connor, 2009b).

Other generic measures of HRQoL have also been used, though they have not attained the widespread usage of the SF-36 (Ware & Sherbourne, 1992). Examples include the SF-12, a 12-question distillation of the 36-question SF-36 (Ware, Kosinski, & Keller, 1996); the Health Assessment Questionnaire, which has been commonly used in rheumatoid arthritis (Fries, Spitz, Kraines, & Holman, 1980); and the Nottingham Health Profile (Hunt & McEwan, 1980).

Utilities

Measurements of utilities can also be used to quantify changes in HRQoL. Utility instruments typically require subjects to score their health in several core domains, then scores are converted into preference-based health state valuations derived from healthy populations. Utility scales define 1 as the "state of perfect or ideal health," and 0 as "death." Advantages of utility measurements include the ability to compare easily health states across different disease states and the simplicity of converting their values into *quality-adjusted life years* (QALYs, defined as utility of health state multiplied by the duration in the health state [in years]), which facilitates cost-effectiveness analyses.

The EuroQol-5 Dimensions (EQ-5D™) seems to be the most commonly used utility measure in chronic pain trials (O'Connor 2009b; Ruchlin & Insinga, 2008), though the Health Utilities Index (Versions 2 and 3) and Short Form 6-D Health Survey (SF-6D) are also used somewhat commonly (Coons et al., 2000; Harrison et al., 2008). The EQ-5D requires subjects to provide scores in five domains: Mobility, Self-Care, Usual Activity, Pain, and Anxiety/Depression, then the combined scores are converted into utilities. It has been used in cross-sectional studies to measure health states of patients with, for example, chronic neuropathic pain, with representative scores provided by patients with "mild," "moderate," and "severe" pain being 0.7, 0.5, and 0.2, respectively (Table 24.2). The EQ-5D has also been used as a secondary outcome measure in some chronic pain clinical trials (O'Connor 2009b; Ruchlin & Insinga, 2008). Several neuropathic pain clinical trials have found statistically significant improvement in the EQ-5D in response to treatment (O'Connor, 2009b).

While certainly useful, utilities are not without disadvantages. A recent systematic review of utility assessment in patients with osteoarthritis found substantial variability from one utility instrument to another within the same patient populations. In addition, while utility values and measures of HRQoL tend to change in tandem, a recent systematic review of the use of utilities in osteoarthritis concluded that "there can potentially be divergent findings with respect to clinical and statistical significance of changes in utility measures and corresponding measures of health status" (Ruchlin & Insinga, 2008, p. 926). One comparison of utility instruments in patients with rheumatoid arthritis

concluded that the EQ-5D had lower test–retest reliability and responsiveness than the Health Utilities Index, Version 3 and SF-6D (Marra et al., 2005), though a more recent review concluded that the EQ-5D and Health Utilities Index, Version 3 have been the most extensively studied and have shown validity and responsiveness in patients with rheumatoid arthritis (Harrison et al., 2008). As with other HRQoL measures, additional research is required to define the best methods of measuring utilities and the appropriate use of utility assessments.

Disease-Specific Measures of HRQoL

As described earlier, disease-specific measures of HRQoL are recommended when they are available. Examples of disease-specific HRQoL scales derived for diseases commonly producing pain are the Western Ontario and McMaster Osteoarthritis Index (WOMAC; Bellamy, Buchanan, Goldsmith, Campbell, & Stitt, 1988) and the Roland–Morris Disability Questionnaire (Roland & Morris, 1983), which have been recommended for osteoarthritis and back pain clinical trials, respectively (Dworkin et al., 2005). In general, disease-specific HRQoL instruments have been found to be more sensitive to changes than generic HRQoL instruments for patients with a specific disease, though exceptions exist; a recent review, for example, found that the results from the WOMAC correlate closely with the generic SF-36 (Strand & Kelman, 2004). However, validated disease-specific HRQoL instruments do not exist for many diseases.

Two scales that measure the effects of pain on HRQoL are the Brief Pain Inventory (BPI, Cleeland & Ryan, 1994) Interference scale and the Multidimensional Pain Inventory (MPI, Kerns, Turk, & Rudy, 1985) Interference scale. There are seven items in the BPI Interference scale, including three for pain interference with physical functioning, three for pain interference with emotional functioning, and one for sleep interference. Several chronic neuropathic pain clinical trials have used the BPI Interference scale as an outcome measure. These trials have typically reported statistically significant improvement in one or more of the BPI subscales, with treatment despite not being powered specifically for this outcome measure (O'Connor,

TABLE 24.2. Average Pain Scores and EQ-5D Utilities for Different Neuropathic Pain States

Study	Subjects	Study location	Average pain severity	Average EQ-5D	EQ-5D of patients with mild pain (%)[a]	EQ-5D of patients with moderate pain (%)[a]	EQ-5D of patients with severe pain (%)[a]
Undifferentiated neuropathic pain							
McDermott et al. (2006)	602	Europe[b]	4.8/10	0.44	0.67 (21%)	0.46 (54%)	0.16 (25%)
Gordon et al. (2006)	126	Canada	NA	NA	0.7 (NA)	0.5 (NA)	0.2 (NA)
Painful diabetic neuropathy							
Tolle, Xu, & Sadosky (2006)[c]	140	Europe[b]	5.0/10	0.41	0.59 (16%)	0.43 (57%)	0.20 (25%)
Gore et al. (2005)	255	United States	5.0/10	0.5	0.7 (27%)	0.5 (45%)	0.2 (26%)
Postherpetic neuralgia							
Oster et al. (2005)	385	United States	4.6/10	0.61	0.69 (35%)	0.58 (43%)	0.25 (20%)
van Seventer et al. (2006)[c]	84	Europe[b]	4.2/10	0.60	0.72 (NA)	0.63 (NA)	0.27 (NA)
Trigeminal neuralgia							
Tolle, Dukes, & Sadosky (2006)[c]	82	Europe[b]	4.2/10	0.56	0.70 (27%)	0.54 (50%)	0.30 (15%)

Note. The EQ-5D utility estimates do not adjust for the patients' coexisting medical illnesses, which would also contribute to the utility values. Utilities are measured on a scale with anchors of 0 ("death") and 1 ("perfect health"). NA, not available. From O'Connor (2009b). Adapted with permission from Wolters Kluwer Health. All rights reserved.
[a]Percentage of subjects in the survey with pain of "mild," "moderate," or "severe" intensity.
[b]Patients from France, Germany, Italy, The Netherlands, Spain, and the United Kingdom.
[c]Results are for the subset of patients from the larger McDermott study (2006) with the described neuropathic pain diagnosis.

2009b). A systematic review of HRQoL in six types of chronic neuropathic pain concluded that pain-specific instruments, such as the BPI or MPI Interference scales, seem to produce more consistent associations with other outcome measures than generic HRQoL scales such as the SF-36 (Jensen, Chodroff, & Dworkin, 2007).

Measures of Physical Functioning

The SF-36 summary score of physical function can be used with any disease, whether painful or not, and its results may be compared with results for other painful and nonpainful illnesses. Interference with sleep is a common and distressing result of chronic pain and is therefore an important component of an assessment of the effects of chronic pain treatment of HRQoL (Dworkin et al., 2005). There is a sleep interference item in the BPI but not in the MPI, so if the MPI is used to assess physical functioning, then an additional sleep interference assessment is recommended (Dworkin et al., 2005).

Measures of Emotional Functioning

As with physical functioning, the SF-36 mental functioning summary score is a generic assessment that can be contrasted with specific measures of emotional functioning. Examples of specific emotional functioning instruments used in chronic pain clinical trials are the Beck Depression Inventory (BDI; Beck, Ward, Mendelson, Mock, & Erbaugh, 1961), which quantifies the severity of depressed mood, and the Profile of Mood States (POMS; McNair, Lorr, & Droppleman, 1971), which measures six different mood states: Tension-Anxiety, Depression-Dejection, Anger-Hostility, Vigor-Activity, Fatigue-Inertia, and Confusion-Bewilderment (Dworkin et al., 2005). Both the BDI and POMS have been found to be responsive to treatment in chronic pain clinical trials (Dworkin et al., 2005). IMMPACT recommends the use of the original versions of the BDI and POMS, which do not adjust for somatic symptoms (Dworkin et al., 2005). The BDI and POMS seem to be more sensitive for detecting associations between pain and emotional functioning in chronic neuropathic pain compared to the mental function summary score of the SF-36 (Jensen et al., 2007).

ADDITIONAL CORE OUTCOME DOMAINS RECOMMENDED BY IMMPACT

Participant Ratings of Global Improvement

A summary rating of global improvement allows patients to rate their overall impression of the effects of treatment. In theory, this rating can incorporate a variety of different factors, such as pain relief, side effects, other beneficial effects of treatment (e.g., improved sleep or physical function), and convenience, along with individuals' valuation of those changes. However, single-item measures of change have potential limitations. To estimate change, subjects must accurately remember their baseline state and perform a mental "subtraction." It is also impossible to assess the internal consistency of single-item scales (Turk et al., 2003). Nevertheless, the simplicity, potential inclusion of diverse effects, and incorporation of patient preferences make patient rating of global impression of change a very appealing type of measure, and it was therefore recommended as a core outcome domain for chronic pain clinical trials (Turk et al., 2003).

IMMPACT recommended the use of the Patient Global Impression of Change (PGIC) rating scale based on its frequent use in recent chronic pain clinical trials. The PGIC is a single question that asks subjects to rate their improvement during the trial on a 7-point scale, with anchors of "very much worse" and "very much improved" on the ends and "no change" as the midpoint of the scale (Dworkin et al., 2005). The PGIC has been used in many chronic pain clinical trials and has proven to be responsive and easily interpretable (Dworkin et al., 2005; Farrar et al., 2001).

Other global measures used less than the PGIC have included ratings of overall satisfaction with treatment, ratings of disease state, and single-item ratings of change in specific domains, such as physical functioning. Additional research defining the uses of the PGIC and these other types of global impression scales is needed.

Symptoms and Adverse Events

Adverse events or side effects that develop during treatment are a critical outcome domain of clinical trials (Turk et al., 2003) and are expected to adversely affect HRQoL. However, there is some evidence that improvements in pain have a larger impact on HRQoL and global impression of change than the development of side effects in patients with moderate or severe chronic neuropathic pain (Deshpande, Holden, & Gilron, 2006; Farrar, Dworkin, Griesling, Murphy, & Emir, 2006).

Two primary methods exist for capturing adverse events during a clinical trial: active or passive assessment. With *active assessment*, subjects are asked specifically about the presence of prespecified likely adverse events. This approach is more sensitive for detecting specific adverse events, since subjects are asked specifically about the presence of those events. However, adverse events that are not explicitly assessed will, in all likelihood, be relatively underreported. *Passive assessment* involves asking open-ended questions of subjects, such as "Did you develop any side effects or new symptoms since your last visit?" In theory, this ascertainment method is less sensitive to detecting relatively mild adverse events but will detect those events that are particularly disturbing to subjects, and will not bias subjects' reporting toward adverse events that are specifically assessed when active capture is used. Regardless of the method of ascertainment, the frequency of individual adverse events and the total frequency of adverse events in treatment and control arms should be reported. The severity of all adverse events should be graded, and the frequency of the more severe or distressing adverse events reported. Blinded investigators can also be used to evaluate the likelihood that an adverse event is attributable to treatment, and this, too, should be reported (Dworkin et al., 2005).

Patient Disposition

Patient disposition in clinical trials is critical to the interpretation of results, and detailed guidelines for reporting patient disposition have been developed (Moher, Schultz, & the CONSORT Group, 2001). The IMMPACT authors recommended detailed reporting of the reasons for subject withdrawals due to adverse events and the reasons for subject withdrawal of consent, since these can be very important considerations in assessing results in a chronic pain clinical trial and evaluating missing data (Dworkin et al., 2005).

CONCLUSIONS

The measurement of pain and quality of life in clinical trials has evolved tremendously in the past three decades. Standardizing assessment and reporting these outcomes in clinical trials also seem to have improved significantly in the past decade, and efforts such as IMMPACT bode well for the future of clinical trials of treatments for chronic pain and their effects on HRQoL.

Additional research is needed. Better-validated and more sensitive measures of HRQoL are needed. In many ways, an assessment of overall HRQoL should be an ideal outcome measure for clinical trials of pain treatment, since it should incorporate and aggregate all changes of importance to patients, including pain improvement, side effects, ancillary benefits (e.g., improvement in physical and emotional functioning), and inconveniences of the treatment. However, current HRQoL instruments do not seem sufficiently sensitive and responsive to treatment effects to serve as primary outcomes. For the time being, separate measures of changes in pain intensity and HRQoL, in-cluding physical and emotional functioning, global improvement, and adverse events, are required to capture changes adequately in response to treatment in chronic pain clinical trials.

REFERENCES

Beck, A. T., Ward, C. H., Mendelson, M., Mock, J., & Erbaugh, J. (1961). An inventory for measuring depression. *Archives of General Psychiatry, 4*, 561–571.

Bellamy, N., Buchanan, W. W., Goldsmith, C. H., Campbell, J., & Stitt, L. W. (1988). Validation study of WOMAC: A health status instrument for measuring clinically important patient relevant outcomes to antirheumatic drug therapy in patients with osteoarthritis of the hip or knee. *Journal of Rheumatology, 15*, 1833–1840.

Brooks, P., Hochberg, M., for ILAR and OMERACT. (2001). Outcome measures and classification criteria for the rheumatologic diseases: A compilation of data from OMERACT (Outcome Measures for Arthritis Clinical Trials), ILAR (International League of Associations for Rheumatology), regional leagues, and other groups. *Rheumatology (Oxford), 40*, 896–906.

Carville, S. F., & Choy, E. H. (2008). Systematic review of the discriminating power of outcome measures used in clinical trials of fibromyalgia. *Journal of Rheumatology, 35*, 2094–2105.

Cleeland, C. S., & Ryan, K. M. (1994). Pain assessment: Global use of the Brief Pain Inventory. *Annals of the Academy of Medicine (Singapore), 23*, 129–138.

Coons, S. J., Rao, S., Keininger, D. L., & Hays, R. D. (2000). A comparative review of generic quality-of-life instruments. *Pharmacoeconomics, 17*, 13–35.

Deshpande, M. A., Holden, R. R., & Gilron, I. (2006). The impact of therapy on quality of life and mood in neuropathic pain: What is the effect of pain reduction? *Anesthesia and Analgesia, 102*, 1473–1479.

Dworkin, R. H., Turk, D. C., Farrar, J. T., et al. (2005). Core outcome measures for chronic pain clinical trials: IMMPACT recommendations. *Pain, 113*, 9–19.

Dworkin, R. H., Turk, D. C., Revicki, D., et al. (2009). Development and initial validation of an expanded and revised version of the Short-Form McGill Pain Questionnaire (SF-MPQ-2). *Pain, 144*, 35–42.

Dworkin, R. H., Turk, D. C., Wyrwich, K. W., et al. (2008). Interpreting the clinical importance of treatment outcomes in chronic pain clinical trials: IMMPACT recommendations. *Journal of Pain*, 9, 105–121.

Farrar, J. T., Dworkin, R. H., Griesling, T., Murphy, T. K., & Emir, B. (2006, November). *Investigation of possible predictors of patient global impression of change response in peripheral neuropathic pain: Results from an analysis of 10 trials with pregabalin*. Poster presented at the Southampton, Bermuda 9th International Conference on the Mechanisms and Treatment of Neuropathic Pain.

Farrar, J. T., Young, J. P., LaMoreaux, L., Werth, J. L., & Poole, R. M. (2001). Clinical importance of changes in chronic pain intensity measured on an 11-point numerical pain rating scale. *Pain*, 94, 149–158.

Fries, J. F., Spitz, P., Kraines, G., & Holman, H. (1980). Measurement of patient outcome in arthritis. *Arthritis and Rheumatism*, 23, 137–145.

Gladmann, D. D., Mease, P. J., Strand, V., et al. (2007). Consensus on a core set of domains for psoriatic arthritis. *Journal of Rheumatology*, 34, 1167–1170.

Gordon, A., Choinière, M., Collet, J.-P., Rousseau, C., & Tarride, J.-E. (2006). The humanistic burden of neuropathic pain in Canada. *Journal of Outcomes Research*, 10, 23–35.

Gore, M., Brandenburg, N. A., Dukes, E., et al. (2005). Pain severity in diabetic peripheral neuropathy is associated with patient functioning, symptom levels of anxiety and depression, and sleep. *Journal of Pain and Symptom Management*, 30, 374–385.

Harrison, M. J., Davies, L. M., Bansback, N. J., et al. (2008). The validity and responsiveness of generic utility measures in rheumatoid arthritis: A review. *Journal of Rheumatology*, 35, 592–602.

Herr, K., Bjoro, K., & Decker, S. (2006). Tools for assessment of pain in nonverbal older adults with dementia: A state-of-the-science review. *Journal of Pain and Symptom Management*, 31, 170–192.

Hunt, S. M., & McEwan, J. (1980). The development of a subjective health indicator. *Sociology of Health Illness*, 2, 231–246.

Jensen, M. P., Chodroff, M. J., & Dworkin, R. H. (2007). The impact of neuropathic pain on health-related quality of life: Review and implications. *Neurology*, 68, 1178–1182.

Kerns, R. D., Turk, D. C., & Rudy, T. E. (1985). The West Haven–Yale Multidimensional Pain Inventory (WHYMPI). *Pain*, 23, 345–356.

Li, D., Puntillo, K., & Miaskowski, C. (2008). A review of objective pain measures for use with critical care adult patients unable to self-report. *Journal of Pain*, 9, 2–10.

Marra, C. A., Rashidi, A. A., Guh, D., et al.

(2005). Are indirect utility measures reliable and responsive in rheumatoid arthritis? *Quality of Life Research*, 14, 1333–1344.

McDermott, A. M., Toelle, T. R., Rowbotham, D. J., Schaefer, C. P., & Dukes, E. M. (2006). The burden of neuropathic pain: Results of a cross-sectional survey. *European Journal of Pain*, 10, 127–135.

McGrath, P. J., Walco, G. A., Turk, D. C., et al. (2008). Core outcome domains and measures for pediatric acute and chronic/recurrent pain clinical trials: PedIMMPACT recommendations. *Journal of Pain*, 9, 771–783.

McNair, D. M., Lorr, M., & Droppleman, L. F. (1971). *Profile of Mood States*. San Diego, CA: Educational and Industrial Testing Service.

Mease, P., Arnold, L. M., Bennett, R., et al. (2007). Fibromyalgia syndrome. *Journal of Rheumatology*, 34, 1415–1425.

Moher, D., Schultz, K. F., Altman, D., & CONSORT Group (Consolidated Standards of Reporting Trials). (2001). The CONSORT statement: Revised recommendations for improving the quality of reports of parallel-group randomized trials. *Journal of the American Medical Association*, 285, 1987–1991.

O'Connor, A. B. (2009a). The need for improved access to FDA reviews. *Journal of the American Medical Association*, 302, 191–193.

O'Connor, A. B. (2009b). Neuropathic pain: A review of the quality of life impact, costs, and cost-effectiveness of therapy. *Pharmacoeconomics*, 27, 95–112.

Oster, G., Harding, G., Dukes, E., Edelsberg, J., & Cleary, P. D. (2005). Pain, medication use, and health-related quality of life in older persons with postherpetic neuralgia: Results from a population-based survey. *Journal of Pain*, 6, 356–363.

Roland, M. O., & Morris, R. W. (1983). A study of the natural history of back pain: Part 1. Development of a reliable and sensitive measure of disability in low back pain. *Spine*, 8, 141–144.

Ruchlin, H. S., & Insinga, R. P. (2008). A review of health-utility data for osteoarthritis: Implications for clinical trial-based evaluation. *PharmacoEconomics*, 26, 925–935.

Russel, A. S. (2008). Quality-of-life assessment in rheumatoid arthritis. *PharmacoEconomics*, 26, 831–846.

Strand, V., & Kelman, A. (2004). Outcome measures in osteoarthritis: Randomized controlled trials. *Current Rheumatology Reports*, 6, 20–30.

Tait, R. C., Chibnall, J. T., & Kalauokalani, D. (2009). Provider judgments of patients in pain: Seeking symptom certainty. *Pain Medicine*, 10, 11–34.

Tolle, T., Dukes, E., & Sadosky, A. (2006). Patient burden of trigeminal neuralgia: Results from a cross-sectional survey of health state impairment and treatment patterns in six European countries. *Pain Practice, 6,* 153–160.

Tolle, T., Xu, X., & Sadosky, A. B. (2006). Painful diabetic neuropathy: A cross-sectional survey of health state impairment and treatment patterns. *Journal of Diabetes Complications, 20,* 26–33.

Turk, D. C., Dworkin, R. H., Allen, R. R., et al. (2003). Core outcome domains for chronic pain clinical trials: IMMPACT recommendations. *Pain, 106,* 337–345.

van Seventer, R., Sadosky, A., Lucero, M., & Dukes, E. (2006). A cross-sectional survey of health state impairment and treatment patterns in patients with postherpetic neuralgia. *Age and Ageing, 35,* 132–137.

Ware, J. E. (2009). SF-36 Health Survey update. Retrieved March 29, 2009, from *www.sf-36.org/tools/sf36.shtml.*

Ware, J. E., Kosinski, M., & Keller, S. D. (1996). A 12-Item Short-Form Health Survey: Construction of scales and preliminary tests of reliability and validity. *Medical Care, 34,* 220–233.

Ware, J. E., & Sherbourne C. D. (1992). The MOS 36-Item Short-Form Health Survey (SF-36): I. Conceptual framework and item selection. *Medical Care, 30,* 473–483.

World Health Organization. (2009). International Clinical Trials Registry Platform (ICTRP). Retrieved from April 3, 2009, *www.who.int/ictrp/en.*

CONCLUSION

CHAPTER 25

Trends and Future Directions

DENNIS C. TURK
RONALD MELZACK

The chapters in this volume attest to the breadth and depth of attention given to the issues involved in assessment and evaluation of people experiencing pain. A diverse array of newly developed instruments, methods, and procedures have become available, and refinements of older instruments have appeared since the previous edition of this volume. Many commonly used instruments have been refined and revised, for example, the Short-Form McGill Pain Questionnaire (SF-MPQ-2; Dworkin et al., 2009); the Beck Depression Inventory (BDI-II; Beck, Steer, Ball, & Ranieri, 1996); the Fibromyalgia Impact Questionnaire (FIQ-R; Bennett et al., 2009); the Survey of Patient Attitudes (SOPA–Short Form; Jensen, Turner, & Romano, 2002); the Multidimensional Pain Readiness to Change Questionnaire (MPRCQ2; Nielson, Jensen, Ehde, Kerns, & Molton, 2008), and new instruments, methods, and procedures have been developed.

PAIN > SENSORY INTENSITY

It is evident from the chapters in this volume that major advances have been made in developing and refining sophisticated instruments and procedures designed to quantify the subjective experience of pain. The question most frequently asked by physicians when a patient complains of pain is some variation of "How much does it hurt?" Historically, clinical investigators focused almost exclusively on some subjective rating of change in pain intensity following treatment. A great deal of attention has been given to the fact that pain*is a multidimensional perception and not a simple sensation (see Turk & Robinson, Chapter 10, this volume). It is the person's perception of pain rather than solely the nociceptive stimulus that determines the extent of pain experienced, levels of adaptation, and responses to nociception. Thus, appropriate measurement of pain needs to include motivational–affective and cognitive–evaluative, along with sensory contributions as proposed by Melzack and Casey over 40 years ago (1968; see Katz & Melzack, Chapter 3, this volume). The impact of pain on physical and emotional functioning, along with general concepts captured under the rubric of health-related quality of life (HRQoL) and patient satisfaction have begun to receive much more attention (see DeGood & Cook, Chapter 4, this volume). It is not only the question "How much does it hurt?" but also "What is the impact of the pain on your life?"

QUANTIFICATION OF PAIN VERSUS ASSESSMENT OF THE PERSON WHO EXPERIENCES PAIN

It is apparent that the experience and report of pain are influenced by multiple factors, including cultural conditioning, expectancies, current social contingencies, treatments received, adverse effects of treatments, and the like. Physical pathology and the resulting nociception thus constitute only one, albeit a very important, contributor to the experience of and subsequent response to pain. Rather than focusing exclusively on the assessment of pain, many clinicians and investigators have urged that adequate assessment, especially of patients with pain, needs to be comprehensive. There has been an urgent plea to "assess the patient and not just the pain" (Turk, 1993), and this admonition appears to have been heard. As is reflected in all of the chapters is this volume, regardless of type of pain (acute, chronic noncancer, cancer-related), age and ability to communicate, and specific diagnoses (myofascial, nociceptive), greater attention has been given to patients' beliefs, attitudes, coping resources, mood states, and behaviors as they relate to the impact of pain on daily life, as well as physical pathology. The emphasis has been shifting to the patient and not just the physical pathology, and subsequent nociception that is ultimately perceived by the individual as pain. To understand a person's pain obviously requires knowledge of the various domains that influence it.

Even though measures that are not solely dependent on self-report have been developed, there continue to be concerns about the meaning of the results based on indirect measures and how they can be incorporated within clinical practice. Some require expensive equipment (sophisticated imaging, quantitative sensory testing [QST], psychophysiological recording), and others, particularly training and expertise (observation and quantification of pain behaviors and facial expressions). They create a particular clinician burden that has hindered their addition to the clinical assessment armamentarium. Demonstration of their value as sufficient to warrant the expense and investment is needed, and it will be necessary to adapt the technology for practical use in the clinic if we hope to see the advantages of the methods adopted—an extension from research to practice (e.g., for an application of QST to clinical practice, see Walk et al., 2009).

SUBJECTIVITY VERSUS OBJECTIVITY

Pain is a subjective experience. However, investigators have attempted to develop surrogate measures, such as performance tests to assess strength, lifting capacity, and trunk muscle function. Such measures may provide information about physical capacity but not specifically about pain. Other indirect methods have included assessment of physiological correlates, including advanced imaging techniques and electrophysiology and facial expressions, and other behaviors. However, there is limited evidence demonstrating that each of these is correlated highly with the experience of pain, related disability, or HRQoL.

A problem that has not been addressed adequately concerns the psychometric properties of "objective" measures. In contrast to the careful attention given to the reliability and validity of self-report measures, physical assessment measures, imaging, and other technologies have rarely studied the properties of these measures and methods. For example, what is the interrater reliability of physical assessment? The results from the handful of studies that have reported on this are not particularly encouraging (e.g., Hunt et al., 2000; Nitschke, Nattrass, & Disler, 1999). Yet the entire basis for determining impairments and subsequently awarding disability benefits to millions of people, using the American Medical Association's *Guides for the Evaluation of Permanent Impairment* (Cocchiarella & Andersson, 2001), is predicated on the reliability of the assessment procedures recommended, not one of which has been demonstrated to be reliable (Nitschke et al., 1999; Robinson, Turk, & Loeser, 2004). It is also important to acknowledge that many physical measurements that are viewed as "objective" are in fact influenced by a patient's motivation, effort, and psychological state (see Polatin Worzer, Brede, & Gatchel, Chapter 9, this volume). Fear of pain may be more disabling that pain itself (Crombez, Vervaet, Lysens, Eelen, & Baeyerns, 1996; Crombez, Vlaeyen, Heuts, & Lysens, 1999).

The association between psychophysiological parameters and pain has not been demonstrated. As Sternbach (1968, p. 57) noted,

> Because of the variability of responses elicited by different pain stimuli, and because of the additional variance contributed by individual differences in response-stereotype, it is difficult to specify a pattern of physiological responses characteristic of pain.

It is also true that studies of the association between observable pain behaviors and self-reports of pain have provided equivocal results. These efforts have not produced the objective measures of pain that many researchers and clinicians have desired from the beginning of the systematic study of pain and well before that. Clinicians' continue to rely on, to depend on, and to be frustrated by the problems inherent in the patient's self-report. As McCaffery (1979, p. 3) suggested many years ago, "Pain is what the patient tells us it is"; but apparently it is much more: There are both neurophysiological and psychological bases for the self-report and individual response.

"Methodolatry"

Other fundamental questions about newly developed methods abound. Are physiological responses displayed by functional magnetic resonance imaging (fMRI) and measured to determine diffuse noxious inhibitory control (DNIC) stable over time? Are the procedures standardized, and is there agreement on how to conduct the assessment and interpret the results of test of DNIC and QST? How will the information obtained with electronic, real-time data capture be analyzed and interpreted? Despite calls for standardization (e.g., Pud, Granovsky, & Yarnitsky, 2009) and attempts to develop consensus (Cruccu et al., 2004; Stone & Shiffman, 2002), little available evidence contributes to confident affirmative conclusions to these questions. Sometimes it appears that we suffer from "methodolatry," research that is so enamored by the technical aspects of the equipment and the promise they hold that it neglects essential studies to increase confidence in the meaningfulness of results reported.

In Chapter 2 in this volume, Jensen and Karoly suggest that temporal measures of pain have validity and represent a distinct dimension of pain, and a number of assessment strategies can be utilized to measure this aspect of pain. Much of the research on pain has focused on patients' retrospective self-reports. Several problems with self-reports may bias responses and impede the validity of our understanding of pain (see Mason, Fauerbach, & Haythornthwaite, Chapter 14, this volume; however, see Von Korff, Chapter 23, this volume). Most notably, they rely on patients' memory and their ability to average information over periods of time. Retrospective recall is influenced by patients' current mood and pain severity. Current state serves as an anchor for retrospective recall. Consider your own response if we asked you to provide a rating of your average fatigue over the past month. Most likely you would use your current level of fatigue as the basis for your reflections, recall, and estimate of your average fatigue. Thus, the question is how accurate your recall and subsequent estimate would actually be. One way to examine this question is to compare the average ratings collected daily over a month with the retrospective recall.

People with pain can be asked to rate their pain over a specific time period (e.g., past week, month) or several times each day (e.g., on waking, at meals, bedtime) for several days or weeks using daily diaries, which can provide an opportunity to note when and in what situations a person's pain increases or decreases. In this way, identified patterns of pain may indicate whether pain intensity is highest in the morning versus other times of the day. People can, of course, be asked to rate their mood, sleep, activities, and so forth, as well as their pain in self-report diaries.

Self-report diaries have both advantages and disadvantages. They can be completed on a daily or more frequent basis and do not rely on peoples' retrospective recall and anchoring biases. However, some individuals may "fill forward" (complete the entire diary at the onset of the trial rather than on a daily basis) or "fill backward" (complete the entire diary at once, immediately prior to submission to the clinician or investigator). If they maintain diaries for some time period before submitting them to the investigator or clinician, they may use prior ratings as the basis for current decisions, thereby providing invalid information (e.g., Gendreau, Hufford, & Stone, 2003; Stone, Shiffman, Schwartz, Broderick, & Hufford, 2003).

An alternative that obviates several of these problems has followed from the advent of electronic technology. Palm-top computers, two-way pagers, and *voice-over Internet protocols* (VOIPs; a technology in which phone calls can be made using a broadband Internet connection) have been used to prompt people to record their pain ratings, thus avoiding the problems noted with paper-and-pencil diaries. A number of commentators have advocated the use of electronic devices that can prompt patients for ratings and "time stamp" the actual ratings, thus facilitating real-time data capture.

The use of such electronic data acquisition methods may be particularly useful in studying the lagged effects of pain, mood, activity, and so forth, on each other (Turk, Burwinkle, & Showlund, 2007). For example such time-stamped data collected multiple times during the course of the day and week can permit determination of the effects of previous ratings on subsequent ratings repeated multiple times, permitting replication of the effects (e.g., Affleck et al., 1999; Sorbi et al., 2006).

Although real-time, electronic strategies have sufficient advantages to warrant the investment, it can be a costly endeavor. Moreover, problems with technology and methods that can be categorized as operator, software, and hardware problems have been noted (Turk et al., 2007). The incremental validity of real-time compared retrospective methods has not been consistently demonstrated (e.g., Broderick et al., 2008; Jamison, Raymond, Slawsby, McHugo, & Baird, 2006). Moreover, only preliminary results of the utility of these approaches over extended periods have been reported (Jamison et al., 2001). An additional problem with paper-and-pencil diaries and technological methods that request frequent ratings is that they have the potential to sensitize people to symptoms by repeatedly and frequently requesting ratings of events and features to which they might not normally attend. Such reactivity has been investigated with electronic diaries, but the results, although promising, need to be viewed as preliminary

(Stone, Shiffman, et al., 2003). The question of interest should guide the selection of methods used and not just a technology that is appealing.

Impact of Psychological Variables on Physical Performance

Motivational and cognitive factors affect performance on these tests and cannot be separated from a person's responses. It is important to acknowledge that we will probably never be able to evaluate pain without some reliance on patients' subjective reports. These reports are also important, because they influence how patients are responded to by significant others, including health care providers. Moreover, patients' self-reports of their beliefs, moods, coping strategies, and expectations have been shown to be related to the following:

- Functional behavior (see, e.g., Jensen, Romano, Turner, Good, & Wald, 1999; Vlaeyan, & Linton, 2000).
- Return to work following injury (see, e.g., Waddell, 2004).
- Adaptation (Jensen et al., 2002).
- Physical functioning (Jensen, Turner, & Romano, 2007)
- Disability (see, e.g., Dobkin et al., 2010; Turner, Jensen, & Romano, 2000).
- Use of the health care system (e.g., Flor & Turk, 1988).
- Premature termination from treatment (e.g., Richmond & Carmody, 1999).
- Adherence to treatment regimens (e.g., Cipher, Fernandez, & Clifford, 2002).
- Response of patients with diverse pain syndromes to treatment (e.g., Burns, Kubilus, Bruehl, Harden, & Lofland, 2003; Jensen, Nielson, Turner, Romano, & Hill, 2004; Olsson, Bunketorp, Carlsson, & Styf, 2002).

Of course, it is not just individual differences that affect this set of responses. Socioeconomic factors also make important contributions to adjustment and disability following injury (see Robinson, Chapter 21, and Watson, Chapter 15, this volume). Regardless of the treatment received (e.g., surgery, rehabilitation), compensation issues seem to play a role, such that the outcomes are poorer for those receiving disability payments. To put it succinctly, "Money matters" (Rohling, Binder, & Langhinrichsen-Rohling, 1995). However, other factors may contribute to the poorer outcomes observed, not the least of which is that the type of work and increased risk for injury may be more physically demanding and may preclude return following injury. Most people live in a social context. Failure to consider the influence of social supports and contacts contribute to an incomplete understanding of people experiencing pain. Family and social supports have direct impacts on perceptions of pain, along with adjustment and adaptation (see Romano, Cano, & Schmaling, Chapter 5, this volume).

We also need to remember that all of us have learning histories that precede the development of pain. For example, many patients with chronic pain have extensive histories. One review noted that the average age of patients treated in multidisciplinary pain clinics is 44 years old and the mean duration of pain exceeds 7 years (Flor, Fydrich, & Turk, 1992). These data should remind us that people with chronic pain have been exposed to innumerable life experiences prior to the development of the pain that influence their responses. Moreover, they have had over 7 years to adapt to their pain and over this period will have evolved to accommodate their lives to their circumstances. Thus, at the time of assessment, many factors are involved in the response to the questions about how much they hurt and the impact of pain on their lives.

Research to date suggests that patients' performances on physical and biomechanical measures are not associated with the risk of acute pain evolving into chronic pain (Carragee, Alamin, Miller, & Carragee, 2005) or their return to work (e.g., Klenerman et al., 1995). Thus, the hope that objective measurement based on type of performance, using a sophisticated apparatus designed to assess functional capacity, will predict disability or identify malingering is unlikely. Furthermore, the relationship between this performance and their return to work has yet to be demonstrated. Investigators and clinicians must be cautious in not overselling these expensive pieces of equipment and advanced technologies.

In a number of chapters in this volume (e.g., Polatin et al., Chapter 9; Robinson, Chapter 21; and Watson, Chapter 15, this volume), authors have emphasized that greater attention must be given to the combination of sets of physical information and the processes whereby decisions are made about the extent of pathology, the amount of impairment, the degree of disability, and the appropriateness of different treatment alternatives. Additional research is needed to demonstrate the interrelationships among pathology, impairment, disability, and pain. It is essential that research address how individual characteristics of patients and their social environments influence responses to impairment, development of disability, and differential responses to alternative treatment interventions (e.g., Thieme, Turk, & Flor, 2007; see Romano et al., Chapter 5, this volume).

PSYCHOMETRIC PROPERTIES OF INSTRUMENTS AND ASSESSMENT PROCEDURES

The importance of psychometric characteristics has long been acknowledged, and careful attention to reliability, validity, utility, and normative data is required for any new assessment instrument. Detailed recommendations have described the required steps in the development of any new self-report measure for pain (Turk et al., 2006).

One feature that is included in instrument development is input from the population for whom the measure is being developed (Acquadro et al., 2003; Turk, Dworkin, Revicki, et al., 2008). Representative samples should be included in the early stages to help instrument developers incorporate questions that address meaningful issues and that are important to future respondents (for a recent example that followed these recommendations, see Dworkin et al., 2008).

Validity of Instruments and Procedures

Many chapters in this volume focus on the reliability of instruments. Considerably less attention has been given to the issue of validity: Is the instrument or procedure appropriate, meaningful, and useful for making specific inferences? The question is whether the test is valid for the purposes and samples for which it is to be used.

It is essential that the association between psychological measures and meaningful behaviors be established. For example, it is commonly believed that physical deconditioning is prevalent in patients with back pain; however, this assumption has been challenged (Wittinik, Michel, Wagner, Sukiennik, & Rogers, 2000). So before debating the reliability of various procedures to assess aerobic capacity, muscle strength, and spinal flexibility in patients with back pain (Wittinik, Michel, Kulich, et al., 2000) we need to examine the validity of the assumption. Similarly, surrogate or indirect measures, such as physical examinations and imaging, should be demonstrated to be related to meaningful outcome criteria (e.g., patients' pain reports, health care utilization, return to work, response to treatment). The relationships in physical pathology, as measured by sophisticated imaging, and subsequent pain and disability are being challenged (Carragee, Barcohana, Alamin, & Van den Haak, 2004; Carragee et al., 2005; Jarvik et al., 2005). More effort is needed to demonstrate that assessment instruments and procedures are clinically valid.

Translations

Assessment instruments originally developed in one language are often translated into other languages. The fact that questions constituting the instruments can be translated, however, does not mean that the concepts being measured are equivalent in different cultures. The fact that an instrument is valid for one sample of patients does not guarantee that it is valid for another sample with different characteristics. Over 20 years ago, Deyo (1984) showed the pitfalls of simply translating an assessment instrument into another language and assuming that the validity of the instrument in the two languages (English and Spanish) is comparable. The nonprofit Mapi Institute and Research Trust (*www.mapi-institute.com*) has a set of standards detailing a rigorous methodology that should be followed to create each linguistic version of instruments.

Normative Information

The appropriateness of tests' norms has rarely been considered in the pain litera-

ture (for a recent exception, see Nicholas, Asghari, & Blyth, 2008). In the absence of normative information, the raw score on any test is meaningless. To observe that a patient with migraine headaches scores a 10 on a visual analogue scale (VAS) of pain intensity conveys little or no information. However, we know that the average VAS pain severity score for 100 patients with migraine headache is 5.4, with a standard deviation of 1.0, then this information permits the conclusion that this patient is signifying a very high level of pain relative to other such patients. If, on the other hand, the only available normative evidence is based on patients with cancer, and their mean is 5.4, with a standard deviation of 1.0, then we do not know how the patient rated his or her pain relative to a group of patients with migraine. Is the patient's pain report atypical for sufferers from migraine? Without appropriate normative information, it is not possible to answer this question.

In all areas of pain assessment, it is important to know the type(s) of patients for whom normative information is available, and thus the appropriateness of generalizing from the original sample(s) used to establish reliability. In many cases, instruments developed for use with physically healthy or psychiatrically impaired people have been used for patients with chronic pain. This can lead to erroneous conclusions.

Before using the norms of an instrument, it is important to demonstrate the invariance of the factor structure of the new instrument for the new population. For example, Turk and Rudy (1988) demonstrated that subgroups of patients with pain can be identified based on their responses on the West Haven–Yale Multidimensional Pain Inventory (MPI; Kerns, Turk, & Rudy, 1985). The original sample was a heterogeneous group of patients evaluated at a pain clinic. Would the same subgroups generalize to other medical diagnoses, or were the results idiosyncratic to the original sample of patients? Turk and Rudy (1990) demonstrated that although the mean scores on different scales of the MPI and the percentage of patients comprising each subgroup differed among patients with low back pain, headache, and temporomandibular pain, the correlation matrices among the scales were invariant. Thus, although different normative values should have been used for different diagnoses, the subgroups identified transcended medical and dental diagnoses, thus validating the generalizability of the patterns of the scales that characterize the subgroups.

As many chapters in this volume illustrate, measures that were never developed for samples of patients with pain but were used because of their availability, are being replaced by measures specifically developed for and standardized (normed) for patients with specific types of pain. Future research needs to demonstrate that these pain-specific measures are both psychometrically acceptable and clinically useful. However, there may be circumstances in which the use of general measures may be warranted and even desirable. For example, when disease-specific measures are not available or there is a desire to compare across populations, use of generic measures may be appropriate (Turk et al., 2003).

The incremental validity of any new instrument should also be considered; that is, do the new instruments add anything to existing measures, or do they place less demand upon the patient? Patient burden is a considerable and growing problem. As more and more detailed measures are developed, this can lead not only to patient burden but to reduce quality as respondents become fatigued and the validity of their responses decline. When two measurement instruments are shown to be measuring the same thing, the one that requires the least time and therefore places the least burden on the patient to complete may be preferred, all others things being equal.

PROLIFERATION OF MEASURES

The development of new assessment instruments and procedures is a laborious task requiring large samples of patients, extensive amounts of time, and substantial expense. It is all too easy to avoid this task by using published instruments that appear to measure constructs related to our interests (Tukey, 1979). It is also possible that the availability of instruments may shape the research questions we ask.

The wealth of available pain assessment measures and procedures described throughout this volume can be both a blessing and a curse. Not only must the clinician or investigator choose a set of procedures to use, but he or she must also decide how to integrate the large amount of information obtained, and how to adjust for the quantity of data acquired in clinical research (Turk, Dworkin, McDermott, et al., 2008). Many questions should be considered in determining an assessment battery. What measures should be included in the assessment of a patient with pain? Have the measures been shown to be psychometrically sound? Can the information be aggregated into a single score? Are these measurements reproducible and sensitive enough to detect clinical response to therapy? Does each measure, regardless of its name, assess a unique variable, or does it merely duplicate an existing measure that has a different label but assesses the same domain? What norms are available, and are they appropriate?

Those who select from the array of assessment instruments must also ask themselves, "Assessment for what purpose—classification, diagnosis, treatment planning, decision making, quality improvement, prediction, or outcome?" Although some criteria for evaluating the appropriateness of a specific instrument encompass these different purposes, this is not always the case. For example, if an investigator or clinician wishes to evaluate the efficacy of a treatment based on changes from pretreatment to posttreatment, he or she needs to be concerned about whether the instruments selected to evaluate success are subject to change. Related to this is the ability of an instrument to detect small changes. For example, the diagnostic criteria for fibromyalgia syndrome include the presence of 11 of 18 specific tender points. Positive tender points are based on the patient's dichotomous response ("yes" or "no") when asked whether he or she feels pain on palpation at each location. The range of response is quite limited on such a simple rating system, and the system may not be sensitive to small but significant changes following treatment.

Another important question concerns what to assess. In clinical areas there should be some relation between the instruments selected and treatment. It is unfair to ask a patient to complete a lengthy assessment battery or to submit to a large number of laboratory tests if the information collected is simply entered in the patient's file but has no impact on treatment. Insufficient attention has been devoted to customizing treatments to important characteristics of patients (Turk, 2005). The new measures described in this volume may help to answer questions about customizing treatment. Several studies have identified subgroups of patients with the same medical diagnosis on the basis of psychosocial and behavioral characteristics (e.g., Bergstrom, Jensen, Bodin, Linton, & Nygren, 2001; Jensen et al., 2004; Kerns, Wagner, Rosenberg, Haythornthwaite, & Caudill-Slosberg, 2005). Efforts to develop methods to predict opioid misuse (Turk, Swanson, & Gatchel, 2008) and differential responses of patients to treatment for various chronic pain syndromes (e.g., Junghaenel, Schwartz, & Broderick, 2007; Olsson et al., 2002; Thieme et al., 2007) have been receiving additional attention.

FEASIBILITY

There is a growing concern about feasibility of various assessment procedures for different samples. There may be an ideal measure, but one that is not appropriate. For example, it may not be possible to administer a lengthy pain questionnaire on a frequent basis to terminal-stage patients with pain. Young children and patients with limited communication skills may be unable to respond to questions in the same way that "normal" adults can (see Ruskin, Amaria, Warnock, & McGrath, Chapter 11, and Hadjistavropoulos, Breau, & Craig, Chapter 13, this volume). Older people display different "pain behaviors" than do younger adults and may not be able to engage in some biomechanical tests (see Gauthier & Gagliese, Chapter 12, this volume).

The behaviors of patients with different pain syndromes may be influenced by the nature of their diseases, and it may be inappropriate to generalize from one disease to another (Wilkie, Keefe, Dodd, & Copp, 1992). Particular consideration must be given to the special characteristics of different populations in determining what assessment procedures can reasonably be used—for example, for patients with cancer versus low back pain. The comparability of measures ostensibly designed to measure the same things, but in demographically very different samples, needs to be demonstrated.

HANDBOOK OF PAIN ASSESSMENT REDUX

It is almost 30 years since Melzack's (1983) volume on pain assessment first appeared, and almost 20 years since the first edition of this text was published. In the time since the publication of these volumes, there has been a veritable explosion of research devoted to the development of systematic techniques for measuring pain and for evaluating people who experience it. The chapters contained in this volume present the state of the art at this point in time.

As we noted in the two previous editions of this book, it is precarious to predict how pain assessment will evolve. In that edition we enumerated a nine-item "wish list." At this juncture it seems appropriate that we review the progress made on our list.

1. We hoped that trends in developing appropriate psychometrics for instruments and procedures for assessment of people in pain would escalate. Over the past decade, investigators and clinicians have adopted our concern; much more information has been published on the reliability, validity, utility, and normative data for existing and new assessment methods. In the area of physical assessment, however, there continues to be much less attention given to psychometrics, especially the intra- and interjudge reliability of physical examination procedures, imagining methods, and other technologies (DNIC, QST).

2. We indicated that new instruments and procedures should be developed in an effort to measure domains believed to be important in understanding pain and the person who experiences it. Many new procedures and measures have been developed, with greater attention given to prediction of disability (e.g., Turner, Franklin, & Turk, 2000); readiness for treatment (Nielson et al., 2008); response to treatment (e.g., Jensen et al., 2004; Thieme et al., 2007); misuse or abuse of medication (Turk, Swanson, & Gatchel, 2008); and the role of fear of increased pain, further injury, or reinjury

associated with activity (Turk, Robinson, Sherman, Burwinkle, & Swanson, 2008; Vlaeyen & Linton, 2000).

3. We called for the consolidation of instruments that might be measuring similar concepts, as well as the replacement of some by new approaches demonstrated to be more appropriate (reliable, valid, less demanding on patients). Although some effort has been devoted to this call (De Gagne, Mikail, & D'Eon, 1995; Mikail, DuBreuil, & D'Eon, 1993), and there continue to be a large number of measures that are likely to be highly correlated. Recently, Davidson, Tripp, Fabrigar, and Davidson (2008) conducted an evaluation to demonstrate the interrelationship among many of the most commonly used self-report measures in assessing patients with chronic pain. Based on a factor analysis of 32 empirically derived pain subscales, they demonstrated that a set of factors (i.e., pain and disability, pain description, affective distress, support, positive coping strategies, negative coping strategies, and activity) appeared to underlie these measures. Of course, we must be cautious in the interpretation of the results of these analyses, because they are directly related to the selection of the measure included in the study. The availability of overlap often leads to confusion in investigators who have to select from among the diversity of measures assessing similar constructs. If the results of the Davidson and colleagues study are replicated with other commonly used sets of measures, then efficient use might reduce the number necessary to provide a generic and comprehensive assessment battery for chronic pain. No comparable effort has been made in the assessment of acute pain, or pain with infants, children, and adolescents.

4. We suggested that greater emphasis should be placed on relating assessment instruments and procedures to important behavioral outcomes. As we have noted in this chapter, there is no question that investigators have begun to move beyond instrument development to evaluate the utility of measures and procedures in assessing important outcomes.

5. We noted that more attention needs to be given to innovative strategies for integrating diverse sets of information. Unfortunately, the issue of information integration has not received sufficient attention and continues to be an area greatly in need of research (Turk, Dworkin, McDermott, et al., 2008).

6. We recommended that greater emphasis should be given to prescribing treatments based on patient characteristics derived from assessment data, rather than treating all patients with pain as basically the same, or matching treatment exclusively to medical diagnosis. Increased research in this area has shown promise for obtaining better outcomes. Initial attempts (e.g., Burns et al., 2003; Jensen et al., 2004; Olsson et al., 2002) have been reported; however, the emphasis has continued to be on identification of subgroups, without taking the next step of relating subgroups to treatments. Statistical procedures can easily be used to identify clusters or profiles of patients, but these groupings may have little clinical utility. We hope that more treatment-matching studies will be conducted to demonstrate the additive value of knowing the characteristics of patient subgroups.

7. We suggested that there was a need to demonstrate the generalizability of different instruments to new populations rather than to assume that such instruments can be used with samples that differ from the original sample. Several studies have begun to evaluate the appropriateness of generalizing the use of the instruments originally developed on one population of patients with chronic pain to others (e.g., Mendoza, Mayne, Rublee, & Cleeland, 2006; Widerström-Noga, Duncan, & Turk, 2004), but much more research is needed to demonstrate the appropriateness of using measures across diagnoses.

8. We suggested use of recent advances in test theory (e.g., item response theory) in evaluating pain assessment instruments and procedures. On this point, we have seen a great deal of progress with the National Institutes of Health patient-reported outcomes measurement information system (PROMIS) project (e.g., Cell, Gershon, Lai, & Choi, 2007). There continues to be a tendency to rely on classical psychometric methods.

9. We expected to see major advances in the use of sophisticated imaging procedures to advance our understanding of pain and responses to treatment. There has been an

explosion of interest in brain imaging (Stephenson & Arneric, 2008), but there continue to be few studies reporting changes in brain activity as a result of treatments, and the relationship between images and patient experiences is still to be determined.

SOME NEW DIRECTIONS

The development and refinement of advanced imaging procedures (e.g., single-photon emission tomography [SPECT] and fMRI have begun to provide new insights into the processing of noxious information associated with pain (Stephenson & Arneric, 2008; see Flor & Meyer, Chapter 8, this volume). For example, recent studies have shown that when acute noxious stimuli are administered to normal individuals, there is activation of cerebral blood flow in multiple brain areas. The fact that many different areas respond to the same noxious stimuli supports the view that the pain experience, rather than being a distributive process based exclusively in one location, results from interaction among a number of distinct brain regions. Interestingly, imaging studies suggest that the patterns of activation of regions of the brain are different for chronic pain syndromes (e.g., Cesaro et al., 1991; Di Piero et al., 1991).

A great deal of what we know about people with chronic pain is based on patients who are treated at multidisciplinary pain centers. Yet only a small proportion of people with chronic and recurring pain are treated in such facilities. Consequently, these samples are highly selective and may not be representative of people with persistent pain. For example, epidemiological studies comparing patients treated at specialized pain clinics and community-dwellers with chronic pain indicate that those treated at pain centers had greater psychological distress, greater psychiatric morbidity, and lower levels of education, and that they were more likely to have experienced work-related injuries (Crook, Weir, & Tunks, 1989). Realization of the limitations of samples from pain clinics has resulted in an increasing number of efforts to learn more about people with persistent pain in the general community by national surveys (e.g., National Center for Health Statistics, 2006; Von Korff et al., 2005) and cross-national surveys (e.g., Elliott, Smith, Penny, Smith, & Chambers, 1999; Gureje, 1998), in primary care settings (Gureje, 1998; Harstall, 2003; Von Korff, Ormel, Keefe, & Dworkin, 1992), and in community settings (see, e.g., Drossman et al., 1988). Von Korff (Chapter 23, this volume) describes the basic features of epidemiological and survey methods that are likely to expand our understanding of chronic pain beyond the usual setting of tertiary care. One tradeoff with large-scale epidemiological studies that can tell us about the prevalence of pain and treatments received is the balance between the large sample and the amount of detail that can be acquired. To learn more about the experience of pain in the community, including impact on physical and emotional functioning and HRQoL, will require more in-depth study of community samples.

Meaningfulness of Change

An issue of growing concern in clinical trials is the importance or meaningfulness of changes in outcome measures. Commonly, in results of clinical trials, researchers report mean differences between various intensities (e.g., quantity or frequency of physical exercise, dosages of medication), types of treatments, and "inactive treatments" (placebo). However, statistical significance reflects the magnitude and variability of the treatment effect, as well as the sample size; it is not necessarily an indication of a meaningful change. Even treatment conditions that differ significantly from each other on some statistical analyses do not confirm that the treatment has an important or meaningful effect, but they do demonstrate the magnitude of the change. Depending on the specific outcome, clinical importance and meaningfulness can be assessed by patients, clinicians, significant others, and representatives of society at large (Frost, Bonomi, Ferrans, Wong, & Hays, 2002) for example, third-party payers.

The use of effect sizes has been suggested as a method for demonstrating meaningfulness of the results (Busse & Guyatt, 2009). Another important method for reporting meaningfulness responder rates (Busse & Guyatt, 2009). There are many approaches for performing such "responder analyses," and for evaluating treatment effect sizes more generally, including calculating the number needed to treat (NNT) or harm (H). The NNT is the reciprocal of the absolute risk reduction and reflects the "number of patients who must be treated to generate one more success or one less failure than would have resulted had all persons been given the comparison treatment; that is, what percentage of patients in each group in an outcome study demonstrate change at a predetermined level deemed to be important. The level specified as important is referred to as the *minimal important difference or minimal clinically important difference* (Jaeschke, Singer, & Guyatt, 1989).

Two general methods, either anchor-based or distribution-based, have been used to establish what change is minimally important (Lydick & Epstein, 1993). *Anchor-based methods* relate changes in scores on a measure to a standard that is different from the specific measure itself, whereas *distribution-based methods* use statistical parameters associated with the measure (e.g., effect size, standard error of measurement) to interpret the magnitude of changes in the measure's scores over time (Sloan, Symonds, Vargas-Chanes, & Fridley, 2003).

It is has been recommended that all chronic pain clinical trials report a cumulative proportion of responders analysis (Farrar, Dworkin, & Max, 2006). In this approach, the entire distribution of treatment response is depicted in a graph of the proportion of responders for all percentages of pain reduction from 0 through 100%. Using such a graph, it is possible to compare treatment groups with respect to patients achieving any percentage of pain reduction, not only the benchmarks discussed earlier but also any others that might be more informative depending on the specific circumstances. Such an analysis can also be extended to include percentages of patients whose pain has increased over the course of the clinical trial, which makes it possible to compare the extent to which worsening has occurred in the different treatment groups.

The Patient Global Impression of Change scale (PGIC; Guy, 1976) consists of a single-item rating of participants' responses during a clinical trial using a 7-point rating scale, with the options "very much improved," "much improved," "minimally improved," "no change," "minimally worse," "much worse," and "very much worse." There has been widespread use of the PGIC in recent chronic pain clinical trials (Dworkin et al., 2003; Wernicke et al., 2006), and the measure provides a responsive and readily interpretable assessment of participants' evaluations of the importance of their improvement or worsening; however, it is reported at a single point in time and stability of response must be confirmed (Senn, 2008).

The PGIC has been used as an anchor in determining the clinical importance of improvement in pain ratings and other measures, which assumes that the importance of the different patient ratings on this measure is self-evident. Ratings of "much improved" and "very much improved" (or "very much worse") clearly reflect what patients consider to be important changes, and it appears likely that ratings of "minimally improved" (or "minimally worse") reflect changes that patients consider less substantial but minimally important. How important a *minimal* improvement or worsening is to patients must depend, at least in part, on factors such as treatment convenience and cost, as well as any aspects of the side-effect burden that are not considered by patients in rating their overall change. When using the PGIC in a clinical trial, it is therefore recommended that the percentage of patients endorsing each of the seven response options in each treatment group be analyzed and reported separately, and that ratings of "minimally improved" (or "minimally worse") not be combined with the other ratings of improvement (or worsening) or the ratings of "unchanged."

Establishing the minimally important difference (MID) for the different measure use to assess outcomes in clinical trials has received growing attention in the pain field. We expect that this important concept will become the hallmark of future research, particularly on patient-reported outcomes (Dworkin et al., 2008).

Technology

A number of innovative technologies have raised the potential for improvements or at least extensions of opportunities for assessment of important components of the pain experience. Several of these have been noted, along with their limitations. There are other technologies that will likely be tapped in the future. The availability of the Internet creates assessment opportunities to acquire general information about pain, the impact of pact, efficacy of treatments, and so forth, in general surveys (e.g., Bennett, Jones, Turk, Russell, & Matallana, 2007). There will be opportunities to increase assessment of individual patients from their homes.

Portable devices that are being developed can be incorporated into assessment plans. For example, there is a growing recognition of the impact of sleep on the experience of pain. It is reasonable to assume that poor sleep quality will contribute to greater fatigue and impaired daytime functioning, but relationships between objective measures of poor sleep quality and fatigue have not been well-documented. However, one small study did confirm a significant association (Landis et al., 2003). Subjective perceptions of poor sleep are often out of proportion to and do not match modest changes in polysomnography (PSG). PSG is considered the most valid, objective means for measuring sleep stages, although it is a cumbersome, resource-intensive procedure that requires patients to spend several nights in a sleep laboratory.

Recent technological advances in the development of portable and unobtrusive actigraphic recording devices can be used as an unobtrusive measure of sleep in the home environment. The actigraph is used to measure daily sleep–wake patterns based on the assumption that wakefulness is associated with arm movements and sleep is not. Disturbed sleep patterns have been observed with the use of actigraphy, an objective indicator of sleep in fibromyalgia (Korszun et al., 2002). Actigraphy has been shown to be highly correlated with PSG (all $rs > .85$) and to be a valid means of assessing sleep problems (Sadeh, Sharkey, & Carskadon, 1994). It is being used more frequently as a behavioral indicator of sleep quality in the evaluation of sleep problems (Sadeh, Hauri, & Kripke, 1995). Actigraphic recordings have the added advantage of being objective measures that are not solely dependent on patients' reports of sleep quality. Increas-

ingly in sleep research, data derived from sleep diaries and from actigraphy are used to validate sleep patterns. Actigraphy has been shown to correlate well with both the use of sleep logs and PSG (Hauri & Wisbey, 1992). This technology holds promise for use in assessing both sleeping and waking activity, without relying on self-report. Moreover, actigraphy is a useful method for studying activity in an objective, naturalistic way, with individuals following their usual routine in their home environments. When used to measure activity, actigraphy is an objective measure that occurs in real time and does not rely on self-reports that can be biased by a number of variables (Stone & Shiffman, 2002).

Although the actigraphic recording devices are convenient to use, about the size of a large wristwatch, and can be worn at all times except in the shower or bath, there are some limitations related to cost, extensive quantity of data, and number of parameters. Moreover, basic studies, such as differential effects based on the limb on which the device is worn and the absence of normative information across populations and samples with different pain location, there are no data on the MID for such activity recordings.

The Promise of PROMIS

There have been a number of criticisms of classical test theory with use of reliability and validity, and its dependence on large number of items and, consequently, excessive patient burden. An alternative, item response theory (IRT), was developed to address these and other concerns. IRT models express the probability of a particular response to a scale item as a function of the quantitative attribute (unobservable, latent trait) of the person and certain characteristics (parameters) of an item (Chang & Reeve, 2005). IRT is designed to describe explicitly the functional relationship between individuals' responses at the item level and the characteristics (parameters) of the items on the test. Because there is a nonlinear relationship between response to an item and the *latent variable* (i.e., the concept the item is intended to measure), estimates based on IRT are not sample-dependent, redundant items are unnecessary and possibly detrimental (e.g., in small multi-item scales, redundant items can hurt the validity of a scale), and scales and items can be evaluated for having comparable characteristics on the outcome of interest (Reeve & Fayers, 2005).

The aim of IRT models is to make predictions about constructs such as health status and functional abilities of individuals from as few items as possible. In contrast, classical test theory does not focus on the person but is applied at the level of the scale or test (the psychometric properties of the scale or test). IRT-based measures have important properties that provide advantages over classical test theory for health outcomes measurement: (1) Each question in a scale is characterized with a set of properties that describes its relationship with a measured construct and how the item functions within a study population; (2) IRT item properties are relatively invariant with respect to the sample of respondents, and respondent scores are relatively invariant with respect to the set of items used; and (3) scores can be compared or combined despite individuals receiving different sets of IRT-calibrated questions. The advantage of IRT-based measures is that not every item needs to be administered to an entire sample; hence, IRT provides a potentially more efficient method of data collection and reduced respondent burden. This makes IRT an important analytical tool to evaluate items, to scale the performance of a questionnaire, to evaluate the equivalence of content for an instrument used for different populations or in different settings, and to link two or more instruments on a common metric (Chang & Reeve, 2005). IRT requires the development of large pools of well-characterized items and uses computer algorithms to present the smallest number of items that will produce the most valid assessment of a particular outcome domain for a given patient (Fries, Bruce, & Cella, 2005).

The National Institutes of Health has undertaken a major initiative to fund the PROMIS network to develop improved measures of pain, function, quality of life, and participation in activities. PROMIS was created to examine the application of IRT in areas related to pain and to physical and emotional functioning.

This project is in its early, formative stages. IRT is a promising approach that will require further refinements before it can be recommended for use in clinical trials. Most likely, the approach will be of use in measurements of physical functioning but probably less so for symptoms such as pain and fatigue, because IRT assumes an underlying dimension (e.g., the pain experience) that may not be valid. IRT models are not panaceas that resolve all problems identified with classical test theory. Turk and colleagues (2006) have presented a direct comparison of the features, advantages, and disadvantages of both classical test theory and IRT.

Are We There Yet?

On the whole, it appears that important strides have been made since publication of the first edition of this volume. There remain areas in our list that have not yet received sufficient attention, and that we hope will be addressed in the next decade.

One primary goal in this volume has been to provide practical and useful information for clinical investigators and health care providers. It is our hope that the discussions initiated throughout this volume serve to inspire additional research and improve clinical practice by increasing understanding of people who are experiencing pain, not just their pain. The continuing evolution of human pain assessment is essential for success in the search for treatments for those who experience pain, regardless of causes, diagnoses, and ages.

ACKNOWLEDGMENT

Preparation of this chapter was supported in part by Grant No. AR/AI44724 from the National Institute of Arthritis and Musculoskeletal and Skin Diseases to Dennis C. Turk.

REFERENCES

Acquadro, C., Benson, R., Dubois, D., Leidy, N. K., Marquis, P., Revicki, D., et al. (2003). Incorporating the patient's perspective into drug development and communication: An ad hoc task force report of the patient-reported (PRO) harmonization group meeting at the Food and Drug Administration: February 2001. *Value in Health, 6,* 522–531.

Affleck, G., Tennen, H., Keefe, F. J., Lefebvre, J. C., Kashikar-Zuck, S., Wright, K., et al. (1999). Everyday life with osteoarthritis or rheumatoid arthritis: Independent effects of disease and gender on daily pain, mood, and coping. *Pain*, *83*, 601–609.

Beck, A. T., Steer, R. A., Ball, R., & Ranieri, W. F. (1996). Comparison of Beck Depression Inventories -IA and -II in psychiatric outpatients. *Journal of Personality*, *67*, 588–597.

Bennett, R. M., Friend, R., Jones, K., Ward, R., Han, B. K., & Ross, R. L. (2009). The revised Fibromyalgia Impact Questionnaire (FIQR): Validation and psychometric properties. *Arthritis Research and Therapy*, *11*, R120.

Bennett, R. M., Jones, J., Turk, D. C., Russell, J., & Matallana, L. (2007). An Internet survey of 2,596 people with fibromyalgia. *BMC Musculoskeletal Disorders*, *8*, 27.

Bergstrom, K. G., Jensen, I. B., Bodin, L., Linton, S. J., & Nygren, A. L. (2001). The impact of psychologically different patient groups on outcome after a vocational rehabilitation program for long-term spinal pain patients. *Pain*, *93*, 229–238.

Broderick, J. E., Schwartz, J. E., Vikingstad, G., Pribbernow, M., Grossman, S., & Stone, A. A. (2008). The accuracy of pain and fatigue items across different reporting periods. *Pain*, *139*, 146–157.

Burns, J. W., Kubilus, A., Bruehl, S., Harden, R. N., & Lofland, K. (2003). Do changes in cognitive factors influence outcome following multidisciplinary treatment for chronic pain?: A cross- lagged panel analysis. *Journal of Consulting and Clinical Psychology*, *71*, 81–91.

Busse, J. W., & Guyatt, G. H. (2009). Optimizing the use of patient data to improve outcomes for patients: Narcotics for chronic noncancer pain. *Expert Review of Pharamcoeconomics and Outcomes Research*, *9*, 171–179.

Carragee, E. J., Alamin, T. F., Miller, J. L., & Carragee, J. M. (2005). Discography, MRI and psychosocial determinants of low back pain disability and remission: A prospective study in subjects with benign persistent back pain. *Spine Journal*, *5*, 24–35.

Carragee, E. J., Barcohana, B., Alamin, T., & Van den Haak, E. (2004). Prospective controlled study of the development of lower back pain in previously asymptomatic subjects undergoing experimental discography. *Spine*, *29*, 1112–1117.

Cella, D., Gershon, R., Lai, J.-S., & Choi, S. (2007). The future of outcomes measurement: Item banking, tailored short forms, and computerized adaptive testing. *Quality of Life Research*, *16*, 133–141.

Cesaro, P., Mann, M. W., Moretti, J. L., Defer, G., Roualdes, B., Nguyen, J. P., et al. (1991). Central pain and thalamic hyperactivity: A single photon emission computerized tomographic study. *Pain*, *47*, 329–336.

Chang, C.-H., & Reeve, B. B. (2005). Item response theory and its applications to patient-reported outcomes measurement. *Evaluation and the Health Professions*, *28*, 264–282.

Cipher, D. J., Fernandez, E., & Clifford, P. A. (2002). Coping style influences compliance with multidisciplinary pain management. *Journal of Health Psychology*, *7*, 665–673.

Cocchiarella, L., & Andersson, G. B. J. (2001). *Guides to the evaluation of permanent impairment* (5th ed.). Chicago: AMA Press.

Crombez, G., Vervaet, L., Lysens, R., Eelen, P., & Baeyerns, F. (1996). Do pain expectancies cause pain in chronic low back patients?: A clinical investigation. *Behaviour Research and Therapy*, *34*, 919–925.

Crombez, G., Vlaeyen, J. W. S, Heuts, P. H. T. G., & Lysens, R. (1999). Fear of pain is more disabling that the pain itself: Further evidence on the role of pain-related fear in chronic back pain disability. *Pain*, *80*, 529–539.

Crook, J., Weir, R., & Tunks, E. (1989). An epidemiological follow-up survey of persistent pain sufferers in a group family practice and specialty pain clinic. *Pain*, *36*, 49–61.

Cruccu, G., Anand, P., Attal, N., Garcia-Larréa, L., Haanpää, M., Jerum, E., et al. (2004). EFNS guidelines on neuropathic pain assessment. *European Journal of Neurology*, *11*, 147.

Davidson, M. A., Tripp, D. A., Fabrigar, L. R., & Davidson, P. R. (2008). Chronic pain assessment: A seven-factor model. *Pain Research and Management*, *13*, 299–308.

De Gagne, T. A., Mikail, S. F., & D'Eon, J. L. (1995). Confirmatory factor analysis of a 4-factor model of chronic pain evaluation. *Pain*, *60*, 195–202.

Deyo, R. A. (1984). Pitfalls in measuring the health status of Mexican Americans: Comparative validity of the English and Spanish Sickness Impact Profile. *American Journal of Public*, *6*, 560–573.

Di Piero, V., Jones, A. K. P., Iannotti, F., Powell, M., Perani, D., Lenzi, G. L., et al. (1991). Chronic pain: A PET study of the central effects of percutaneous high cervical cordotomy. *Pain*, *46*, 9–12.

Dobkin, P. L., Liu, A., Abrahamowicz, M., Ionescu-Ittu, R., Bernatsky, S., Goldberger, A., et al. (2010). Predictors of disability and pain six months after the end of treatment of fibromyalgia. *Clinical Journal of Pain*, *26*, 23–29.

Drossman, D. A., McKee, D. C., Sandler, R. S., Michell, C. M., Cramer, E. M., Lowman, B. C., et al. (1988). Psychosocial factors in the irritable bowel syndrome: A multivariate study of patients and non-patients with irritable bowel syndrome. *Gastroenterology, 95,* 701–708.

Dworkin, R. H., Corbin, A. E., Young, J. P., Sharma, U., LaMoreaux, L., Bockbrader, H., et al. (2003). Pregabalin for the treatment of postherpetic neuralgia: A randomized, placebo-controlled trial. *Neurology, 60,* 1274–1283.

Dworkin, R. H., Turk, D. C., Revicki, D. A., Harding, G., Coyne, K. S., Peirce-Sandner, S., et al. (2009). Development and initial validation of an expanded and revised version of the Short-Form McGill Pain Questionnaire (SF-MPQ-2). *Pain, 144,* 35–42.

Dworkin, R. H., Turk, D. C., Wyrwich, K. W., Beaton, D., Cleeland, C. S., Farrar, J. T., et al. (2008). Interpreting the clinical importance of treatment outcomes in chronic pain clinical trials: IMMPACT recommendations. *Journal of Pain, 9,* 105–121.

Elliott, A. M., Smith, B. H., Penny, K., Smith, W. L., & Chambers, W. A. (1999). The epidemiology of chronic pain in the community. *Lancet, 354,* 1248–1252.

Farrar, J. T., Dworkin, R. H., & Max, M. B. (2006). Use of the cumulative proportion of responders analysis graph to present pain data over a range of cut-off points: Making clinical trial data more understandable. *Journal of Pain and Symptom Management, 31,* 369–377.

Flor, H., Fydrich, T., & Turk, D. C. (1992). Efficacy of multidisciplinary pain treatment centers: A meta-analytic review. *Pain, 49,* 221–230.

Flor, H., & Turk, D. C. (1988). Chronic pain and rheumatoid arthritis: Predicting pain and disability from cognitive variables. *Journal of Behavioral Medicine, 11,* 251–265.

Fries, J. F., Bruce, B., & Cella, D. (2005). The promise of PROMIS: Using item response theory to improve assessment of patient-reported outcomes. *Clinical and Experimental Rheumatology, 23,* S53–S57.

Frost, M. H., Bonomi, A. E., Ferrans, C. E., Wong, G. Y., & Hays, R. D. (2002). Patient, clinician, and population perspectives on determining the clinical significance of quality of life scores. *Mayo Clinic Proceedings, 77,* 488–494.

Gendreau, M., Hufford, M. R., & Stone, A. A. (2003). Measuring clinical pain in chronic widespread pain: Selected methodological issues. *Best Practice and Research Clinical Rheumatology, 17,* 575–592.

Gureje, O. (1998). Persistent pain and well-being: A World Health Organization study in primary care. *Journal of the American Medical Association, 280,* 147–151.

Guy, W. (1976). *ECDEU assessment manual for psychopharmacology* (DHEW Publication No. ADM 76-338). Washington, DC: U.S. Government Printing Office.

Harstall, C. (2003). How prevalent is chronic pain? *Pain: Clinical Updates, 11,* 1–4.

Hauri, P. J., & Wisbey, J. (1992). Wrist actigraphy in insomnia. *Sleep, 15,* 293–301.

Hunt, D. G., Zuberbier, O. A., Kozolowski, A. J., Robinson, J., Berkowitz, J., Schultz, I. Z., et al. (2000). Reliability of the lumbar flexion, lumbar extension and passive straight leg raise test in normal populations embedded within a complete physical examination. *Spine, 26,* 2714–2718.

Jaeschke, R., Singer, J., & Guyatt, G. H. (1989). Measurement of health status: Ascertaining the minimal clinically important difference. *Controlled Clinical Trials, 10,* 407–415.

Jamison, R. N., Raymond, S. A., Levine, J. G., Slawsby, E. A., Nedeljkovic, S. S., & Katz, N. P. (2001). Electronic diaries for monitoring chronic pain: 1-year validation study. *Pain, 91,* 277–285.

Jamison, R. N., Raymond, S. A., Slawsby, E. A., McHugo, G. J., & Baird, J. C. (2006). Pain assessment in patients with low back pain: Comparison of weekly recall and momentary electronic data. *Journal of Pain, 7,* 192–199.

Jarvik, J. G., Hollingworth, W., Heagerty, P. J., Haynor, D. R., Boyko, E. J., & Deyo, R. A. (2005). Three-year indicence of low back pain in an initially asymptomatic cohort: Clinical and imaging risk factors. *Spine, 30,* 1541–1548.

Jensen, M. P., Ehde, D. M., Hoffman, A. J., Patterson, D. R., Czerniecki, J. M., & Robinson, L. R. (2002). Cognitions, coping and social environment predict adjustment to phantom limb pain. *Pain, 95,* 133–142.

Jensen, M. P., Nielson, W. R., Turner, J. A., Romano, J. M., & Hill, M. L. (2004). Changes in readiness to self manage pain are associated with improvement in multidisciplianry pain treatment and pain coping. *Pain, 111,* 84–95.

Jensen, M. P., Romano, J. M., Turner, J. A., Good, A. B., & Wald, L. H. (1999). Patient beliefs predict patient functioning: Further support for a cognitive-behavioral model of chronic pain. *Pain, 81,* 95–104.

Jensen, M. P., Turner, J. A., & Romano, J. M. (2002). Pain belief assessment: A comparison of the short and long version of the Survey of Pain Attitudes. *Journal of Pain, 1,* 138–150.

Jensen, M. P., Turner, J. A., & Romano, J. M. (2007). Changes after multidisciplinary pain treatment in patient pain beliefs and coping are associated with concurrent changes in patient functioning. *Pain, 131,* 38–47.

Junghaenel, C. U., Schwartz, J. E., & Broderick, J. E. (2007). Differential efficacy of written emotional disclosure for subgroups of fibromyalgia patients. *British Journal of Health Psychology, 13*(Pt. 1), 57–60.

Kerns, R. D., Turk, D. C., & Rudy, T. E. (1985). The West Haven–Yale Multidimensional Pain Inventory (WHYMPI). *Pain, 23,* 345–356.

Kerns, R. D., Wagner, J., Rosenberg, R., Haythornthwaite, J., & Caudill-Slosberg, M. (2005). Identification of subgroups of persons with chronic pain based on profiles on the Pain Stages of Change Questionnaire. *Pain, 116,* 302–310.

Klenerman, L., Slade, P. D., Stanley, I. M., Pennie, B., Reilly, J. P., Atkinson, L. E., et al. (1995). The prediction of chronicity in patients with an acute attack of low back pain in a general practice setting. *Spine, 4,* 345–56.

Korszun, A., Young, E. A., Engleberg, N. C., Brucksch, C. B., Greden, J. F., & Crofford, L. A. (2002). Use of actigraphy for monitoring sleep and activity levels in patients with fibromyalgia and depression. *Journal of Psychosomatic Research, 52,* 439–443.

Landis, C. A., Frey, C. A., Lentz, M. J., Rothermel, J., Buchwald, M., & Shaver, J. L. F. (2003). Self-reported sleep quality and fatigue correlates with actigraphy in midlife women with fibromyalgia. *Nursing Research, 52,* 140–147.

Lydick, E., & Epstein, R. S. (1993). Interpretation of quality of life changes. *Quality of Life Research, 2,* 221–226.

McCaffery, M. (1979). *Nursing management of the patient with pain* (2nd ed.). Philadelphia: Lippincott.

Melzack, R. (Ed.). (1983). *Pain measurement and assessment.* New York: Raven Press.

Melzack, R., & Casey, K. L. (1968). Sensory, motivational, and central control determinants of pain: A new conceptual model. In D. Kenshalo (Ed.), *The skin senses* (pp. 423–443). Springfield, IL: Thomas.

Mendoza, T., Mayne, T., Rublee, D., & Cleeland, C. (2006). Reliability and validity of a modified Brief Pain Inventory-Short Form in patients with osteoarthritis. *European Journal of Pain, 10,* 353–362.

Mikail, S. F., DuBreuil, S. C., & D'Eon, J. L. (1993). A comparative analysis of measures used in the assessment of chronic pain patients. *Psychological Assessment, 5,* 117–120.

National Center for Health Statistics. (2006). *Health, United States, 2006 with chartbook on trends in the health of Americans.* Hyattsville, MD: National Center for Health Statistics.

Nicholas, M. K., Asghari, A., & Blyth, F. M. (2008). What do the numbers mean?: Normative data in chronic pain measures. *Pain, 134,* 158–173.

Nielson, W. R., Jensen, M. P., Ehde, D. M., Kerns, R. D., & Molton, I. R. (2008). Further development of the Multidimensional Pain Readiness to Change Questionnaire: The MPRCQ2. *Journal of Pain, 9,* 552–565.

Nitschke, J. E., Nattrass, C. L., & Disler, P. B. (1999). Reliability of the American Medical Association Guides' model for measuring spinal range of motion. *Spine, 24,* 262–268.

Olsson, I., Bunketorp, O., Carlsson, S. G., & Styf, J. (2002). Prediction of outcome in whiplash-associated disorders using West Haven–Yale Multidimensional Pain Inventory. *Clinical Journal of Pain, 18,* 238–245.

Pud, D., Granovsky, Y., & Yarnitsky, D. (2009). The methodology of experimentally induced diffuse noxious inhibitory control (DNIC)-like effect in humans. *Pain, 144,* 1–19.

Reeve, B. B., & Fayers, P. (2005). Applying item response theory modeling for evaluating questionnaire item and scale properties. In P. Fayers & R. D. Hays (Eds.), *Assessing quality of life in clinical trials: Methods of practice* (2nd ed., pp. 55–73). New York: Oxford University Press.

Richmond, R. L., & Carmody, T. P. (1999). Dropout from treatment for chronic low-back pain. *Professional Psychology: Research and Practice, 30,* 51–55.

Robinson, J. P., Turk, D. C., & Loeser, J. D. (2004). Pain, impairment, and disability in the AMA Guides. *Journal of Law, Medicine and Ethics, 32,* 315–326.

Rohling, M. L., Binder, L. M., & Langhinrichsen-Rohling, J. (1995). Money matters: A meta-analytic review of the association between financial compensation and the experience and treatment of chronic pain. *Health Psychology, 14,* 537–547.

Sadeh, A., Hauri, P. J., & Kripke, D. F. (1995). The role of actigraphy in the evaluation of sleep disorders. *Sleep, 18,* 188–202.

Sadeh, A., Sharkey, K. M., & Carskadon, M. A. (1994). Activity-based sleep–wake identification: An empirical test of methodological issues. *Sleep, 17,* 201–207.

Senn, S. (2008). Subgroups, significance, and circumspection. *Biomedical Statistics and Clinical Epidemiology, 2,* 11–21.

Sloan, J., Symonds, T., Vargas-Chanes, D., & Fridley, B. (2003). Practical guidelines for assessing the clinical significance of health-related quality of life changes within clinical trials. *Drug Information Journal, 37,* 23–31.

Sorbi, M. J., Peters, M. L., Kruise, D. A., Maas, C. J., Kerssens, J. J., Verhaak, P. F., et al. (2006). Electronic momentary assessment in chronic pain I: Psychological pain responses as predictors of pain intensity. *Clinical Journal of Pain, 22,* 55–66.

Stephenson, D. T., & Arneric, S. P. (2008). Neuroimaging of pain: Advances and future prospects. *Journal of Pain, 9,* 567–479.

Sternbach, R. (1968). *Pain: A psychophyiological analysis.* New York: Academic Press.

Stone, A. A., Broderick, J. E., Schwartz, J. E., Shiffman, S., Litcher-Kelly, L., & Calcanese, P. (2003). Intensive momentary reporting of pain with an electronic diary: Reactivity, compliance, and patient satisfaction. *Pain, 104,* 343–351.

Stone, A. A., & Shiffman, S. (2002). Capturing momentary, self-report data: A proposal for reporting guidelines. *Annals of Behavioral Medicine, 24,* 236–243.

Stone, A. A., Shiffman, S., Schwartz, J. E., Broderick, J. E., & Hufford, M. R. (2003). Patient compliance with paper and electronic diaries. *Controlled Clinical Trials, 24,* 182–199.

Thieme, K., Turk, D. C., & Flor, H. (2007). Responder criteria for operant and cognitive-behavioral treatment of fibromyalgia syndrome. *Arthritis Care and Research, 57,* 830–836.

Tukey, J. W. (1979). Methodology and the statistician's responsibility for both accuracy and relevance. *Journal of the American Statistical Association, 74,* 786–793.

Turk, D. C. (1993). Assess the *person,* not just the pain. *Pain: Clinical Updates, 1,* 1–4.

Turk, D. C. (2005). The potential of matching treatments to characteristics of chronic pain patients: Lumping vs. splitting. *Clinical Journal of Pain, 21,* 44–55.

Turk, D. C., Burwinkle, T., & Showlund, M. (2007). Assessing the impact of chronic pain in real-time. In A. Stone, S. Shiffman, A. Atienza, & L. Nebeling (Eds.), *The science of real-time data capture: Self-reports in health research* (pp. 204–228). New York: Oxford University Press.

Turk, D. C., Dworkin, R. H., Allen, R. R., Bellamy, N., Brandenburg, N., Carr, D. B., et al. (2003). Core outcomes domains for chronic pain clinical trials: IMMPACT recommendations. *Pain, 106,* 337–345.

Turk, D. C., Dworkin, R. H., Burke, L., Gershon, R., Rothman, M., Scott, J., et al. (2006). Developing patient-reported outcome measures for pain clinical trials: IMMPACT recommendations. *Pain, 125,* 208–215.

Turk, D. C., Dworkin, R. D., McDermott, M. P., Bellamy, N., Burke, L. B., Chandler, J. M., et al. (2008). Analyzing multiple endpoints in clinical trials of pain treatments: IMMPACT recommendations. *Pain, 139,* 485–493.

Turk, D. C., Dworkin, R. H., Revicki, D., Harding, G., Burke, L. B., Cella, D., et al. (2008). Identifying important outcome domains for chronic pain clinical trials: An IMMPACT survey of people with pain. *Pain, 137,* 276–285.

Turk, D. C., Robinson, J. P., Sherman, J. J., Burwinkle, T. M., & Swanson, K. S. (2008). Assessing fear in patients with cervical pain: Development and validation of The Pictorial Fear of Activity Scale-Cervical (PFActS-C). *Pain, 139,* 55–62.

Turk, D. C., & Rudy, T. E. (1988). Toward an empirically derived taxonomy of chronic pain patients: Integration of psychological assessment data. *Journal of Consulting and Clinical Psychology, 56,* 233–238.

Turk, D. C., & Rudy, T. E. (1990). The robustness of an empirically derived taxonomy of chronic pain patients. *Pain, 43,* 27–35.

Turk, D. C., Swanson, K. S., & Gatchel, R. J. (2008). Predicting opioid misuse by chronic pain patients: A systematic review and literature synthesis. *Clinical Journal of Pain, 24,* 497–508.

Turner, J. A., Franklin, G., & Turk, D. C. (2000). Predictors of long-term disability in injured workers: A systematic literature synthesis. *American Journal of Industrial Medicine, 38,* 707–722.

Turner, J. A., Jensen, M. P., & Romano, J. M. (2000). Do beliefs, coping, and catastrophizing independently predict functioning in patients with chronic pain? *Pain, 85,* 115–125.

Vlaeyan, J. W. S., & Linton, S. J. (2000). Fear-avoidance and its consequences in chronic musculoskeletal pain: A state of the art. *Pain, 85,* 317–332.

Von Korff, M., Crane, P., Lane, M., Miglioretti, D. L., Simon, G., Saunders, K., et al. (2005). Chronic spinal pain and physical–mental comorbidity in the United States: Results from the National Comorbidity Survey Replication. *Pain, 113,* 331–339.

Von Korff, M., Ormel, J., Keefe, F., & Dworkin, S. F. (1992). Grading the severity of chronic pain. *Pain, 50,* 133–149.

Waddell, G. (2004). *The back pain revolution* (2nd ed.). Edinburgh, UK: Churchill Livingstone.

Walk, D., Sehgal, N., Moeller-Bertram, T., Edwards, R. R., Wasan, A., Wallace, M., et al. (2009). Quantitative sensory testing and mapping: A review of nonautomated quantitative methods for examination of the patient with neuropathic pain. *Clinical Journal of Pain, 25,* 632–640.

Wernicke, J. F., Pritchett, Y. L., D'Souza, D. N., Waninger, A., Tran, P., Iyengar, S., et al. (2006). A randomized controlled trial of duloxetine in diabetic peripheral neuropathic pain. *Neurology, 67,* 1411–1420.

Widerström-Noga, E. G., Duncan, R., & Turk,

D. C. (2004). Psychosocial profiles of people with pain associated with spinal cord injury: Identification and comparison with other chronic pain syndromes. *Clinical Journal of Pain, 20,* 261–271.

Wilkie, D. J., Keefe, F. J., Dodd, M. J., & Copp, L. A. (1992). Behavior of patients with lung cancer: Description and associations with oncologic pain variables. *Pain, 51,* 231–240.

Wittinik, H., Michel, T. H., Kulich, R., Wagner, A., Sukiennik, A., Maciewicz, R., et al. (2000). Aerobic fitness testing in patients with chronic low back pain: Which test is best? *Spine, 25,* 1704–1710.

Wittinik, H., Michel, T. H., Wagner, A., Sukiennik, A., & Rogers, W. (2000). Deconditioning in patients with chronic low back pain—fact or fiction? *Spine, 25,* 2221–2228.

Author Index

507

Subject Index

Page numbers followed by *f* indicate figure, *t* indicate table